# Abbreviated H-2 Regions of Mouse Strains Discussed

| | K | $A_\beta$ | $A_\alpha$ | $E_\beta$ | $E_\alpha$ | D | H-2 Haplotype Designation |
|---|---|---|---|---|---|---|---|
| | | | | I | | | |
| C57BL/6, C57BL/10, C3H.SW | b | b | b | b | b | b | b |
| BALB/c, DBA/2, B10.D2, NZB | d | d | d | d | d | d | d |
| CBA, C3H, AKR, B10.BR | k | k | k | k | k | k | k |
| A, A/J, B10.A | k | k | k | k | k | d | a |
| AQR | q | k | k | k | k | d | y1 |
| A.TL, B10.TL | s | k | k | k | k | d | t1 |
| B10.A(3R) | b | b | b | b | k | d | i3 |
| B10.A(4R) | k | k | k | k | b | b | h4 |
| B10.A(5R) | b | b | b | b | k | d | i5 |
| B10.M | f | f | f | f | f | f | f |
| B10.MBR | b | k | k | k | k | q | bq1 |
| B10.S(24R) | s | s | s | s | s | d | t6 |
| B10.T(6R) | q | q | q | q | q | d | y2 |
| C3H.OH | d | d | d | d | d | k | o2 |
| D2.GD | d | d | d | d/b | b | b | g2 |

# Chromosome Location of Some Genes of Immunological Interest

| Genes | Human | Mouse |
|---|---|---|
| Antibody heavy (H) chains | 14 | 12 |
| Antibody kappa ($\kappa$) light chains | 2 | 6 |
| Antibody lambda ($\lambda$) light chains | 22 | 16 |
| Major histocompatibility complex (MHC) | 6 | 17 |
| $\alpha$ chain of T cell receptor | 14 | 14 |
| $\beta$ chain of T cell receptor | 7 | 6 |
| c-myc | 8 | 15 |

# Introduction to
# Immunology

# Introduction to Immunology

SECOND EDITION

## John W. Kimball

**Macmillan Publishing Company**
New York
**Collier Macmillan Publishers**
London

To
## A. M. Pappenheimer, Jr.
### Professor of Biology *Emeritus*, Harvard University

Macmillan Publishing Company
866 Third Avenue, New York, New York 10022
Collier Macmillan Canada, Inc.

**Library of Congress Cataloging in Publication Data**
Kimball, John W.
  Introduction to immunology.
  Includes bibliographies and index.
  1. Immunology. I. Title. [DNLM: 1. Immunity.
QW 504 K49i]
QR181.K49  1986        616.07'9        85-10607
ISBN 0-02-363830-3

Printing:      5 6 7 8      Year:      8 9 0 1 2 3 4 5

ISBN 0-02-363830-3

# Preface
## to the Second Edition

Many important advances in our knowledge of the immune system have been made since the first edition was completed. The nature of the T cell receptor for antigen, the interactions between *myc* and immunoglobulin genes in Burkitt's lymphoma, and the accumulating evidence of a network of idiotype–anti-idiotype interactions in the immune system are just three of many examples. The rapid progress in the field fully justifies a new edition.

However, I have also used this opportunity to rework other parts of the book in the hope of improving them pedagogically. In general, I have tightened up the organization of topics, retreating somewhat from my earlier tendency to keep returning to a topic for another look. For example, some of the formerly scattered material on H-2 has been brought together in Chapter 3 where it should provide a sounder basis for much that follows.

Users of the first edition will find that the major changes in organization occur in Part IV. The first three chapters of this part (8–10) now examine, respectively, the cellular, protein, and genetic bases of humoral immunity. The same sequence is followed for T lymphocytes in Chapter 11. Chapter 12 is devoted largely to the interaction of T helper cells and their products with B cells, and Chapter 13 examines the ways in which T cells interact with other cells in cell-mediated immune responses. The final chapter in Part IV examines the complement system and various other effector mechanisms in immunity.

One of the greatest hazards in revising a textbook is the temptation to add new material without subtracting old. While this edition has grown somewhat in size, I have reduced the coverage of certain topics to compensate partially for the many additions. For example, much of the earlier material on the suppressor cell cascade has been eliminated to make room for a more comprehensive treatment of network theory. While I find it painful to discard worthy material, I suspect that by doing so a clearer story often emerges.

I hope that the book's pedagogical value will also be enhanced by the

v

addition of summaries at the end of those chapters in which the major points of the story may have been obscured by the multitude of details presented. A glossary has also been added to this edition.

I am deeply indebted to the following who took time from their busy schedules to evaluate parts (in some cases, all) of the manuscript: Joseph M. Davie and Julian B. Fleischman, Washington University School of Medicine; Philippa Marrack, National Jewish Hospital in Denver; John Martinko, Southern Illinois University; John R. Preer, Jr., Indiana University; Lloyd Y. Quinn, Iowa State University; Fred S. Rosen, Harvard University Medical School; Gary Splitter, University of Wisconsin, Madison; and Walter Schoenholz, California State University, Hayward. Lisa A. Steiner of M.I.T. provided many valuable suggestions for the glossary as well as once again carefully critiquing the entire manuscript.

I am grateful to my students in Biology 169 at Harvard who by their suggestions as well as by their questions and puzzled expressions showed me ways in which the book needed improvement. Finally, my thanks to all those at Macmillan who labored so hard and patiently to convert my manuscript and rough art into a finished product.

J. W. K.

## Acknowledgments

The following figures were reproduced from *The Journal of Experimental Medicine* by copyright permission of The Rockefeller University Press: 2.1 & 2.2 (1953, **98**:21); 2.5 (1946, 84:387); 7.7 (1973, 138:488); 7.5 (1967, **126**:291 & 1973, **137**:504); 7.23 (1979, **149**:1); 8.9 (1974, **140**:904); 8.18 (1973, 137:1024); 12.12 (1984, **160**:858); 15.1 (1973, **138**:1426); 15.3 (1966, **124**:953); 17.7 (1978, 148:46); 18.9 (1953, **97**:257); 20.14 (1980,**151**:69).

The following figures were reprinted by permission from *Nature,* Macmillan Journals Limited: 4.19 (**256**:495 © 1975); 6.1 (**285**:340 © 1980); 17.5 (**252**:503 © 1974); 17.8 (**273**:613 © 1978); 3.14 (**291**:35 © 1981).

The following figures were reproduced from *Science,* copyright by the American Association for the Advancement of Science: 5.5 (© 1980); 10.26 (© 1978); 14.13 (© 1981); 16.2 (© 1971).

The following figures were reproduced from *The Journal of Immunology,* copyright by The Williams & Wilkins Co., Baltimore: 2.7 (© 1971); 3.4 (© 1964); 5.19 (© 1980); 8.16 (© 1979); 14.10 (© 1980); 20.8 (© 1961).

The following figures were reprinted with permission from *Immunochemistry,* copyright Pergamon Press, Ltd.: 4.5 (3:213, 1966); 8.12 & 15.2 (9:1169, 1972).

Figure 9.3 was reproduced with permission from R. C. Valentine and N. M. Green, *Journal of Molecular Biology,* **27**:615, 1967. Copyright: Academic Press Inc. (London) Ltd.

Copyright to Figure 10.11 is held by M.I.T.

# Preface
## to the First Edition

This book has grown out of a semester-long course in immunology that I taught for a number of years at Tufts University and presently teach at Harvard University. A course in genetics and one in biochemistry were prerequisites for the course at Tufts and are strongly recommended at Harvard. Because of these requirements, the course has been populated chiefly by advanced undergraduate biology majors and graduate students. But even with prerequisites, any class represents a considerable spectrum of ability and current preparation, and I often find it necessary to review topics in genetics, biochemistry, and physiology. In writing this book, therefore, I decided not to assume any prior knowledge on the part of the reader other than the terminology and concepts one would expect to find in a reasonably rigorous introductory biology text. Specifically, I have used the contents of my own text, *Biology* (5th edition, Addison-Wesley, 1983) as the criterion by which to decide what additional background information is needed for the discussion of each topic. This should not suggest that a year of introductory biology is adequate preparation for this book. The serious student will need more background to properly appreciate the material. However, the inevitable lapses in memory ought to be able to be filled by referring to a comprehensive introductory text.

A glance at the table of contents will reveal the basic organization of topics. One of my aims in choosing this way of organizing the material was to reinforce the importance and distinctiveness of cell-mediated immune responses. Perhaps this approach will reduce the number of students who, even at the end of their course, still think of antibodies as the sole expression of immunity.

The virtually exponential growth in our knowledge of the immune system makes the writing of a text that is both manageable in size and accessible to the beginning student a challenging task. One approach to the task is to set out our current thinking as a series of succinct conclusions. But such an approach misses, I believe, not only the essence of the subject but the excitement as well. I have chosen instead to develop most of the topics around the experimental evidence for such tentative conclusions as we can now draw. This approach requires, of course, more lines of text than would a strict didactic presentation. Of necessity, then, I have had to be selective not only in what topics to include but what experiments to describe to support them. Sometimes I have chosen the classic work that laid the foundations of the topic; sometimes recent work that provides a more complete view of the topic in a single set of experiments. In any case, I hope that you will not find my choices overly idiosyncratic.

It has been my experience that beginning students profit more from reading original research papers than from reading reviews. The majority of the experiments I describe are illustrated by figures, and the citations to the original work appear in the legend accompanying the illustration. Therefore, the list of references at the end of each chapter is not by any means to be considered comprehensive, but simply represents other material I felt appropriate that was not cited earlier in the chapter. A number of the papers cited are readily available to students in the excellent reprint collection prepared by Vicki L. Sato and Malcolm L. Gefter (*Cellular Immunology,* Addison-Wesley, 1981).

Another recurring problem is how close to approach the advancing edge of each subject. I have usually, perhaps rashly in some cases, carried the discussion into recent, less well-tested areas. I have done this because (1) I want students to sense the excitement of the new directions that the field is taking and (2) I want to prepare students to be able to read the current literature. Surely one of the greatest satisfactions of a teacher is to work with students to the point where they can sit down with a current journal article and be able to understand and evaluate it.

I am indebted to many people for the help that they have given me in preparing this book. Each of the following read large sections of the manuscript and gave many valuable suggestions for its improvement: Duane W. Sears, University of California, Santa Barbara; William D. Baxter, Bowling Green State University; Cynthia V. Sommer, University of Wisconsin, Milwaukee; Edward M. Hoffman, University of Florida; Charles A. Janeway, Jr., Yale University; David W. Thomas, Washington University; John Clausz, Carroll College; Roderick MacLeod, University of Illinois (who also tested some of the material with his students); and Ray L. Bratcher, Syracuse University. Although in some cases I decided not to follow a particular piece of advice, I assure them that I paid close attention to all their suggestions and, of course, absolve them of any responsibility for the final product. I am especially indebted to Lisa Steiner (MIT) for her meticulous and thoughtful appraisals and for steering me away from many pitfalls both syntactic and scientific.

I also want to thank all the students who took my course at Tufts in 1980–81. They were the guinea pigs for Chapters 1–12 and helped me greatly by returning the manuscript chapters marked with suggestions for improvement.

Despite the best efforts of all concerned, I am sure that errors—of fact, of interpretation, of proofreading—still remain. I do hope that those who examine and/or use the book will communicate to me any suggestions that they have for its improvement.

All the drawings were prepared by Cynthia Phillips. Working under imminent deadlines, she carefully and speedily turned my rough ideas into clear and, I believe, pedagogically effective illustrations. I also wish to thank the many colleagues who supplied me with their photographs and electron micrographs. Their names appear in the legend accompanying their work.

Every book is the product of a partnership between the author and the publisher. I am grateful to the many people at Macmillan involved in the creation of this book for the skill and spirit of cooperation that they brought to their tasks.

And, finally, my special thanks to A. M. Pappenheimer, Jr. ("Pap"), now Professor *Emeritus* at Harvard, who not only taught me how to do immunology, but taught me —by example rather than by precept—so much about standards and style in any scientific undertaking. This book is dedicated to him with the hope that it will partially balance the debt I owe to him.

J. W. K.

# Contents

PART **V**

**Regulation of Immune Responses**

PART **VI**

**Immunity and Disease**

# PART I

# Introduction

# CHAPTER 1

# The Nature of Immunity

## 1.1  What Is an Immune Response?

An immune response can be defined as "altered reactivity to a specific molecular configuration that develops following contact with it." The altered reactivity might take the form of, for example, resistance to a second infection by measles virus or an allergic response to grass pollen. The specific molecular configuration would be the surface structure of a specific molecule, such as one found on a virus particle or a pollen grain. This definition contains two critically important concepts. One is the concept of **specificity**. The other is the concept of **memory**.

3

## Specificity

In order to qualify as immune, the response must meet the criterion of specificity. The investigator must be able to demonstrate that the altered response occurs *only* with respect to the *same* molecular configuration encountered before.

Consider what happened in 1977 to people who encountered the influenza virus called A/Texas/77 for the first time. Following their recovery from the infection, these people were no longer susceptible to a second infection by the same virus. They were now immune. However, they were still fully susceptible to the "Russian" flu virus (A/USSR/77) circulating throughout the world at the same time. Their *selective reactivity* to one virus and not the other demonstrates specificity and qualifies their response as immune.

If, on the other hand, they had been exposed to the Russian flu virus while their illness was still in progress or in early convalescence, the second virus would not have caused disease. This is because when certain kinds of cells (e.g., lymphocytes) become infected with a virus, they synthesize and secrete a protein called *interferon*. *Interferon* inhibits viral replication in cells and is thus an important antiviral agent. But interferon exerts its inhibitory effect on the multiplication of *all* types of viruses. Therefore, the interferon response fails to meet our definition of an immune response.

## Memory

In order to qualify as immune, any subsequent response to an agent must be measurably different in its qualities from the initial response. The immunity that follows a bout with A/Texas/77 does not mean that the virus can never again enter the body. But if a second infection by the virus should occur, the defensive responses will be so swift that the virus will be unable to cause enough tissue damage to create noticeable symptoms. Only laboratory tests will be able to reveal the telltale traces of its re-entry. On the other hand, if phagocytic cells in the body proceed to scavenge invading microorganisms with the same speed and efficiency they displayed on their first encounter with that microorganism, then immunity has played no role in their response.

A third feature is often—but not always—a hallmark of immunity. Immunity to a specific molecular configuration will normally occur only if that configuration is not found in the body of the responding animal. In other words, the immune system usually responds only to "foreign" molecular configurations. Thus the immune system discriminates between "nonself" and "self." We shall, however, examine a number of violations of this principle in the following chapters. Immune response to "self" creates a state of *autoimmunity*. Autoimmunity may result in pathological effects on the organism, as we shall see in Chapter 18.

You may have noticed that the terms "immune response" and "immunity'' have not been used in precisely the same way. This is because some immune responses lead to a state of **immunological tolerance.** Immunological tolerance is a specific *hypo*responsiveness to a particular molecular configuration. It is also induced by contact. Thus immune responses can lead either to immunity (enhanced reactivity) or to tolerance (sharply decreased reactivity). Both show specificity and memory. Immunological tolerance is the topic of Chapter 16.

As you read the literature of immunology, you will occasionally encounter the expressions *natural immunity* and *nonspecific immunity.* ''Natural immunity'' is sometimes used to describe the innate lack of susceptibility of humans to many animal diseases. The basis of this innate protection is often obscure, but no evidence exists that it involves immunity as we have defined it. If you accept our definition of immune responses, then ''nonspecific immunity'' is a contradiction in terms. It refers to defense mechanisms, like interferon and some examples of phagocytosis, that are effective against a broad range of agents. Nonspecific host defense mechanisms such as these are important, but they fail to meet the criteria that we have established for immune responses.

No one knows just when humans first became aware of the existence of immunity. In his history of the Peloponnesian Wars, Thucydides wrote of a plague that swept Athens some 2500 years ago. He mentions that whatever attention the sick received was ''tended by the pitying care of those who had recovered, because they were themselves free of apprehension. For no one was ever attacked a second time. . . . '' Today we cannot tell what the pestilence was; perhaps it was typhus, perhaps plague. Regardless, these words, written two and a half millenia ago, express the central concept of immunity.

## 1.2 The Duality of the Immune System

Two kinds of effector mechanisms mediate immune responses. Some immune responses are mediated by specific molecules, called **antibodies,** that are carried in the blood and lymph. The synthesis of antibodies occurs in a subset of lymphocytes called **B lymphocytes** or B cells. Antibody-mediated immunity is called **humoral immunity.** Other immune responses are mediated by cells. All the leukocytes (white cells) of the blood participate in **cell-mediated immunity** (CMI). However, the *specificity* of the response depends upon a subset of lymphocytes called **T lymphocytes** or T cells. Most immune responses involve the activity and interplay of both the humoral and the cell-mediated branches of the immune system.

This duality of function in the immune system recurs as a theme throughout this book. It in fact provides a major organizational pattern to the topics discussed. Chapter 2 deals largely with humoral immunity. The basic features of cell-mediated immunity are considered in Chapter 3.

On October 26, 1977, Ali Maow Maalin came down with smallpox (variola) in the town of Merka in Somalia. Within a few weeks he was fully recovered. Since that time, not a case of smallpox (except as a result of one laboratory accident) has been discovered anywhere in the world. By May of 1980, the World Health Organization (WHO) felt that it could confidently announce that smallpox had been completely eradicated. Smallpox certainly qualified as one of the greatest scourges of humanity. It regularly killed 25% and sometimes as many as 50% of its victims. Introduced into Europe around the sixth century A.D., smallpox rivaled plague in its ability to decimate entire populations. Introduced into the New World in the sixteenth century, smallpox devastated the native populations and played a far greater role than weaponry in the Spanish Conquest.

How was such a pestilence eradicated? Four factors were decisive.

1. The variola virus, which causes the disease, attacks only humans; no animal reservoirs have been found (as they have for, e.g., the yellow fever virus and the plague bacillus).
2. With recovery from the disease, the virus is completely eliminated from the body. There are no smallpox "carriers" as there are for such diseases as typhoid fever and malaria.
3. An effective vaccine was available. The vaccine could quickly establish a strong (and reasonably long-lasting) immunity. Thus the chain of contagion could quickly be broken by vaccinating all possible contacts associated with a new case.
4. The WHO and the countries involved provided personnel, money, and the determination to do the job. An effective vaccine had, as we shall see, been available since 1796 and had already rendered many parts of the world free of the disease during the first half of this century. But still the disease smouldered in Asia, Indonesia, Brazil, and Africa. Only a heroic public health effort—a campaign that began in 1967—finally eliminated it worldwide.

### Variolation

The first effective attempts to cope with smallpox were made in some of the same regions—Asia, India, Africa—that were the last freed of the disease. The technique was deliberately to inoculate susceptible individuals (i.e., those with no pockmarks to indicate that they had survived an earlier epidemic) with material taken from the pustules of victims having a mild case of the disease. This practice, called *variolation*, induced an active case in the recipient, but usually the case was less severe than if the disease had been contracted in the normal way (by inhalation as it turned out). Variolation was introduced into England and the American colonies early in the eighteenth century. For many years, the practice was accompanied by violent controversy. For one thing, it was not an entirely safe

| | Year | | |
|---|---|---|---|
| | 1721 | 1764 | 1792 |
| Population | 10,700 | 15,500 | 19,300 |
| Natural smallpox | | | |
|   Cases | 5,759 | 699 | 232 |
|   Deaths | 842 | 124 | 69 |
|   Deaths/1000 cases | 146 | 177 | 298 |
| Smallpox caused by variolation | | | |
|   Cases | 130 | 4,977 | 9,152 |
|   Deaths | 2 | 46 | 179 |
|   Deaths/1000 cases | 15 | 9 | 20 |

**Figure 1.1** Smallpox in Boston. [From J. B. Blake, *Public Health in the Town of Boston, 1630–1832.* Harvard University Press, 1959.]

procedure. The variolated person often became quite ill and the mortality rate, although only a fraction of that for people who contracted the disease in the normal way, was nonetheless appreciable (Figure 1.1). But far more significant in terms of public acceptance was the fact that the variolated individual was fully contagious to others during the period of his brief, hopefully mild illness. Thus a family electing variolation could serve as the starting point of a fresh smallpox epidemic. Nonetheless, the practice gradually gained favor (Figure 1.1) until it was replaced by vaccination.

## Vaccination

Edward Jenner (Figure 1.2), was a Gloucestershire physician who introduced the practice that led to the elimination of smallpox. Jenner's success was grounded on two observations.

1. The regional folk belief that if a milkmaid had ever contracted cowpox, she would not contact smallpox.
2. The inability to variolate successfully those who had had an earlier case of cowpox. Cowpox is a disease characterized by pustules on the teats and udders of cows. Persons in close contact with cows frequently contracted the disease and suffered a mild and transient infection.

Jenner systematically exploited these observations. First he deliberately induced cowpox in his human subjects by inoculating them with material from cowpox pustules. Then he showed that these individuals could not be variolated. Jenner's procedure, which we call *vaccination* (L. *vacca*, cow) quickly replaced variolation as a public health measure because

1. Any reaction it induced was far milder than the disease induced by variolation.
2. The vaccinated subject was not contagious to others.

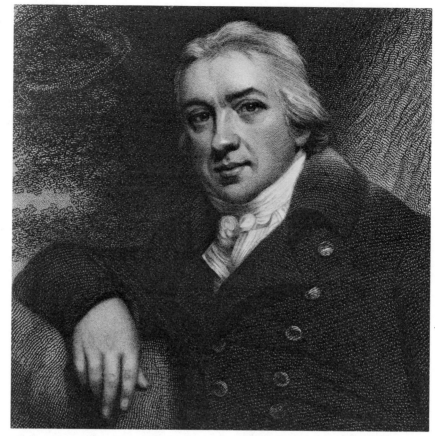

**Figure 1.2** Edward Jenner, 1749–1823. Engraved by J. R. Smith. [Courtesy of the Boston Athenaeum.]

Jenner's was the first safe and successful attempt to artificially induce an active immunity. Many successful attempts have followed since Jenner's day, but the principles that guided him are still followed: to develop a harmless (or as harmless as possible) preparation that will, upon introduction into the body, induce a response that will protect the individual from a harmful pathogenic agent. Because of Jenner's priority and his success, the term *vaccine* is used today for all such preparations. The administration of a vaccine is called *immunization*.

The virus used in today's smallpox vaccine is called the *vaccinia virus.* It is probably not cowpox virus. Possibly it is a highly attenuated form of smallpox (variola) virus. Just when the switch occurred is lost in the obscurity of the years since Jenner's day.

Jenner knew nothing of viruses, lymphocytes, or antibodies. His success was based on empirical methods of observation and clinical trials. Today we know a great deal more about the machinery of immunity. And much of this knowledge intersects with fundamental knowledge about the properties of cells and molecules. But as you read the chapters that follow, never lose sight of the incalculable benefits that the ability to manipulate the immune system has brought to humanity. Jenner himself wrote of vaccination: "the annihilation of smallpox must be the final result of this practice." One hundred and eighty-two years later, his prediction appears to have been fulfilled at last.

9

*Section 1.4*
*Antigens*

Other afflictions await. For some, such as polio and tetanus, the knowledge and tools are already at hand. What is now needed are money and commitment. For other goals, such as a vaccine for malaria, successful organ transplants, perhaps even specific and effective tumor therapy, more knowledge is needed.

## 1.4 Antigens

An antigen is a substance that when introduced into an animal with a functioning immune system, can elicit a specific immune response. If the response leads to a state of immunity, the antigen is said to be *immunogenic*. An antigen that produces a state of specific tolerance is called a *tolerogen*.

Proteins are highly immunogenic when injected into an animal for whom they are not normal ("self") constituents. Thus bovine serum albumin (BSA), which is a normal component of cow serum, is strongly immunogenic in mice but not in cows. Chicken ovalbumin (OVA), the major protein in the white of the egg, and keyhole limpet hemocyanin (KLH), the oxygen-carrying pigment of this marine gastropod, are other examples of protein antigens frequently used in immunological studies.

Polysaccharides and nucleic acids can also serve as antigens, although nucleic acids tend to be only weakly immunogenic. Conjugated proteins, such as nucleoproteins, glycoproteins, and lipoproteins, are strongly immunogenic, thanks largely to the protein portion of the molecule. Conversely, most small molecules, those with molecular weights below about 2000, *by themselves* do not elicit the formation of antibodies. For example, injections of steroid hormones like testosterone, drugs like digitalis and morphine, or nucleotides like cyclic AMP do not induce antibody formation. But if these same molecules are first coupled with an immunogenic antigen such as a protein, antibodies will be elicited to the complex, and a *subset* of these antibodies will bind specifically to the small molecule. Thus while only macromolecules are immunogenic, the antibodies produced in response to the antigen react with (bind to) only certain portions of the antigen. These portions are called **antigenic determinants** (or "epitopes"). Covalently bound to a macromolecular "carrier," small molecules such as testosterone and morphine can serve as — or be part of — an antigenic determinant.

To take another example, dinitrobenzene is not by itself immunogenic. However, when covalently coupled to a protein (to the epsilon amino groups of its lysine residues), the resulting dinitrophenyl complex (for example, DNP–BSA) is immunogenic. Injections of DNP–BSA into a rabbit induce the formation of a broad spectrum of antibody molecules, subsets of which react with different antigenic determinants on the mole-

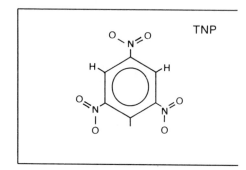

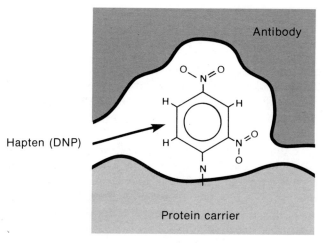

**Figure 1.3** The dinitrophenyl (DNP) group makes up a major part of the antigenic determinant to which the antibody binds. The antibody will also bind to the hapten coupled to a different protein carrier. *Top:* The structure of the related trinitrophenyl (TNP) group. Most anti-DNP antibodies will also bind to TNP and vice versa.

cules, and *one* subset of which binds specifically to ("recognizes") those determinants of which DNP is a part (Figure 1.3). This latter subset of antibody molecules will also bind to molecules of DNP that have been coupled to ovalbumin (DNP–OVA), but none of the antibodies will bind to OVA alone. A molecule that is not immunogenic by itself but can serve as part of an antigenic determinant on an immunogenic molecule (the "carrier") is called a **hapten.**

The universe of antigenic determinants is immense, perhaps limitless. Probably no molecular configuration exists that when presented to the appropriate animal in an appropriate fashion, cannot elicit the formation of antibodies directed against itself. This should not suggest, however, that the ability to produce different kinds of antibodies is limitless. Although the number is still uncertain, we can probably synthesize $10^6$–$10^7$ different kinds of antibody molecules. This means, then, that a given antibody molecule must be able to combine with more than one kind of antigenic determinant. Thus the specificity of antibodies is not absolute.

Antigenic determinants occur on parasites. Those that occur on the surface of the parasite usually play a major role in stimulating the immune defenses of the host. But immunity is a far broader phenomenon than protection against disease agents. Our environment is filled with noninfectious—but foreign and thus immunogenic—macromolecules with the potential to induce an immune response. A protein (called antigen E) in ragweed pollen, certain proteins in shellfish, proteins in bee venom, and the "D" antigen on the surface of Rh-positive red cells are just a few examples of antigens that, while noninfectious, play important roles in human disease. Each of these is discussed at greater length in Chapter 18 where the various kinds of allergies are examined.

## 1.5 Vaccines

At present vaccines are certainly the greatest practical benefit immunology has given humanity. Earlier we saw how, after 182 years, what is still essentially Jenner's vaccine against smallpox appears to have eliminated the disease. Since Jenner's time, a number of other vaccines have been developed, several of which have had a dramatic impact on human morbidity and mortality (Figure 1.4). The principles underlying their development are the same: to introduce into the body an immunogenic agent that is harmless (or as harmless as possible) but shares antigenic determinants with the intact, fully virulent disease agent. Immunity to the vaccine then results in the production of antibodies and/or specifically immune lymphocytes capable of inactivating the pathogenic agent if it should gain access to the body.

**Figure 1.4** Decline in the incidence of paralytic poliomyelitis in the United States since the introduction of the polio vaccines. [U.S. Public Health Service.]

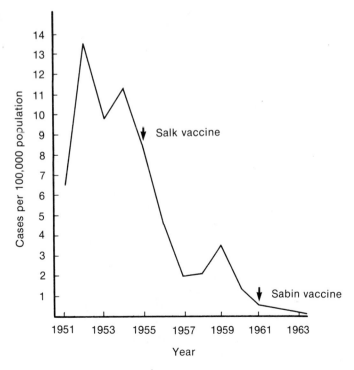

Almost a century elapsed before Jenner's vaccine was followed by others when Louis Pasteur ushered in the modern era of immunology. A crucial observation occurred during his studies of fowl cholera, a bacterial disease plaguing the French poultry industry. A group of chickens inoculated with an aged culture of the bacteria failed to become ill. Correctly surmising that the old culture had lost its virulence, Pasteur directed that a fresh culture be prepared and administered to the animals. But the animals still remained healthy. This was the critical observation. Pasteur deduced, again correctly, that the first inoculation with attenuated bacteria had induced an immunity in the chickens that protected them from fully virulent organisms. In due course this realization led to a vaccine against anthrax (in this case, the organisms were rendered harmless by heating them to 42°C) and against rabies, one of the most dreaded of diseases. The "Pasteur treatment," which has only recently been replaced by safer vaccines, was first given to Joseph Meister, a boy of nine years, who had been badly bitten by a rabid dog. The boy remained healthy. Fifty-five years later, with the Nazis occupying Paris, the same Meister — for many years a custodian at the Pasteur Institute in Paris — took his own life rather than hand over the keys to Pasteur's crypt to the Nazis.

For certain infectious diseases, the danger stems not from the rapid proliferation of the organism but from the great toxicity of the protein toxin liberated by the bacteria. This is true for tetanus and for diphtheria. In each case, a protective vaccine is made by destroying the toxin's toxicity while leaving some of its antigenic determinants intact. The resulting material is called a **toxoid**. Both tetanus and diphtheria toxoids are made by treating the native toxin with formaldehyde, a protein-denaturing agent.

Formaldehyde treatment was also used by Jonas Salk to render the three types of poliovirus noninfectious and, as a result, to produce the first effective vaccine against poliomyelitis. The polio vaccine developed by Albert Sabin exploited the alternate approach of creating attenuated strains of the types 1, 2, and 3 viruses. The attenuated strains are still infective for the cells of the intestine but no longer threaten the tissues of the central nervous system.

With the eradication of smallpox, routine immunization with vaccinia virus has ceased. However, further triumphs may yet be achieved with vaccinia virus. Workers in several laboratories have succeeded in introducing selected antigen-encoding genes from other pathogens into the vaccinia virus genome. These genes are expressed by the virus and appear to provide a potent immunogenic stimulus to animals inoculated with the altered virus. By means of genetically engineered vaccinia, experimental animals have been successfully immunized against hepatitis B, influenza, rabies, and other diseases.

There are several advantages to this approach. Introducing just one gene from a pathogen avoids some of the dangers inherent in vaccines made from the entire organism (such as incomplete inactivation or, for attenuated vaccines, reversion to full virulence). Furthermore, it should be possible to engineer vaccinia virus with genes from several pathogens, thus providing immunization against several diseases in a single vaccine.

As we have defined it, immunity is a vertebrate trait. Antibodies can be induced in vertebrates of all classes, including the most primitive of living vertebrates, lampreys and hagfish. However, the speed and complexity of humoral immune responses is greatest in birds and mammals.

Cell-mediated immune responses also occur throughout the vertebrate classes. One easily tested manifestation of cell-mediated immunity is the ability to reject grafts of foreign tissue. Almost all animals, invertebrates as well as vertebrates, have this ability. Even animals as simple as the colonial cnidarians are able to recognize and reject foreign tissue. However, rejection alone is not enough to meet our criteria of immunity. In order for its response to qualify as immune, the animal must reject the foreign tissue more vigorously on a second or any subsequent encounter with it. All vertebrates do this. And there have been a number of interesting reports of memory responses in annelid worms and in echinoderms. In these animals, however, the second response is sometimes slower, not faster, than the first.

Just because most invertebrates show no evidence of immune responses does not mean that they live their lives at the mercy of environmental pathogens. Far from it. A variety of effective defense mechanisms exist among the various invertebrates. These defense mechanisms include the secretion of antimicrobial substances, tissue reactions to wall off invading microorganisms, and phagocytic cells to engulf such invaders. But these are nonspecific defense mechanisms that fail to qualify as immune. And these same mechanisms coexist with immune responses in vertebrates. As comparative studies continue, we shall surely find precursors of the machinery of immunity among the invertebrate descendants of the ancestors of the vertebrates. However, the full expression of immunity is a vertebrate achievement.

## 1.7 The Ontogeny of Immune Responsiveness

The ability to mount immune responses depends upon an interacting system of cells, tissues, and organs. These constitute the immune system. Like all body systems, it emerges during embryonic development as the outcome of complex, precisely orchestrated patterns of morphogenesis and differentiation. (Chapter 7 examines the anatomy and some details on the development of the immune system.) As the system develops, it begins to become functional. At this time, the organism has gained **immunocompetence.**

Immunocompetence does not develop in an all or none fashion. The development of the ability to mount humoral responses may not coincide with the development of the ability to mount cell-mediated responses. The ability to respond to certain antigens develops before the ability to respond to others.

The period during which the animal gains immunocompetence varies from species to species. The human fetus is able to mount a humoral immune response as early as the second trimester of pregnancy, although it usually does not need to. Sheep also develop immunocompetence well before birth. Mice, however, are unable to mount humoral responses until several days after birth.

## Self vs. Nonself

Whatever the time frame, the development of immunocompetence represents a watershed in the life of the animal. At this time the organism learns to discriminate between "self" and "nonself." Whatever molecular configurations the developing immune system encounters before it becomes immunocompetent will henceforth be regarded as self. This includes most, but perhaps not all, of the normal constituents of the body. From that time, the animal will be incapable of mounting an immune response to these molecular configurations (at least for as long as they remain within the body). The mechanism by which this "self-tolerance" is established is still not understood. Chapter 16 examines some possibilities. Whatever the mechanism, the phenomenon is profoundly important to the animal and is also extremely valuable to the experimental immunologist. In later chapters, we shall see examples of the experimental induction of tolerance to "foreign" molecules by their administration to the animal before it develops immunocompetence.

Molecular configurations encountered for the first time *after* the development of immunocompetence are regarded as nonself and are potentially capable of eliciting an immune response. The molecular configuration does not have to be truly "foreign" in order to be considered nonself. Let us look at two examples. There are a number of rare genetic disorders that are characterized by an inability to synthesize one or another plasma protein. When these individuals mature, injections of that *human* protein are as immunogenic for them as injections of bovine serum albumin (BSA) are for you and me (and for them). Some of the autoimmune disorders may also illustrate the point. Evidence exists that some components of the body are not ordinarily "seen" by the developing immune system. This appears to be the case for certain proteins in the eye and in the central nervous system. If the immune system accidentally encounters these proteins at a later time, perhaps as a result of trauma or infection, they may generate an immune response. This could account for some of the examples of autoimmunity discussed in Chapter 18.

## ADDITIONAL READING

1. Cooper, E. L., *Comparative Immunology*, Foundations of Immunology Series, Prentice-Hall, Englewood Cliffs, NJ, 1976. Discusses both the phylogeny and the ontogeny of immune responsiveness.

2. Henderson. D. A., "The Eradication of Smallpox," *Scientific American* **235**:25, October, 1976. Describes the strategy and procedures of the WHO campaign.

3. Jenner, E., *An Inquiry into the causes and effects of the variolae vaccinae, a disease discovered in some of the western counties of England, particularly Gloucestershire, and known by the name of The Cow Pox*, London, 1798. [Portions reprinted in T. D. Brock (ed.), *Milestones in Microbiology*, American Society for Microbiology, 1975.]

4. Kabat, E. A., *Structural Concepts in Immunology and Immunochemistry*, 2nd ed., Holt, Rinehart and Winston, New York, 1976. Chapter 2 discusses the types of antigens and the addition of haptens to protcins.

5. Moss, B., et al., "Live Recombinant Vaccinia Virus Protects Chimpanzees Against Hepatitis B," *Nature* **311**:67, 1984.

6. Pasteur, L., "De l'attenuation du virus du cholera des poules," *Comptes rendus des seances de l'Academie des Sciences* **91**:673, 1880. [Reprinted, along with a translation, in T. D. Brock (ed.), *Milestones in Microbiology*, American Society for Microbiology, 1975.]

CHAPTER **2**

# Humoral Immunity

## 2.1 Pneumococcal Pneumonia

Before the development of sulfa drugs and antibiotics, one of the most worrisome of infectious diseases humans are prey to was lobar pneumonia. The agent causing this disease is a bacterium, *Streptococcus pneumoniae*. It often lives harmlessly in our nasopharyngeal passages. But, on occasion, the organism descends into one or more lobes of the lungs where it proliferates rapidly. In response to this invasion, tissue fluids begin to accumulate in the bronchioles and alveoli. As the lungs fill with fluid, the surface area available for gas exchange is reduced. In fatal cases, death results from asphyxiation.

If one cultures the organisms taken from a patient, the colonies that grow on the agar have a characteristic sheen (Figure 2.1). The light microscope reveals (Figure 2.2) that the organisms occur in pairs (accounting for an earlier name for the genus, *Diplococcus*). A thick gela-

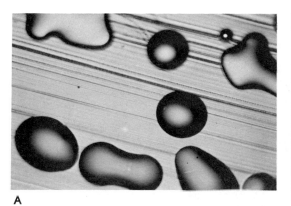 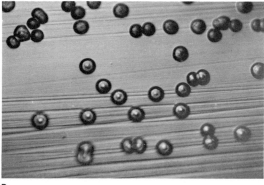

A                                                          B

**Figure 2.1**  Smooth (A) and rough (B) colonies of *Streptococcus pneumoniae*. Rough colonies appear after prolonged cultivation in vitro when the organisms cease producing a capsule (and lose their virulence). [Courtesy of Robert Austrian, *J. Exp. Med.* **98**:21, 1953.]

tinous capsule composed of a polysaccharide coats the cell wall of the organism. This capsule causes the glistening appearance of the colonies.

   *Streptococcus pneumoniae*, often called the pneumococcus, occurs in a large number (about 80) of "types." The chemical composition of the polysaccharide capsule that surrounds the organism distinguishes one type from another. In a number of cases, the nature of the polysaccharide has been established. Figure 2.3 shows the structure of the capsular polysaccharides of type 3 and type 8 pneumococci. The type 3 pneumococcal polysaccharide is an unbranched polymer of alternating units of glucose and glucuronic acid. The repeating unit in the type 8 polysaccharide is the tetramer [glucuronic acid – glucose – glucose – galactose]. In each case, the polymers are of indeterminate but enormous (thousands of residues) length.

   Humans who survive an attack of lobar pneumonia caused by, say, type

**Figure 2.2**  Encapsulated (A) and nonencapsulated (B) pneumococci. The encapsulated forms produce smooth colonies. [Courtesy of Robert Austrian, *J. Exp. Med.* **98**:21, 1953.]

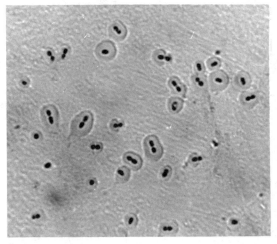 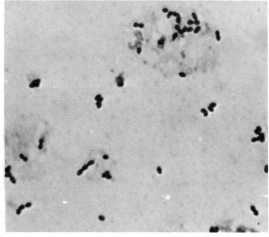

A                                                          B

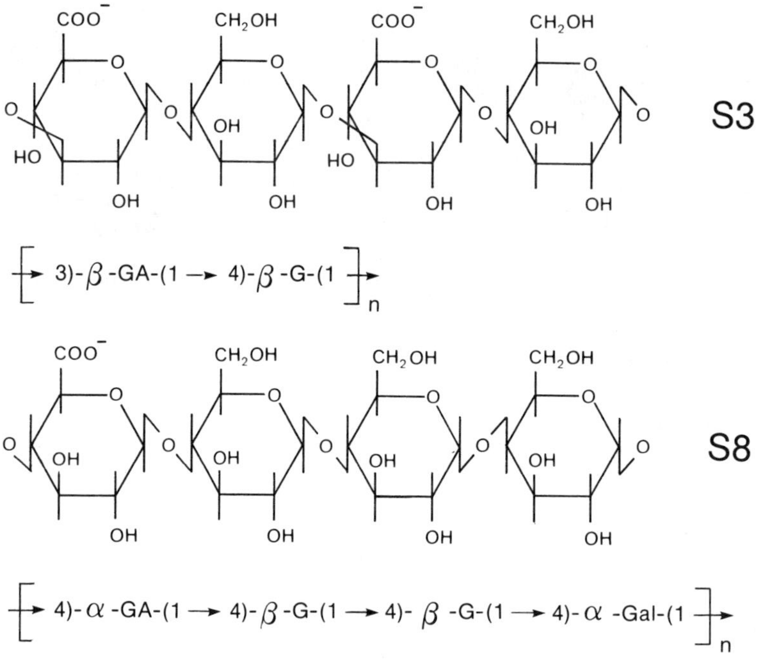

Figure 2.3 The structures of the type 3 and type 8 pneumococcal polysaccharides. (GA = glucuronic acid, G = glucose, Gal = galactose.)

$$[\rightarrow 3)\text{-}\beta\text{-GA-}(1 \rightarrow 4)\text{-}\beta\text{-G-}(1 \rightarrow]_n$$

$$[\rightarrow 4)\text{-}\alpha\text{-GA-}(1 \rightarrow 4)\text{-}\beta\text{-G-}(1 \rightarrow 4)\text{-}\beta\text{-G-}(1 \rightarrow 4)\text{-}\alpha\text{-Gal-}(1 \rightarrow]_n$$

3 pneumococci, will not be afflicted by that organism again. They are immune. As a result of exposure to the organism, they have gained future protection from it. And this protection is specific. That is to say, while immune to future attacks by type 3 pneumococci, they are still fully susceptible to invasion by pneumococci of the other types. What is the nature of this protection?

Although normally an inhabitant of human airways, the pneumococcus is extremely pathogenic for mice. Injected into the peritoneal cavity, just a few living, encapsulated, type 3 pneumococci will quickly multiply. In 24 hours or so, the mouse will die of an overwhelming septicemia, its body teeming with billions of pneumococci.

Knowing this, let us now inject several million living, fully virulent pneumococci into a mouse and, at the same time, a drop or two of serum (blood plasma minus fibrinogen and other clotting factors) taken from a human who has recently recovered from type 3 pneumonia. This time the mouse remains healthy despite its injection of a dose of pneumococci over a million times larger than what is needed to kill a normal mouse. But if we vary the experiment by injecting living type 3 pneumococci along with a little serum from a patient who has recovered from pneumonia of another type, say type 1 or 2, or from a person who has never had pneumonia at all, the mouse succumbs promptly. This simple experiment tells us a great deal. We have found that the *serum* of a patient recovering from an infection by type 3 pneumococci has acquired the capacity to protect another mammal (as well as the patient) against pneumonia of the *same type*. This protection stems from the presence of antipneumococcal antibodies in the serum. A serum that contains a particular set of antibodies is called an *antiserum*. The effect of the antiserum is specific; i.e., antibodies against type 3 pneumococci give no protection against type 1 or 2 or (with occasional exceptions) any of the other 80-odd types (and vice versa). The reason for this specificity is that the capsular polysaccharide, which distinguishes the various types, is the major antigen of the invading organisms to be recognized by the immune system.

The capsular polysaccharide can be removed from pneumococci and purified. If we mix a solution of purified type 3 polysaccharide with serum from a person immune to type 3 (i.e., serum containing anti-type 3 antibodies), a dense white precipitate quickly forms (Figure 2.4). If we have chosen the relative concentrations of polysaccharide and antiserum properly, the supernatant can now be shown to be completely devoid of antibodies (by adding more polysaccharide to a portion of it) and also devoid of polysaccharide (by adding additional anti-type 3 antibodies to another portion of the supernatant). Evidently, both activities now reside in the precipitate. Chemical analysis of the precipitate does, in fact, reveal the polysaccharide in the precise amount we had introduced into the test tube. The remaining material in the precipitate is protein. Thus these antipneumococcal antibodies are proteins.

The ability of anti-type 3 antibodies and the type 3 polysaccharide to interact and precipitate is more than a laboratory curiosity. In the infected animal, the interaction of these two materials provides immunity. For reasons not yet fully known, the capsular polysaccharide interferes with phagocytosis by such scavenging cells as macrophages and neutrophils. It is, in fact, their ability to resist phagocytosis that allows encapsulated pneumococci to proliferate so rapidly. If pneumococci are grown for a period of time on synthetic culture medium, they eventually cease to produce the capsule. These organisms now produce rough-surfaced colonies instead of the glistening "smooth" colonies of the encapsulated forms (Figure 2.1). And these organisms are no longer virulent. When introduced into a mouse, they are quickly destroyed by phagocytes.

**Figure 2.4**   Precipitation in liquid. The tube at A contains diluted serum from a rabbit immunized with killed type 3 pneumococci. A solution of the type 3 polysaccharide is added (B), and the formation of insoluble antigen–antibody complexes is revealed by the almost instantaneous appearance of turbidity (C). After an hour, the complexes settle out as a precipitate (D). If the proportion of antigen to antibodies in the mixture was selected properly, the supernatant will contain neither.

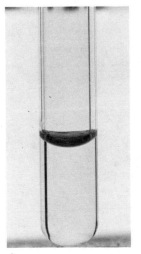 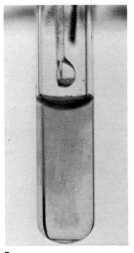 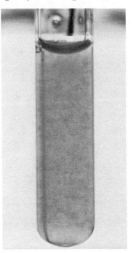 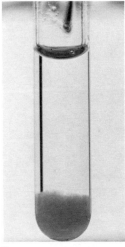

A                    B                    C                    D

Figure 2.5 shows several encapsulated pneumococci being engulfed by a neutrophil. The process proceeds efficiently despite the presence of a capsule around the bacteria. This is because a few drops of antiserum — i.e., serum containing antibodies capable of binding to the capsular polysaccharide — were added to the medium containing the predator and prey. Evidently, the interaction of antibodies with the polysaccharide altered the surface of the bacteria so that they could then be readily engulfed. The process is called *opsonization*. We may assume that the same phenomenon, occurring in the infected animal, shifts the tide in favor of the host and brings recovery. The time of the first appearance of antipneumococcal antibodies does in fact determine the resolution of the "crisis," one of the most characteristic features of lobar pneumonia. Before therapy with antibiotics became available, the progress of the disease culminated after around five days in the so-called crisis. Over a period of a few hours, the victim either reached a life-threatening stage of oxygen deprivation or began to make a dramatic recovery. In the latter case, the fever dropped quickly and, in a matter of hours, the patient was well on the road to recovery. We know now that the crisis represented a race between the suffocating progression of the disease and the first appearance of antipneumococcal antibodies. Extrapolating from our in vitro demonstration (Figure 2.5), a successful resolution of the crisis represented a shift in the balance between the rate of bacterial proliferation and the rate of bacterial engulfment and destruction by phagocytes. And now we can appreciate why immunity to pneumococcal infection is type specific. The major antigen of each type is its surface polysaccharide, the single feature that distinguishes each type from the others.

**Figure 2.5** A: A neutrophil extends a pseudopod toward two pneumococci. B: These bacteria have now been engulfed by phagocytosis (arrows), and the neutrophil is beginning to engulf four more pneumococci at the upper right. C: Antibodies to the polysaccharide capsule surrounding the pneumococci were added to enhance phagocytosis ("opsonization"). [From W. B. Wood, M. R. Smith, and B. Watson, *J. Exp. Med.* 84:387, 1946.]

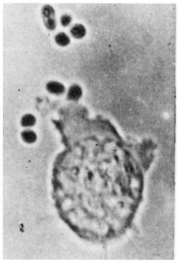 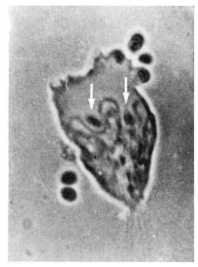 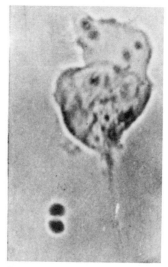

A                                   B                                   C

In addition to its content of water, salts, and a variety of small molecules, blood serum contains a heterogeneous collection of proteins. Some of the major protein components of the serum can be separated by *electrophoresis*. A drop of serum is applied to a paper-like matrix soaked in a buffer at a pH of 8.6. At this pH, all the serum proteins carry a net negative charge. Passing a direct current through the matrix causes the protein molecules to move in the electric field and separates them on the basis of their charge. Serum albumin, the most negatively charged protein, migrates most rapidly toward the anode (Figure 2.6). It is followed by proteins collectively called *alpha globulins*. Next come the beta globulins, one of the most distinct members of which is transferrin, an iron-transport protein. The most weakly charged proteins, the gamma globulins, come last. (In fact, the charge is so weak on some of the gamma globulins that they may be swept a short distance back toward the cathode, carried in the flow of buffer toward that electrode.) After a period of time (e.g., 20 minutes), the current is turned off and the now-separated proteins are fixed in the matrix and stained. Figure 2.7 shows the pattern of bands produced by electrophoresis of serum samples taken from several rabbits, all but one of which had been injected many times with killed type 3 pneumococci. The serum of these "hyperimmune" rabbits contained anti-type 3 antibodies in concentrations ranging from 3 to 41 mg/ml. While the gamma globulin region in the unimmunized rabbit is light and diffuse, the gamma regions of the hyperimmune rabbits reveal high concentrations of protein. Are these gamma globulins the antibodies? To find out, we perform electrophoresis on hyperimmune serum before and after precipitating out all the anti-type 3 antibodies (remembering to compensate for the dilution of the serum samples). The answer is clear: the removal of antibody activity coincides with the removal of a large part of the protein in the gamma region (Figure 2.8). In fact, the serum from which the anti-type 3 antibodies have been removed contains no higher concentration of gamma globulins than that of nonim-

**Figure 2.6** Separating serum proteins by electrophoresis. The albumin molecules migrate most rapidly in the electric field. The slowest moving proteins are the *γ*-globulins. Only the transferrin band can be seen without staining.

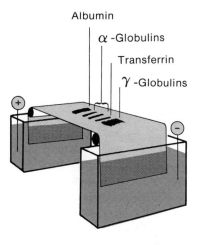

Albumin

α -Globulins

Transferrin

γ -Globulins

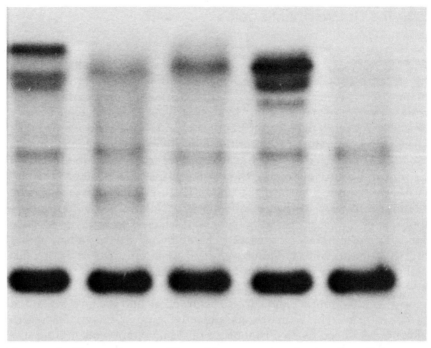

**Figure 2.7** Electrophoresis of five rabbit serum samples (anode at the bottom). Each rabbit (except the one represented on the extreme right) had been intensively immunized with killed type 3 pneumococci. The concentrations of anti-type 3 antibodies were (from left to right) 20, 3, 11, 41, and 0 (mg/ml). [From J. W. Kimball et al., *J. Immunol.* **106:**1177, 1971.]

mune animals. These antibodies are, then, gamma globulins. However, some antibodies migrate more rapidly than those shown here, and antibody activity can sometimes be detected in the beta and, on occasions, the alpha regions. Therefore, it is now common practice to describe all proteins with antibody activity as "immunoglobulins."

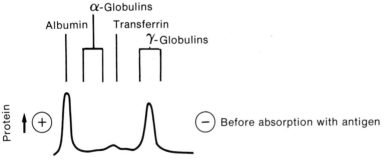

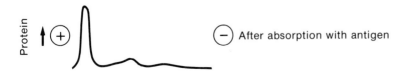

**Figure 2.8** Densitometric tracings of the electrophoretograms of a rabbit antipneumococcal serum before and after absorption with the polysaccharide. Most of the gamma globulins were antipneumococcal antibodies. [Adapted from J. H. Pincus et al., *J. Immunol.* **104:**1143, 1970.]

The basic unit out of which all immunoglobulins are constructed is a dimer containing four polypeptides. Two of these, each containing an identical sequence of over 200 amino acid residues, are called the light (L) chains. The other two each contain an identical sequence of 400–500 residues. These are the heavy (H) chains (Figure 2.9). Each L chain is attached to an H chain by a disulfide bridge linking cysteine (Cys) residues and *also* by the mutual attraction of some of their hydrophobic amino acids. The two H chains are held together by one or more disulfide bridges.

The sequence of amino acids in the amino terminal ("N terminal") half of the light chains differs substantially between different molecules. In other words, the N terminal of the L chains of an antibody molecule that binds to DNP would be expected to have a different sequence from that in the L chains of a molecule that binds KLH. This region of the L chains is called the variable (V) region.

The carboxyl terminal of L chains shows far less sequence variability from one kind of molecule to another. This region is thus called the constant (C) region.

A similar pattern is found in H chains. The V region occupies the N terminal of the chain. The remainder of the chain makes up the C region (Figure 2.9).

**Figure 2.9** Chain structure of a human IgG molecule. The numbers indicate the number of amino acid residues (counting from the amino terminal). The two light chains are identical, as are the two heavy chains. In the intact molecule, the chains are folded so that each intrachain cysteine is brought close to the partner with which it forms a disulfide (S–S) bond. In a given species, different antibody molecules (of any one type) have the same or almost the same sequence of amino acids in their constant regions but show marked differences in their variable regions. These differences are especially pronounced in the hypervariable regions. Other classes of antibody molecules (e.g., IgM, IgA) differ in the construction of the constant region of the heavy chain.

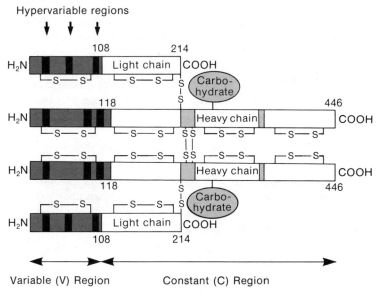

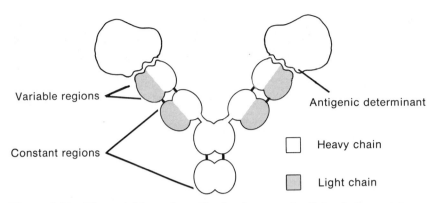

Variable regions

Antigenic determinant

Constant regions

Heavy chain

Light chain

**Figure 2.10** The variable region of both a heavy and a light chain participate in forming the antigen-binding site. All of the sites on a single antibody molecule (two in this case) are identical because all of the H chains, as well as all of the L chains, are identical.

The antigen-binding specificity of an antibody molecule resides in its variable regions. The folding of the V regions of one H and L chain forms a groove or cavity into which the antigenic determinant fits (Figure 2.10). The contours of the site provide a surface that is complementary to the surface of the antigenic determinant capable of being bound at that site. This complementarity involves more than simple topography. The precise location of particular amino acids (whether charged, hydrophobic, etc.) also dictates what antigenic determinants can be bound. Thus the binding specificity of antibody molecules depends on the same sort of lock and key mechanism that exists for the binding of an enzyme to its substrate.

Because a binding site is constructed from one H and one L chain, this dimeric structure has two sites. Because the two L chains are identical as are the two H chains, the two binding sites are identical. Thus the molecule is *bivalent* (Figure 2.10).

Five distinctly different kinds of constant regions are found in the heavy chains of human immunoglobulins (as well as in those of other mammals like mice). These five types of H chain establish five distinct *classes* of immunoglobulins. The most abundant is called *immunoglobulin G* (IgG). The other four are IgM, IgA, IgD, and IgE. The heavy chains, which establish the class to which the molecule is assigned, are called **gamma** ($\gamma$), **mu** ($\mu$), **alpha** ($\alpha$), **delta** ($\delta$), and **epsilon** ($\epsilon$) chains, respectively (Figure 2.11). Two light chain classes, called **kappa** and **lambda,** are also found, but these are associated indiscriminately with all five classes of heavy chains.

Why do so many kinds of constant regions exist? The different heavy chain constant regions differ in their biological properties. For example, only IgG molecules are able to traverse the placenta from the mother's circulation to that of her fetus. IgE molecules, another example, are able to bind to specific receptors on the surface of basophils and mast cells and, as a result, mediate certain allergic responses. In each case, these properties are a function of the constant region of the heavy chain (gamma and epsilon, respectively).

The basic dimer structure described here is found in IgG, IgD, and IgE

| Class | H chain | L chain | Structure | Concentration in serum (mg/ml) | Notes |
|-------|---------|---------|-----------|-------------------------------|-------|
| IgG | $\gamma$ | $\kappa$ or $\lambda$ | $H_2L_2$ | 13 | Transferred across placenta |
| IgM | $\mu$ | $\kappa$ or $\lambda$ | $(H_2L_2)_5$ +J | 0.5–2.5 | First antibodies to appear after immunization |
| IgA | $\alpha$ | $\kappa$ or $\lambda$ | $(H_2L_2)_{1-2}$ +J | 0.5–3 | Higher concentrations in secretions |
| IgD | $\delta$ | $\kappa$ or $\lambda$ | $H_2L_2$ | 0.03 | Function uncertain |
| IgE | $\epsilon$ | $\kappa$ or $\lambda$ | $H_2L_2$ | 0.0003 | Binds to basophils and mast cells sensitizing them for certain allergic reactions |

Figure 2.11 The immunoglobulin classes. The concentrations are those normally found in human serum. $J$ = joining chain.

molecules. IgA molecules contain one or two of these units. IgM molecules contain five of them: $(H_2L_2)_5$. But note that IgM molecules are *not* simply pentamers of five molecules of IgG. The structure of the H chains in IgM (mu chains) is quite different from those in IgG (gamma chains).

Over the past 30 years, a wealth of information has been gained about the structure of antibody molecules. Much of this knowledge, and the discoveries that led to it, will be examined in Chapter 9. However, this brief introduction should provide a basis for understanding the following chapters. It should also give you a glimpse of one of the most remarkable features of humoral immunity: the extraordinary diversity of the molecules that comprise any set of antibodies. Let us now pursue the subject of antibody diversity by quite a different approach. We will study the various kinds of antigenic determinants expressed on the surface of antibody molecules.

## 2.3   The Diversity of Antibodies

Antibodies are proteins and when introduced into an animal for which they are foreign, they — like any other protein — elicit the formation of antibodies ("anti-antibodies"). Thus antibodies can be antigens.

### Isotypes

When human immunoglobulins are injected into a rabbit, the rabbit recognizes these proteins as foreign and develops antibodies against them. The resulting antiserum will, when mixed with human serum, form a copious precipitate. However, this precipitate is not a simple two-component aggregate. It actually contains a variety of types of human immunoglobulin molecules. If we subject a sample of human serum to electro-

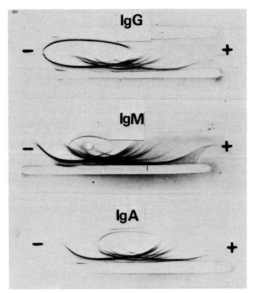

**Figure 2.12** Identification of IgG, IgM, and IgA. Identical serum samples were placed in the three central wells and subjected to electrophoresis. For each electrophoretogram, a polyvalent antiserum (raised against whole serum) was placed in the lower trough and an antiserum specific for a single isotype of heavy chain (for IgG, for IgM, and for IgA) placed in the upper trough. (This technique, called immunoelectrophoresis, is described more fully in Section 5.4.) Note that each H-chain-specific antiserum produces a single arc that corresponds to one of the arcs produced by the polyvalent antiserum. In the examples shown here, the serum samples were from a rabbit and the antiserum raised in a goat. [From Justine S. Garvey, Natalie E. Cremer, and Dieter H. Sussdorf, *Methods in Immunology*, 3rd ed. W. A. Benjamin, Inc., Advanced Book Program, 1977.]

phoresis and then expose the separated proteins to the rabbit antiserum, we get some idea of the complexity of the response. The rabbit antiserum precipitates with a number of distinct components in the human serum. Each of these lines of precipitate defines a separate *isotype* of antibody molecule (Figure 2.12). *Each of these isotypes corresponds to one of the classes* of antibody described in the previous section. The dominant isotype is IgG. The antiserum also forms separate precipitin arcs with IgM and IgA antibodies. The concentration of IgD and IgE in the serum is too low to be detected by the method used here.

Isotypic (*iso* = same) determinants are shared by all members of a species. For this reason, the rabbit antiserum will reveal the same isotypes in any sample of human serum. And because all the members of a species "see" isotypic determinants as "self," anti-isotypic antisera must be raised in another (heterologous) species.

## Allotypes

Antibody *allotypes* (*allo* = other) are antigenically distinct kinds of antibody molecules that are found in some members of the species but not in others. They are inherited as simple Mendelian traits.

The ABO blood groups in humans provide a rough analogy. You will recall that human blood is assigned to blood groups A, B, AB, or O, depending on whether the red cells carry the A antigen, the B antigen, both of, or neither of these antigens. Humans of blood group B will respond to injections of A red cells by producing anti-A antibodies. They do not produce anti-B antibodies because the B antigen is not foreign to them. However, both the A and the B antigen are foreign to group O individuals, and they can produce antibodies against each. The ABO phenotype is governed by a single locus. Three alleles are present in the

26

| Blood group | Antigens on RBCs | Antibodies in serum | Genotypes |
|:---:|:---:|:---|:---|
| A | A | Anti-B | *AA or AO* |
| B | B | Anti-A | *BB or BO* |
| AB | A and B | Neither | *AB* |
| O | Neither | Anti-A and Anti-B | *OO* |

**Figure 2.13** The Landsteiner (ABO) blood groups and the genotypes that give rise to each. Allotypic variants of antibodies are inherited in the same manner.

human population: *A*, *B*, and *O*. The blood group of a single individual is determined by which pair of these alleles is inherited (Figure 2.13).

Allotypic differences associated with antibody molecules behave in much the same fashion. For example, rabbit IgG molecules exist in two allotypic forms: d11 and d12. A homozygous d11 rabbit (*d11/d11*) will produce anti-d12 antibodies when injected with the IgG molecules of a d12 rabbit. The resulting antiserum can be used to identify all rabbits that express the d12 allotype.

The expression of allotypes is inherited as a single gene trait controlled by codominant alleles. Therefore, both the d11 and d12 allotypes are found (in roughly equal amounts) in the serum of heterozygous (*d11/ d12*) animals (Figure 2.14).

Anti-allotype antisera are usually raised in the same species. One could use a different species to secure anti-d12 antibodies, but the procedure is not efficient. A goat, for example, would recognize not only the allotypic determinant(s) as foreign but also all those isotypic determinants that distinguish rabbit IgG antibodies from goat IgG antibodies. In order to make it specific for a given allotype, the goat antiserum would have to

**Figure 2.14** Inheritance of allotypes. The *d11/d12* allotypes are genetic variants of rabbit gamma chains that are inherited as a single-gene trait controlled by codominant alleles.

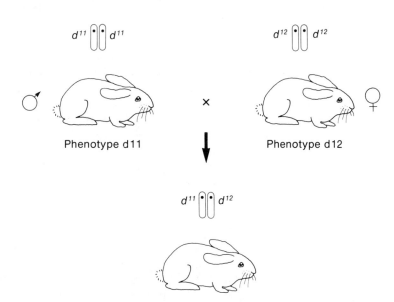

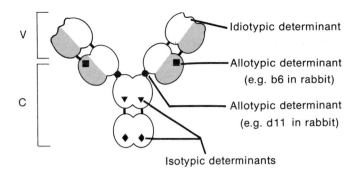

Figure 2.15 Characteristic locations of idiotypic, allotypic, and isotypic determinants. Both H and L chains express their own isotypic and allotypic determinants most of which are located in their constant (C) regions. Idiotypic determinants are expressed by V regions and often the expression of the determinant requires the participation of both the H and the L chain.

Idiotypic determinant

Allotypic determinant (e.g. b6 in rabbit)

Allotypic determinant (e.g. d11 in rabbit)

Isotypic determinants

first be absorbed with pooled rabbit immunoglobulins (of some other allotype) to remove antibodies directed against isotypic determinants. As anti-isotypic antibodies would most likely have dominated the immune response, the anti-allotypic activity remaining is likely to be slight. For this reason, anti-allotypic antisera are usually raised in members of the same species.

Allotypic determinants associated with a given isotype (for example, d11 and d12 on rabbit IgG) are found on all molecules of that isotype regardless of their antigen-binding specificity. For example, anti-DNP, anti-BSA, and anti-KLH antibodies (of the IgG isotype) from a homozygous d12 rabbit would all carry the d12 allotypic determinant.

A number of antibody allotypes have been identified in other animals, including humans and mice. Each is associated with one particular class of H chain (e.g., a gamma chain) or L chain. With a few exceptions (such as a set of allotypes, the "a" allotypes, associated with the V region of rabbit H chains), allotypic determinants are located in constant regions (Figure 2.15).

## Idiotypes

A rabbit IgG molecule capable of binding DNP must differ in its structure from one capable of binding KLH. We might well expect that this difference in structure would produce one or more antigenic determinants unique to that portion of the IgG molecule responsible for recognizing DNP. Injected into another rabbit, these determinants should be seen as foreign (especially if the second rabbit is not making any anti-DNP antibodies of its own). If the second rabbit has all the same allotypes of the first rabbit, then only these anti-DNP-associated determinants should be seen as foreign. The resulting antiserum defines an *idiotype* (*idios* = one's own). An idiotypic determinant is thus one that is associated with antibody molecules of a particular antigen-binding specificity. And, in fact, a given idiotype is usually found only on that subset of antibodies that share an identical antigen-binding site.

Anti-idiotypic antisera are usually raised in animals of the same species that have been matched with the donor for all known allotypes. If matching is not done or if another species is used, then extensive absorptions must be carried out to remove anti-isotypic and anti-allotypic antibodies.

How can one be sure that the antiserum elicited in a rabbit ("B") is not simply detecting a previously unknown allotype in the donor rabbit ("A")? The test is simple. The antiserum should react with the specific (e.g., anti-DNP) antibodies from rabbit A that were used for immunization but not with the "pre-immune" serum from rabbit A. In other words, the anti-idiotypic antibodies should not recognize any IgG molecules that were present in rabbit A before it was immunized against DNP.

As Rodkey so simply and brilliantly demonstrated in 1974, anti-idiotypic antibodies can even be elicited in the same rabbit that produced the idiotype. He immunized rabbits with hapten–protein conjugates; then isolated, purified, and *stored* the resulting antihapten antibodies. Sixteen months after the last injection of antigen, the animals were injected with their own antibodies. In due course, the animals produced antibodies against these antibodies, that is, "auto-anti-idiotypic" antibodies.

**Figure 2.16**  Graph showing inhibition by the hapten DNP-L-lysine of the precipitation of a homogenous DNP-binding protein (MOPC-315) by its anti-idiotypic antibodies. Competition between the hapten molecules and the anti-idiotypic antibodies for the same site (schematic) could account for this. Alternatively, binding of hapten could cause a conformational change in the anti-DNP molecule, altering its idiotypic determinants. [Data from B. W. Brient et al., *Proc. Natl. Acad. Sci. USA* **68**:3136, 1971.]

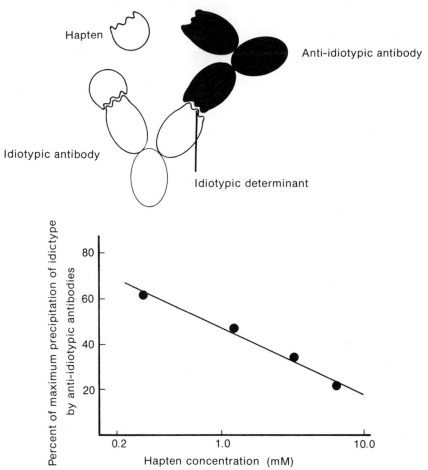

It is generally more difficult to elicit anti-allotypic and, especially, anti-idiotypic antibodies than anti-isotypic antibodies. In the first two cases, most of the molecule is seen as "self." Usually, the molecules must be administered in an especially immunogenic way: (1) complexed with antigen, (2) aggregated, and/or (3) with the use of immuno-enhancing agents called *adjuvants.*

Idiotypes are usually associated with antibody molecules of a particular antigenic specificity. Thus we find that they can be absorbed from serum by exposing the serum to the antigen. Neither isotypic nor allotypic specificities can be totally removed by absorbing with antigen.

As the word suggests, the idiotype of an anti-DNP antibody molecule made by one rabbit should be different from that made by another rabbit. For outbred animals (like rabbits) this is usually the case. However, in inbred mouse strains immunized with certain antigens, a particular idiotype may occur in most or all of the animals. Such a shared idiotype is called a cross-reacting or public idiotype. These probably occur because all the members of an inbred strain share an identical inherited set of antibody-forming genes.

Idiotypic determinants are localized in the V regions of antibodies and thus near the part of the molecule that binds to antigen (Figure 2.15). Therefore V regions are capable of binding two distinct entities: an antigenic determinant (such as hapten) and an anti-idiotypic antibody molecule. In some cases, the two activities interfere with each other. The interaction of idiotype with anti-idiotype is frequently inhibited by the presence of hapten (Figure 2.16). Such idiotype – antiidiotype interactions are said to be "hapten modifiable."

Isotype, allotype, and idiotype are three broad categories reflecting the diversity of antibodies. We have examined this diversity as it is revealed by antisera directed against particular sets of antigenic determinants. But whether isotypic, allotypic, or idiotypic, these antigenic determinants must reflect particular configurations of the antibody molecule. Antibodies are proteins, and thus we should be able to find that each of these categories of antigenic determinant can be correlated with a distinct structure or structures in the protein molecule. As we shall see in later chapters, this has turned out to be true in many cases.

## 2.4 The Primary and Secondary Responses

When first exposed to a novel antigen, the immune system may need a considerable period of time before it begins making appreciable amounts of antibodies against the antigen. Recall that a pneumococcal infection can proceed unchecked for five days or so before the first appearance of the antipneumococcal antibodies that turn the tide of the disease. Then, for a period of days, the concentration of antipneumococcal antibodies rises in the serum. A decline follows and may continue until antibodies are no longer detectable. This entire response pattern is called the *primary response* (Figure 2.17).

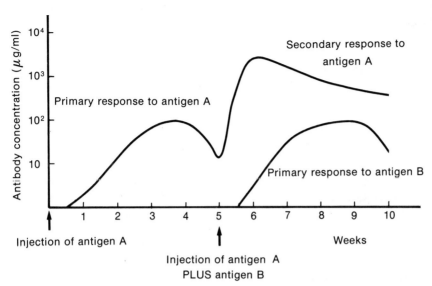

**Figure 2.17** The primary and secondary humoral responses. The altered kinetics and magnitude of the second response to antigen A shows memory. The response to antigen B demonstrates the specificity of the secondary response to A. Note the logarithmic scale on the ordinate.

When the primary response is over and antibodies are no longer present, is the individual once again susceptible to the disease? In many cases, no. Re-exposure to the same antigen produces a different response pattern. Now after a period of hours, not days, specific antibodies appear in the serum. Their concentration rises to greater levels than before, and the response wanes more slowly. This pattern is called the *secondary response*. It is the manifestation of memory in humoral immunity. And, as you can see from Figure 2.17, this memory response is specific: another antigen administered at the same time, dose, etc., as the second dose of the first antigen produces a primary, not a secondary, response.

The speed of the secondary response is such that an infection (against which humoral immunity is effective) may be brought under control before any signs of the illness become evident. Closed communities, like prisons and orphanages, are often repeatedly swept by hidden epidemics: epidemics of infectious agents spreading from one "primed" and thus immune individual to another. The only clear evidence of such hidden epidemics is a sudden rise in antibody levels against the agent involved.

In Section 1.4, we noted that some of the *antibodies* raised to DNP–BSA will also bind to DNP when it is coupled to another carrier, e.g., OVA. However, a *secondary response* to DNP–BSA requires that the DNP be once again administered coupled to BSA. DNP–OVA will not work. The reason for this "carrier specificity" of the secondary response is that B cells ready to mount a secondary response to DNP must receive help from T cells ready to respond a second time to, in this case, BSA. Given DNP–OVA in the second injection, the animal has no T cells primed to the new carrier. Further details of the interaction of T and B cells in the secondary response are presented in Chapter 12.

## 2.5   Active vs. Passive Immunity

The development of humoral immunity in response to stimulation by antigen is called *active immunity*. The production of circulating antibodies against the antigen characterizes active immunity. The response is specific; i.e., the antibodies recognize (are able to bind to) the particular antigenic determinants present on the immunizing antigen. Once formed, the protection afforded by circulating antibodies or — as we shall see — any phenomenon mediated by antibodies can be passively transferred to another animal by the injection of antiserum. The recipient of the antiserum is said to be passively immunized.

The clinical use of tetanus antitoxin provides an instructive case. Tetanus antitoxin is an antiserum that has been produced by actively immunizing an animal, such as a horse, with tetanus toxoid. Its therapeutic value arises when a human is at risk from an infection by tetanus bacilli (perhaps introduced in a dirty wound) and has never, or not for a long time, been actively immunized with tetanus toxoid. Fearing that the race between the liberation by the bacteria of tetanus toxin and the development of an active immune response on the part of the host may go badly, the physician injects tetanus antitoxin in order to provide immediate protection. This protection is, however, short-lived. It remains effective only until the last of the injected gamma globulins have been catabolized by the host.

Horse proteins are foreign to the human patient and will, in due course, elicit an active immune response. This response may take the form of a damaging allergic reaction (such as anaphylaxis — Section 18.2 — or serum sickness — Section 18.6). For this reason, humans are increasingly used as the source of antibodies for passive immunization. Immune globulin (IG) is prepared from the gamma globulin fraction of pooled plasma from the outdated blood of several thousand blood donors. The assumption is that such a large pool of donors will reflect the immune status of the general population. IG prepared in this way is used to protect persons exposed to hepatitis A or to measles. Preparations of immune globulin harvested from selected hyperimmune human donors are used to provide immediate protection against rabies, tetanus, and chicken pox.

The great advantage of using human immune globulins rather than horse antitoxins is that many irrelevant proteins are omitted and those that remain, being human proteins, are far less immunogenic than horse proteins. Thus the risk of unpleasant active immune reactions is minimized. And, in addition, passively administered human antibodies are catabolized far more slowly than horse antibodies.

### ADDITIONAL READING

1. Kindt, T. J., "Rabbit Immunoglobulin Allotypes: Structure, Immunology, and Genetics," *Adv. Immunol.* **21**:35, 1975.

2. Robbins, J. B., "Vaccines for the Prevention of Encapsulated Bacterial Diseases: Current Status, Problems, and Prospects for the Future," *Immunochemistry* **15**:839, 1978. Includes a discussion of pneumococcal disease.

3. Rodkey, L. S., "Studies of Idiotypic Antibodies: Production and Characterization of Autoantiidiotypic Antisera," *J. Exp. Med.* **139**:712, 1974.

# CHAPTER 3

# Cell-Mediated Immunity

## 3.1 Delayed-Type Hypersensitivity (DTH)

Pasteur's triumphs in the late nineteenth century ushered in a period of intense activity to identify the agents of infectious disease and to find methods—immunological and otherwise—to combat diseases. A major cause of human suffering in those days was tuberculosis. The causative agent is the tubercle bacillus, *Mycobacterium tuberculosis,* and the organs most commonly affected are the lungs.

Attempting to isolate an antigen to serve as the basis of a vaccine, Robert Koch prepared crude extracts of cultures of the organism. This material was called tuberculin. It never fulfilled Koch's hopes for a vaccine, but it did make available an important diagnostic tool still in use today. This is the Mantoux test. It is used to determine if an individual has ever been exposed to, and thus mounted an immune reaction against, the tubercle bacillus. In the United States, a positive Mantoux test is strong evidence of exposure to the tubercle bacillus — from an active or subclinical case of tuberculosis. In many other countries, however, a positive Mantoux test is simply a reflection of prior vaccination with an attenuated strain of *Mycobacterium bovis,* the organism that causes tuberculosis in cattle. The attenuated strain is called the bacillus of Calmette – Guerin (BCG).

The test is performed by introducing into the skin a tiny amount (about 0.1 microgram) of tuberculin (or a somewhat more pure protein extract of the tubercle bacilli called "purified protein derivative" or PPD). If the individual has been sensitized (i.e., has mounted a prior response to the antigen), a characteristic lesion appears at the site of injection. The area becomes red, slightly swollen, and firm to the touch. The lesion first appears in about 10 hours and reaches a peak in 48 – 72 hours. Because the response takes so much longer to appear than certain rapid, antibody-mediated responses (discussed in Chapter 18), it is called delayed-type hypersensitivity (DTH). Microscopic examination of the lesion reveals a densely packed collection of lymphocytes and macrophages. The response meets the criteria of immunity: individuals with no prior exposure to either the disease or the vaccine produce no reaction. However, if one examines the serum of the responders for the presence of antibodies against the antigens in tuberculin, more often than not none can be detected. And even if antibodies are present, they cannot passively transfer this immune response to another individual.

The tuberculin reaction (and DTH reactions, in general) can also be studied in guinea pigs. In 1945, Chase reported that tuberculin immunity could be transferred to a "naive" guinea pig by injecting it with a suspension of living "lymphoid" cells (which are primarily lymphocytes and macrophages) taken from an immune guinea pig. The response could not be passively transferred by an injection of serum alone. The cells responsible for the transfer of DTH ultimately turned out to be a particular subset of lymphocytes called **T lymphocytes.** We shall use the designation $T_D$ for these cells. The passive acquisition of immunity by an injection of lymphocytes from an immunized ("primed") donor is called **adoptive immunity.**

The DTH reaction is, then, a response that meets all the criteria of an immune response: it displays memory and specificity. Since it is not mediated by antibodies, it cannot be passively transferred by injections of serum. Mediated instead by cells — a subset of T lymphocytes — it is properly described as a "cell-mediated" immune (CMI) reaction.

## 3.2  In Vitro Correlates
## of Cell-Mediated Immunity

Skin testing platoons of guinea pigs is an expensive (and sometimes rather unreliable) business. So an early goal of cellular immunologists was the development of in vitro assays to measure cell-mediated immunity.

### Lymphocyte Proliferation

If one takes a lymphoid cell population capable of transferring a DTH reaction to tuberculin, for example, and places the cells in culture along with the antigen, *some* of the lymphocytes will be stimulated to undergo mitosis. One can determine this by supplying radioactive (tritiated) thymidine ($^3$H-TdR) to the culture medium. During the S phase of the cell cycle, the stimulated lymphocytes incorporate the radiolabeled thymidine in their freshly synthesized DNA. The uptake of the radioactive label by the cells can easily be measured by removing the cells from the culture (by filtration or centrifugation) and measuring their radioactivity. The specificity of the proliferative response can be shown by culturing batches of lymphocytes from an antigen-sensitized animal with sev-

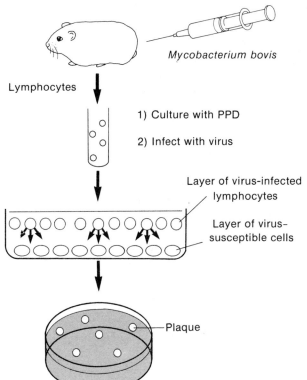

**Figure 3.1**  Enumeration of antigen-specific lymphocytes by their capacity to support virus replication [Based on the work of B. R. Bloom et al., *J. Exp. Med.* **132**:16, 1970.]

*Mycobacterium bovis*

Lymphocytes

1) Culture with PPD

2) Infect with virus

Layer of virus-infected lymphocytes

Layer of virus-susceptible cells

Plaque

eral different antigens. Only the original sensitizing antigen will stimulate a marked increase in the uptake of tritiated thymidine.

The population of lymphocytes that mediate DTH to a particular antigen is only a minor fraction of the total lymphocyte pool in the animal. To evaluate the size of this fraction, we can take advantage of another distinguishing feature of activated lymphocytes. This is their ability to support the proliferation of RNA viruses such as measles virus and poliovirus. RNA viruses do not proliferate successfully in small, resting lymphocytes. So only those lymphocytes specifically sensitized to a particular antigen will support viral replication when cultured with the antigen and exposed to the virus (Figure 3.1). We can determine the number of infected lymphocytes by plating the cell culture on a sheet of cells (e.g., mouse cells) that can be infected and lysed by the same virus. As each infected lymphocyte releases progeny virus, the virus infects and lyses the mouse cells directly beneath it. The result is a clear zone or plaque. The results of such experiments reveal that only 0.1% of the lymphocytes in a sensitized guinea pig responds specifically to the sensitizing antigen.

**Figure 3.2** Demonstration that most of the cells in a DTH lesion are not specific for the antigen. Presumably a small population of antigen-specific cells recruits a large population of nonspecific cells to the site. This recruitment is mediated by lymphokines—substances released by antigen-sensitized lymphocytes exposed to the antigen.

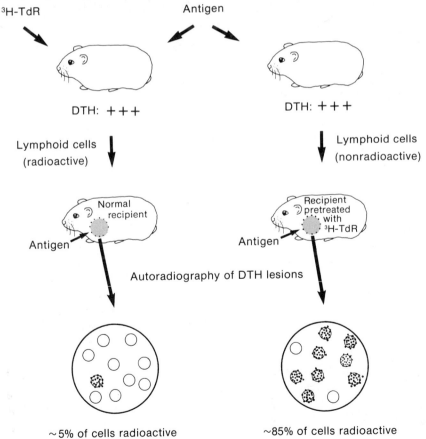

Are these activated cells the ones that are found in a DTH lesion? To answer this question, we induce DTH to an antigen (such as PPD) in a group of guinea pigs. Some of these animals are given $^3$H-TdR along with additional antigen in order to label their active lymphocytes. The lymphoid cells from the isotope-treated animals are then injected into normal recipients — the classic method of transferring CMI. The recipients are then injected intradermally with the antigen. When the resulting DTH lesions are examined by autoradiography, only 4–5% of the cells in the lesion turn out to be radioactive (Figure 3.2). On the other hand, when recipient guinea pigs have been injected for several days with $^3$H-TdR before receiving *unlabeled* cells from immunized donors, as many as 85% of the cells in the resulting DTH lesions are radioactive (Figure 3.2). Furthermore, *most* of the 4–5% labeled donor cells in the first experiment are not antigen-specific cells. If labeled lymphocytes from a PPD-sensitized donor are given to an OVA-sensitized recipient, the same percentage of labeled donor cells will appear in the DTH lesion induced in the recipient by an intradermal injection of OVA. We must conclude, therefore, that the great majority of the cells participating in a DTH reaction are nonspecific cells. In these examples, the lesions are mostly filled with host lymphocytes and macrophages along with a small number of donor lymphocytes (of which only a very few are responsible for the specificity of the response).

The implication of these findings is that a DTH reaction is mediated by a tiny population of specifically sensitized cells that — following recognition of the sensitizing antigen — recruits a large population of nonspecific cells into the area where the antigen is present.

## Lymphokines

While not all the details are yet known, the mechanism of this recruitment process is becoming established. Macrophages are actively motile cells. However, in the early 1930s, it was observed that when a mixture of white blood cells taken from a tuberculin-sensitized guinea pig was cultured with tuberculin, the normal motility of the macrophages was inhibited. This observation led to a valuable in vitro test with which to assess DTH.

The test material consists of capillary tubes packed with lymphoid cells from antigen-sensitized animals. A convenient source of cells is the peritoneal exudate — containing chiefly macrophages and lymphocytes — produced following injection of an irritant into the peritoneal cavity. Placed in a culture medium lacking the sensitizing antigen (Figure 3.3), the mobile macrophages migrate out from the ends of the capillary tubes. However, if the sensitizing antigen is present in the culture medium, migration is inhibited (Figure 3.4). The specificity of the response is dependent on the lymphocytes, not the macrophages. Lymphocytes from antigen-sensitized donors cultured with the sensitizing antigen inhibit the migration of *normal* (i.e., unsensitized) guinea pig macrophages. The inhibition is mediated by a soluble molecule, a glycoprotein,

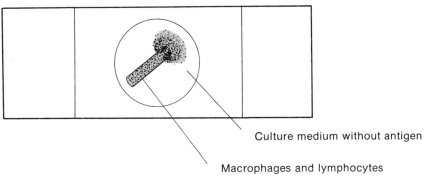

Culture medium without antigen

Macrophages and lymphocytes

**Figure 3.3**  Assay method for migration inhibition factor (**MIF**). Macrophages migrate out of the open end of the capillary tube unless inhibited by the presence of **MIF**. **MIF** is released by antigen-specific lymphocytes upon contact with the antigen in the surrounding medium.

**Figure 3.4**  Results of an assay for migration inhibition factor (MIF). Culturing peritoneal exudate cells from a guinea pig sensitized to ovalbumin (middle row) or diphtheria toxoid (bottom row) with the sensitizing antigen inhibits the migration of macrophages out of the open end of the capillary tube (*e* and *i*). The specificity of the response depends only on the lymphocytes: lymphocytes from antigen-sensitized donors will also inhibit the migration of macrophages from normal (unsensitized) guinea pigs: [Courtesy of Dr. John R. David; from J. R. David et al., *J. Immunol.* 93:264, 1964.]

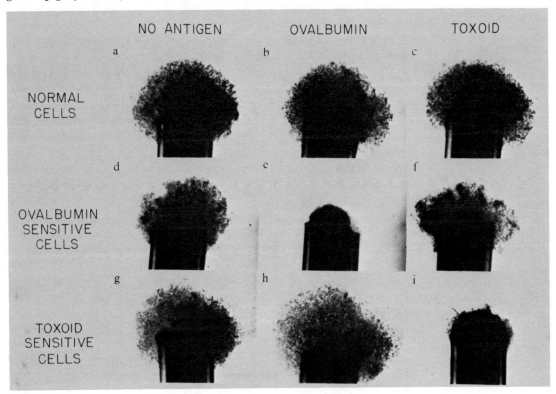

called **migration inhibition factor** (MIF), which is liberated into the medium by the stimulated lymphocytes.

MIF is only one of a number of factors that are released by sensitized lymphocytes upon encountering the sensitizing antigen. Collectively, these substances are known as lymphokines. They possess a number of activities, such as a chemotactic stimulus for macrophages, which suggest that their role in vivo is the recruitment and activation of nonspecific cells—chiefly macrophages—to the regions of interaction between sensitized lymphocytes and the sensitizing antigen.

## 3.3 Transplantation Immunity

For centuries, people have dreamed of and, on occasions, attempted the transplantation of living tissues and organs from one animal to another. But only recently have the rules governing the feasibility of such procedures been worked out. It will aid us in our discussion to distinguish between four categories of transplants.

1. **Autografts** are grafts from one part of an animal's body to another. If performed with proper care, they succeed. For example, burn victims can be greatly helped by the grafting of sheets of skin from an undamaged part of the body to the burned area. Coronary patients may benefit from bypassing a partially blocked coronary artery with a section taken from one of the leg veins.

2. **Isografts or syngeneic grafts** are grafts between two genetically identical (syngeneic) individuals. A graft between monozygotic ("identical") twins is an isograft. It, too, succeeds for, as we shall see, the recipient's immune system sees the graft as "self." Grafts between members of the same inbred mouse strain are also isografts. Inbred strains of mice are produced by brother–sister matings through sufficient generations that the animals become homozygous—and identical—at the vast majority (>98%) of their gene loci. Except, then, for the genetic differences associated with sex, the members of an inbred strain have virtually identical genomes, and grafts between them are successful. A large number of inbred mouse strains are available for experimental work. Some inbred strains of rats and two of guinea pigs have also been produced.

3. **Allografts** are grafts between nonsyngeneic members of the *same* species. Thus most cases of human transplantation involve allografts. The success of allografting rests upon blocking the immune system of the recipient from rejecting the graft it recognizes as nonself. Allografts are also called *homografts*.

4. **Xenografts** are grafts of tissues or organs from one species to another. A few attempts have been made to transplant such organs as the liver from a pig to a human. The immune system recognizes xenografts as nonself, foreign, but its attempts at rejection are not necessarily any more vigorous than for allografts. Xenografts are sometimes called *heterografts*.

If we transplant a piece of skin from an inbred mouse of, for example, the CBA strain to an inbred mouse of the BALB/c strain, the following events occur. At first all goes well. The blood vessels of the host revascularize the graft; it takes on a healthy appearance and begins to heal nicely. After some 10–14 days, however, matters take a turn for the worse. The graft becomes heavily infiltrated by inflammatory cells (including macrophages), and the blood supply to the graft breaks down. In a few more days, the graft shrivels into a scab and is sloughed off. The graft has been rejected.

Now let us repeat the process, transplanting a fresh piece of CBA skin to another site on the *same* recipient. This time, the rejection process is much swifter. In most cases, a blood supply does not become established and in five or six days the second graft is rejected. This more rapid response to the second graft is called the "second-set" reaction. It is specific. That is, if instead of (or even along with) the second CBA graft we place a graft of skin from a third mouse strain (e.g., C57BL), the third-party graft is rejected in 10–14 days, not the 5–6 days characteristic of the second-set response (Figure 3.5). Thus, we have met the

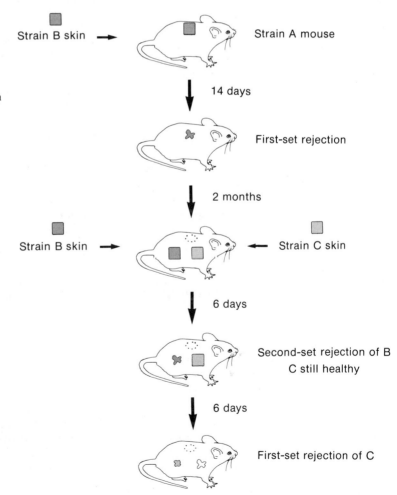

**Figure 3.5** Demonstration that graft rejection is an immune response. The first set rejection of C skin by a mouse that is giving a second-set response to B skin shows that the rejection response displays specificity as well as memory.

Strain B skin ⟶

Strain A mouse

14 days

First-set rejection

2 months

Strain B skin ⟶ ⟵ Strain C skin

6 days

Second-set rejection of B
C still healthy

6 days

First-set rejection of C

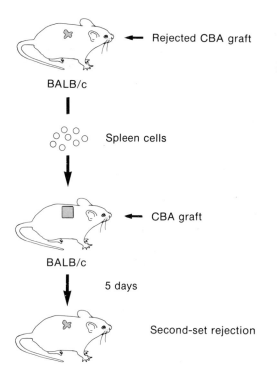

BALB/c

Rejected CBA graft

Spleen cells

CBA graft

BALB/c

5 days

Second-set rejection

**Figure 3.6** Adoptive transfer of the second-set response. Serum alone cannot confer the ability to mount a second-set response showing that graft rejection is a cell-mediated response. However, the transfer of antibodies directed against antigens on the graft can produce immediate damage to the graft.

criteria of immunity: specificity and memory. Graft rejection is an immune phenomenon.

Antibodies can be, and often are, produced in response to foreign transplants. In most cases, however, these antibodies do not play a significant role in the rejection process. The second-set response cannot be passively transferred by injection of antiserum. On the other hand, if we inject *lymphocytes* from a BALB/c mouse that has received a single CBA graft into a fresh BALB/c mouse, the recipient will mount a second-set response against a graft of CBA skin (Figure 3.6). The ability to mount a second-set response has thus been adoptively transferred by lymphocytes. So, graft rejection is another example of cell-mediated immunity (**CMI**).

## 3.4 The Genetics of Histocompatibility

The antigens that trigger graft rejection are called *transplantation antigens*. They are glycoproteins encoded by genes called **histocompatibility genes.** The grafts between two male and two female mice or from a female to a male of the same inbred strain are not rejected because these animals share the same histocompatibility genes. (Grafts from males to females will eventually be rejected because the Y chromosome carries a gene that allows for the expression of a transplantation antigen not expressed in females.)

If we cross a CBA mouse with a BALB/c mouse, the $F_1$ offspring

(CBA × BALB/c) will accept grafts from *either* parent, but neither parent will accept a graft from its $F_1$ offspring. The offspring are heterozygous for all the histocompatibility genes that differ in the two inbred strains, and their cells express both sets of transplantation antigens. Thus, parental → $F_1$ grafts succeed because the parental transplantation antigens are seen as "self" by the immune system of the $F_1$ recipient. On the other hand, $F_1$ → parental grafts fail because the $F_1$ skin expresses one set of transplantation antigens foreign to, and thus antigenic to, the recipient (Figure 3.7).

Interbreeding $F_1$ animals produces an $F_2$ generation. How will these animals respond to grafts of homozygous, parental skin? The answer depends upon the number of loci carrying different histocompatibility genes in the original two strains. If only a single locus is involved, we would expect that 75% of the $F_2$ generation would accept grafts of skin from *either* parental type (Figure 3.8). This is because one-half of the $F_2$ generation will be heterozygous, like the $F_1$ generation, and one-quarter will be homozygous for the histocompatibility antigens of the donor. However, one-quarter will be homozygous for the histocompatibility antigens of the other parental type and will reject the graft as nonself.

If, on the other hand, the two mouse strains differ at two (unlinked) loci, then 56% [9/16 or $(3/4)^2$] of the $F_2$ generation will accept grafts from either parent (Figure 3.8). This is simply a problem in classical Mendelian genetics. If three unlinked loci are involved, the fraction accepting

**Figure 3.7** Fate of skin grafts between two inbred strains of mice (A and B) and their $F_1$ offspring. The parental types reject each other's skin and also skin from their offspring because in each case it expresses foreign transplantation antigens. The hybrids, however, will accept skin grafts from either parental strain because they have inherited the histocompatibility genes, and thus express the antigens, of both.

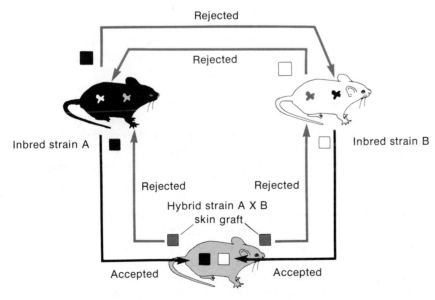

Rejected

Rejected

Inbred strain A

Inbred strain B

Rejected    Rejected

Hybrid strain A X B
skin graft

Accepted    Accepted

Hybrid strain A X B

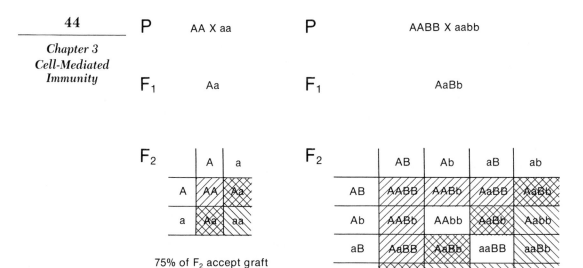

**Figure 3.8** Expected results of grafting P skin on $F_2$ animals if rejection is controlled by a single histocompatibility locus *(left)* or two unlinked loci *(right)*.

parental type grafts drops to 42% [27/64 or $(3/4)^3$]. Thus the fraction of the $F_2$ generation that will accept parental grafts is $(0.75)^n$ where $n =$ the number of unlinked histocompatibility loci.

As early as 1916, Little and Tyzzer used this approach to estimate the number of histocompatibility loci in mice. Although carefully defined inbred strains were a thing of the future, these workers used as one parental strain the so-called Japanese waltzing mouse that had been bred as a pure strain for many generations. They also had available a carcinoma (epithelial cancer) which had arisen in Japanese waltzing mice and could be successfully transplanted from one member of the strain to another. They crossed a Japanese waltzing mouse with a "common" mouse. Interbreeding the offspring ($F_1$), they produced an $F_2$ generation. The members of this generation were then challenged with an inoculation of the carcinoma. In principle, this was no different from grafting skin from the Japanese waltzing mice onto $F_2$ animals except that acceptance of the graft was scored as death from the tumor; graft rejection meant survival. Only 1.6% of the $F_2$ mice died from the tumor. This showed that the two parental mice differed at 14 or 15 histocompatibility loci: $0.016 = (0.75)^{14.3}$.

In the ensuing years, additional histocompatibility loci have been discovered in mice. The number now stands at over 30.

The genetics of histocompatibility goes beyond simple multiplicity of loci. Each locus probably is, and some certainly are, highly polymorphic as well. In other words, several to many alleles have been identified in the species at a number of these different loci. (But a single mouse, being diploid, can have at most two alleles at a single locus.)

## 3.5 Congenic Mouse Strains

Much of the recent analysis of histocompatibility loci and alleles has depended upon the development of congenic strains of mice. Congenic strains have, in fact, played such a crucial role in the development of our understanding of how the immune system works that we should examine how they are produced. The procedure is diagrammed in Figure 3.9. Like the procedure of Little and Tyzzer, a mouse of an inbred strain ("A") is bred with a different mouse ("B"). It does not matter whether mouse B is from an inbred strain or not. In either case, their offspring ($F_1$) will accept a graft from the A parent (which was homozygous at all histocompatibility loci), but they will accept a graft from the B parent only if it, too, was from an inbred—hence homozygous—strain. Members of the $F_1$ generation are interbred and their offspring ($F_2$) challenged with a tumor that grows in strain A. *Most* of the $F_2$ generation will survive because they will be homozygous for strain-B alleles at at least one histocompatibility locus and therefore will reject the strain-A tumor as foreign. Next, the survivors are backcrossed to additional strain-A mice, introducing into their offspring a fresh, complete set of strain-A genes. If the offspring were challenged with the tumor, they all would die because they have at least one A allele at every locus (including all the histocompatibility loci). So another intercross is performed to allow Mendelian segregation, and the new batch of offspring is challenged with the tumor (Figure 3.9). Then the survivors in this group are once again backcrossed to the A strain. This procedure gradually restores

**Figure 3.9** Original procedure for developing congenic strains of mice. Today, by using antisera, rather than a potentially lethal tumor, to detect the histocompatibility antigens, the need for intercrossing is eliminated. The heterozygous members of each backcross generation (who would die if challenged with the tumor) are simply backcrossed again to the strain donating the background genes (A in this case). After a dozen or so more such backcrosses, the progeny are bred together and those offspring homozygous for the desired allele are selected as founders of the congenic strain.

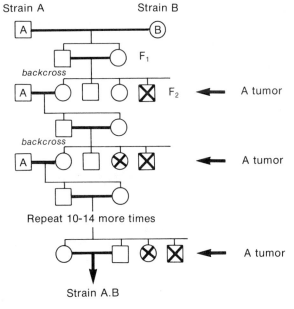

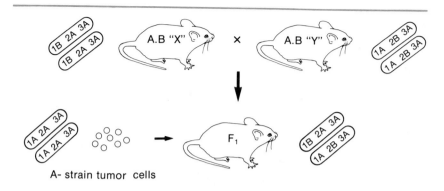

**A**     Tumor not rejected- one "A" allele at each locus - mouse dies.

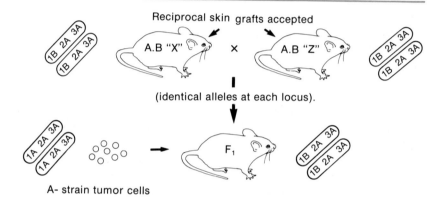

**B**     Tumor rejected - no "A" allele at locus 1 - mouse lives.

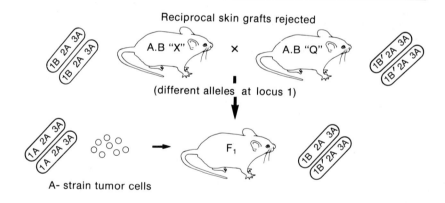

**C**     Tumor rejected - no "A" allele at locus 1 - mouse lives.

**Figure 3.10**   Methods for analyzing the histocompatibility relationships of four independently derived congenic strains. A: The two congenic strains carry B-derived histocompatibility genes at *different* loci. B: The two strains carry identical B-derived histocompatibility alleles at the *same* locus. C: The two strains carry *different* B-derived alleles at the *same* locus.

homozygosity at all strain-A loci *except* for one (usually) strain-B histocompatibility locus that is being selected for by backcrossing only the survivors, i.e., those that reject the strain-A tumor.

After repeating the process 10 or more times, the mice will have over 99% of their genes derived from strain A ("background genes"). But the survivors from the final intercross will be homozygous for one histocompatibility locus derived from strain B. Inbreeding two survivors of the process begins the congenic strain (Figure 3.9).

Congenic strains are designated as follows: a designation for the background strain, followed by a period, followed by a designation for the strain that contributed the new histocompatibility locus. Thus a CBA.B10 mouse represents a congenic strain carrying background genes of the CBA strain and a homozygous pair of histocompatibility loci derived from the C57BL/10 strain.

The development of a series of independently derived congenic strains provides the tools for learning more about the genetic basis of histocompatibility. Let us take mice of several different congenic strains, say A.B"X," A.B"Y," and so forth. We cross these in various combinations and, for each cross, challenge the $F_1$ with the strain-A tumor. If the $F_1$ offspring succumb to the tumor, we have established that the two congenic strains owe their resistance to the tumor to histocompatibility genes at *different* loci. Figure 3.10A shows why this is so. These $F_1$ mice carry at least one strain-A gene at each histocompatibility locus and thus "accept" the tumor as "self." Conversely, if the $F_1$ mice survive the challenge, then we know that the two congenic strains share a strain-B-derived histocompatibility gene at the *same* locus (Figure 3.10B). In this case, we can carry the analysis further. We exchange skin between the two congenic strains. If the grafts are accepted (A.B"X" and A.B"Z"), the two strains share the same histocompatibility alleles at that locus. If they reject each other's skin (A.B"X" and A.B"Q"), the alleles at that locus are different (Figure 3.10C).

## 3.6 H-2: The Major Histocompatibility Complex (MHC) of Mice

Graft rejection in mice is controlled by histocompatibility (H) genes of which over 30 have been identified so far. These are numbered H-1, H-2, H-3, etc. For all but one of these loci, a difference in alleles results in the slow rejection of skin grafts. The process may take 20–300 days to complete. These loci are called **minor histocompatibility loci.** However, allelic differences at one "locus," called H-2, results in a rapid (about 11 days) first-set rejection of the graft. As we shall see, H-2 is, in fact, a set of closely linked genes involved in a variety of immune phenomena. For this reason, the H-2 region is called the major histocompatibility complex (MHC). It is located on chromosome 17 of the mouse haploid set of 20 chromosomes.

In analyzing the nature of the H-2 complex, it might be wise to remember the procedures used and their limitations. Until recently, almost all of our knowledge of the H-2 complex has come from the methods of classical genetics: breeding animals to study the pattern of inheritance of particular traits (phenotypes). If two traits are inherited in the classic Mendelian ratios and independently of each other, we conclude that they are under the control of separate, unlinked loci. If two phenotypic traits are *invariably* inherited together, we conclude that both are the manifestations of a single gene locus. However, if the two traits can be inherited independently, even if rarely, then we conclude that they are under the control of separate but tightly linked genes on the same chromosome. This is the situation observed with several traits that are associated with H-2. By examining the frequency of recombinants in several types of crosses, the order and relative spacing of the genes can be mapped on the chromosome. Let us take a specific example.

Although graft rejection is primarily a cell-mediated immune response, histoincompatible skin grafts or the transfusion of histoincompatible cells will induce antibody formation in the recipient. The antisera that result can be used to identify antigenic determinants ("specificities") associated with cell surface molecules of particular strains of mice. The H-2 "locus" has been particularly well studied in this respect. Different mouse strains possess certain specificities that are unique to that strain. These are called "private" specificities. In some cases, however, strains that have different private specificities may share certain other specificities. These are called "public" specificities. They probably reflect shared antigenic determinants on the molecules encoded by the alleles.

The H-2 specificities, whether public or private, are designated by number. Scores of different antigenic specificities encoded by genes in the H-2 complex have been identified and can be used to characterize different strains of mice.

If we mate mice that express, for example, specificities 31 and 4 to mice that express 33 and 2, the $F_1$ offspring express all four specificities (Figure 3.11). This shows codominant expression of the responsible gene or genes. If these $F_1$ animals are then backcrossed to one of the parental strains (e.g., 33/2), there are three possible outcomes depending on the relationship of the controlling genes. If specificities 31 and 4 are under the control of unlinked genes (e.g., located on separate chromosomes), then four possible combinations would be seen in roughly equal numbers. On the other hand, if the two specificities are two phenotypic manifestations of the *same* gene (representing, e.g., different determinants on the same molecule), then only the original combinations will be seen: 31 always with 4 and 33 always with 2. In this particular case, most of the backcross generation animals do express the original combinations. However, approximately 0.25% express 31 without 4 and the same number express 4 without 31 (Figure 3.11). The occurrence of these *recombinants* tells us immediately that specificities 31 and 4 are controlled by separate loci. In this case, the loci are designated K and D (Figure 3.12). The recombination frequency of 0.5% tells us that H-2K and H-2D are separated by approximately 0.5 centiMorgans (map units) on the chromosome.

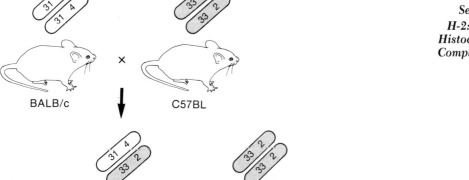

BALB/c × C57BL

F₁ × C57BL

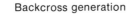

Backcross generation

~0.25%   ~0.25%   ~49.75%   ~49.75%

**Figure 3.11** Recombination in the H-2 region. While the inheritance of certain specificities of histocompatibility antigens is closely linked (e.g., 31 and 4, 33 and 2), the occurrence of occasional recombinants shows that these specificities are controlled by separate loci. These are designated H-2K for specificities 31 and 33; H-2D for 4 and 2. The frequency of recombination (0.005) gives a map distance between these loci of 0.5 centiMorgan.

The inheritance of a number of other genetic "markers" (=phenotypic traits) has been shown to be linked to the histocompatibility genes of H-2. The genes controlling these and other traits are thus located on chromosome 17 and relatively close to the H-2K and H-2D loci. For example, the ability of a particular mouse strain to mount an immune

**Figure 3.12** The H-2 region of mice. The order of loci above the horizontal bar has yet to be established.

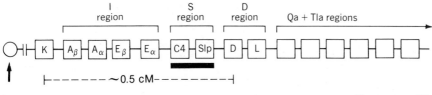

Centromere                                                    Chromosome 17

response to certain synthetic polypeptide antigens is under genetic control, and the inheritance of this trait is tightly linked to the inheritance of H-2. These genes are called *immune response* (Ir) *genes.* Several have been identified. Gene mapping by the analysis of recombinants has placed the Ir loci between the K and D loci in the so-called I region of the MHC (Figure 3.12). In the chapters ahead, we shall discover a number of other vital roles that I region genes play in the induction, regulation, and expression of immune responses.

Although recombination occurs within the H-2 region, the frequency is very low; that is, the linkage is very tight. Most of the time, all the alleles in this region are inherited as a single block. The block of alleles found in a given mouse strain is called its **haplotype** ("haploid genotype"). A particular haplotype is defined by the collection of phenotypic traits, for example the H-2D and H-2K specificities associated with a particular strain of mouse. The alleles of that haplotype are designated by lowercase letters. Thus, the C57BL/10 mouse is assigned the haplotype designation H-2$^b$, and each of the alleles in its H-2 region is designated with a *b* (Figure 3.13). The haplotype of the BALB/c mouse is H-2$^d$ and that of the CBA mouse is H-2$^k$. An F$_1$ mouse produced by the mating of a BALB/c and a CBA mouse would carry the designation H-2$^{d/k}$.

A number of structural genes have also been localized in the I region. For this reason, the antigens encoded by these genes are often called Ia ("I associated") antigens. It is now quite clear that many of the functional properties (e.g., the failure to respond to certain antigens) that map to the I region do so because these properties are mediated by the Ia antigens encoded there.

Three distinct types of molecules are encoded by the loci in H-2. They are called class I, class II, and class III molecules. The class I and class II molecules are integral membrane glycoproteins. Class I molecules are encoded by H-2K, H-2D, H-2L, as well as the Qa and Tla loci (Figure 3.12). The class II molecules are encoded by loci in the I-A and I-E subregions of the I region. The class III molecules are encoded in the S region.

Humans also have a major histocompatibility complex, which is called HLA. It, too, contains a large number of genetic loci encoding molecules of all three classes. As is the case for mice, the human major histocompat-

**Figure 3.13**  The H-2 haplotypes of representative mouse strains. BALB.B10 and B10.A(5R) are congenic strains for certain loci in H-2.

| Strain | Haplotype | K | A$_\beta$ | A$_\alpha$ | E$_\beta$ | E$_\alpha$ | D | |
|--------|-----------|---|-----------|------------|-----------|------------|---|---|
| C57BL/10("B10") | H-2$^b$ | b | b | b | b | b | b | |
| BALB/c, DBA/2, NZB | H-2$^d$ | d | d | d | d | d | d | |
| CBA, C3H | H-2$^k$ | k | k | k | k | k | k | |
| (BALB/c × CBA)F$_1$ | H-2$^{d/k}$ | d/k | d/k | d/k | d/k | d/k | d/k | (hybrid) |
| BALB.B10 | H-2$^b$ | b | b | b | b | b | b | (congenic) |
| A | H-2$^a$ | k | k | k | k | k | d | (recombinant) |
| B10.A(5R) | H-2$^{i5}$ | b | b | b | b | k | d | (double recombinant) |

The I region spans the A$_\beta$, A$_\alpha$, E$_\beta$, E$_\alpha$ columns.

ibility complex plays a dominant role in the success or failure of tissue and organ allografts. A detailed examination of HLA is presented in Chapter 19.

Although class I and class II molecules (but not class III) are the major histocompatibility antigens, they surely have not been retained in the genome to enable allografts to be rejected. However, it turns out that all of these molecules have vital roles to play in normal immune reactivity.

**Figure 3.14** Schematic representation of the H-2K$^b$ transplantation antigen (class I). (The single letter code of amino acids is given on the inside front cover of the book). The molecule of $\beta_2$-microglobulin is associated by noncovalent interactions only. The disulfide bonds are indicated with black bars. Cleavage with papain releases the exterior domains (N, C1, C2) from the cell membrane and cleaves some of these fragments between C1 and C2. [Courtesy of T. J. Kindt from J. E. Coligan, et al., *Nature* **291**:35, 1981.]

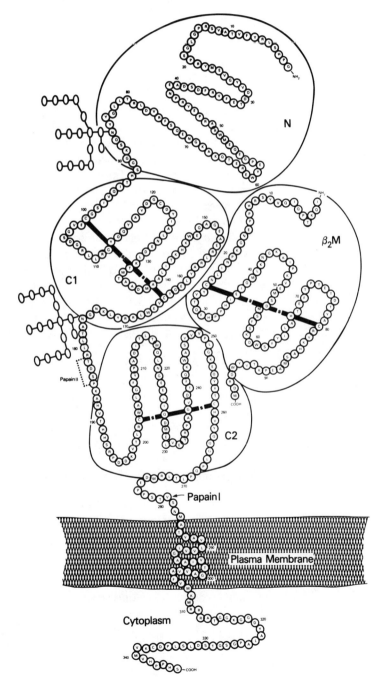

One example is presented in Section 3.7, and many other examples will appear elsewhere in the book. But before we look at these, let us examine the H-2 complex in a systematic way.

## The K Region

The only functional gene assigned to this region, H-2K, encodes one chain of a class I antigen that is expressed on the surface of almost all the cells of the mouse's body. This chain has a molecular weight of approximately 45,000. It is associated noncovalently with a smaller chain of 12,000 daltons called $\beta_2$-microglobulin (Figure 3.14). The gene for $\beta_2$-microglobulin is not in the MHC but located on chromosome 2.

The H-2K$^b$ molecule has been completely sequenced. It contains 346 amino acid residues grouped into five distinct regions. Three of these extend above the surface of the cell membrane; one spans the membrane; and the carboxyl terminal region extends into the interior of the cell (Figure 3.14). Two of the three exterior domains have carbohydrate residues attached to them. As is true of other integral membrane proteins, the portion of the chain that traverses the lipid bilayer of the membrane is rich in hydrophobic amino acids as befits its hydrophobic surroundings.

Some dozen different alleles have been identified at H-2K among the standard inbred strains of mice. Each is characterized by at least one unique ("private") antigenic specificity that is revealed by particular antibodies. Thus H-2K in the C57BL mouse (H-2K$^b$) carries private specificity 33 (Figure 3.11). Studies of wild mice reveal some of these same specificities and others besides. It has been estimated that 100 or more different H-2K alleles will eventually be discovered. This is an extraordinary degree of polymorphism. Most of the structural genes of a species exist in only a few allelic forms.

In view of the genetic polymorphism of H-2K molecules, we would expect to find evidence of sequence differences that could account for this diversity. Comparison of the sequences of several different class I molecules reveals the presence of such sequence diversity primarily in the outer two domains. Almost two dozen mutant forms of H-2K have also been discovered, and for some of these the amino acid substitutions in the molecule have been identified.

## The I Region

The I region was established by mapping genes (Ir genes) controlling the ability of the mouse to respond to certain antigens. The study of recombinant mice has revealed several distinct loci within the region.

*I-A.* Three structural genes have been located in the I-A subregion. These are designated $A_\beta$, $A_\alpha$, and $E_\beta$. Each encodes a polypeptide that is used to construct a so-called class II antigen.

Two kinds of class II molecules are produced by most mice. Both are integral membrane glycoproteins. Each consists of two polypeptide chains (Figure 3.15). The alpha chain has a molecular weight of approximately 32,000. The beta chain, which has less carbohydrate attached, has a molecular weight of some 28,000.

Three of the 4 genes encoding these polypeptides are located in the I-A subregion. One entire Ia antigen ($A_\alpha + A_\beta$) is controlled exclusively here. The I-A subregion also encodes the $\beta$ chain of a second Ia molecule, but its $\alpha$ chain is encoded in I-E (Figure 3.15).

The primary structure of these polypeptides varies from strain to strain. This polymorphism is particularly evident in the $\beta$ chains. The diversity of Ia antigens is further enhanced by the ability of the controlling genes to be expressed in *trans* as well as in *cis* combination. Thus a mouse that is heterozygous for the genes controlling both $A_\alpha$ and $A_\beta$ synthesizes 4 kinds of $A_\alpha A_\beta$ molecules: $A_\alpha A_\beta$, $A_\alpha A'_\beta$, $A'_\alpha A_\beta$, and $A'_\alpha A'_\beta$. A similar permutation occurs for the $E_\alpha E_\beta$ molecules.

In contrast to the class I molecules, which are found on virtually every cell of the body, class II molecules are found only on cells of the immune system, primarily B lymphocytes and cells, such as macrophages, that "present" antigen to lymphocytes. The role that class II molecules play in the interactions of the cells of the immune system are examined in Chapter 12 and 13.

*I-E.* This subregion contains a gene that encodes $E_\alpha$, a polypeptide that associates with the $E_\beta$ polypeptide (encoded in the I-A subregion) to form an Ia antigen. Mice of certain haplotypes, e.g., H-2$^b$, do not express $E_\alpha E_\beta$ antigens.

## The S Region

This region includes a gene that encodes the fourth component (C4) of the complement system (Section 14.2).

**Figure 3.15** Structure and genetic control of Ia (class II) antigens in mice. These loci display *trans* as well as *cis* complementation. Thus, for example, an outbred mouse heterozygous at both $E_\alpha$ and $E_\beta$ produces 4 different kinds of these class II molecules. The association of the I-A and I-E loci with immune responsiveness (Ir genes) is discussed in Section 12.9

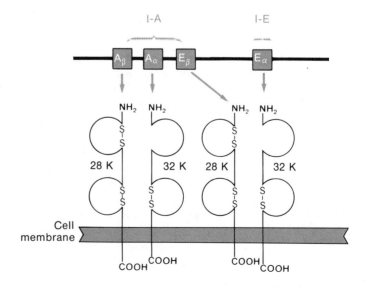

## The D Region

Like the K region, the D region encodes a class I glycoprotein that is expressed on most of the cells of the body. This locus is also extremely polymorphic: over 40 alleles have been detected by the use of antisera directed against specificities controlled by the D region. The true number of alleles may be greater than 100.

At least one other class I antigen, designated H-2L, is encoded in the D region of some strains of mice. Genetic analysis of a rare recombinant between H-2D and H-2L has established that H-2L is located to the right of H-2D (Figure 3.12).

## The Qa and Tla Regions

Analysis of the DNA in these regions reveals some 36 closely related genes in the BALB/c mouse. However, only a few gene products have as yet been identified for this region. These include (1) several Qa antigens, which are expressed — often at very low levels — on lymphocytes, and (2) a Tla antigen. A Tla antigen is expressed on the surface of certain kinds of leukemic cells and is also found on immature T cells in the thymus of certain mouse strains (Section 7.7). This tissue distribution is the basis for the name: *t*hymus – *l*eukemia *a*ntigen. Both Qa and Tla antigens are class I molecules consisting of a large polypeptide ($\sim$45,000 daltons) associated with $\beta_2$-microglobulin. The function of the Qa and Tla antigens is unknown.

## Other I Region Loci?

Several other loci have been assigned to the I region.

1. I-B, located between I-A and I-E, was thought to control the immune response to certain antigens. However, no polypeptide product has been detected for such a gene. Furthermore, the phenomena associated with I-B are probably the result of the combined effects of the two flanking subregions, and thus I-B may not exist.
2. I-C was assigned to the interval between the I-E and S subregions. However, it has been difficult to distinguish the supposed properties of I-C from those of I-E, and many workers now lump the two together as the "I-E/C" subregion.
3. I-J. This locus has been placed between the $E_\beta$ and $E_\alpha$ loci. The I-J locus is thought to encode a polypeptide found on cells that suppress the immune response (T suppressor cells) and factors produced by them. However, analysis of the DNA in this region has failed to detect a candidate for such gene, and the reason why I-J molecules appear to be encoded here has yet to be discovered. The distribution and properties of I-J molecules are examined in Chapter 15.

## 3.7 Adoptive Transfer of DTH is Restricted by Class II Antigens of the MHC

**55**

*Section 3.7*
*Adoptive Transfer*
*of DTH is Re-*
*stricted by Class II*
*Antigens of the MHC*

Delayed-type hypersensitivity is an in vivo response. It can be adoptively transferred from a sensitized animal to a naive (unsensitized) animal by the transfer of T lymphocytes. If a mouse is sensitized to, for example, fowl gamma globulin (FGG), a suspension of its lymphocytes will transfer its hypersensitivity to the antigen to a naive syngeneic recipient, i.e., a syngeneic mouse that has had no prior exposure to FGG. After the cell transfer, an intradermal injection of FGG produces the characteristic lesion of DTH in the recipient.

In a sense, the $T_D$ cell is both a responding cell and an effector cell. When transferred to a naive recipient, it is capable of responding to the antigen used to sensitize the donor. In the course of its response, it liberates a variety of lymphokines. These recruit nonspecific cells (e.g., macrophages) of the host to produce the tissue damage characteristic of DTH.

However, the ability of transferred $T_D$ cells to respond in the new host requires that the antigen-presenting cells of the new host have a MHC similar to that of the donor. As Miller and his colleagues have demonstrated, it is not possible to transfer DTH to an allogeneic recipient. For example, FGG-sensitized lymphocytes from a CBA mouse will not transfer DTH to a C57BL/10 recipient (Figure 3.16). This, in itself, tells us that something other than simple recognition of FGG is at work. If T cells primed in one strain to FGG (or any other conventional antigen) needed only to encounter that antigen again in order to mediate a DTH

**Figure 3.16** Role of the H-2 region in the adoptive transfer of delayed-type hypersensitivity (DTH). The donor mice were sensitized to fowl gamma globulin (FGG). Five days later, their lymph node cells were injected into naive (unsensitized) recipients. The recipients were then challenged with FGG and any DTH response measured 24 hours later. The alleles listed for each haplotype are for the K, $A_\beta$, $A_\alpha$, $E_\beta$, $E_\alpha$, and D loci in that order. [From J. F. A. P. Miller et al., *Proc. Natl. Acad. Sci. USA* 72:5095, 1975.]

| Donor | Recipient | DTH response | Interpretation |
|-------|-----------|--------------|----------------|
| CBA *kkkkkk* | CBA *kkkkkk* | + | Syngeneic transfer works |
| CBA *kkkkkk* | C57BL/10 *bbbbbb* | – | Allogeneic does not |
| CBA *kkkkkk* | B10.BR *kkkkkk* | + | Different background, same H-2 — works |
| C57BL *bbbbbb* | B10.BR *kkkkkk* | – | Similar background, different H-2 — does not work |
| CBA *kkkkkk* | A.TL *skkkkd* | + | Identity at K and D not needed |
| CBA *kkkkkk* | B10.A(4R) *kkkkbb* | + | Identity at $A_\beta A_\alpha$ — works |

reaction, then they should be able to do so in allogeneic as well as syngeneic surroundings. But this is not the case.

Further, as Miller's group went on to show, the ability of FGG-sensitized T cells to respond in a new environment requires only that the H-2 region of the donor and recipient be the same. $T_D$ cells from a CBA mouse can successfully mount a DTH response in a B10.BR mouse (Figure 3.16) that has the same H-2 haplotype as CBA but on a different background.

By using recombinant strains, these workers were able to show that it is the I subregion of H-2 that determines whether or not successful transfer of DTH takes place (Figure 3.16). $T_D$ cells sensitized to FGG can respond again to FGG only if they encounter the antigen associated with either (or both) the same $A_\alpha A_\beta$ or $E_\alpha E_\beta$ molecules as before. Thus the response of $T_D$ cells to a conventional antigen like FGG is said to be "restricted" by the MHC. In later chapters we shall see that the response of most T cells to antigen is restricted by the MHC, but in some cases class I, rather than class II, molecules are responsible.

## 3.8 The Biological Significance of Cell-Mediated Immunity

Delayed-type hypersensitivity and allograft rejection are clear examples of cell-mediated immune responses. Both have been of enormous value to immunologists in their search for a better understanding of immunity. But both are certainly artifacts of the endeavors of the immunologist. Neither skin testing nor skin grafting represent normal events in the life of an animal. Of what value is cell-mediated immunity to the normal organism?

Several lines of evidence lead to the conclusion that at least one major function of CMI is to defend the host against parasites that can live *within* cells. All viruses and some bacteria reside within the cells of their host. Viruses invade and replicate in a variety of kinds of cells. Some species of bacteria are able to survive phagocytosis by macrophages and continue to replicate within the cytoplasm of the macrophage. This ability to survive within macrophages is characteristic of mycobacteria (such as the tubercle bacillus), *Listeria monocytogenes,* and a number of other microorganisms. As long as they remain tucked inside a macrophage, antibodies cannot reach intracellular pathogens. But the cell-mediated branch of the immune system appears to be equipped to cope with the problem. Let us examine the evidence supporting this. In later chapters, we shall examine possible mechanisms by which immune cells bring about the destruction of intracellular pathogens.

Humans are occasionally born with or develop defects in their ability to mount cell-mediated immune responses. These defects are usually first revealed by repeated infections with viruses and fungi. These persons are generally able to cope with infections by bacteria like streptococci that remain outside of cells. The deficiency in cell-mediated immunity in these patients can be demonstrated directly by their failure to develop DTH to antigens, such as PPD and dinitrochlorobenzene

(DNCB), used for skin testing. Attempts to immunize such persons with live virus vaccines (e.g., vaccinia, mumps) are extremely dangerous. Although these viruses are so attenuated that they cause only a mild, transient infection in normal individuals, they become life threatening in individuals with defective CMI.

In the early 1960s, Mackaness secured direct evidence of the importance of CMI in protecting animals against those bacteria that can live within macrophages. Mice given small doses of *Listeria monocytogenes* survive the infection and develop immunity against the organism. When challenged with a 100-fold larger dose of bacilli, a dose that would kill an unimmunized mouse, they remain well. At first glance, this seems no different from the immunity induced by pneumococci (see Section 2.1). But there is a major difference between the two. Antipneumococcal immunity can be passively transferred with serum. Immunity to *Listeria* cannot. However, Mackaness demonstrated that immunity to *Listeria* can be transferred by an injection of lymphocytes (T lymphocytes) from an immune donor (Figure 3.17). Here, then, is a direct demonstration of a cell-mediated immune response that also is clearly of protective value to the host.

Curiously, when a mouse that is immune to *Listeria* is subsequently challenged with *Listeria*, its immunity extends to other intracellular bacteria (e.g., the tubercle bacillus) as well. In other words, the mouse remains healthy when *simultaneously* given large doses of both *Listeria* and tubercle bacilli. You might argue that this response violates our rule of specificity, and in one sense it does. But the specific component of the response is revealed by injecting the tubercle bacilli alone. In this case, the animal becomes ill and dies. It is the specific response of *Listeria*-primed T lymphocytes to subsequent challenge by *Listeria* that confers on macrophages their ability to effectively dispose of all types of intracellular bacteria. The mechanism at work in this response — which involves a lymphokine — is examined in Section 14.8.

The evidence is quite clear that cell-mediated immunity plays a vital

**Figure 3.17**  Adoptive transfer of anti-*Listeria* immunity. The lymphocytes that mediate this immunity are T lymphocytes. [Based on the work of G. B. Mackaness.]

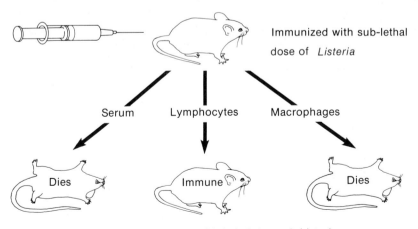

Immunized with sub-lethal dose of *Listeria*

Serum   Lymphocytes   Macrophages

Dies   Immune   Dies

All recipients challenged with lethal dose of *Listeria*

role in protecting the host against intracellular parasites. In Chapter 20, we shall examine the evidence for another possible role for CMI: the defense against neoplastic (cancerous) cells that arise in the host. So while most of the *examples* of CMI that you will meet in this book will represent manipulations of experimental immunologists, do not let this cause you to lose sight of the importance of CMI in the normal life of an animal.

## ADDITIONAL READING

1. Hood, L., et al., "Genes of the Major Histocompatibility Complex of the Mouse," *Ann. Rev. Immunol.* **1**:529, 1983.

2. Klein, J., et al., Genetics of the Major Histocompatibility Complex: The Final Act," *Ann. Rev. Immunol.* **1**:119, 1983. The H-2 region of mice.

3. Mackaness, G. B., "Cellular Resistance to Infection," *J. Exp. Med.* **116**:381, 1962. Demonstrates that resistance of mice to *Listeria monocytogenes* is not mediated by antibodies.

4. Marchal, G., et al., "Local Adoptive Transfer of Skin Delayed-Type Hypersensitivity Initiated by a Single T Lymphocyte," *J. Immunol.* **129**:954, 1982.

5. Snell, G. D., "Studies in Histocompatibility," *Science* **213**:172, July 10, 1981. Snell's Nobel Lecture (1980) gives a succinct historical account of the elucidation of the MHC of mice.

# PART II

# Immunoassays

Measurement is the basis of all knowledge.
—LORD KELVIN

# CHAPTER 4

# The Interaction of Antibodies and Antigens

## 4.1 Precipitation in Liquid

In Chapter 2, we examined the reaction that occurs when a solution of type 3 pneumococcal polysaccharide and antibodies directed against that antigen are mixed. The result is a precipitate of antigen–antibody complexes. As the test was presented, it was purely qualitative. However, this reaction can be used to determine the concentration of antibodies in a solution, e.g., serum. This is the basis of the quantitative precipitation assay. It is usually performed as follows.

Increasing amounts of antigen are added to a series of tubes containing equal amounts of antiserum or a solution of purified antibodies (Figure 4.1). The mixture is incubated (e.g., at 37°C) for a time and then transferred for a day or two to the cold (4°C). The precipitates, which have formed in the tubes, are separated from the supernatants by centrifugation and *both* are saved. The precipitates are washed in cold saline or a

61

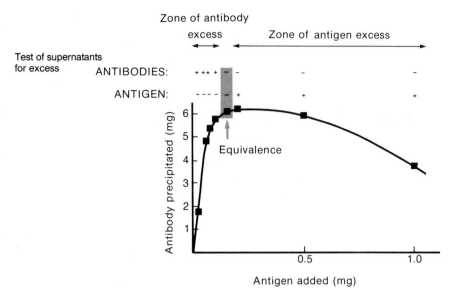

**Figure 4.1**   Quantitative precipitation. The antigen is the type 3 pneumococcal polysaccharide; the antibodies are from a rabbit immunized with killed type 3 pneumococci. At equivalence, no residual antigen or antibody is found in the supernatant. With protein antigens, the ascending limb (antibody excess) tends to be less steep and the descending limb (antigen excess) more steep than is the case here. [Based on M. Heidelberger and F. E. Kendall, *J. Exp. Med.* **65**:647, 1937.]

buffer (to remove all irrelevant serum proteins) and redissolved in a fixed volume of dilute acid or alkali (such as 0.1 *N* NaOH). The concentration of protein in each sample is determined by a standard protein assay, for example, the colorimetric assay of Lowry or by measuring the absorbance of ultraviolet light at 280 nm. In this particular case, the antigen is a polysaccharide, so all the protein measured represents anti-type 3 antibodies.

If we graph the weight of a precipitated protein as a function of the amount of antigen added, a characteristic curve is produced (Figure 4.1). At first, the addition of increasing amounts of antigen precipitates increasing amounts of protein in the tubes until a maximum is reached. In the later tubes, however, further increases in antigen concentration result in the precipitation of *smaller* amounts of protein. The resulting curve thus has three zones. The ascending limb of the curve describes the zone of **antibody excess.** If we examine the supernatants that were saved, we find (by adding antigen to them) that the supernatants from the tubes in antibody excess still contain anti-type 3 antibodies. The supernatants from the tube or tubes giving maximal precipitation show neither residual antibody nor residual antigen. This portion of the curve is described as the zone of **equivalence.** The supernatants from the tubes on the descending limb of the curve reveal (by adding antibodies to them) the presence of additional antigen. Thus this portion of the curve is described as the zone of **antigen excess.**

Knowing the maximum amount of antibody precipitated, it is a simple calculation to determine the concentration of specific antibody in the

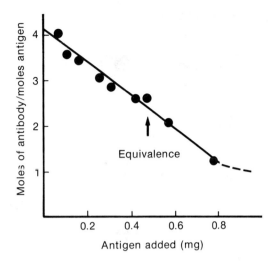

**Figure 4.2** Decline in antibody/antigen mole ratio in the precipitates formed in the presence of increasing amounts of antigen. The antigen is ovalbumin (OVA) and the anti-OVA antibodies were raised in a rabbit. At extreme antigen excess, the mole ratio reaches a limiting value close to 1. Aggregates with ratios less than 1 (e.g., $Ab_2Ag_3 = 0.67$) are formed in extreme antigen excess, but these are soluble and remain in the supernatant. [Based on M. Heidelberger and F. E. Kendall, *J. Exp. Med.* **62**:697, 1935.]

starting material such as a serum sample. This is the goal of the quantitative precipitation test: a determination of the concentration (e.g., in mg/ml) of specific antibody in the sample being examined.

What accounts for the descending limb of the quantitative precipitation curve? In other words, why should less antibody be precipitated by an excess of antigen? We can gain a clue to this puzzle by measuring the ratio of moles of antibody to moles of antigen in the collected precipitates (Figure 4.2). We must, of course, know the molecular weights of both antibody and antigen. In the pneumococcal system described here, the antigen—a polymer of varied lengths—has no definable molecular weight. But we can determine this ratio if we do a quantitative precipitation analysis on, for example, a rabbit anti-OVA antiserum, where the antibodies have a molecular weight of approximately 160,000 and the molecular weight of the antigen is approximately 43,000. Doing so, we discover that with increasing amounts of antigen in the reaction mixture, the antibody/antigen mole ratio in the precipitate declines. At extreme antigen excess, it reaches a limiting value slightly greater than 1 (Figure 4.2). Antibody–antigen complexes with mole ratios less than one are also formed in the zone of antigen excess, but these complexes are soluble and hence remain in the supernatant. These phenomena can be explained by assuming that the antibodies are at least bivalent (that is, they have two antigen-binding sites) and the antigen is multivalent. (We shall see in Section 4.4 that IgG antibodies are indeed bivalent.) Thus the crosslinking of antigen molecules by antibody molecules can build large insoluble aggregates that form the precipitate (Figure 4.3). With increasing amounts of antigen in the reaction mixture, the large, insoluble aggregates reach a limiting structure of alternating antigen–antibody molecules. This accounts for the limiting antigen–antibody mole ratio of approximately 1. In the region of extreme antigen excess, only one determinant on some antigen molecules may be bound by antibody, resulting in the formation of small, soluble complexes such as $Ab_2Ag_3$ or $AbAg_2$ (the limiting size) that remain in the supernatant (Figure 4.3).

It frequently happens that the maximum amount of precipitated antibody is found in the tube containing a slight excess of antigen in the

Precipitating complexes     Soluble complexes

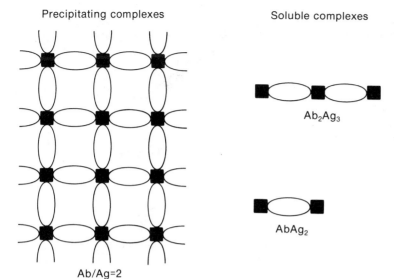

**Figure 4.3** Structures of representative complexes of antigen and bivalent antibodies. These structures can be formed with antigens carrying several identical determinants or—as shown in Figure 4.4—through the cooperative action of antibodies of different specificities binding to determinants on the antigen that occur singly. The limiting structure for precipitating complexes has an antibody/antigen mole ratio close to 1. Complexes with ratios less than 1 are soluble.

Ab/Ag≅1

supernatant rather than in the tube in which neither residual antibody nor residual antigen is present *(equivalence)*. But the absence of antibody in the supernatant at equivalence is only apparent. Antibody molecules are there, but these molecules bind so weakly to the antigen that, by themselves, they are not precipitated when antigen is added to the supernatant. They can, however, become incorporated in the aggregate that precipitates in the zone of slight antigen excess (Figure 4.1). The strength with which an antibody binds to a macromolecular antigen is called its **avidity**.

The theory of aggregate formation requires that the antigen as well as the antibody be at least bivalent. If, for example, we take a population of anti-DNP antibodies and mix them with a protein that is substituted with only one DNP group per molecule of protein, no precipitation occurs. No opportunity for cross-linking of the antigen exists. Does this mean, then, that only antigens that bear two or more identical determinants can be precipitated? The answer is no, and the explanation was provided by the work of Pauling, Pressman, and Campbell in 1944. They raised an antiserum to the hapten *p*-azobenzenearsonate ("A") and another antiserum to the hapten *p*-azobenzenecarboxylate ("C") (Figure 4.4). Each of these antisera was then checked for its ability to precipitate a synthetic antigen consisting of a single A group coupled to a single C group. In neither case did any appreciable precipitate form. But when the synthetic antigen was added to a *mixture* of the two antisera, a copious precipitate formed. Figure 4.4 shows the explanation: the development of large, insoluble aggregates through the cooperative binding of antibody molecules of the two different specificities. And this is the way it

64

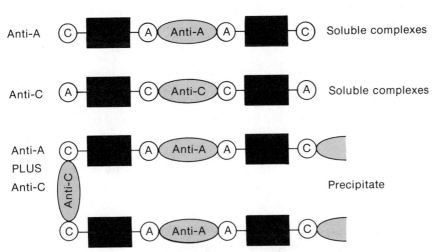

Figure 4.4  Formation of precipitating complexes by the cooperative action
of antibody molecules of two different specificities binding to a synthetic
antigen carrying one of each determinant. [Based on L. Pauling, D. Pressman,
and D. H. Campbell, *J. Am. Chem. Soc.* **66**:330, 1944.]

goes for many, if not most, protein antigens. Protein molecules invariably
carry a number of different antigenic determinants, but often each determinant occurs only once in the molecule. Each of these determinants
induces the formation of antibodies specific for it, and it is the cooperative action of the resulting antibodies that provides the cross-linking that
makes precipitation possible.

What about antibodies? Could not the same phenomenon occur if
antibodies carried one binding site of one specificity and a second binding site of another? The answer is yes, but that is not how it works in
nature. We can show with a simple test that the binding sites on antibodies do not differ in their specificity. Immunizing an animal with two
antigens, A and B, gives rise to an antiserum containing antibodies of both
specificities. First, let us assume that one-third of this pool of antibodies
consists of antibody molecules with both binding sites capable of binding
A; one-third have both sites directed against B; and one-third have one
site for A and the second for B. If we add antigen A to this antiserum,
two-thirds of the antibody activity should be precipitated. Adding antigen B to the supernatant should precipitate the remaining antibodies. If
we reverse the order in which we add the antigen, we should get the
same results: two-thirds upon the first addition, one-third on the second.
Now let us predict the results if we assume that two-thirds of the original
antiserum contained molecules with both sites directed against A and the
remaining molecules had both sites directed against B. Now the order of

addition of the reagents should change the results. If A were added first, two-thirds of the molecules would be precipitated and the remaining third would be precipitated by B. But if B were added first, only one-third of the antibody molecules would be precipitated; the remaining two-thirds would be brought down by A. When the experiment is performed, the second result is always found. Thus we must conclude that the two binding sites on naturally produced bivalent antibody molecules are of identical specificity. (It is, however, possible in the laboratory to synthesize "hybrid" antibody molecules, i.e., molecules with two different binding sites. These are useful reagents for several immunological procedures.)

The binding of an antigen molecule by an antibody molecule occurs at discrete sites on each: an antigenic determinant of the antigen and the binding site on the antibody molecule. In the following sections, we shall examine the nature of this interaction in several aspects: (1) the area involved in the interaction, (2) the forces of attraction between the two sites, (3) the total strength of binding, and (4) the specificity of binding, i.e., the ability of an antibody molecule to discriminate between similar antigenic determinants.

## 4.2   The Size of Antigenic Determinants

How large is an antigenic determinant? Or, to put the question another way, how large is the antigen-binding site on an antibody molecule? The availability of such simple polymeric antigens as the type 3 pneumococcal polysaccharide provides one way to answer these questions. First we determine the equivalence zone for an anti-type 3 pneumococcal antiserum reacting with the type 3 polysaccharide. We prepare, by hydrolysis of the polysaccharide and exclusion chromatography, oligosaccharide fragments of varying lengths. We then set up a row of tubes containing identical amounts of antibody and antigen, picking a concentration for each so that they will be at or close to equivalence. We add increasing amounts of one of the oligosaccharide fragments to the tubes (Figure 4.5). A competition is set up between the macromolecular antigen and its

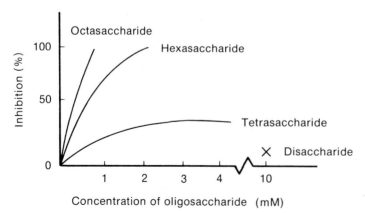

**Figure 4.5**   Inhibition of the precipitation of the type 3 pneumococcal polysaccharide by fragments of the polysaccharide. The anti-type 3 serum was raised in a rabbit. The results suggest that anti-type 3 antibodies bind to a determinant on the polysaccharide that encompasses 6–8 hexose residues. [From J. H. Campbell and A. M. Pappenheimer, Jr., *Immunochemistry.* 3:213, 1966.]

oligosaccharide fragments for the antigen-binding sites on the antibody molecules. With increasing concentration of the oligosaccharide, it becomes increasingly favored to occupy the binding site. But if the fragments are small enough to be *monovalent*, they will not be precipitated. Instead, they will inhibit the precipitation of the macromolecular antigen. When this test is run using a disaccharide (glucuronic acid–glucose) prepared from the type 3 polysaccharide, little inhibition is observed, even at high concentrations of the inhibitor (Figure 4.5). The tetrasaccharide is a somewhat more effective inhibitor, the hexasaccharide much better. The octasaccharide is only slightly more effective an inhibitor than the hexasaccharide (Figure 4.5). From these results we conclude that an oligosaccharide of 6–8 hexose units competes on equal terms with the intact polysaccharide. This tells us that the antibody is recognizing — binding to — a portion of the polysaccharide spanning 6–8 hexose units. This represents a length of approximately 30 angstroms. The pioneering studies by Kabat on the inhibition of dextran (poly-D-glucose) by small polymers of glucose gave similar results. The precipitation of antipolythymidine antibodies is maximally inhibited by oligonucleotides 6–7 nucleotides in length. The precipitation of antipolyalanine antibodies is maximally inhibited by oligomers of polyalanine containing 6–8 residues. Thus, for each of these antigen–antibody systems, the results are roughly concordant: antigenic determinants span a distance on the order of 30 angstroms. Such a distance provides many opportunities for the various atomic interactions that contribute to antigen–antibody binding.

## 4.3 The Forces That Bind Antigens to Antibodies

The binding of an antibody to the appropriate antigenic determinant is achieved by noncovalent forces. These are of three principal kinds (Figure 4.6).

*1. Ionic Interactions.* At any given pH, antibodies and, often, antigens have charged groups that may participate in the binding of one to the other. For example, the negatively charged carboxyl groups of aspartic and glutamic acid residues on a protein antigen may be attracted by the positively charged free amino groups of lysine (Figure 4.6) and arginine residues on the antibody (or vice versa). The presence of such interactions can be detected by altering the pH of the reaction medium thus adding (when the pH is lowered) or removing (when the pH is raised) protons to and from these residues. Increasing the salt concentration of the reaction medium reduces the strength of binding by providing competing ions for the sites. Both of these manipulations are apt to have substantial effects on the binding of the type 3 pneumococcal polysaccharide to anti-type 3 antibodies, for example, suggesting that the carboxyl group on the glucuronic acid residues plays a major role in the molecular interaction.

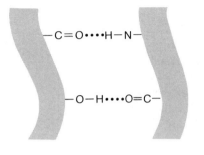

Ionic interactions

Asp
or
Glu

Lys
or
Arg

**Figure 4.6** Some types of noncovalent interactions that bind antibodies to antigens (and enzymes to their substrates).

Hydrogen bonds

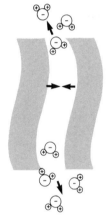

Hydrophobic interactions

**2. Hydrogen Bonds.** The protein nature of antibodies provides many opportunities for establishing hydrogen bonds. For example, the carboxyl group at peptide bonds can be hydrogen-bonded to (a) the amide nitrogen of the peptide bonds on a protein antigen (Figure 4.6), (b) the hydroxyl groups of serine and threonine residues of proteins, and (c) the hydroxyl groups of sugars. Hydrogen bonds are sensitive to small changes in temperature. If a slight increase in temperature reduces the strength of antigen–antibody binding, we may conclude that hydrogen bonds participate in the molecular interaction of the two.

**3. Hydrophobic Interactions.** The R groups of such amino acids as phenylalanine and leucine are nonpolar and hence interact poorly with polar molecules like water. For this reason, most of the nonpolar residues in globular proteins are directed toward the interior of the molecule while such polar groups as aspartic acid and lysine are on the surface exposed to the solvent. However, nonpolar residues may be found in the binding site of antibodies. Brought into close proximity with a nonpolar portion of an antigenic determinant, it is energetically more favorable for the two "oily" nonpolar areas to approach each other closely (Figure 4.6), displacing the polar molecules of solvent from between them. If sufficiently large areas are involved, the mutual attraction of complementary hydrophobic regions can provide substantial strength of antigen–antibody binding. In general, antigens with nonpolar antigenic determinants are bound more tightly than those with polar determinants. The strength of hydrophobic interactions is not appreciably affected by changes in pH, or salt concentration of the reaction medium.

In each of the cases discussed above, the strength of the interactions are individually weak (on the order of 5 kcal/mole) as compared with a covalent bond (with its 90–100 kcal/mole of bond energy). Furthermore, the strength of these interactions is dependent on the closeness with which the interacting groups can approach each other. Separated by more than an angstrom or so, these forces are negligible. These two observations lead to two important conclusions about antigen–antibody binding (and enzyme–substrate binding for that matter). These are (1) a number of such noncovalent interactions usually participate in the binding of an antibody molecule to an antigenic determinant, and (2) the topography of the surface of the antigenic determinant, including its distribution of polar and nonpolar atomic groups, must be complementary to the topography of the binding site on the antibody molecule; i.e.,one must make a close fit with the other.

## 4.4  Antibody Affinity

The tightness with which an antigenic determinant is bound to the antigen-binding site of an antibody molecule depends upon the types and number of the noncovalent interactions that occur between the atomic groups of each. The *total* strength with which the site on the antibody molecule binds to the antigenic determinant is called the **affinity** of the antibody. It can be quantitated. One relatively simple and reproducible technique for measuring antibody affinity is the method of *equilibrium dialysis.*

In this procedure, we measure the strength of binding between a macromolecule — the antibody molecule — and a small monovalent **ligand** (a molecule that can bind to the antibody). The ligand might be the hapten of the hapten-carrier conjugate used to produce the antiserum. It could be a short oligosaccharide or polypeptide encompassing a determinant present on the immunizing antigen. However, the ligand must be small enough to diffuse freely through a differentially permeable membrane through which the antibody molecules cannot pass. There must also be some method of accurately measuring the concentration of ligand at the concentrations that will be used in the procedure.

Small oligosaccharides derived from the pneumococcal polysaccharides meet these criteria. The hexasaccharide of the type 3 pneumococcal polysaccharide has a molecular weight of 1,032 and passes easily through the pores of cellophane, which exclude molecules with molecular weights ranging above 12,000. The hexasaccharide can be easily radiolabeled with tritium, and its concentration measured accurately in the micromolar range.

We set up two compartments separated by a dialysis membrane. Into one compartment ("F," see Figure 4.7) we place a solution of the radiolabeled hexasaccharide dissolved in a suitable buffer. Into the other compartment ("B"), we place a solution (in the same buffer) of pre-immune rabbit serum; serum from a rabbit that has not been immunized against the type 3 polysaccharide. Over the next few hours, we periodically withdraw portions from each side and measure their radioactivity. At first, all the radioactivity is in F, none in B. But as diffusion proceeds, the radioactivity (and thus the concentration of ligand) declines in F and rises in B at the same rate. Eventually, the concentrations of ligand in the two chambers become equal and remain so. Equilibrium has been reached.

Now we repeat the experiment, substituting in chamber B a solution of anti-type 3 antibodies. This could be a solution of purified antibodies or simply a sample of suitably diluted and buffered antipneumococcal antiserum. This time, the concentration of ligand in B rises to an equilibrium value higher than its concentration in F (Figure 4.7). The difference

**Figure 4.7** Equilibrium dialysis. The contents of each chamber are shown after equilibrium has been reached. In the second case, the concentration of ligand is higher in B than in F because of binding to the antibody molecules. Salts are added to the medium in which equilibrium dialysis is performed to minimize Donnan effects. Nonspecific binding of the ligand may be compensated for by adding enough normal serum to the ligand solution in F to achieve a protein concentration equal to that in the antibody preparation.

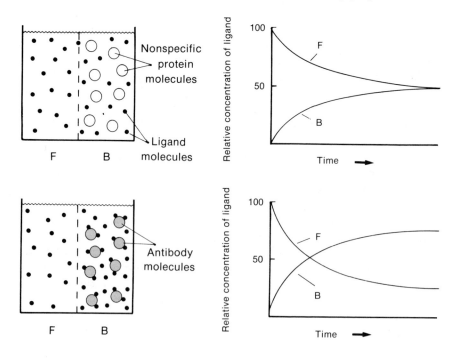

between the two values represents the ligand which has been bound by antibody molecules and, while bound, is unable to diffuse back into chamber F.

For a given concentration of antibody molecules, the greater the fraction of ligand bound by them, the greater their affinity for the ligand. This value can be expressed as an association constant, $K$. At equilibrium,

$$K = \frac{[Ab-Lg]}{[Ab][Lg]}$$

where the terms in brackets represent the concentrations of antibody–ligand complexes [Ab–Lg], unbound antibody [Ab], and unbound ("free") ligand [Lg]. Note that this is the reciprocal of the classical *dissociation* constant. A more convenient form of this equation is

$$K = \frac{r}{(n-r)(c)}$$

where $r$ = the *ratio* of the concentration of *bound* ligand to the concentration of antibody molecules placed in the system; $n$ = the number of ligand-binding sites on the antibody molecules, their valence; and $c$ = the concentration of unbound ("free") ligand.

To determine $K$, we set up a series of equilibrium dialysis chambers to which we add varying concentrations of ligand and a constant concentration of antibody. While it is convenient to place the ligand in one chamber, F, and the antibody in the other, B, it is not necessary to do so. The final equilibrium value will be reached even though both ingredients are initially present together in one chamber.

Figure 4.8 gives the results of equilibrium dialysis performed on a rabbit anti-pneumococcal antiserum diluted in buffered saline to a final antibody concentration of $1.82\ \mu M$ $(10^{-6}\ M)$. Solutions of the hexasaccharide derived from the type 3 polysaccharide were added to each chamber at concentrations ranging from 0.2 to $6.4\ \mu M$. The hexasacchar-

**Figure 4.8**  Results of equilibrium dialysis performed on a solution of rabbit antibodies elicited by the type 3 pneumococcal polysaccharide. The ligand was the hexasaccharide produced by the hydrolysis of the type 3 polysaccharide and labeled with tritium ($^3H$). The expressions in parentheses at the top of columns A, F, G, and J are the units in which the values in those columns are to be expressed.

| A Ligand added $(\times 10^{-6}\ M)$ | B "F"ront cpm | C "B"ack cpm | D (B + C) Total cpm | E (C − B) Bound cpm | F[1] Bound ligand $(\times 10^{-6}\ M)$ | G[2] Free ligand (c) $(\times 10^{-6}\ M)$ | H[3] $r$ | I $r/c$ $(\times 10^6)$ | J[4] $K$ $(\times 10^6\ M^{-1})$ |
|---|---|---|---|---|---|---|---|---|---|
| 0.2 | 182 | 1044 | 1226 | 862 | 0.14 | 0.03 | 0.08 | 2.6 | 1.4 |
| 0.4 | 367 | 2021 | 2388 | 1654 | 0.28 | 0.06 | 0.15 | 2.5 | 1.4 |
| 0.8 | 739 | 3923 | 4662 | 3184 | 0.55 | 0.13 | 0.30 | 2.4 | 1.4 |
| 1.6 | 1616 | 7394 | 9010 | 5778 | 1.0 | 0.29 | 0.57 | 2.0 | 1.4 |
| 3.2 | 3952 | 14347 | 18299 | 10395 | 1.8 | 0.69 | 1.0 | 1.5 | 1.4 |
| 6.4 | 11341 | 27028 | 38369 | 15687 | 2.6 | 1.9 | 1.4 | 0.8 | 1.4 |

"B"ack chamber contained anti-type-3 antibodies at a concentration of $1.8 \times 10^{-6}\ M$.

[1] (E/D) × A.
[2] (B/D) × A.
[3] F/$1.8 \times 10^{-6}\ M$.
[4] $r/((2-r) \times c)$.

ide was radiolabeled with tritium ($^3$H). When equilibrium was reached, the radioactivity in the chambers containing antibody (B) was, in every case, greater than in the chambers without antibodies (F). The radioactivity in B represents (1) a concentration of unbound ligand equal — given diffusion to equilibrium — to that in the other chamber (F) plus (2) a concentration of ligand bound to the antibody molecules in B. To determine the first value (free ligand, $c$), we multiply the concentration of ligand that was initially added to the system by the ratio of the radioactivity (in counts per minute, *cpm*) in chamber F to the total radioactivity. To determine the second value (bound ligand), we first subtract the radioactivity in F from that in B, giving a value for bound radioactivity. The ratio of bound radioactivity to total radioactivity is then multiplied by the concentration of ligand initially added to the system. This yields a value for the concentration of bound ligand. To determine $r$, we simply divide this value by the concentration of antibody molecules (in this case, 1.82 $\mu$M).

A useful way to present the resulting data is to plot the ratio $r/c$ as a function of $r$. Such a plot is called a Scatchard plot. If $K$ is truly a constant, the plot should produce a straight line, the slope of which is $-K$. Inspection of the graph (Figure 4.9) shows that this antibody population is indeed homogeneous with respect to its affinity for the ligand. The value for $K$ in this case is $1.4 \times 10^6$ liters/mole ($M^{-1}$).

The second valuable piece of information revealed by the Scatchard plot is that the maximum value for $r$ (the x intercept) is 2. At infinitely high concentrations of ligand, each antibody molecule can bind a maxi-

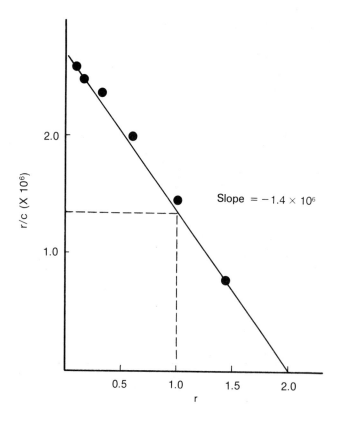

**Figure 4.9** Scatchard plot of the results in Figure 4.8. The straight line indicates that the antibodies were homogeneous with respect to the strength with which they bound the ligand, i.e., their affinity. The value for $K$ of these antibody molecules is the negative of the slope of the line; that is, $K = 1.4 \times 10^6$ liters/mole (or $M^{-1}$).

Slope $= -1.4 \times 10^6$

| A Ligand added ($\times 10^{-6}$ M) | B "F"ront cpm | C "B"ack cpm | D (B + C) Total cpm | E (C − B) Bound cpm | F[1] Bound ligand ($\times 10^{-6}$ M) | G[2] Free ligand (c) ($\times 10^{-6}$ M) | H[3] r | I r/c ($\times 10^6$) | J[4] K ($\times 10^6$ M$^{-1}$) |
|---|---|---|---|---|---|---|---|---|---|
| 5. | 400 | 4144 | 4544 | 3744 | 4.1 | 0.44 | 0.52 | 1.2 | 0.80 |
| 10 | 1262 | 8006 | 9268 | 6744 | 7.3 | 1.4 | 0.92 | 0.68 | 0.63 |
| 15 | 2702 | 11348 | 14052 | 8644 | 9.2 | 2.9 | 1.2 | 0.40 | 0.49 |
| 25 | 6648 | 18159 | 24807 | 11511 | 12. | 6.7 | 1.5 | 0.22 | 0.41 |
| 40 | 13693 | 27380 | 41073 | 13687 | 13. | 13. | 1.7 | 0.13 | 0.40 |
| 50 | 19286 | 34091 | 53377 | 14805 | 14. | 18. | 1.8 | 0.10 | 0.40 |

"B"ack chamber contained anti-type-3 antibodies at a concentration of $7.9 \times 10^{-6}$ M.

[1] (E/D) × A.
[2] (B/D) × A
[3] F/7.9 × 10$^{-6}$ M.
[4] r/((2 − r) × c).

**Figure 4.10** Results of equilibrium dialysis performed on another solution of rabbit antibodies directed against the type 3 pneumococcal polysaccharide. See the legend to Figure 4.8 for additional details.

mum of two ligand molecules. In other words, the valence of these antibody molecules is 2.

The fact that all the antibody molecules in this experiment have the same affinity for the ligand turns out, as we shall see, to be unusual. In this respect, this particular population of antibodies resembles a population of enzyme molecules, which always have a fixed affinity for their substrate.

Figure 4.10 presents the data produced when equilibrium dialysis was performed on another rabbit antipneumococcal (again type 3) antiserum. The results differ from those in Figure 4.8 in one striking way: $K$ is no longer a constant, but ranges from a value of $0.8 \times 10^6 M^{-1}$ in the chambers to which 5 $\mu$M ligand was added to $0.4 \times 10^6 M^{-1}$ in the chambers to which 50 $\mu$M ligand was added. This shows that the antibodies in this particular antiserum are not homogeneous with respect to their affinity for the ligand. At low ligand concentrations, the binding of ligand is being carried out by a subpopulation of high affinity antibodies. As the concentration of ligand is increased, an increasingly large population of antibodies of lower affinity binds the ligand.

The heterogeneity of binding in this system is clearly revealed by the Scatchard plot of the data (Figure 4.11). Now the slope of the line is continuously changing as the concentration of ligand in the chambers increases. Scatchard plots of this sort are the norm, not the exception, for antisera. In other words, the antibodies elicited by most antigens using most immunization schedules constitute a diverse population of molecules of varying affinity for the antigenic determinants on the antigen. Here, then, is another important aspect of the heterogeneity of antibodies. Not only does immunization with a single antigen give rise to antibodies directed against different determinants on the antigen, but even that subset of antibodies directed against a single determinant possesses a spectrum of affinities.

Despite the heterogeneity of affinity displayed by most antibody populations, it is convenient to be able to characterize such a population with respect to its affinity. We do this by defining an **average affinity** ($K_0$) as the value of $K$ when the ligand concentration is such that one-half the

73

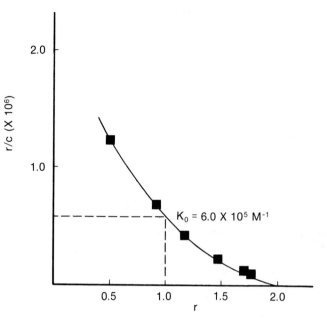

**Figure 4.11** Scatchard plot of the results in Figure 4.10. Although this population of antibodies was heterogeneous with respect to its affinity for the ligand, we can define an average association constant, $K_0$, which is the reciprocal of the concentration of free ligand $(c)$ at which one-half of all the binding sites are filled $(r = 1)$. In this case, $K_0 = 6.0 \times 10^5 \, \text{M}^{-1}$.

$K_0 = 6.0 \times 10^5 \, \text{M}^{-1}$

antigen binding sites are filled. For the bivalent antibodies discussed here, this would occur when $r = 1$. Thus,

$$K_0 = \frac{1}{(2-1)c} \quad \text{or} \quad \frac{1}{c}$$

Thus the average affinity is the reciprocal of the concentration of free ligand $(c)$ when $r = 1$. This value can be read directly from a Scatchard plot because when $r = 1$, $r/c = 1/c = K_0$. For the antiserum represented in Figure 4.11, $K_0 = 6.0 \times 10^5 \, \text{M}^{-1}$.

Average affinity constants for antibody populations vary over a considerable range. Antibodies directed against hydrophobic determinants like DNP may have association constants as high as $10^9 \, \text{M}^{-1}$ and occasionally even higher. A $K_0$ of $10^7 \, \text{M}^{-1}$ represents the high end of the range for antipolysaccharide antibodies, which are largely dependent upon ionic interactions and hydrogen bonds for their affinity. Antipolysaccharide antibodies may have a $K_0$ as low as $5 \times 10^2 \, \text{M}^{-1}$.

The data presented in Figure 4.8 and 4.10 and plotted in Figure 4.9 and 4.11 can be transformed according to the Sips equation.

$$\log[r/(2-r)] = a \log K + a \log c$$

where $r$, $K$, and $c$ retain their earlier definitions.

Plotting $\log[r/(2-r)]$ as a function of $\log c$ yields a straight line (Figure 4.12). Once again, the value for $K_0$ can be read directly from the plot. When $r = 1$, $\log[r/(2-r)] = 0$. Therefore, $K_0$ is the reciprocal of that value of $c$ where the $\log[r/(2-r)] = 0$ (Figure 4.12).

The coefficient $a$ is a constant called the heterogeneity index. It represents the dispersion of $K$ values about $K_0$. In a population of antibodies displaying homogeneous binding (Figure 4.9), $a = 1$, and the slope of the Sips plot is 1. Antisera containing antibodies representing a spectrum of affinities have values for $a$ of less than 1. The second antipneumococcal

**Figure 4.12** Sips plot of the results given in Figure 4.8 (upper line) and 4.10 (lower line). The slope of the upper line is 1, showing homogeneous binding. The slope of the lower line is 0.8, showing that this population of antibody molecules is heterogeneous with respect to its affinity for the ligand. The value of the slope, *a*, is called the heterogeneity index.

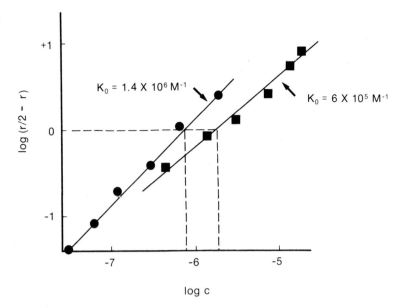

antiserum, which we have already seen is heterogeneous with respect to affinity, has a heterogeneity index of 0.8 (and the slope of its Sips plot is likewise 0.8).

If we are justified in assuming that the dispersion of individual $K$ values in the population of antibody molecules is distributed symmetrically around $K_0$, then the coefficient $a$ becomes a measure of the breadth of the resulting bell-shaped curve. For the example given ($a = 0.8$), roughly 75% of the antibody molecules in the preparation have affinities between $1.6 \times 10^5$ and $2.2 \times 10^6$ $M^{-1}$.

In many, perhaps most, antisera, there are good reasons to believe that the distribution of affinities does *not* follow a normal statistical distribution, i.e., would not yield a bell-shaped curve. Despite this, Sips plots remain a useful way of comparing different antibody preparations with respect to their average affinities and—subject to the qualification mentioned—their relative heterogeneity of affinities.

## 4.5   The Specificity of Antibodies

The specificity of an antibody molecule is its ability to discriminate between the antigenic determinant against which it was elicited and other antigenic determinants of related structure. The antigenic determinant, for example, a hapten like the dinitrophenyl group (DNP), present on the immunogen is called the *homologous determinant*; related structures (e.g., the trinitrophenyl group, TNP) are said to be *heterologous*.

The ability of an antibody molecule to discriminate between homologous and heterologous determinants can be detected by any assay that measures the binding between the two. If the antibody reacts measurably with a heterologous determinant, it is said to show a cross reaction.

**75**

IMMUNOGEN:

HAPTENS OF TEST ANTIGENS:

| | ortho | meta | para |
|---|---|---|---|
| $R = SO_3^-$ | $+$ $\pm$ | $+$ $+$ $\pm$ | $\pm$ |
| $R = AsO_3H^-$ | $0$ | $+$ | $0$ |
| $R = COO^-$ | $0$ | $\pm$ | $0$ |

Figure 4.13 Antibody specificity. Relative amounts of precipitation of rabbit antibodies directed against the homologous hapten (*m*-azobenzenesulfonate) and a variety of heterologous haptens. The antibodies were elicited by immunizing with the homologous hapten coupled to horse serum proteins. The tests were performed with all the haptens coupled to chicken serum proteins thus restricting the reaction to antibodies directed against the haptens. [From K. Landsteiner, *The Specificity of Serological Reactions*, 2nd ed., reprinted by Dover Publications, New York, 1962.]

The earliest systematic studies of antibody specificity were carried out by Karl Landsteiner and his colleagues. They used precipitation in liquid as a semiquantitative assay with which to compare homologous and heterologous reactions. In one series of experiments, antibodies were elicited (in rabbits) to a mixture of horse serum proteins that had been conjugated with the hapten *m*-azobenzenesulfonate (Figure 4.13). The resulting antisera were tested for reactivity with chicken serum proteins that had been conjugated with (1) the same hapten or (2) haptens in which the sulfonate group was in the ortho or para position or (3) azobenzenearsonate or azobenzenecarboxylate, in each case either ortho, meta, or para. The results are shown in Figure 4.13. As you can see, the antibodies reacted with the homologous hapten on the new carrier proteins (as we would predict from the discussion in Section 1.4). The most copious precipitate was formed when the sulfonate group was located in the meta (the homologous) position, although measurable precipitation occurred when its position was either ortho or para. Neither azobenzenearsonate nor azobenzenecarboxylate produced any precipitation except when the charged group was present in the meta position. So, while these antibodies do show cross-reactivity, the reduced reaction with heterologous ligands reveals a substantial degree of specificity.

Equilibrium dialysis provides a method by which antibody specificity can be assessed in a more quantitative manner. With this procedure, a value for $K_0$ can be determined for the homologous ligand as well as for related ligands. The greater the difference between the $K_0$ for the homologous ligand and that for a heterologous ligand, the greater the specificity of the antibody molecule for the homologous ligand. The data in Figure 4.14 show the results of equilibrium dialysis performed on a population of antibodies elicited by a protein carrying DNP groups covalently bound to the epsilon amino groups of lysine residues. As is generally the case, these antibodies had the highest $K_0$ for the homologous ligand ($\epsilon$-DNP–L-lysine). However, they also displayed substantial affinity for related ligands, even to dinitrobenzene itself. On occasions, an antigen will elicit antibodies that bind *more* strongly to a heterologous

| IMMUNOGEN | HAPTENS | | | |
|---|---|---|---|---|
| H O<br>····-N-C-C-····<br>H (CH₂)₄<br>NH<br>NO₂<br>NO₂<br>DNP-BGG | H<br>⁺H₃N-C-COO⁻<br>(CH₂)₄<br>NH<br>NO₂<br>NO₂<br>ε DNP lysine | H<br>⁺H₃N-C-COO⁻<br>(CH₂)₃<br>NH<br>NO₂<br>NO₂<br>δ-DNP-ornithine | NH₂<br>NO₂<br>NO₂<br>2,4-dinitroaniline | NO₂<br>NO₂<br>m-dinitrobenzene |
| $K_0$: | **23** | **9** | **2** | **0.6** $(\times 10^6 \ M^{-1})$ |

**Figure 4.14** Antibody specificity revealed by equilibrium dialysis. A rabbit was immunized with a hapten–carrier conjugate consisting of DNP groups coupled to the ε-amino groups of the lysine residues of bovine gamma globulin (DNP–BGG). The resulting antiserum had an affinity for ε-DNP-lysine of $2.3 \times 10^7 \ M^{-1}$ but less than half that affinity for δ-DNP-ornithine which has one less carbon atom in the chain. The degree to which an antibody population discriminates between the homologous and heterologous ligands is a measure of the specificity of that population. [From H. N. Eisen and G. W. Siskind, *Biochemistry* 3:996, 1964.]

**Figure 4.15** The shift of the hydroxyl group on carbon 17 from the beta position (extending above the plane of the molecule) to the alpha position (extending below) lowers by 1000-fold the affinity of the molecule for antibodies raised against a 17 β-estradiol-BSA conjugate. In each case the binding was measured by radioimmunoassay (see Section 5.9). [From W. M. Hunter, "Radioimmunoassay" in *Handbook of Experimental Immunology*, 3rd ed., Vol. 1, D. M. Weir (ed.), Blackwell, 1978.]

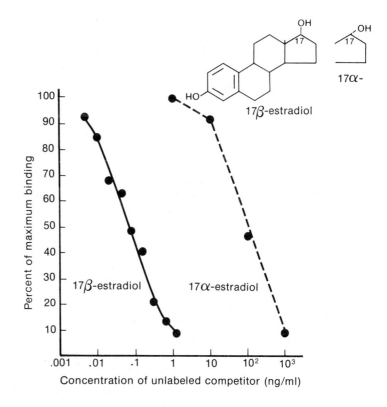

determinant than to the homologous determinant. Such antibodies are said to be *heteroclitic.*

The specificity of antibodies extends to their being able to discriminate between stereoisomers of the same molecule. $17\beta$-Estradiol is the major estrogen found in women of reproductive age. Antibodies elicited by a $17\beta$-estradiol – BSA conjugate bind strongly to the homologous hapten. When presented with $17\alpha$-estradiol, however, the binding efficiency is reduced over 1000-fold (Figure 4.15). The single change in the orientation of the hydroxyl group at carbon 17 from the beta configuration (projecting above the plane of the molecule) to the alpha configuration (projecting below the plane) is responsible for this sharp drop in affinity.

## 4.6 The Specificity of Antisera

The concept of specificity as applied to individual antibody molecules differs somewhat from the concept as applied to **antisera.** Most antisera represent complex mixtures of antibody molecules. These antisera usually display many specificities. This multispecificity arises in two ways.

1. If an animal is immunized with two or more different antigens, the resulting antiserum will react independently with each. Thus Landsteiner's rabbits produced not only anti-azobenzenearsonate antibodies but also antibodies against the many different proteins present in horse serum (which is why he had to use substituted chicken proteins for his assays of antihapten activity).

An antiserum that is specific for a single antigen can be produced in several ways. One is to immunize the animal with a preparation of the antigen that has been sufficiently purified so that no contaminating molecules remain in immunogenic concentrations. For example, we can produce a rabbit antiserum specific for human albumin by immunizing the rabbit with the purified protein rather than with whole human serum.

2. Often the problems of multispecificity cannot be solved simply by immunizing with pure antigen. For example, an antiserum raised against purified human IgG will also react with human IgA and IgM because each of the classes of immunoglobulin uses the same light chains ($\kappa$ and $\lambda$). However, this antiserum can be made specific for IgG by exposing it to an appropriate **immunoadsorbent:** particles to which other molecules containing the light chains (e.g., IgA or IgM) have been attached. Those antibodies directed against determinants on the light chains will bind to the immunoadsorbent and can be removed from the antiserum. The antibodies that remain will now be specific for IgG, i.e., specific for its heavy ($\gamma$) chains. So even if we produce an antiserum that is specific for a single antigen molecule (i.e., human albumin), this specificity is still only relative. Most antigens display several different antigenic determinants, each of which can elicit the formation of a population of antibodies directed against it. Thus an antigen bearing determinants A, B, C, and D will give rise to four separate sets of antibodies, each set directed against one of the determinants. When such an antiserum is presented to an

antigen displaying some—but not all—of these determinants, for example, A and C, the anti-A and anti-C antibodies will still be able to precipitate the molecule. This, then, is cross-reactivity of a different kind: the interaction of an antiserum with a heterologous antigen because of certain determinants *shared* by both antigens.

## 4.7  Purification of Antibodies

In the preceding section we saw how an immunoadsorbent can be used to remove cross-reacting antibodies from an antiserum. In that case, we were interested in what was left behind. But immunoadsorbents provide a tool of great general usefulness in "purifying" antibodies of a desired specificity.

The procedure involves four steps.

*Step 1.*  The immunoadsorbent is prepared by coupling the antigen (e.g., DNP) to a solid matrix. Agarose, sephadex, derivatives of cellulose, or other polymers can be used.

*Step 2.*  The antiserum is passed over the immunoadsorbent (Figure 4.16). As long as the capacity of the column is not exceeded, those antibodies in the mixture specific for the antigen will bind and be retained. Antibodies of other specificities and other serum proteins will pass through unimpeded.

*Step 3.*  Elution. A reagent is passed into the column to release the antibodies from the immunoadsorbent. Buffers containing a high concentration of salts and/or a low pH are often used to disrupt the noncovalent interactions between the antibodies and antigen. A denaturing agent, such as 8 M urea, will also break the interaction by altering the configuration of the antigen-binding site. Another, gentler, approach is to elute with a soluble form of the antigen. In our example, a solution of DNP–lysine run into the column will compete with the immunoadsorbent for the antigen-binding sites of the antibodies and transfer the antibodies to the fluid phase.

*Step 4.*  Dialysis. The eluate is then dialyzed against, for example, buffered saline in order to remove the reagent used for elution.

The result of this procedure, which is called **affinity chromatography**, is a preparation of antibodies of a single specificity. Although such a preparation is "pure" with respect to antigen specificity, it is by no means pure with respect to the structure of the antibody molecules contained in it. Electrophoresis of these purified antibodies will normally reveal as broad a range of mobilities as were present in the original

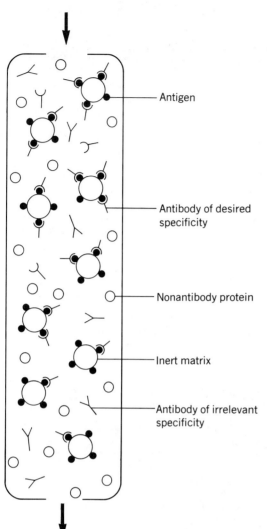

Antigen

Antibody of desired
specificity

Nonantibody protein

Inert matrix

Antibody of irrelevant
specificity

**Figure 4.16** Affinity chromatography. Antibodies with sufficient avidity for the antigen bind to the immunoadsorbent while other molecules pass through the column. The desired antibodies can later be released from the immunoadsorbent by adding an agent that reduces the strength of their binding.

antiserum. By the same token, equilibrium dialysis will reveal a range of association constants.

So while antibody purification by affinity chromatography is useful for some purposes, it is of no value for others. The purified antibodies represent far too heterogeneous a population for such important tasks as determining primary structure or preparing crystals for x-ray analysis. Fortunately, there are ways to secure homogeneous populations of a single kind of antibody molecule, i.e., monoclonal antibodies.

## 4.8 Monoclonal Antibodies

An antibody-secreting cell, like any other cell, can become cancerous. The unchecked proliferation of such a cell is called a *myeloma*. Because a myeloma begins as a single cell, all of its progeny constitute a clone. One

**Figure 4.17** Electrophoretic separation in agarose gel of (top to bottom) normal human serum, serum from a patient with an IgG multiple myeloma, serum from a case of Waldenström's macroglobulinemia (IgM), and an IgA myeloma. Anode at the right. [Courtesy of Beckman Instruments, Inc.]

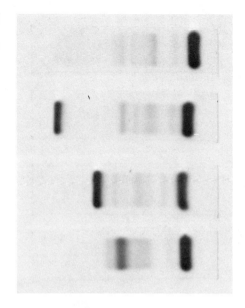

of the remarkable features of antibody-secreting cells is that a single cell secretes only a single kind of antibody molecule. This rule generally holds true for myeloma cells as well. Thus the serum of an animal with a myeloma contains substantial amounts of one kind of immunoglobulin (Figure 4.17).

Myelomas occur spontaneously in a number of species (including humans). They can also be induced (by injecting mineral oil or similar materials) in inbred mice of the BALB/c strain. Because these mice are so highly inbred, they are virtually identical genetically, almost like "identical twins." This makes it possible to propagate the myeloma cells that originated in one mouse in as many other BALB/c mice as one wishes and for periods long after the original mouse would have died of its tumor. Myeloma cells, like other malignant cells, grow indefinitely in tissue culture.

The product of a given myeloma is a homogeneous immunoglobulin (Figure 4.17). Presumably this immunoglobulin is a *bona fide* antibody. But the induction of a myeloma appears to be a totally random event, and thus one cannot determine for what antigen the myeloma protein might be an antibody. Sometimes screening a myeloma protein against a panel of different antigens reveals one to which it binds with a reasonably high value of $K$ (not $K_0$, myeloma proteins are homogeneous — see Section 4.4). Despite many attempts, it has not been possible to induce myelomas specific for a particular antigen.

In 1975, Köhler and Milstein found a way out of this dilemma. They developed a technique for combining the growth potential of myeloma cells with the predetermined antibody specificity of normal immune spleen cells. They did this by literally fusing a myeloma cell with an antibody-secreting spleen cell from an immunized mouse (Figure 4.18). The technique is called somatic cell hybridization. The result is a "hybridoma."

They mixed both kinds of cells with an agent to facilitate fusion of

81

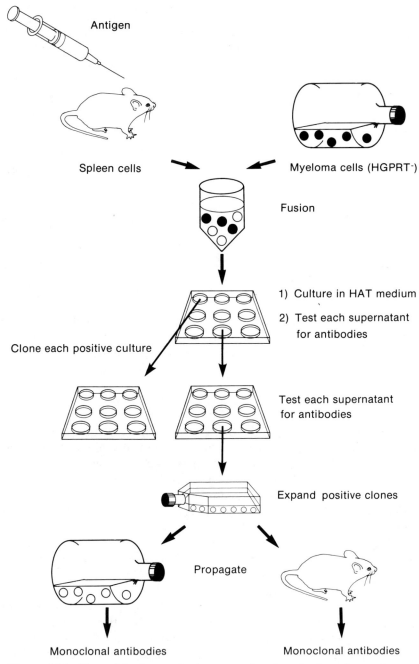

Antigen

Spleen cells

Myeloma cells (HGPRT⁻)

Fusion

1) Culture in HAT medium

2) Test each supernatant
   for antibodies

Clone each positive culture

Test each supernatant
for antibodies

Expand positive clones

Propagate

Monoclonal antibodies

Monoclonal antibodies

**Figure 4.18** Procedure for producing monoclonal antibodies of a predetermined specificity. This technique was developed by Köhler and Milstein. In 1984, they shared a Nobel Prize for this work.

adjacent cell membranes. The rate of successful hybrid formation is quite low (on the order of one in several hundred thousand cells in the culture). This necessitates a technique with which to select for those rare successful fusions. The standard technique is to use a myeloma cell that has lost the capacity to synthesize hypoxanthine–guanine–phosphoribosyltransferase (HGPRT). This enzyme enables cells to synthesize nucleotides using an extracellular source of hypoxanthine as a precursor. Ordinarily, the absence of HGPRT is no great problem because cells have an alternate pathway that they can use. However, when cells are exposed to aminopterin (a folic acid analog), they are unable to use this other pathway. Thus they become fully dependent upon HGPRT.

These properties are exploited by transferring the cell fusion mixture to a culture medium containing hypoxanthine, aminopterin, and thymidine (HAT medium). Unfused myeloma cells are unable to grow in the medium because they lack HGPRT. When a normal cell fuses with a myeloma cell, however, the hybrid is able to grow in HAT medium because the normal cell supplies the enzyme. Of course, unfused normal spleen cells are also able to grow in the medium, but, like all normal cells, their capacity for proliferation is limited and they eventually die out.

Having selected for hybrid cells, it now is necessary to screen them for the production of the desired antibody. After all, the spleen of a mouse — even a mouse actively immunized with a single antigen — contains cells secreting many different specificities of antibodies. So some form of assay technique must be used to look for the presence of the desired antibody. Usually this means removing some of the supernatant from each culture and testing it for antibodies using one of the sensitive assays described in Chapter 5.

A single culture, even though positive for antibody production, can contain the progeny of two or more successful fusions. Therefore, it is necessary to dilute positive cultures so that fresh cultures can be started with a single hybridoma cell. When successful, such cultures are truly monoclonal.

Although the *cultures* are now monoclonal, their products may not be. In other words, a single hybridoma might secrete several different immunoglobulins. If its myeloma parent was secreting an immunoglobulin (with 1 H and 1 L chain), this would continue to be produced along with the antibody of the spleen cell parent. Because H and L chains are synthesized separately, the hybridoma can also produce hybrid molecules containing the H chain from one parent with the L chain from the other. During their early period of culture, all somatic cell hybrids tend to lose chromosomes. Thus it is possible to eventually recover cells that are reduced to secreting only the desired antibody. A more rapid and efficient way to achieve this goal is to use mutant myeloma cells that have lost the ability to secrete an immunoglobulin while still retaining their cancerous growth properties.

In the end (usually after several months of hard work), success is a clone of cells that secretes a single kind of antibody molecule (a monoclonal antibody) directed against a single determinant on a preselected antigen (Figure 4.19). Now all that is needed is to propagate these cells in large numbers. They can be grown in tissue culture where they will secrete their antibody into the medium. Although the concentration of the antibody in these cultures is low (10–60 $\mu$g/ml), the use of large culture vessels can provide sizeable amounts of material. Alternatively, the hybridoma can be propagated in mice. Here the antibody concentration (in the serum and other body fluids) can reach 1–10 mg/ml. The more mice you use, the more monoclonal antibody you can harvest.

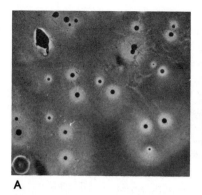 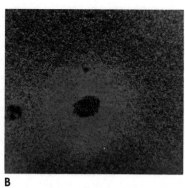

**A**                                          **B**

Figure 4.19   A: Hybridoma clones secreting antibodies against sheep
red blood cells (SRBC). B: A single clone at higher magnification.
Hybridoma cells are first plated individually. After a period of
growth, the resulting clones are covered with a layer of agarose
containing SRBC and complement. The formation of a halo reveals
that the clone is secreting anti-SRBC antibodies. [Courtesy of C.
Milstein, *Nature* **256**:495, 1975.]

Although monoclonal antibodies are homogeneous, they may not be
truly monospecific. They will react with different antigens that happen
to share the determinant against which they are directed or even that
simply carry structurally related determinants (like DNP and TNP).
Nonetheless, monoclonal antibodies have made it possible to avoid many
of the problems of multispecificity inherent in most conventionally produced antisera. In later chapters, we shall find repeated examples of what
valuable scientific, diagnostic and — we hope — therapeutic tools these
monoclonal antibodies can be.

## ADDITIONAL READING

1. Kabat, E. A., *Structural Concepts in Immunology and Immunochemistry*, 2nd
ed., Holt, Rinehart and Winston, New York, 1976. Thorough treatments of specificity (Ch. 1), the quantitative precipitin reaction (Ch. 4), equilibrium dialysis
(Ch. 5), and the size of antigenic determinants (Ch. 6).

2. Kohler, G., and C. Milstein, "Continuous Cultures of Fused Cells Secreting
Antibody of Predefined Specificity," *Nature* **256**:495, 1975. (Reprinted in V. L.
Sato and M. L. Gefter, *Cellular Immunology*, Addison-Wesley Publishing Co.,
Inc., Reading, MA, 1982.

3. Mishell, Barbara B., and S. M. Shiigi (eds.), *Selected Methods in Cellular Immunology*, W. H. Freeman and Company, San Francisco, 1980. Contains a detailed description of the procedures for making hybridoma clones.

4. Weir, D. M. (ed.), *Handbook of Experimental Immunology*, 3rd ed., Vol. 1,
Blackwell, Oxford, 1978. Includes a detailed description of equilibrium dialysis
and the preparation of immunoadsorbents.

CHAPTER **5**

# Antibody – Antigen Assays

## 5.1 Introduction

In this chapter, we examine a number of laboratory techniques with which antibodies are detected and, often, quantitated. In Chapter 6 we consider assays with which cell-mediated immune responses can be measured. If at times you feel that you are simply wading through a long catalog, remember the central importance of these assays to the development of immunology as a science and a health tool. How can one discover the machinery of immunity without techniques for measuring the expression of the immune response? As you examine this material, note also the critical roles that immunoassays play in such areas as (1) assessing the level of immunity in patients, (2) diagnosing illness, and (3) verifying the safety of donated blood, among others. Each of the assays to be described in this chapter and the next will reappear again and again as the source of the data upon which our knowledge of the immune system has been built.

The assay methods described in this chapter are used to detect and quantitate the presence of antibodies of a particular specificity. Therefore, each method depends upon the use of the antigen for which these antibodies are specific; that is, to which they bind. Our chief concern will be the ways in which antigens are used to detect antibodies. However, the complementarity of the interaction of antigens with antibodies allows many of these assay methods to be used to detect antigens as well. In such cases, *antibodies* are used as highly specific reagents to detect the presence of other molecules of scientific or medical interest, such as hormones, drugs, and tumor antigens.

As we examine each assay method, we will consider one or more examples of its use. In most cases, the examples selected not only illustrate the technique but also yield important pieces of immunological information that provide valuable groundwork for the material in later chapters.

## 5.2 The Interfacial Test

Section 4.1 described the quantitative precipitation assay. This technique enables us to determine the concentration of precipitating antibodies in an antiserum. The test takes a few days to complete and is somewhat cumbersome.

Sometimes we need only to establish the presence or absence of antibodies in an antiserum. One good example is as an adjunct to the quantitative precipitation test itself. In order to determine the equivalence point (Figure 4.1), the supernatant of each tube is checked to see if it contains residual antigen or antibody. To determine the equivalence point, a simple, rapid qualitative test is needed. The *interfacial test* (also called the ring test) is ideal for this.

A set of narrow bore tubes is partially filled with one component, for example, the antiserum. A solution of the second component, the antigen, is layered on top, without mixing the two solutions. (If the two solutions differ in density, the more dense solution is placed at the bottom of the tube to avoid accidental mixing.) If the appropriate antibodies and antigens are present, a ring of precipitate forms within a few minutes at or close to the interface between the two solutions (Figure 5.1). When testing for the presence of antigen, an antiserum of known specificity is

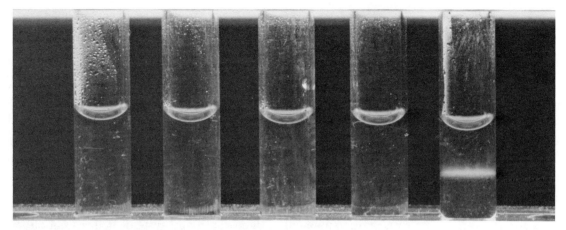

Figure 5.1  The interfacial (or ring) test. A layer of precipitate has formed between the antiserum (bottom) and the antigen solution (top) in the tube at the extreme right. The other four tubes are various controls, such as antiserum with buffer and normal serum with antigen. [Courtesy of Justine S. Garvey from J. S. Garvey, N. E. Cremer, and D. H. Sussdorf, *Methods in Immunology*, 3rd ed., W. A. Benjamin, Inc., Advanced Book Program, 1977.]

placed in the bottom of the tube and the unknown antigen is layered on top. When testing for the presence of antibodies in a serum, a solution of the antigen is layered on top of the serum. When the antibodies are present in a dilute solution, e.g., the supernatant test, adding gelatin or a similar agent helps to increase the density of the bottom layer.

## 5.3  Two-Dimensional Double Immunodiffusion (The Ouchterlony Technique)

Antibody molecules and soluble antigens can diffuse through such semi-solid media as agar or through the interstices of a wetted matrix such as a sheet of cellulose acetate soaked with buffer. Interaction of antigen and antibodies is revealed by a visible line of precipitate that forms in the gel or matrix.

The procedure is technically quite simple. When using agar, wells are cut in the agar (e.g., in a petri dish) and each is filled with the appropriate antigen solution or antiserum. For example, if one well is filled with BSA and a second with a rabbit antiserum raised against BSA, BSA molecules and anti-BSA antibodies will each begin to diffuse out *in all directions* from their respective wells. A line of precipitate forms where the advancing fronts meet and reach equivalence (Figure 5.2).

The rate at which each component diffuses from the wells increases with increasing concentration and decreases with increasing size of its molecules. Therefore, the line of precipitate forms closer to the well containing the lower concentration and/or larger of the reacting molecules.

The procedure, developed by Orlan Ouchterlony, has two great advantages over precipitation in liquid. First, it makes it easier to distin-

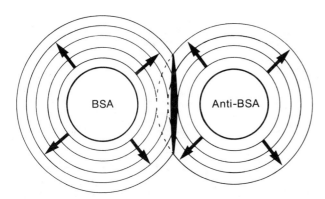

**Figure 5.2** Mechanism of precipitate formation in the Ouchterlony technique.

guish a multicomponent antigen–antibody system. If, for example, a rabbit is immunized with human serum, each component (such as albumin, transferrin, IgG) will elicit antibodies directed against it. When the antiserum is placed in one well and human serum in a second, a number of distinct lines of precipitate form between the two wells (Figure 5.3). Each line represents a different antigen–antibody system, for example, albumin–antialbumin, transferrin–antitransferrin. Quantitative precipitation in liquid would have told us the total weight of reacting materials but would not have so clearly revealed the presence of multiple, distinct antigen–antibody systems.

To identify which line represents which system we need to have available a solution of either purified antigen or monospecific antibodies. If, for example, a solution of human IgG is placed in a well adjacent to the human serum, a *single* line of precipitate will form with the antiserum. In time, this line will fuse with *one* of the lines produced by the whole human serum, thus identifying that line as the IgG–antiIgG reaction (Figure 5.3). The complete fusion of two adjacent precipitin lines is called the *reaction of identity*. Neither antigen nor antibody molecules can diffuse past the line of precipitate, so once these meet, they remain

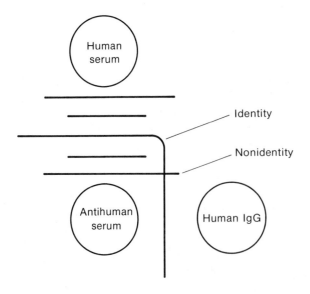

**Figure 5.3** The number of lines of precipitate formed between the two wells indicates the minimum number of *different* antigens being detected by the antiserum. The fusion of the line formed with purified antigen (human IgG) with one of the multiple lines identifies it (reaction of identity).

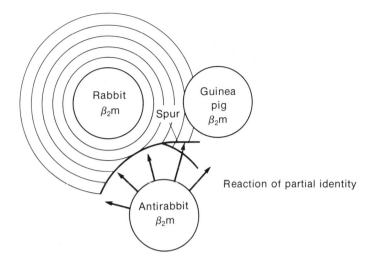

**Figure 5.4** Mechanism of spur formation. The spur represents the reaction of the homologous antigen (rabbit $\beta_2$m) with those antibodies that are *not* precipitated by the heterologous antigen (guinea pig $\beta_2$m).

fused. (However, a line of precipitate can redissolve as diffusing antigen brings it into antigen excess. In such a case, the line of precipitate migrates away from the well containing antigen until diffusion from the well ceases.)

Neither diffusing antigen nor diffusing antibodies are blocked by unrelated lines of precipitate. Thus the line of precipitate formed by one antigen–antibody pair is free to cross any unrelated lines. Such a pattern is called the *reaction of nonidentity* (Figure 5.3).

This technique can also discriminate between an antigen used to elicit the antiserum (the homologous antigen) and related (heterologous) antigens that can also be precipitated by the antiserum. These heterologous antigens are cross-reacting because they *share* some of the determinants found on the homologous antigen. For example, an antiserum raised in goats to rabbit $\beta_2$-microglobulin (r$\beta_2$m) will also precipitate the $\beta_2$-microglobulin of guinea pigs (g$\beta_2$m). If these two antigens are tested by the Ouchterlony technique against the goat antiserum, two lines of precipitate form and fuse (Figure 5.4). However, a projection of precipitate — called a *spur* — forms at the intersection. The spur points toward the well

**Figure 5.5** Reaction of partial identity between the purified serum albumin of the Indian elephant and an extract from the frozen thigh muscle of a 40,000-year-old mammoth found in eastern Siberia. [Courtesy of A. C. Wilson, from E. M. Prager et al., *Science* **209**:287, 1980.]

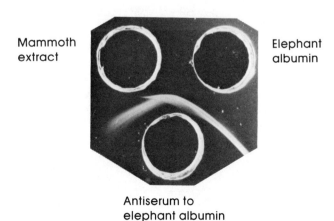

containing the heterologous (in this case, guinea pig) antigen. Spur formation is an indication of *partial identity.* The spur always points toward the well containing the antigen that *lacks* one or more of the determinants present on the homologous antigen. Therefore, the spur represents the reaction between the homologous antigen ($r\beta_2m$) and those antibody molecules that do *not* bind to the heterologous antigen ($g\beta_2m$) and thus are free to diffuse past its band of precipitate. In so doing, they are free to react with the homologous material that continues to diffuse from its well (Figure 5.4). Figure 5.5 provides a vivid illustration of spur formation and the insights it can provide about antigenic relationships.

## 5.4  Immunoelectrophoresis (IEP)

*Immunoelectrophoresis* combines the technique of electrophoresis with that of immunodiffusion. Like those techniques, it is carried out in a semisolid medium (such as, agar), or in a buffered matrix like cellulose

**Figure 5.6**  Technique of immunoelectrophoresis (IEP). Three examples of the use of monospecific antisera to identify arcs developed by a polyvalent antiserum are given in Figure 2.12.

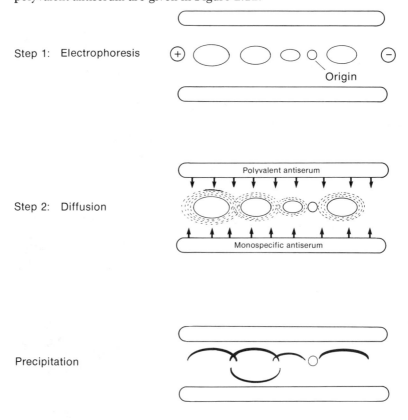

acetate. It is performed in two stages. First, a mixture of antigens is placed in a well and subjected to electrophoresis (Figure 5.6). Then the current is turned off and a trough running parallel to the direction of the electrophoretic separation is filled with the appropriate antiserum. The individual components of the antigen mixture each diffuse out radially from the position where they were left by electrophoresis. The antibody molecules in the antiserum diffuse in a straight advancing front toward the antigens. An arc of precipitate forms where each antigen–antibody component meets (Figure 5.6).

The great advantage of this technique — introduced in 1953 by Grabar and Williams — is its ability to separate the components of complex mixtures. Electrophoresis alone often fails to distinguish proteins of similar electrophoretic mobility. Two-dimensional immunodiffusion of multicomponent systems seldom resolves more than a few lines of precipitate. The combination of techniques exploited in IEP may, on the other hand, resolve as many as 30 individual antigens in a mixture (Figure 5.7). Even if electrophoresis should fail to separate two components completely, their precipitin arcs will be distinct (though, overlapping) if the respective components diffuse from slightly displaced centers of concentration or if their zones of equivalence differ slightly.

Immunoelectrophoresis finds its widest use in the analysis of serum samples. Abnormally low or high concentrations of such serum proteins as albumin, transferrin, IgG, and others are valuable clues in diagnosing a variety of diseases.

If monospecific antisera are available, they can be used to identify individual arcs of precipitate. For example, an antiserum raised against purified IgM will form an arc with that component in electrophoresed serum. This arc will be a mirror image of the IgM arc developed by the polyvalent antiserum. In fact, if the two homologous arcs develop sufficiently, they will fuse to form a reaction of identity (Figure 2.12). Reactions of partial identity can also be detected by immunoelectrophoresis.

**Figure 5.7** Immunoelectrophoretic (IEP) pattern produced by normal human serum reacting with antiserum from a horse immunized with normal human serum. [Courtesy of the Scientific Division of Cooper Biomedical, Inc.]

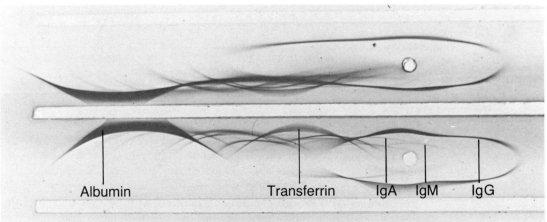

## 5.5 Single Radial Immunodiffusion (SRID)

In this technique, one of the reacting components (usually the antiserum) is incorporated in a gel (e.g., agarose) before it solidifies. The second component, the antigen, is placed in a well cut in the gel. As the antigen diffuses into the gel, it precipitates with the antibody molecules incorporated in the gel, forming a ring or halo. As antigen continues to diffuse from the well, the region close to the well comes into antigen excess, the precipitate dissolves and is redeposited farther out from the well. Thus the halo migrates out from the well. The area of the circle created by the halo is proportional to the initial concentration of antigen. This provides a basis for determining quantitatively the concentration of the antigen in the mixture applied to the well.

Because the absolute area of the halo depends upon other factors such as time, temperature, and the concentration of antibodies in the gel, each assay is run with a set of standards. Several wells are filled with standards containing known amounts of antigen, while other wells are filled with equal volumes of the unknowns. At a selected time the diameters of the halos formed by the standards are determined and plotted as a function of antigen concentration. Concentration values for the unknowns are then read from the plot (Figure 5.8).

The technique of SRID, which was introduced by Mancini, has become widely used. This is because it is a quantitative technique that is simpler to perform than quantitative precipitation in liquid as well as being considerably more sensitive. Antigen concentrations of a few $\mu$g/ml can be routinely measured by SRID. In addition, SRID allows the quantitation of a single antigen in a complex mixture if monospecific antibodies are incorporated in the gel. Earlier techniques required purification of the antigen prior to quantitation.

One common clinical use of SRID is in the determination of immunoglobulin levels in human serum. For example, levels of IgG below the normal range may be an indication of one of the immunodeficiency diseases. Conversely, above normal levels of IgG may indicate a case of multiple myeloma (see Section 4.8).

## 5.6 Electroimmunoassay ("Rocket" Immunoelectrophoresis)

*Electroimmunoassay,* introduced by Laurell in 1966, combines the speed of electrophoresis with the quantification of antigen provided by single radial immunodiffusion (SRID). As in SRID, one of the reacting components (usually the antiserum) is incorporated in the gel. Wells cut in the gel are then filled with the second component (a set of antigen standards and unknowns) and a direct current is applied. The antigen migrates into the gel according to its charge. As the antigen molecules first enter the gel, they form soluble complexes because they are in excess. However, as

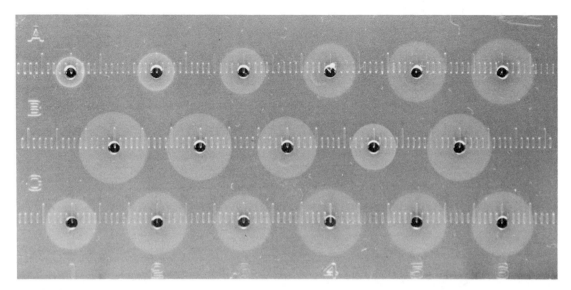

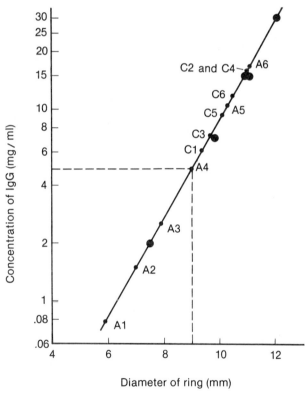

**Figure 5.8** Single radial immunodiffusion (SRID). The agarose gel contains antiserum specific for horse gamma chains. The wells of the middle row (B) were filled with samples of purified horse IgG of known concentration (from left to right: 30, 15, 7, 2, and 15 mg/ml). The wells of row A were filled with doubling dilutions of normal horse serum (A6 → A1: undiluted, 1/2, 1/4, etc.). The wells on the bottom row were filled with other samples of horse sera. A semilog plot is made of the diameter of the halos formed in row B as a function of the concentration of IgG (large circles). From this plot, the concentration of IgG in the serum samples can be determined. [Courtesy of ICN ImmunoBiologicals, Lisle, IL.]

the antigen migrates in the electric field, its concentration declines until, at equivalence, it forms a precipitate in the gel. As additional antigen arrives, the precipitate at the advancing front dissolves, while the precipitate along the sides remains. When no more antigen is left to enter the precipitate at the advancing front, the lines of precipitate converge producing a rocket-shaped appearance (Figure 5.9)(and giving to the procedure its common name of "rocket" electrophoresis). The area en-

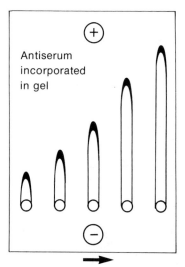

Antiserum
incorporated
in gel

Concentration of antigen in wells

**Figure 5.9** Electroimmunoassay. The area of each rocket is directly proportional to the initial concentration of antigen in the well. Each run should include a set of standards as well as the unknowns.

closed by the precipitin lines or, more roughly, the height of the rocket is directly proportional to the initial concentration of antigen in the well. As in SRID, a series of antigen standards is run in each assay.

The major advantage of this technique is its speed. The migration of antigen through the gel is completed in hours instead of days. The disadvantage of the technique is that the migrating component must carry a different charge from the component in the gel. This means, for example, that electroimmunoassay cannot be used to assay for immunoglobulins (unless they are chemically modified to make them more negatively charged). The sensitivities of electroimmunoassay and SRID are about the same.

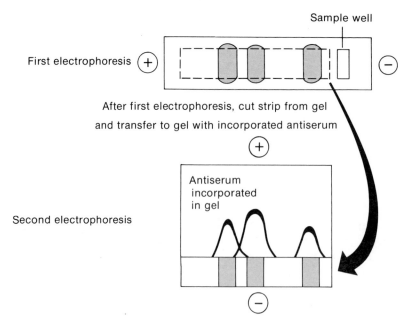

Sample well

First electrophoresis

After first electrophoresis, cut strip from gel
and transfer to gel with incorporated antiserum

Antiserum
incorporated
in gel

Second electrophoresis

**Figure 5.10** Mechanism of two-dimensional immuno-electrophoresis. This procedure combines high resolution with approximate quantitation of the various antigens.

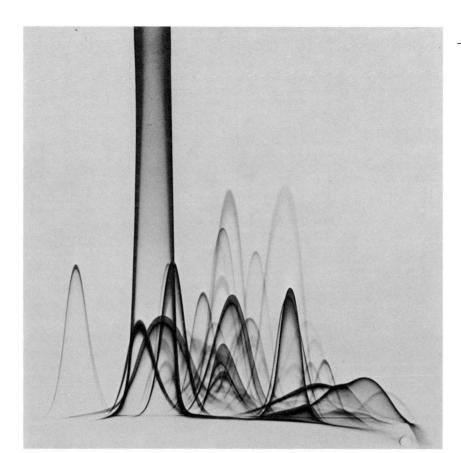

**Figure 5.11** Two-dimensional immunoelectrophoresis of human serum. In the first electrophoretic separation, the sample was placed in the well at the lower right and the anode was at the left. In the second run, the gel contained a rabbit antiserum against whole human serum. The tallest peak represents serum albumin. This procedure is also called *crossed immunoelectrophoresis.* [Courtesy of Pharmacia Fine Chemicals.]

Laurell also developed the technique of **two-dimensional immuno-electrophoresis.** In this technique, a mixture of antigens (e.g., serum proteins) is first separated by electrophoresis just as in the first step of IEP (see Section 5.4). The gel containing the separated components is then placed on or next to an antiserum-containing gel, and a second electrophoretic run is made at right angles to the first (Figure 5.10). The resulting arcs not only provide remarkable resolution of the components (Figure 5.11) but — as with electroimmunoassay — their size provides a rough measure of the concentration of each component.

## 5.7 Agglutination

Particles carrying antigens on their surface may be clumped by appropriate antisera. The major requirements are that the antibodies be multivalent and that the particles be able to approach each other sufficiently

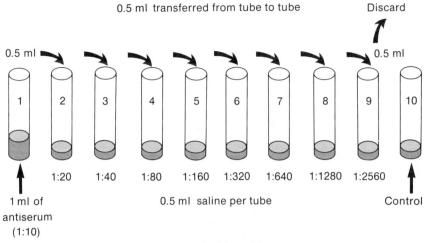

Figure 5.12 Procedure for making doubling dilutions.

closely to be cross-linked by the antibodies. The agglutination phenomenon can serve as a qualitative test, simply indicating the presence or absence of antibodies. It can also serve as a useful semiquantitative measure of the concentration of agglutinating antibodies. The most common procedure in the latter case is to add a fixed amount of the antigen-carrying particles to a series of tubes containing increasing (usually doubling) dilutions of the antiserum (Figure 5.12). The reciprocal of the highest dilution in which agglutination is observed defines the **titer** of the antiserum.

## Bacterial Agglutination

The humoral immune response to bacteria is usually dominated by antibodies directed against antigens present at the surface of the organism. Thus capsular polysaccharides, cell wall components, and flagella elicit antibody production. The presence and titer of these antibodies in an antiserum can often be measured by agglutination of the organisms. For example, the response to pertussis vaccine can be determined by checking the patient's serum for agglutinating antibodies. In this case, a standardized suspension of killed organisms *(Bordetella pertussis)* is added to serial dilutions of the patient's serum and the titer determined.

Bacterial agglutination finds frequent clinical use in diagnosis (usually when the patient is well on the road to recovery). A substantial rise in titer of specific agglutinating antibodies between the time the patient is acutely ill and is convalescing is good evidence of the identity of the pathogen. The Widal test, for example, is an agglutination test used in the diagnosis of typhoid fever. The patient's serum is diluted and mixed with antigens prepared from *Salmonella typhi,* the causative agent.

# Hemagglutination

*Hemagglutination* is the agglutination of red blood cells. At the turn of the century, Landsteiner discovered that antisera raised against red cells would agglutinate the red blood cells of some individuals but not of all. In 1901 he described the ABO system of antigens on human red cells and thus laid the foundation for safe blood transfusions. Figure 2.13 shows the ABO blood groups and the agglutinating antibodies found in the serum of the members of each group. The A and B antigens are inherited as simple Mendelian traits controlled by codominant alleles. The presence in the blood of anti-A and/or anti-B antibodies is not inherited, but is the result of (1) prior exposure to A-like and B-like antigens in the environment (e.g., on the membranes of bacteria) and (2) an immunological response to one or the other or both of these antigens depending on whether they are recognized by the immune system as "nonself."

Typing blood to match donor and recipient with respect to ABO antigens is obviously an important and widely used procedure. A small number of red cells is mixed with a drop of antiserum in a test tube and scored a few minutes later for the presence or absence of agglutination (Figure 5.13).

**Figure 5.13** Human red blood cells before (A) and after (B) addition of serum containing anti-A antibodies. The agglutination reaction indicates the presence of the A antigen on the surface of the cells.

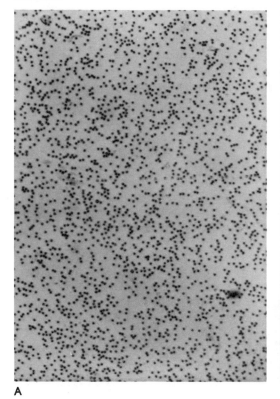

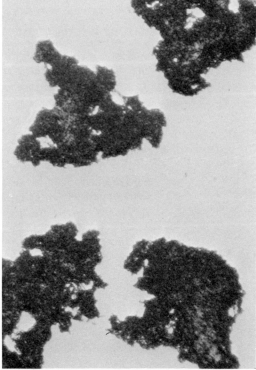

A                                                                 B

Almost four decades after his discovery of the ABO system, Landsteiner (and Wiener) discovered another system of red cell antigens, the rhesus or Rh antigens. Although occasionally responsible for harmful transfusion reactions, their chief clinical significance arises when an Rh-negative mother — previously sensitized (immunized) to the Rh antigen — carries an Rh-positive fetus. Because anti-Rh antibodies are chiefly of the IgG class, they cross the placenta from the mother's to the fetus's circulation. Their presence in the fetal circulation leads to severe — sometimes fatal — red cell destruction.

To avoid such problems as the inadvertent sensitization of an Rh-negative woman, donated blood must be typed for Rh as well as for ABO antigens. This, too, can be accomplished by an agglutination test. However, the number of antigenic determinants on Rh-positive red cells is so low that these cells are difficult to agglutinate. Anti-Rh antibodies are chiefly IgG and are much less efficient at agglutinating these cells than the larger IgM antibodies. However, the IgG antibodies do *bind* to the determinants on the red cells, and with appropriate modifications of the test conditions, can produce agglutination. One of the most reliable (and instructive) of these modifications is to add "antiglobulin" serum to the test mixture. Antiglobulin serum is produced in animals immunized with human IgG. A drop of antiglobulin serum added to the reaction mixture will agglutinate Rh-positive cells by binding to and cross-linking the IgG molecules that have bound to the red cells (Figure 5.14). The antiglobulin reaction was developed by Coombs and is often called the Coombs test.

### Passive Hemagglutination

In *passive hemagglutination*, red cells are agglutinated by antibodies directed against antigens that have been coupled chemically to the red cell surface. Thus the red cell now serves simply as a convenient, visible indicator of an antigen–antibody interaction.

The first step in the assay is to "sensitize" the red cells; that is, to couple the desired antigen to them. Some polysaccharide antigens will adsorb stably onto the surface of red cells. For protein antigens, tannic acid or chromic chloride solutions may be used to couple the antigens to the red cells. The exact mechanisms by which these reagents accomplish this is still uncertain. Bifunctional reagents, such as bisdiazobenzidine, are also used to achieve covalent bonding between the antigen (usually a protein) and the red cell membrane.

The assay is performed by adding a fixed number of the sensitized red cells to doubling dilutions of the antiserum or other antibody preparation. Again, the reciprocal of the highest dilution to give a visible agglutination reaction defines the titer of the antiserum (Figure 5.15).

It is frequently observed in hemagglutination titrations (direct as well as passive) that the first few tubes; that is, the tubes with the most concentrated antiserum, fail to agglutinate the test cells while higher dilutions agglutinate successfully. This phenomenon is called the *prozone effect*. One or more mechanisms may account for the prozone. (1) At high

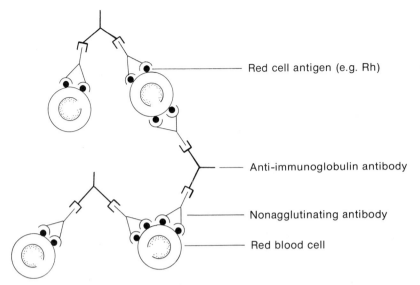

Red cell antigen (e.g. Rh)

Anti-immunoglobulin antibody

Nonagglutinating antibody

Red blood cell

**Figure 5.14** Mechanism of the antiglobulin reaction (Coombs test). The anti-immunoglobulin antibodies are produced in an animal, such as a goat, immunized with human IgG.

concentrations of antibodies, each of the antigenic sites on the red cells may be occupied by an unshared antibody molecule, preventing cross-linking of the cells. (2) Some types of antibody molecules are poor agglutinators, although they bind readily to the surface determinants. For example, an antiserum might contain both IgG, a poor agglutinator, and IgM, an excellent agglutinator. At high concentrations of IgG, many sites will be occupied by the IgG molecules and thus inaccessible to IgM. (3)

**Figure 5.15** Passive hemagglutination. The wells in the top row contain serial dilutions of a human serum mixed with a constant number of human red cells that have been coated with human thyroglobulin. The reaction is strongly positive in the first 5 wells; the bottom of each of these wells is covered with a sheet of agglutinated red cells. Wells 6–9 show increasingly weak reactions. The solid "button" of settled red cells in well 10 is a negative reaction. The control wells in the bottom row contain the same patient's serum mixed with normal, uncoated, red cells. The wells in the middle row contain normal human serum with thyroglobulin-coated red cells. Antithyroglobulin antibodies are often found in patients with such thyroid disorders as Graves' disease (see Section 18.5), myxedema, and chronic thyroiditis. [From P. E. Bigazzi and N. R. Rose in *Manual of Clinical Immunology*, 2nd ed., N. R. Rose and H. Friedman (eds.), American Society for Microbiology, Washington, D.C., 1980, courtesy of Dr. C. Lynne Burek.]

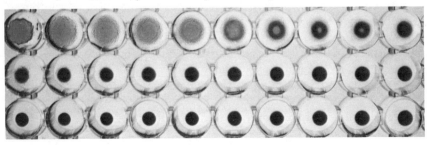

Some of the antibodies in the antiserum may bind the red cell determinants "monogamously," i.e., the bivalent antibody molecule occupies two nearby sites on the *same* red cell. As long as these sites are thus occupied, they cannot provide sites of attachment for cross-linking antibodies. However, as the concentration of these monogamously binding antibodies is lowered in later tubes, their inhibitory effect is diluted out.

Passive hemagglutination is a very sensitive, albeit only semiquantitative, assay. In some systems, antibody concentrations as low as 0.05 $\mu$g/ml can be detected. It should be noted that other types of particles can be substituted for red cells. For example, antigens can be coupled to latex or bentonite particles and used in passive agglutination assays.

Because of its sensitivity and simplicity, passive agglutination (usually hemagglutination) finds widespread use in both research and clinical laboratories. An example of the latter is the reversed passive hemagglutination assay for the surface antigen of the hepatitis B virus. The assay is "reversed" because the titration is for the antigen (HBsAg) and the red cells are coated with anti-HBsAg antibodies. This assay is of great clinical significance because the presence of the antigen (formerly called the Australia antigen) in donated blood indicates that the donor has been infected with live hepatitis B virus and use of the blood could cause posttransfusion hepatitis.

## Inhibition of Agglutination

In this modification of the agglutination test, the reaction between antigen-coated particles (e.g., red cells) and a barely agglutinating concentration of antiserum is inhibited by adding free (soluble) antigen. The free antigen competes with particle-bound antigen for the available antibodies. One popular pregnancy test uses this principle. The test reagents consist of a suspension of latex particles or sheep red cells coated with human chorionic gonadotropin (HCG) and a diluted anti-HCG antiserum just capable of agglutinating the particles. Addition of soluble HCG to the mixture inhibits the agglutination (Figure 5.16). The test is sufficiently sensitive that it can detect the HCG excreted in the urine within a few days after the implantation of the blastocyst. As usually performed, the test is purely a qualitative one. One milliliter of urine is added to the reaction mixture and scored as positive for pregnancy if no agglutination occurs or negative if agglutination does occur. For its purpose, that seems entirely appropriate. However, both this and other agglutination inhibition assays can be made semiquantitative by making serial dilutions of the solutions to be assayed. As before, the titer of the test solution is the reciprocal of the highest dilution which completely inhibits the agglutination reaction.

Agglutination inhibition tests are widely used in both clinical practice and research. In addition to pregnancy testing, this procedure is used to assay for factor VIII (as an aid in the diagnosis of hemophilia and other clotting disorders), to detect the surface antigen of hepatitis B, and to monitor the antibody response to infections by influenza, rubella, and adenovirus.

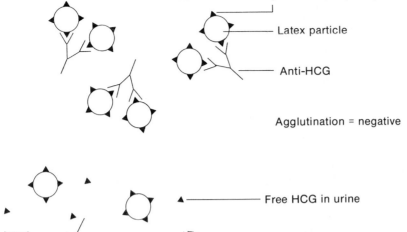

Human chorionic gonadotropin (HCG)

Latex particle

Anti-HCG

Agglutination = negative

Free HCG in urine

No agglutination = positive

**Figure 5.16** Inhibition of agglutination. The presence of HCG in the urine of a pregnant woman inhibits the agglutination of the HCG-coated particles by anti-HCG antibodies.

## 5.8 Cutaneous Anaphylaxis

Shortly after the turn of the century, it became apparent that allergies are immune responses — meeting the criteria of memory and specificity for a sensitizing antigen. But in contrast to immune responses that protect the organism from pathogens, allergies are immune responses that produce damaging effects on the organism. In Chapter 18, we shall examine the various types of allergic responses. But one type — *cutaneous anaphylaxis* — is of special relevance here. Cutaneous anaphylactic responses are allergic responses that occur in skin or on mucous membranes. Thus urticaria (hives), allergic rhinitis (hay fever), and some forms of asthma represent localized responses to environmental antigens, for example, in food or air. These allergic reactions are rapid, occurring within minutes of exposure to the antigen.

In 1921 Prausnitz and Küstner reported a phenomenon that at once provided a glimpse of the immune mechanism underlying these allergic responses, laid the basis for diagnosis of allergies, and provided the methodology for the most sensitive antibody assay available for many years after.

Küstner was exceedingly allergic to fish. But no evidence of antibodies directed against fish antigens could be detected in his serum. [Small wonder, considering that these antibodies, found many years later to be of the IgE class, are present in the serum in concentrations ranging from at most a few micrograms down to only nanograms ($10^{-9}$g) per milliliter.]

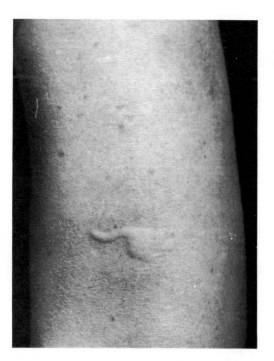

**Figure 5.17** Cutaneous anaphylaxis. In this case, the antigen (0.1 $\mu$g of protein from guinea pig hair) was injected into the skin of the allergic individual. The swelling (wheal) is clearly visible; the reddening (erythema) less so. The same type of response is seen in the P-K test. [Reprinted, with permission, from B. D. Davis et al., *Microbiology*, 3rd ed., Harper & Row, 1980.]

However, when Prausnitz injected a small amount of Küstner's serum into his own skin and the next day followed this with an injection of fish extract into the same site, a rapid reaction occurred. A sharply delineated, soft swelling (a "wheal") quickly appeared at the site of injection (Figure 5.17). The skin surrounding the wheal became reddened (the "flare" or erythema). As we shall see in Section 14.5, this reaction of cutaneous anaphylaxis results from the binding of antigen molecules to IgE molecules present on the surface of mast cells in the skin. The binding of antigen-specific IgE antibodies to their surface is said to "sensitize" the mast cells to that antigen. Interaction of antigen with these sensitized mast cells causes exocytosis of the basophilic granules in their cytoplasm. These granules contain histamine, SRS-A (a mixture of leukotrienes, lipids derived from arachidonic acid), and other vasoactive substances. Release of these materials at the site increases capillary permeability, resulting in the accumulation of fluid (edema) in the tissue spaces. The localized edema of the wheal and flare reaction is the visible outcome.

What Prausnitz did, therefore, was to transfer—with serum—the capacity to display an allergic response. This passive transfer of cutaneous anaphylaxis is, to this day, called the Prausnitz–Küstner or P–K test.

## Skin Testing

With Prausnitz's demonstration that the skin is a suitable site for examining antibody-mediated allergies, this methodology was used to diagnose allergies of unknown cause. By introducing a panel of suspected antigens, called *allergens* (e.g., extracts of grass pollen, ragweed pollen, animal hair, etc.), into the patient's skin and scoring for any wheal and flare responses (Figure 5.17), the offending antigens can be identified. By using graded doses, skin testing can even become a semiquantitative procedure. In some patients, a wheal and flare response can be elicited by as little as 0.1 ng of purified ragweed pollen.

Perhaps it would be wise to note here that the cutaneous anaphylaxis reaction is fundamentally different from the delayed hypersensitivity skin reaction that is described in Section 3.1. A positive Mantoux test takes 24 hours or so to develop after introduction of the antigen, and is passively transferred by cells, not by serum. Cutaneous anaphylaxis occurs within minutes after introduction of the antigen and, as Prausnitz showed, *is* passively transferred by serum. (The nature of the lesion differs as well: a hard, dense infiltrate of macrophages and lymphocytes in DTH; a soft region of localized edema in cutaneous anaphylaxis.)

### Passive Cutaneous Anaphylaxis (PCA)

Antibodies that bind to mast cells and basophils of the same species are known as *homocytotropic*. Thus human IgE is homocytotropic. Curiously, antibodies that are not homocytotropic may nevertheless bind to the mast cells of other species. Such antibodies are called *heterocytotropic*. For example, three of the four subclasses of human IgG (IgGl, IgG3, and IgG4 — see Section 9.6) bind to and thus sensitize the mast cells of guinea pigs. While of no biological significance, this chance phenomenon makes possible a very sensitive in vivo test for such antibodies. The test is called passive cutaneous anaphylaxis (PCA). It is simply a modification of the P–K test. As commonly performed, a sample of the serum to be assayed is injected into the shaved skin of an albino guinea pig. After a period of 24 hours or so (to give the sensitizing antigens time to bind to the mast cells and any noncytotropic antibodies — that could compete for the antigen — to diffuse away from the site), the antigen is injected intravenously along with a marker like Evans blue dye. Evans blue binds to serum albumin and thus is normally retained within the blood vessels. However, where antigen meets sensitized mast cells, the release of vasoactive substances increases capillary permeability so that the dye passes into the tissue spaces, and the reaction site becomes blue.

Positive PCA responses can detect as little as 0.1 µg of antibodies. While this in vivo test is expensive, its great sensitivity made it an important assay technique until relatively recently when such highly sensitive in vitro assays as radioimmunoassay (RIA) became widely available.

## 5.9 Radioimmunoassay (RIA)

The technique of *radioimmunoassay* (RIA) has revolutionized biomedical research as well as clinical practice in such areas as cardiology, blood banking, the diagnosis of allergies, and — preeminently — endocrinology. The technique was introduced in 1960 by Berson and Yalow as an assay for the concentration of insulin in plasma. It represented the first time that hormone levels *in the blood* could be detected by an in vitro assay. Today, radioimmunoassays are available for virtually all the hormones.

The principle of the assay is quite straightforward. A mixture of radiolabeled antigen and the appropriate antibodies is prepared in the region of slight antigen excess. Known amounts of unlabeled ("cold") antigen are added to portions of the mixture. The unlabeled antigen molecules compete for the binding sites on the antibody molecules. At increasing concentrations of unlabeled antigen, an increasing amount of labeled antigen is displaced from the antibody molecules (Figure 5.18). The antibody-bound antigen is separated from the free antigen and the radioactivity of each fraction is determined. From these data, a standard binding curve can be constructed (Figure 5.19). The concentration of antigen in samples to be assayed (the unknowns) is determined by running parallel incubations with the knowns. After determining the ratio of bound

**Figure 5.18** Mechanism of radioimmunoassay (RIA). An alternative procedure for separating bound antigen from free antigen is to couple the first antibody to the walls of the reaction vessel (see Figure 5.20) or to solid particles which can be separated from the mixture by centrifugation or filtration. This modification avoids the need for a second antibody.

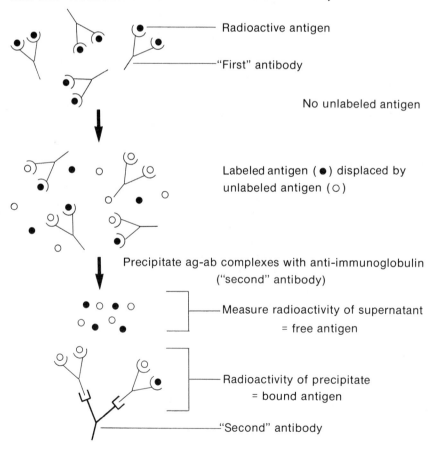

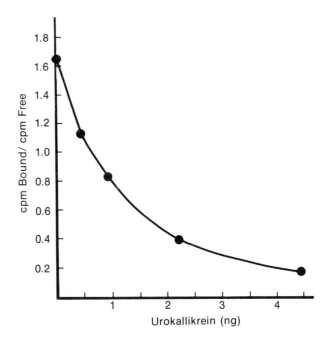

**Figure 5.19** Calibration curve for the radioimmunoassay of urokallikrein (a serine protease found in urine that generates kinins from kininogen). The ratio of bound/free counts was determined in reaction vessels containing unlabeled urokallikrein (abscissa). [From M. R. Silver et al., *J. Immunol.* **125**:1551, 1980.]

to free antigen in each unknown, the antigen concentration can be read directly from the standard curve.

A variety of techniques are used to separate bound from free antigen. One popular technique is to precipitate the bound antigen by adding a second antibody directed against the first. If, for example, a rabbit IgG antibody is used to bind the antigen, then the complex can be precipitated by adding a goat antirabbit-IgG antiserum. It should be noted that the concentrations of antigen and antibodies in the original mixture (in the ng/ml range) are far too low for precipitation to occur even though higher concentrations (mg/ml) would precipitate nicely.

Another convenient separation technique is to couple the antibodies to a solid: e.g., to the inner walls of the reaction vessel or to particles like Sephadex. In the first case, the contents of the tube are removed and counted (giving unbound counts). The tubes are washed and counted to give bound counts. When the antibodies are coupled to particles, centrifugation of the reaction mixture separates the bound counts (in the pellet) from the free counts (in the supernatant). In all of these procedures, it is not really essential to determine *both* free and bound counts so long as you know the total counts placed in the initial incubation mixture (total cpm − bound cpm = free cpm).

Radioimmunoassay has achieved a well-justified popularity. The major reason for this is its great sensitivity. Using antibodies of high affinity ($K_0 = 10^8 - 10^{11}$ M$^{-1}$), it is possible to detect a few picograms ($10^{-12}$g) of antigen in the reaction vessel. The greater the specificity of the antiserum, the greater the specificity of the assay. Figure 4.15 shows the greater than 1000-fold decrease in binding when the —OH group is shifted from the beta to the alpha configuration at the number 17 carbon atom of estradiol. RIA is also popular because multiple samples can be handled with ease, and there is usually no need to purify the unknowns. The main drawbacks to RIA are the expense and hazards associated with preparing and handling the radioactive antigen. Because of the ease with which iodine atoms can be introduced into tyrosine residues, most protein and many peptide antigens are radiolabeled with $^{125}I$ or $^{131}I$. Both of these isotopes emit gamma radiation that requires special counting equipment. These isotopes also pose a special health hazard because the body concentrates them in the thyroid gland where they are incorporated in thyroxin ($T_4$) and triiodothyronine ($T_3$).

Despite these drawbacks, RIA is not only used in research settings but is becoming a major tool in the clinical laboratory. Reagents are now commercially available for assaying virtually all of the human hormones, for monitoring the levels of digitoxin or digoxin in patients receiving this therapy, and for detecting certain abused drugs in body fluids. A radioimmunoassay for the hepatitis B surface antigen (HBsAg) is widely used to screen donated blood. RIA is also used to detect tumor-associated antigens and anti-DNA antibodies (in systemic lupus erythematosus).

## 5.10   Enzyme Immunoassay (EIA)

The recent development of enzyme immunoassay provides a technique with the advantages of RIA (extreme sensitivity, simplicity, and ease of handling multiple samples) with none of the disadvantages associated with handling hazardous isotopes.

The assay depends upon being able to couple highly specific antibodies to (1) an enzyme and (2) a solid such as plastic beads or the inner walls of the tubes in which the assay is run. The antibody – enzyme complex must retain the immunological specificity of the antibody and the catalytic activity of the enzyme. The enzyme used is generally one that produces a colored product upon conversion of its substrate. Alkaline phosphatase, horseradish peroxidase and beta-galactosidase are frequently used for this purpose.

One commonly used procedure for the assay takes place in three steps (Figure 5.20).

*Step 1.*   An antibody-coated solid is incubated with the antigen solution to be assayed. Antigen molecules present in the test solution bind to the immobilized antibody molecules.

*Step 2.*   An antibody – enzyme conjugate is added to the reaction mixture. The antibody portion of the complex binds to any antigen molecules that were bound previously, creating an antibody – antigen – antibody "sandwich" (Figure 5.20).

*Step 3.*   After washing away any unbound conjugate, the substrate solution is added. After a set interval, the reaction is stopped (e.g., by adding 1 N NaOH), and the concentration of colored product formed is

**Figure 5.20** An example of enzyme immunoassay (EIA) procedure. When antibodies specific for the antigen to be assayed are unavailable in the purity and/or quantity needed for coupling to the enzyme, unconjugated antibodies can be used and their binding can be revealed by the addition of enzyme-coupled anti-immunoglobulin antibodies (similar in principle to the *indirect method* of immunofluorescence shown in Figure 5.26). When this is done, however, the antigen-specific antibodies that are coupled to the solid phase cannot be from the same species as the antigen-specific antibodies added during the assay.

Conversion of the substrate is stopped at a fixed time, e.g., by adding NaOH to the reaction mixtures.

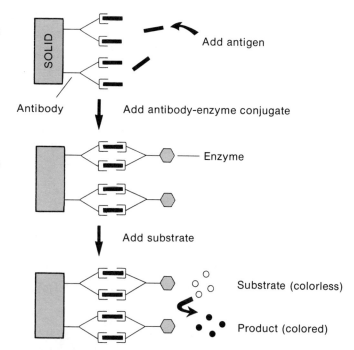

determined in a spectrophotometer. The concentration is proportional to the concentration of bound antigen.

This assay method is also referred to as an *enzyme linked immunosorbent assay* or ELISA. Like RIA techniques, it can routinely detect antigens at concentrations below 1 ng/ml. In fact, using a radioactive rather than a colorproducing enzyme substrate, Harris and his colleagues have been able to detect as little as 0.1 femtogram ($0.1 \times 10^{-15}$g: about 600 molecules!) of cholera toxin.

As described above, EIA is an assay for antigen. It can also be used as a qualitative or quantitative assay for antibodies. In this modification, the appropriate *antigen* is adsorbed to a solid surface and incubated with the test solution. After any antibodies in the test solution have bound to the immobilized antigen, their presence is detected by adding an enzyme-labeled anti-immunoglobulin. After washing away unreacted reagent, the substrate is added. As before, the amount of substrate that is converted is proportional to the amount of enzyme-labeled antibodies bound. This version of the EIA method promises to provide a rapid method of diagnosing a wide variety of viral and fungal infections.

## 5.11 Complement Fixation

Complement is the term applied to an integrated system of 17 distinct serum proteins. When certain classes of antibody molecules, for example, IgM, bind to antigen, they become capable of triggering an elaborate sequence of reactions involving the complement proteins. These reac-

**107**

tions lead to the production of a number of biologically active molecules. The details of the process are presented in Section 14.2. For our purpose here, we need to simply note that (1) if the antibodies are directed toward antigens present on cell membranes (e.g., red cell membranes), the activation of complement leads to the lysis of the cell; and (2) the greater the concentration of antigen–antibody complexes, the greater the consumption of complement proteins, that is, the more complement that is "fixed."

The complement fixation assay requires five components (Figure 5.21).

1. A known concentration of complement. Guinea pig serum is often used as a source of complement.
2. The antigen (or antibody) to be assayed.
3. The appropriate antibody (or antigen) to react with No. 2.
4. Red blood cells, usually sheep red blood cells (SRBC).
5. Anti-SRBC antibodies (commonly called hemolysins).

One typical way of performing the assay is as follows.

*Step. 1.* The sheep red blood cells are treated with anti-SRBC antibodies in the absence of complement. The conditions and concentrations must be such that the antibodies do not agglutinate the red cells. The antibodies do, however, coat the cells by binding to determinants on the

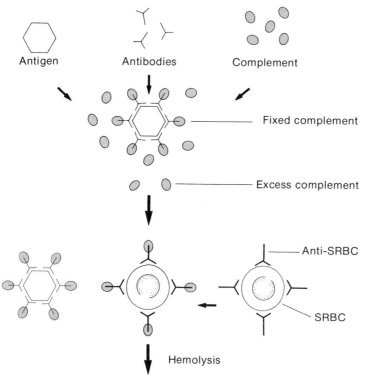

Antigen

Antibodies

Complement

Fixed complement

Excess complement

Anti-SRBC

SRBC

Hemolysis

Free hemoglobin

**Figure 5.21** The complement fixation assay. See text for details.

| Reaction Mixture | 1 | 2 | 3 | 4 | 5 | 6 | 7[1] | 8[2] | 9[3] | 10 |
|---|---|---|---|---|---|---|---|---|---|---|
| Antibody soln, ml | 1.0 | 1.0 | 1.0 | 1.0 | 1.0 | 1.0 | 1.0 | — | — | — |
| Diluent, ml | 3.0 | 3.0 | 3.0 | 3.0 | 3.0 | 3.0 | 4.0 | 4.0 | 5.0 | 6.0 |
| Complement soln, ml | 1.0 | 1.0 | 1.0 | 1.0 | 1.0 | 1.0 | 1.0 | 1.0 | 1.0 | |
| Antigen soln, ml | 1.0 | 1.0 | 1.0 | 1.0 | 1.0 | 1.0 | — | 1.0 | — | — |
| Antigen, $\mu$g/ml after 16–18 hours at 2–4°C | 0.5 | 0.25 | 0.12 | 0.06 | 0.03 | 0.015 | — | 0.5 | — | — |
| EA[4] suspension, ml after 1 hour at 37°C, | 1.0 | 1.0 | 1.0 | 1.0 | 1.0 | 1.0 | 1.0 | 1.0 | 1.0 | 1.0 |
| Hemolysis ($OD_{413\,nm}$)[5] | 0.489 | 0.253 | 0.114 | 0.199 | 0.341 | 0.459 | 0.489 | 0.502 | 0.511 | 0.002 |
| Complement fixation[6] | 0.012 | 0.248 | 0.387 | 0.302 | 0.160 | 0.042 | | | | |
| % complement fixation[7] | 2 | 49 | 77 | 60 | 32 | 8 | | | | |

[1] Antibody control; antibody soln = rabbit antipig hemoglobin, 1:200.
[2] Antigen control; antigen = pig hemoglobin.
[3] Complement control; complement soln = guinea pig serum, 1:260.
[4] EA = sheep red blood cells sensitized with rabbit anti-SRBC serum.
[5] OD = optical density.
[6] Average of control OD's (tubes 7, 8, 9) minus reaction OD.
[7] (4) ÷ control OD × 100.

**Figure 5.22** Protocol and results of a complement fixation assay of known amounts of pig hemoglobin. [From L. Levine, "Microcomplement fixation" in *Handbook of Experimental Immunology*, 3rd ed., Vol. 1, D. M. Weir (ed.), Blackwell, 1978.]

red cell membrane. The antibody-coated red cells are now said to be sensitized and are often designated "**EA**" (erythrocyte antibody).

*Step 2.* A series of test tubes is set up, each tube containing (a) sufficient complement to lyse 90% of a sample of the red cell suspension prepared in step 1; (b) sufficient antiserum to consume ("fix") about 75% of the complement in the tube; (c) a graded series of dilutions of the antigen to be assayed (Figure 5.22).

Because some complement components deteriorate rapidly at room temperature, the test is usually carried out in the cold (2–4°C). After 18 hours or so, equal volumes of the sensitized SRBC suspension are added to each tube. Any unfixed complement that remains in a tube will now bind to the red cell membrane lysing the cell, a process called *hemolysis*. After 30–60 minutes at 37°C, the concentration of hemoglobin released by the lysed red cells is measured with a spectrophotometer (Figure 5.22).

Several control tubes are necessary: antibody alone, antigen alone, complement alone, and diluent alone (Figure 5.22). The antigen and antibody controls are needed to be sure that neither material by itself inhibits (or enhances) complement activity. Thus the amount of lysis in the first three control tubes should be approximately the same and represents the maximum available in the test system. (The control tube containing diluent alone should produce little or no hemolysis.)

The amount of lysis in each tube of the test solutions will be *inversely* proportional to the amount of complement fixed initially. That is, the spectrophotometer measures complement activity that *remains* after the interaction of test antigen with its antibody.

The results can be plotted as complement fixed (optical density, OD, of the control tubes minus the OD of the test solutions) and/or as percent complement fixed. In either case, the resulting curve resembles a quantitative precipitation curve (Figure 5.23).

Complement fixation has been in widespread use since early in the century. There are several reasons for its popularity. One is its sensitiv-

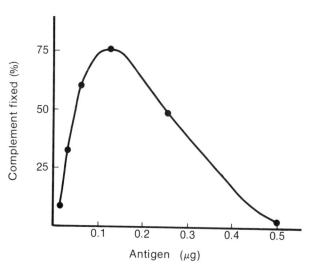

**Figure 5.23** Graph of the percent of complement fixed with increasing amounts of antigen in the assay shown in Figure 5.22. Note the resemblance to a typical quantitative precipitation curve.

ity: it can detect antigen concentrations as low as 0.5 μg/ml. Another is that it can be used successfully with crude preparations of antigens and even with insoluble antigens. The Wassermann test for syphilis is a complement fixation assay. Complement fixation assays are also used in the diagnosis of a number of diseases caused by viruses, protozoan, and metazoan parasites. In most cases, the "antigen" consists of a crude extract of the organisms. Even such particulate matter as platelets—to detect antibodies against histocompatibility antigens—and the microsomal fraction of thyroid cells—to detect antithyroid antibodies—can be used.

## 5.12  The Hemolytic Plaque Assay

For many years, the study of humoral immunity was largely limited to examining the antibodies circulating in the blood or found in other body fluids. In fact, every assay discussed to this point does just that. The population of blood-borne antibody molecules represents a pool of the contribution of the various antibody-secreting sources within the body. Analysis of the antibody activity in serum is also complicated by the fact that different subpopulations of antibody molecules may be catabolized at different rates in the circulation.

In the early 1960s, Jerne and his coworkers in the United States and Ingraham and Bussard in France introduced a technique for examining the antibody production of individual cells. This technique is called the hemolytic plaque assay (or, alternatively, localized hemolysis in gel). This technique has had an immeasurable impact on various lines of immunological inquiry. To cite one example, it made possible the discovery that an antibody-secreting cell normally produces only one kind of antibody molecule (at one time).

Let us examine the procedure as it might be used to determine the response in mice to an injection of sheep red blood cells (SRBC). A group of mice of the same age, sex, and inbred strain are immunized with a standardized dose of SRBC. It is important to use inbred mice because of the greater variability in the response of outbred animals.

Four days after the immunization, the mice are killed and their spleens removed. The spleens are minced and strained to prepare a homogeneous suspension of individual cells. All these operations are performed in cold tissue culture medium in order to inhibit premature release of antibodies from the cells. Appropriate numbers of spleen cells are then mixed with a fixed number of SRBC and suspended in warm agar or agarose. The mixture is poured into a petri dish and the agar allowed to harden. The density of SRBC is sufficient that the agar layer is a uniform red color. The plates are then incubated at body temperature (37°C). The spleen cell suspension contains lymphocytes, macrophages, and plasma cells. Many of the plasma cells will be synthesizing anti-SRBC antibodies, and at 37°C they release these antibodies. As the antibodies diffuse away from the plasma cell, they bind to determinants on the surface of the SRBC in the immediate vicinity. After two hours or so, a preparation of complement (usually dilute guinea pig serum) is poured over the plates. The interaction of complement with the antibodies bound to the red cell antigens results in the lysis of the red cells and causes the area around the antibody-secreting cell to become clear. The clear circular zone in the otherwise red lawn of SRBC is called a plaque (Figure 5.24). Examination under the light microscope reveals a single (usually) white cell at the center of each plaque (Figure 5.25). This is the antibody-secreting cell.

The assay is very sensitive. As few as one in a million spleen cells secreting anti-SRBC antibodies can be detected. And one antibody-secreting cell may form a visible plaque after releasing as few as 1000 antibody molecules.

Four days after immunization with SRBC, most antibody production is confined to the IgM class. This type of antibody is extremely efficient at

**Figure 5.24** Photograph of an agar plate showing the plaques formed by mouse spleen cells secreting antibodies against sheep red blood cells. The plate was stained with benzidine to show the plaques more clearly. [Courtesy of Albert A. Nordin from N. K. Jerne, A. A. Nordin, and Claudia Henry, "The Agar Plaque Technique for Recognizing Antibody-Producing Cells," in *Cell-Bound Antibodies*, B. Amos and H. Koprowski (eds.), The Wistar Institute Press, Philadelphia, 1963.]

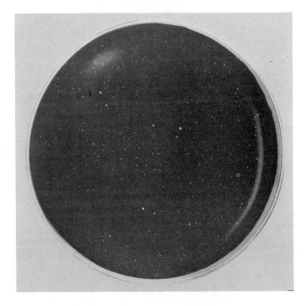

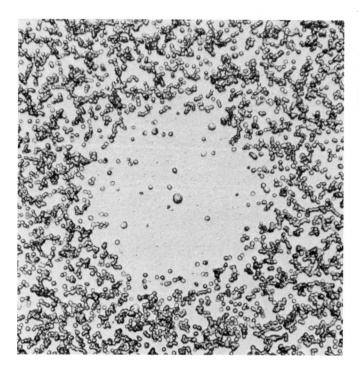

**Figure 5.25** Photomicrograph of a single plaque. Note the clear zone surrounded by unlysed sheep red cells. A single antibody-secreting spleen cell is present in the center of the plaque. [Courtesy of Albert A. Nordin.]

binding complement and thus triggering cell lysis. Probably a single IgM molecule bound to the surface of a red cell is sufficient to bring about its lysis.

Cells secreting antibodies of other classes such as IgG often do not form plaques when the assay is performed as described above. However, these antibody-secreting cells can be detected if the plate is incubated with antimouse immunoglobulin serum (e.g., rabbit antimouse IgG) before the complement is added. The anti-IgG binds to the IgG molecules and this complex does activate complement and bring about cell lysis. Plaques revealed in this way are called "indirect" plaques.

The hemolytic plaque assay is easily modified for use with antigens other than membrane antigens. All that is required is that the antigen be coupled stably to the surface of the indicator red cells. Polysaccharides, proteins, and many haptens can be coupled to the surface of SRBC and antibody activity against these antigens determined. In these cases, the spleen cell donor is immunized only with the antigen or hapten under study, not with sheep red cells.

## 5.13 Cytotoxicity

As we saw in the previous section, antibodies capable of fixing complement can damage a cell membrane bearing determinants to which they can bind. In the case of a red cell (essentially a container of hemoglobin), the result is hemolysis. In the case of white cells, the loss of membrane integrity brings about the death of the cell. This can be determined by several techniques. One of the most commonly used approaches is to see if the cell membrane continues to exclude dyes such as trypan blue or eosin Y. Living cells exclude the dye. Dead cells do not, and the cell contents quickly become stained.

Cytotoxicity can be used to establish the titer of antisera directed against membrane antigens, or it can be used to identify (and destroy) cells bearing particular membrane antigens. Serial dilutions of antiserum are incubated with cell suspensions, often purified suspensions of lymphocytes. Complement and trypan blue are added. Cytotoxicity is assessed by determining the frequency of stained cells in each tube.

Cytotoxicity testing is widely used to identify the major histocompatibility antigens (HLA) on human lymphocytes. This work is of great practical as well as theoretical importance. HLA testing allows the selection of HLA-compatible organ (e.g., kidney) donors (see Section 19.5). HLA testing has also provided valuable data in such fields as human population genetics, anthropology, and led to the discovery of associations between the possession of certain HLA specificities and a predisposition to certain diseases. HLA analysis, primarily by cytotoxicity testing, has shown that the organization of the genes coding for HLA specificities and their pattern of inheritance closely parallels the situation that occurs at the major histocompatibility complex (H-2) in mice (see Section 3.6).

## 5.14  Immunofluorescence

*Immunofluorescence* uses fluorescent antibody molecules to detect antigens or antibodies, usually in association with cells. It is thus a qualitative histological technique, but one of great sensitivity.

The many modifications and applications of this technique stem largely from the work of Albert Coons, who first introduced the method in 1941. There are three major versions of the technique: (1) the direct method, (2) the indirect method, and (3) the "sandwich" method. Each uses a preparation of antibodies, as pure and as specific as possible, covalently coupled to a fluorescent dye. The most widely used of these are fluorescein isothiocyanate (FITC) and rhodamine isothiocyanate (RITC). Each absorbs light of one wavelength and emits it at another. FITC emits a yellow-green light; RITC, orange red. The fluorescence microscope is simply a light microscope equipped with filters that permit the exciting wavelengths to strike the specimen but allow only the emitted wavelengths to reach the eyepiece.

### The Direct Method

In the direct method, the histological specimen is flooded with the fluorescent antibody to permit binding between the antibody molecules and

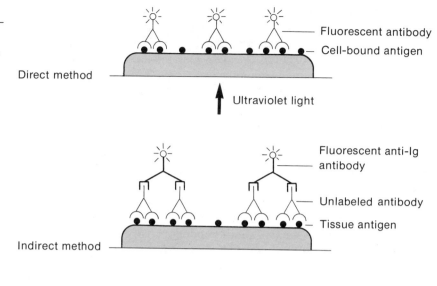

Direct method

Ultraviolet light

Indirect method

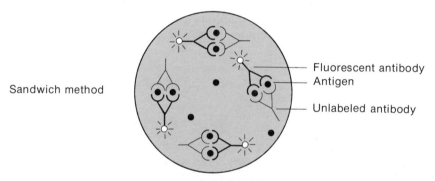

Sandwich method

**Figure 5.26** Three techniques of immunofluorescence. An example of the indirect method is shown in Figure 5.27, of the sandwich method in Figure 5.28.

any cell-bound antigen (Figure 5.26). After washing off any unbound antibodies, the preparation is examined under the fluorescence microscope.

The direct method can be used to identify microbes in tissue preparations. For example, FITC-conjugated antibodies to *T. pallidum* are used to identify the organism in suspected syphilitic lesions.

## The Indirect Method

The indirect method is the most popular technique of immunofluorescence. It is a qualitative serological assay; that is, it is an assay for antibodies. The test consists of treating a tissue known to contain cell-bound antigen with the serum to be assayed. If the appropriate antibodies are present, they will bind to the tissue. Their presence is then revealed by treating the preparation with a fluorescent anti-immunoglobulin (Figure 5.26).

A common clinical use of this procedure is the assay for antinuclear antibodies. These are antibodies directed against a variety of antigens associated with cell nuclei. Such antibodies may be found in several disease conditions and occasionally in healthy people. However, they are always found in victims of systemic lupus erythematosus (SLE). Thus a positive test for antinuclear antibodies *suggests* the possibility of SLE but a negative test almost surely rules it out. Two reagents are needed for the test: (1) fixed tissue slices (those from mouse liver work well) and (2) a preparation of antihuman immunoglobulin antibodies conjugated with FITC. The antiserum is usually raised in a rabbit or a goat.

A drop of the patient's serum is placed on the tissue. The fixation process permits any antibodies present to enter the cells. After washing, the fluorescent antiglobulin antibodies are placed on the tissue. After a second wash, the slide is examined under the fluorescence microscope. Fluorescence around or within the nuclei shows the presence of antinuclear antibodies in the patient's serum (Figure 5.27 and photomicrograph on the cover).

**Figure 5.27**  Antinuclear antibodies revealed by immunofluorescence (the indirect method—see text for details). This pattern of staining is often produced by the serum of patients with rheumatoid arthritis or systemic lupus erythematosus. [Courtesy of Dr. Eng M. Tan.]

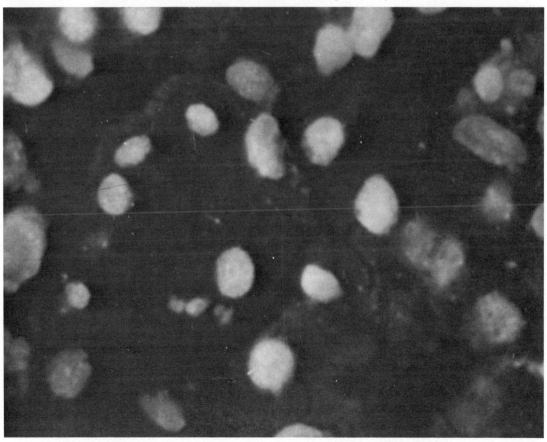

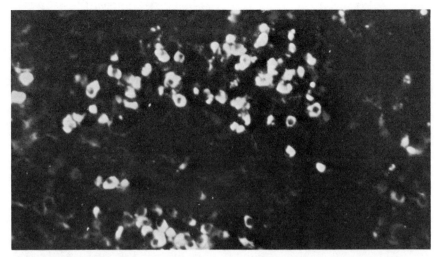

**Figure 5.28** Antibody-containing plasma cells from the spleen of a rabbit immunized with type 3 pneumococci. These cells were first treated with a solution of the purified polysaccharide and then with anti-type 3 antibodies coupled to fluorescein isothiocyanate (an example of the sandwich method — see Figure 5.26). Viewed under ultraviolet light, the cytoplasm of those plasma cells manufacturing anti-type 3 antibodies glows brightly. [Fluorescence micrograph by Dr. Albert H. Coons.]

## The Sandwich Method

The sandwich method uses *antigen* to cross-link cell bound antibody molecules with fluorescent antibody molecules of the same specificity. The technique is useful for locating the tissues and cells that are active in a particular antibody response. The use of the sandwich technique enabled Coons to show that antibody-secreting cells are plasma cells. Figure 5.28 is a fluorescence photomicrograph of spleen cells taken from a rabbit immunized against the type 3 pneumococcal polysaccharide. The cells were treated with the polysaccharide and then with FITC-conjugated anti-type 3 antibodies. The cells containing anti-type 3 antibodies stand out clearly. Note that the fluorescence is confined to the cytoplasm of these cells, in contrast to those in Figure 5.27.

## ADDITIONAL READING

1.  Garvey, J. S., N. E. Cremer, and D. H. Sussdorf, *Methods in Immunology*, 3rd ed., W. A. Benjamin, Inc., Reading, MA, 1977. Includes a wealth of information on such basic procedures as the preparation of antigens, immunization, the purification of antisera, and most of the assays described in this chapter.

2.  Harris, C. C., et al., "Ultrasensitive Enzymatic Radioimmunoassay: Application to Detection of Cholera Toxin and Rotavirus," *Proc. Natl. Acad. Sci. USA*

76:5336, 1979. Describes a procedure using features of ELISA and RIA to achieve a sensitivity 1000-fold greater than possible with either alone.

3. Hudson, L., and F. C. Hay, *Practical Immunology*, 2nd ed., Blackwell, Oxford, 1981. A laboratory guide.

4. Mishell, Barbara B., and S. M. Shiigi (eds.), *Selected Methods in Cellular Immunology*, W. H. Freeman and Company, San Francisco, 1980. Detailed instructions for performing hemolytic plaque assays, cell viability tests, radioimmunoassay, and much more.

5. Rose, N. R., and H. Friedman (eds.), *Manual of Clinical Immunology*, 2nd ed., American Society for Microbiology, Washington, DC, 1980.

6 Weir, D. M. (ed.), *Handbook of Immunology*, 3rd ed., Blackwell, Oxford, 1978. Volume 1 is devoted to a variety of immunochemical methods, including complement fixation, radioimmunoassay, passive hemagglutination, PCA, the Ouchterlony technique, immunofluorescence, and others.

# Assays of Cell-Mediated Immunity

Until quite recently, our knowledge of cell-mediated immune (CMI) responses lagged far behind our understanding of humoral immunity. This was true even though it had been known since the turn of the century that some immune reactions are not mediated by serum-borne factors (antibodies). A major reason for the slow progress was the lack of good assay techniques for cell-mediated immune reactions. In fact, no suitable in vitro assay of CMI existed until the 1960s. Prior to then, only in vivo assays were available. These were skin testing (for DTH) and allograft rejection.

## 6.1 Delayed-Type Hypersensitivity (DTH)

Edward Jenner was the first person to describe the delayed type response to antigen introduced into the skin of an immune recipient. He observed this reaction after revaccinating his patients.

The nature of the DTH reaction was examined in Chapter 3 (Section 3.1). The example described there is the tuberculin reaction. You will recall that its essential features are

1. Introduction of the antigen into the skin of a previously sensitized recipient.
2. The accumulation of lymphocytes and macrophages at the site 24 – 48 hours later.
3. Lymphocytes, but not serum, from sensitized donors can adoptively transfer DTH sensitivity when injected into normal recipients. This was the major justification for classifying the reaction as cell mediated rather than humoral.

The Mantoux test for tuberculin sensitivity (and various modifications of it) are still in wide clinical use. Skin testing for DTH sensitivity is occasionally used to aid in the diagnosis of certain fungal, protozoan and viral infections. Skin testing is also used to aid in the diagnosis of immunodeficiency disorders. The patient is given an intradermal injection of an antigen to which he has previously been naturally or deliberately exposed. Failure to respond to this challenge with a typical DTH lesion suggests a general defect in CMI.

Although in vitro tests for cell-mediated immunity are now available, skin testing is still used in research. Guinea pigs are the most satisfactory animals for this purpose. However, DTH reactions can be studied in mice by injecting the antigen into a footpad and measuring the amount of swelling produced. Many important observations that have clarified the cellular events and the genetic requirements of cell-mediated immunity have been made using DTH responses as the primary assay method. (See, for example, Section 3.7.)

## 6.2 Lymphokine Production

In Section 3.2, we examined an in vitro correlate of cell-mediated immunity. This was the macrophage inhibition assay, the first in vitro assay for cell-mediated immunity. You will recall that when lymphocytes taken from an animal exhibiting DTH to an antigen (such as ovalbumin) are cultured with the antigen, they liberate a factor, MIF, which inhibits the migration of macrophages. The macrophages are inhibited even if they are derived from an unsensitized donor. If as few as 1% of the cells in the capillary tube (Figure 3.4) are lymphocytes from a sensitized animal, migration of the remaining cells is inhibited.

Migration inhibition factor was the first of a large number (about 50) of "factors" found to be released when sensitized T lymphocytes are exposed in vitro to the sensitizing antigen. Often the name given each factor reflects the assay used to detect its activity. Thus antigen-stimulated T lymphocytes release something that *attracts* macrophages ("macrophage chemotactic factor"), something that increases the metabolic activity of macrophages ("macrophage activating factor"), and so on. Collectively, these factors are known as *lymphokines*.

## Interleukin 2 (IL-2)

One of the best characterized lymphokines is one that stimulates the T cells themselves to undergo mitosis. This activity gave rise to the name "T cell growth factor" (TCGF). However, TCGF turned out to be the same substance as the "factor" active in a number of other assays. Therefore, the various earlier designations for this molecule are being abandoned in favor of the term interleukin 2 (IL-2).

In contrast to some lymphokine assays, the measurement of IL-2 production is quite simple. It employs a population of target cells that are incapable of dividing in the absence of IL-2. Several of these IL-2 dependent cell lines have been developed. Samples of the supernatant fluid harvested from the test cultures; i.e., cultures containing antigen-stimulated T lymphocytes, are added to wells containing the IL-2 dependent target cells. If IL-2 is present in the supernatant, the target cells will begin mitosis. The strength of the response can be quantitated by adding tritiated thymidine to the assay cultures and measuring its uptake by the cells.

## 6.3  Allograft Rejection

In Sections 3.3 and 3.4, we saw that the rejection of a graft of foreign skin meets all the criteria of a cell-mediated immune reaction. While a somewhat cumbersome procedure, skin grafting has been one of the most fruitful assays for determining the genetics of histocompatibility.

The donor animal (e.g., a mouse) is killed, shaved, and skinned. After scraping away any adhering underlying tissue, the skin is cut into uniformly sized pieces. The recipient animal is anesthetized and shaved. The graft bed is prepared by removing a piece of skin from the back. A piece of donor skin is then pressed onto the site, treated with antibiotic solution, and held in place with a bandage. In nine days or so, the bandage can be removed and the progress of the graft monitored. The scoring is quite direct: rapid rejection (about 14 days), slow rejection (many weeks), or no rejection.

Let us examine one specific example of the procedure in the hope that it will not only make the methodology clear but also provide further insight into the genetic analysis that grafting between inbred, congenic strains makes possible.

In 1980, Hansen and his colleagues reported the results of a skin-grafting study designed to map the location of two mutations that had been discovered within the H-2 region. In each case, the mutation was detected because the animals rejected skin grafts from their own inbred strain — C57BL/6. The substrains carrying the mutations are designated B6.C-H-$2^{bm1}$ and B6.C-H-$2^{bm12}$, respectively. The haplotype of the C57BL/6 strain is H-$2^b$. Each locus (K, A$_\beta$, A$_\alpha$, etc.) in its H-2 complex carries the "*b*" allele and thus the haplotype is designated *bbbbbb* (Figure 6.1).

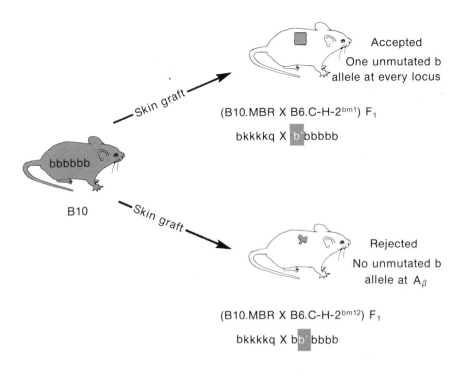

Accepted

One unmutated b allele at every locus

(B10.MBR X B6.C-H-2$^{bm1}$) F$_1$

bkkkkq X b'bbbbb

Rejected

No unmutated b allele at A$_\beta$

(B10.MBR X B6.C-H-2$^{bm12}$) F$_1$

bkkkkq X bb'bbbb

| | H-2 haplotypes | | | | | |
|---|---|---|---|---|---|---|
| | K | A$_\beta$ | A$_\alpha$ | E$_\beta$ | E$_\alpha$ | D |
| B10 | b | b | b | b | b | b |
| B10.MBR | b | k | k | k | k | q |

**Figure 6.1** Procedure for mapping H-2 mutations in two strains of mice derived from the C57BL/6 strain *(bbbbbb)*. The mutant animals were first identified by their failure to accept skin grafts from the ancestral C57BL/6 strain. This method depends upon gene complementation; i.e., the ability of a *b* allele at a locus on one chromosome in the hybrids to supply the missing function of the allele at that locus on the homologous chromosome. Thus, acceptance of the graft showed that the mutation H-2$^{bm1}$ was located at the *K* locus. Rejection of the graft showed that the mutation H-2$^{bm12}$ was located somewhere to the right of *K*. Other studies pinpointed the location of this mutation to the A$_\beta$ gene. [Based on the work of T. H. Hansen et al., *Nature* **285**:340, 1980.]

The "reagent" for pinpointing the location of these two mutations was the congenic strain B10.MBR. This strain has been derived from one of the rare recombinations that occasionally occur as a result of crossing over within the H-2 complex. It carries the "*b*" allele at the K locus but the "*k*" allele at all the identified loci within the I region (A$_\beta$, A$_\alpha$, etc.). The D allele is "*q*" (Figure 6.1).

The experiment consisted of producing F$_1$ hybrids between each of the mutant strains and the B10.MBR strain. These hybrids were then challenged with skin grafts from a C57BL/10 donor with the "pure" *b* haplotype (H-2$^b$) to see if they would be rejected or not.

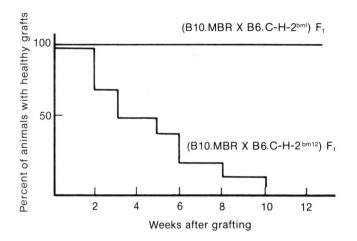

Figure 6.2 Contrasting fates of the skin grafts performed according to the protocol in Figure 6.1. [Adapted from Fig. 1 in T. H. Hansen et al., *Nature* 285:340, 1980.]

If either mutation is located at the K locus, then the graft should survive. This is because in the $F_1$ hybrid there would be at least one "*b*" allele at every locus (Figure 6.1) and thus the H-2$^b$ antigens of the donor skin would be seen as "self." If, on the other hand, the mutation is located anywhere to the right of the K locus, the graft should be rejected. In this case, the mutant locus would be paired with a "*k*" (or, in the case of D, a "*q*") allele (Figure 6.1). Thus the antigen encoded by the "*b*" allele on the donor skin would be seen as foreign and the skin rejected.

The results of this experiment are shown in Figure 6.2. The mice carrying the mutation H-2$^{bm1}$ tolerated the grafted skin indefinitely. On the other hand, all the mice carrying the H-2$^{bm12}$ mutation had rejected the skin transplants by the end of ten weeks following the operation. Thus, these two "*b*" mutations map to different parts of the H-2 complex. H-2$^{bm1}$ is a mutation in the K region while H-2$^{bm12}$ is not. In fact, similar skin grafting studies have shown that the H-2$^{bm12}$ mutation is located in the A$_\beta$ chain.

## 6.4 Graft vs. Host Reaction (GVHR)

As we have seen, an $F_1$ hybrid does not reject skin grafts from either inbred parent (Figure 3.7). Nor does the hybrid reject parental lymphocytes. In each case, the parental tissue bears only "self" antigens. In the second case, however, the injected parental lymphocytes respond to the foreign set of histocompatibility antigens present on the *host* cells (Figure 6.3) and mount an immunological attack against their host. One of the earliest signs of this graft versus host reaction (GVHR) is an enlargement of the host spleen, and this provides a convenient quantitative assay for GVHR.

The donor lymphocytes to be tested are injected into the peritoneal cavity of the $F_1$ hosts. Usually two different doses of test cells are used. Control animals matched for age and sex are injected with fully compatible (that is, $F_1$) lymphocytes. After 8–10 days, each animal is killed,

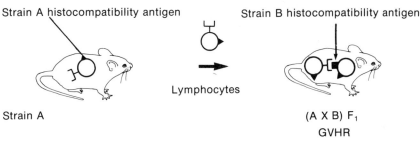

Strain A histocompatibility antigen      Strain B histocompatibility antigen

Lymphocytes

Strain A            (A X B) F$_1$
                     GVHR

**Figure 6.3**   One procedure for generating a graft vs. host reaction. Immunocompetent strain A lymphocytes recognize strain B histocompatibility
antigens on the cells of the hybrid and mount an immune response against
them. The hybrid recipients are generally used for the assay within a few days
of their birth.

weighed, and the weight of its spleen determined. From these data, a
spleen index for each test is calculated.

$$\text{Spleen index} = \frac{\text{Spleen weight/Body weight of test animal}}{\text{Avg. spleen weight/Body weight of controls}}$$

A spleen index of 1.0 thus indicates no response. A spleen index of 1.3 or
more is considered a significant GVHR.

The GVHR has been a valuable tool for analyzing the genetics of
histocompatibility. When using normal (i.e., unsensitized) parental cells,
only differences in the H-2 complex create a GVHR. Furthermore, by
using recombinant strains, it can be shown that the I-region differences
play a more important role in GVHRs than differences at K and D only.
Differences at minor histocompatibility loci can produce GVHR only if
the donor cells have been *pre*sensitized to the antigens.

The GVHR is also of great importance in clinical practice. Bone marrow transplants have been used successfully in some cases of leukemia,
aplastic anemia, and certain immunodeficiency diseases. However, it is
essential that the marrow donor be compatible with the recipient, at least
at the MHC, if a fatal GVHR is to be avoided. Minor incompatibilities will
produce a GVHR, but with immunosuppressive therapy this can usually
be controlled.

## 6.5   The Mixed Lymphocyte Reaction (MLR)

If lymphocytes from two histoincompatible donors are cultured together, each set reacts against the foreign histocompatibility antigens of
the other set. The responding cells become lymphoblasts and begin DNA
synthesis and mitosis. The response usually reaches a peak after four or
five days in culture. If tritiated thymidine ($^3$H-TdR) is added at this time,
it is taken up into the newly synthesized DNA. After 18 hours of exposure to $^3$H-TdR, the radioactivity incorporated in the cells can be determined and this provides a measure of the degree of activity (Figure 6.4).

The assay is most useful when only one set of cells is permitted to

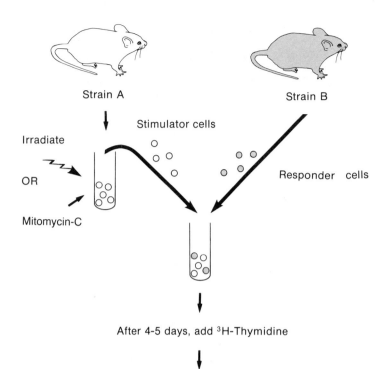

Strain A

Strain B

Irradiate

Stimulator cells

OR

Responder cells

Mitomycin-C

After 4-5 days, add $^3$H-Thymidine

Measure radioactivity in cells 18 hours later.

**Figure 6.4** The one-way mixed lymphocyte reaction (MLR). The assay is *one-way* because the strain A cells have been inactivated and cannot proliferate in response to the strain B cells. However, they still provide a strong proliferative stimulus to the strain B cells.

respond. This is the "one-way" MLR. The stimulator cells are either irradiated or treated with the antibiotic mitomycin C. Either treatment destroys their capacity to undergo mitosis, but they remain otherwise viable. Therefore, in the one-way MLR, the uptake of the isotope is a measure of the degree to which one set of cells — the responding cells — react against the histocompatibility antigens present on the inactivated stimulator cells. The result of each assay can be expressed as a stimulation index (SI).

$$SI = \frac{\text{Avg. cpm in experimental cultures}}{\text{Avg. cpm in control cultures}}$$

Control cultures are those in which the responding cells are cultured with mitomycin-treated cells from the same (or at least a syngeneic) donor.

Differences confined to minor histocompatibility loci do not produce positive MLRs. However, differences at the MHC (H-2 in mice, HLA in humans) do produce strong SIs. By the use of recombinant strains, it has been shown that differences at K and D are not especially effective in producing a large SI. However, when there is identity at K and D but different alleles in the I region, a strong stimulation index is produced (Figure 6.5). As we saw in the previous section, this is also the case for GVH reactions. The antigens encoded in the I region that are responsible for strong MLR and GVH reactions are the class II antigens (Section 3.6).

In a sense, the MLR is simply a special case of the lymphocyte proliferative response described in Section 3.2. Each involves antigen-induced

| Responder | Stimulator and target | H-2 difference | SI[1] | CMC (%) |
|---|---|---|---|---|
| B10.T(6R) qqqqqd | C57BL/10 bbbbbb | Complete | 26.0 | 68 |
| B10.T(6R) qqqqqd | AQR qkkkkd | I region | 16.0 | <1 |
| AQR qkkkkd | B10.A kkkkkd | K only | 1.4 | 22 |

[1] SI = stimulation index.

**Figure 6.5** Effect of differences at the major histocompatibility complex on the mixed lymphocyte reaction and on cell-mediated cytotoxicity (CMC). Histoincompatibility limited to the I region of H-2 provides a more powerful proliferative stimulus in mixed lymphocyte culture than does a difference limited to the K locus. However, antigenic differences at K induce more vigorous cytotoxicity than do differences confined to the I region. Both proliferation and cytotoxicity are strongest when the entire H-2 region is allogeneic. [From Alter and Bach, *J. Exp. Med.* **140**:1410, 1974; Bach, et al., *Nature* **259**:273, 1976.]

stimulation. However, there are several significant ways in which the response to a soluble antigen like OVA or PPD differs from the MLR.

1. The proliferative response to soluble antigens is measurable only if the cells are taken from an animal previously immunized with the antigen. The MLR does not require any priming of the cell donors. This difference is the reflection of the respective frequencies of the cells capable of responding to the antigen. From 0.5 to 10% of the lymphocytes of an immunologically "naive" mouse are capable of responding to a histocompatibility difference in H-2. The frequency in such an unprimed animal of lymphocytes capable of responding to a particular conventional antigen is far lower.
2. The MLR measures the reactivity of T lymphocytes exclusively. Both T lymphocytes (responsible for CMI) and, to a lesser extent, B lymphocytes (responsible for humoral immunity) proliferate when cultured with a soluble antigen they have been primed to.

## 6.6  Cell-Mediated Cytotoxicity (CMC)

If lymphocytes are cultured with cells bearing foreign antigenic determinants, a subset of the lymphocytes develops the capacity to lyse the stimulating cells. These lymphocytes have become cytotoxic. The response is specific in that the sensitized lymphocytes are only cytotoxic for target cells bearing the same antigenic determinants as the stimulating cells. The phenomenon is thus an example of in vitro cell-mediated immunity.

As usually performed, the assay begins like a one-way MLR. A population of viable lymphocytes is cultured with an irradiated (or mitomycin C treated) population of stimulator cells (often lymphocytes as well). After 5 days, the cells are removed from the culture vessels, washed, and resuspended at various cell densities. These cell suspensions are then mixed with a constant number of target cells. After four hours of incubation, the amount of target cell lysis is determined (Figure 6.6).

One of the most convenient ways of measuring target cell lysis is by using target cells that contain an intracellular radioactive label and determining the amount of this label that is released into the culture supernatant after four hours of exposure to the cytotoxic cells. The amount of radioactivity released into the supernatant is proportional to the degree of cytotoxicity. The most widely used radioactive label is chromium-51. For reasons only partly understood, living cells rapidly take up chromate ions into their cytoplasm but do not release appreciable amounts of the ion as long as they remain viable. By incubating the target cells for 45 minutes with $Na^{51}CrO_4$, they become internally labeled and ready to use in the assay.

Two controls must be included in each assay. "Control release" cul-

**Figure 6.6**  Procedure for measuring cell-mediated cytotoxicity (CMC). Mitogen-stimulated lymphocytes (as shown here) or certain types of tumor cells can serve as target cells.

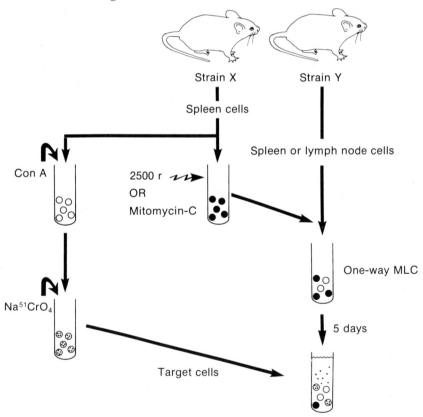

tures are those containing target cells but no cytotoxic cells. The target cells spontaneously release a certain amount of isotope which must be subtracted from the experimental values. "Maximum release" controls are cultures in which the cells have been completely lysed by chemical or physical means (e.g., freezing and thawing). These controls indicate the maximum amount of isotope that can be released by that density of target cells.

The results of the assay are expressed as percent CMC, where

$$\% \text{ CMC} = \frac{\text{Experimental release} - \text{Control release}}{\text{Maximum release} - \text{Control release}} \times 100$$

The sensitization phase of the CMC assay is identical to that of the MLR assay. Are, then, these two assays measuring the same aspect of cell-mediated immunity? Probably not. The cells active in CMC do undergo a phase of proliferation during the culture period and thus would take up $^3$H-TdR. However, one-half or more of the cells responding in the MLR are probably quite distinct from those capable of mediating CMC. You will recall that MLR responses are particularly vigorous where I region differences occur between the stimulating and responding cell populations. However, studies with recombinant strains clearly show that the cytotoxic lymphocytes act primarily against antigens encoded in the K and, to a lesser extent, D regions of H-2. Differences confined to the I region fail to generate significant cytotoxicity (Figure 6.5). Later we shall find other distinctions between the lymphocytes active in MLR and those active in CMC.

Is the CMC assay merely a laboratory phenomenon? It is clearly an example of a cell-mediated immune reaction, but does it reflect cell-mediated immune responses that occur in the living organism? The answer is not yet certain. We know that cytotoxic lymphocytes can be induced in vivo as well as in vitro. And there is evidence that these cytotoxic lymphocytes can attack virus-infected cells in the host and, possibly, tumor cells and allogeneic cells (i.e., those present in an allograft). We shall examine the evidence for these natural expressions of cytotoxicity later. Whatever its biological significance may or may not be, the CMC assay has been a valuable research tool. As we shall see in later chapters, it has, for example, revealed much valuable information about the interactions that occur between different cells of the immune system.

## ADDITIONAL READING

1. Garvey, J. S., N. E. Cremer, and D. H. Sussdorf, *Methods in Immunology*, 3rd ed., W. A. Benjamin, Inc., Reading MA, 1977. Includes directions for eliciting and adoptively transferring DTH reactions and for measuring the inhibition of macrophage migration.

2. Hudson, L., and F. C. Hay, *Practical Immunology*, 2nd ed., Blackwell, Oxford, 1981. Includes instructions for eliciting graft versus host reactions.

3. Mishell, Barbara B., and S. M. Shiigi (eds.), *Selected Methods in Cellular Immunology*, W. H. Freeman and Company, San Francisco, 1980. Detailed instructions are provided for performing skin grafting (of mice), cell-mediated cytotoxicity assays, and the mixed-lymphocyte reaction.

4. Rose, N. R., and P. E. Bigazzi (eds.), *Methods in Immunodiagnosis,* 2nd ed., John Wiley & Sons, New York, 1980. Includes serological assays as well as assays of cell-mediated immunity.

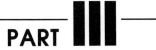

# The Immune System

# The Tissues and Cells of the Immune System

## 7.1 Introduction

The immune system consists of an interconnecting network of organs and tissues (Figure 7.1) between which moves a heavy and ceaseless traffic of cells. This cellular traffic is borne along in the flow of blood and lymph.

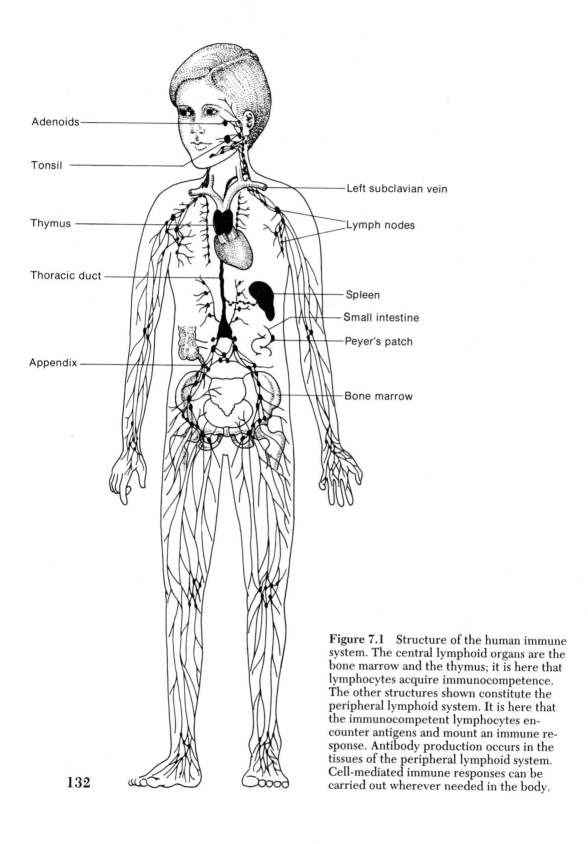

Adenoids

Tonsil

Thymus

Thoracic duct

Appendix

Left subclavian vein

Lymph nodes

Spleen

Small intestine

Peyer's patch

Bone marrow

**Figure 7.1** Structure of the human immune system. The central lymphoid organs are the bone marrow and the thymus; it is here that lymphocytes acquire immunocompetence. The other structures shown constitute the peripheral lymphoid system. It is here that the immunocompetent lymphocytes encounter antigens and mount an immune response. Antibody production occurs in the tissues of the peripheral lymphoid system. Cell-mediated immune responses can be carried out wherever needed in the body.

Each structure in the immune system has a relatively fixed architecture into and out of which flow the mobile cells of the system: lymphocytes and monocytes. These mobile cells are produced in the organs and tissues of the immune system, and they interact with antigen and each other while within the system. The synthesis and release of antibodies occurs in the tissues of the system. Cell-mediated immune responses, however, can occur anywhere within the body.

Lymphocytes (Figure 7.2) are the dominant cell type in most of the organs and tissues of the immune system. For this reason, such tissues are described as *lymphoid*. They include all the body's lymph nodes, the spleen, the adenoids and tonsils, small clusters of lymphoid tissue in the wall of the intestine called Peyer's patches (Figure 7.1), and the thymus. All except the thymus constitute the so-called *peripheral lymphoid system*.

Immune responses are generated in the structures of the peripheral lymphoid system. These structures serve as filters, trapping circulating lymphocytes, phagocytic cells, and antigens. Thus the cells needed to mount an immune response to an antigen are brought into close proximity to that antigen. While the structures of the peripheral lymphoid system are centers of immune reactivity, they are peripheral in the sense that they are absolutely dependent for their development and function on cells generated in the thymus as well as on cells manufactured in the bone marrow.

**Figure 7.2** Transmission electron micrographs ($\times 10,500$) of a small lymphocyte (A) and a plasma cell (B). Most of the lymphocyte is occupied by its nucleus. No endoplasmic reticulum and only a single mitochondrion are visible in this section. The cytoplasm of the plasma cell reveals a well-developed rough endoplasmic reticulum, a Golgi apparatus, and several mitochondria. [Courtesy of Dr. Carlo E. Grossi.]

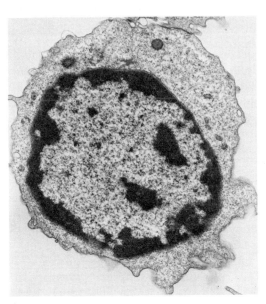

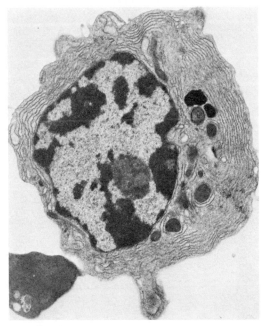

A                                              B

134

*Chapter 7*
*The Tissues and*
*Cells of the Immune*
*System*

7.2  Bone Marrow

All the cells of the blood are produced in bone marrow. In most mammals and under most circumstances, bone marrow is the major source of the red cells, platelets and granulocytes. Bone marrow also manufactures lymphocytes and monocytes.

If an animal such as a mouse is given a lethal dose of radiation (about 950 rads), the animal can be restored to health by fresh bone marrow cells. This can be demonstrated in two ways.

1. If a tiny portion of its own bone marrow is shielded from the radiation, cells from the protected region are able to repopulate all the irradiated lymphoid tissue.
2. Alternatively, a totally irradiated animal can be given a suspension of syngeneic marrow cells and, in this way, restored to health. Injections of syngeneic lymphocytes alone will repopulate the tissues of the immune system, but the animal will die from a deficiency of red cells and granulocytes.

Shortly after lethal irradiation, the spleen becomes grossly depleted of cells. However, after reconstitution with bone marrow cells, nodules or colonies appear in the spleen (Figure 7.3). If the *donor* of the bone marrow cells is given a moderate dose (about 700 rads) of radiation, many of its bone marrow cells will suffer chromosomal damage such as breaks and translocations. These are often not lethal, but the process is so random that they can serve as unique identifying markers for the cell. When the cells of a given spleen colony are induced to undergo mitosis and blocked at metaphase, all the cells reveal the same chromosomal aberration. All the cells in an adjacent colony will share a different pattern. This suggests then that all the cells in one colony are descended from a single precursor cell.

What cells are found in a colony? The precursors of red cells, the three types of granulocytes and megakaryocytes are regularly found. In addition, a cell suspension from a spleen colony can also form spleen colonies in a second lethally irradiated recipient. This tells us that the single cell that gave rise to the original colony produces daughter cells like itself as well as the cells destined to enter the various pathways of blood cell differentiation. We use the term **stem cell** for a cell with these properties.

Over a period of weeks, the individual colonies fuse and the spleen regains its normal appearance. During the period while the colonies remain distinct, it has not been possible to demonstrate lymphocytes within them. Later, however, lymphocytes appear in the spleen, thymus and elsewhere in the lymphoid system. When cultured and stimulated to undergo mitosis, they often show the same pattern of chromosome abnormalities found in the other blood cells. This strongly indicates that a single stem cell has given rise to all the cells of the blood (Figure 7.4). It remains uncertain whether this "pluripotent" stem cell gives rise directly to the spleen colonies or whether they are produced by a "sub" stem cell that has already diverged from the pluripotent stem cell along a

**Figure 7.3** Colonies of cells in the spleen of a mouse that had been lethally irradiated and then reconstituted with $8 \times 10^4$ syngeneic bone marrow cells. All of the cells in a given colony—and several types of blood cells may be present—are descended from a single precursor cell, a stem cell called a colony-forming unit–spleen (CFU–S). [Courtesy of E. A. McCulloch, from E. A. McCulloch, "The Origin of the Cells of the Blood," in *The Physiological Basis of Medical Practice*, 8th ed., C. H. Best and N. B. Taylor (eds.), Williams & Wilkins, Baltimore, 1966.]

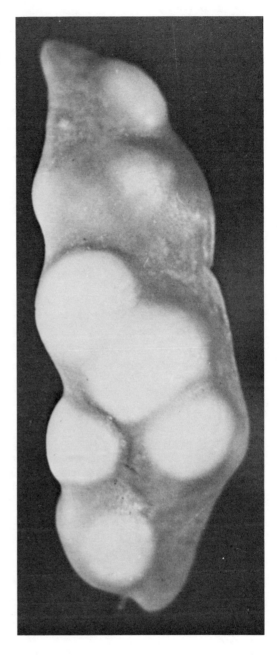

pathway restricted to red cells, granulocytes, monocytes, and megakaryocytes.

Although the bone marrow is the source of all the blood cells, it cannot fully restore an irradiated animal unless the thymus is also present. This is only one bit of evidence we shall examine that leads to the conclusion that although bone marrow is the *source* of the cells destined to participate in CMI, these cells do not gain competence to do so until they have been exposed to the influence of the thymus.

135

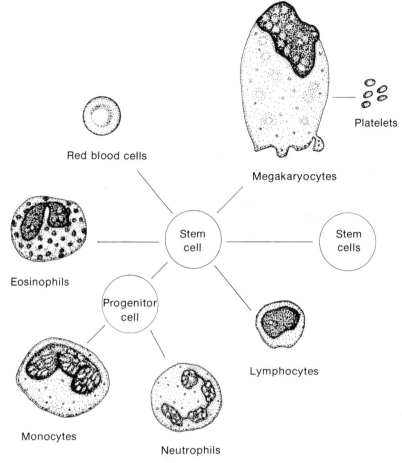

**Red blood cells**

**Megakaryocytes**

**Platelets**

**Eosinophils**

**Stem cell**

**Stem cells**

**Progenitor cell**

**Lymphocytes**

**Monocytes**

**Neutrophils**

**Figure 7.4** Hypothetical pathways of differentiation of the blood cells. In addition to the progenitor cell that gives rise to both monocytes and neutrophils, some of the other blood cells may share a common progenitor cell (not shown) descended from the pluripotent stem cell. The morphology of the pluripotent stem cell is uncertain; in both rats and mice, cells able to form spleen colonies are quite similar to lymphocytes in appearance.

## 7.3 The Thymus

In mammals, the thymus is a bilobed, grayish organ located high in the thoracic cavity. Until the late 1960s, the thymus' function was uncertain, and more or less by default, it was usually lumped together with the endocrine glands. If one suspects that one is dealing with an endocrine gland, the first thing to do is to remove it and look for the onset of physiological abnormalities. This was often done with the thymus, but without clear-cut results. Surgical removal of the thymus (thymectomy) in mature animals produces no discernible problems.

Not until 1961 did Miller in Australia and Good in Minnesota reveal the crucial importance of this organ to proper immune function. They succeeded where others had failed because they removed the thymus close to the time of birth, a procedure known as *neonatal thymectomy* (NTx). The thymus in a newborn mouse is a prominent organ—almost the size of the heart. Its removal at the time of birth leads to a dramatic series of consequences. A profound lymphopenia occurs; i.e., the number of circulating lymphocytes declines to very low levels. The animal fails to develop normal cell-mediated immune responses: it does not reject allografts and it fails to develop DTH responses.

The picture with respect to humoral immunity is not so clear-cut. The animal's humoral immune response to some antigens is normal or even higher than normal (we will look at the latter phenomenon again later). For example, NTx mice respond well to purified pneumococcal polysaccharide. On the other hand, their response to such antigens as sheep red blood cells (SRBC) and soluble protein antigens (such as OVA) is seriously impaired. This dichotomy has, in fact, led to the classification of antigens like OVA and SRBC as thymus dependent (TD) and antigens like the pneumococcal polysaccharides as thymus independent (TI).

All the experiments to elucidate these facts must be done promptly after birth or hatching because after a few weeks, these neonatally thymectomized (NTx) animals become strikingly unhealthy. They begin to lose weight, they suffer from diarrhea, their general appearance is poor, and they soon succumb to what is called "wasting disease." However, wasting disease can be avoided by rearing the animals in a germ-free environment. This suggests that those immune functions provided by the thymus are needed to enable the animal to cope with the microorganisms that normally inhabit its tissues harmlessly.

Why, then, does neonatal thymectomy generate such profound consequences while adult thymectomy seems inconsequential? One clue is provided by accompanying adult thymectomy with heavy doses of radiation to the rest of the immune system, including the bone marrow. Such treatment is fatal unless the animal is reconstituted with a suspension of syngeneic bone marrow cells. Such reconstitution is only partial, however. Without a thymus, this bone marrow reconstituted animal suffers the same defects as the neonatally thymectomized animal. However, bone marrow reconstitution *plus* a thymus graft restores complete immune function. This evidence suggests that the functions of the thymus are carried out early in the animal's life, and the thymus becomes less important as long as the remaining parts of the immune system remain functional. In fact, if one thymectomizes adult animals and monitors their progress long enough, a slow deterioration of cell-mediated immunity (e.g., DTH) eventually becomes apparent.

The thymus gland develops from the third and fourth pairs of pharyngeal pouches in the vertebrate embryo. It thus begins as an epithelium of endodermal origin. Into this epithelium migrate cells of mesodermal origin. The most abundant of these are lymphocytes.

The thymus is divided into two anatomically distinct compartments: an outermost **cortex** and an inner **medulla.** Both regions are densely packed with lymphocytes, called **thymocytes** while they reside within the thymus. In the mouse, approximately 85% of the thymocytes are in the cortex. Almost all of these cortical thymocytes are immature cells that are unable to carry out immune functions. However, a few cortical thy-

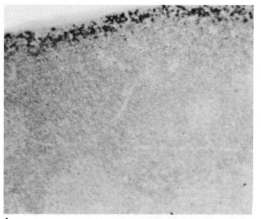

**A**

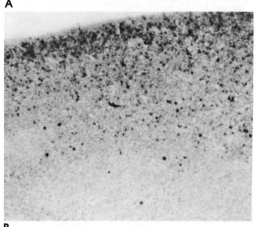

**B**

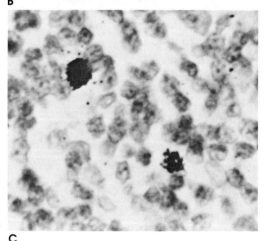

**C**

**Figure 7.5** (A) Autoradiograph of the thymus from a 5-day-old mouse sacrificed 3 hours after the application of tritiated thymidine to the surface of its thymus. The cells in the outermost cortex have taken up the label. (B) Mouse thymus 24 hours after the application of tritiated thymidine. Note that labeled cells now appear deep in the cortex and close to the medulla. (C) Three days after the application of tritiated thymidine to the thymus, labeled cells can be found in peripheral lymphoid tissue, such as the spleen shown here. [Courtesy of Irving L. Weissman from I. L. Weissman, *J. Exp. Med.* **137**:504, 1973 (A and B) and *J. Exp. Med.* **126**:291, 1967 (C).]

mocytes and most of the thymocytes in the medulla are mature, immunocompetent cells.

The cortex is a region of intense mitotic activity (Figure 7.5). Curiously, though, most ( > 97%) of the cells produced by mitosis in the thymus are destined to die there. Nonetheless, there is a steady export of thymocytes to the peripheral lymphoid tissues. These cells — now called

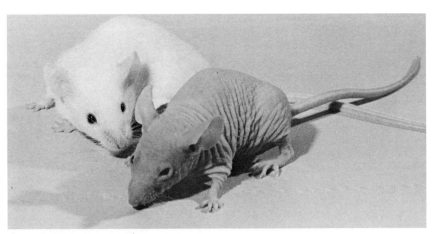

**Figure 7.6** A nude mouse (*nu/nu*) and its phenotypically normal, heterozygous littermate (*nu/+*). [Jackson Laboratory Photo.]

T lymphocytes—are immunocompetent and are able to carry out cell-mediated immune responses.

The "nude" mouse is one of the most useful animals in which to study thymus function. As its name suggests, this animal has no hair (Figure 7.6). But far more interesting from our perspective is the fact that it is also born without a thymus. These defects are the pleiotropic·effects of a single gene locus. They occur when the animal is homozygous for the recessive mutant gene *nu*. This gene has been bred into several inbred mouse strains. Like NTx mice, these animals become unhealthy and die unless reared under very clean conditions.

Nude mice are unable to reject grafts. Even xenogeneic grafts are retained indefinitely (Figure 7.7). Nude mice mount no humoral responses to thymus-dependent antigens but make normal, or even supranormal, humoral responses to thymus-independent antigens.

In humans (as well as in other mammals), the thymus reaches its maximum size at about the time of puberty. Thereafter, it shrinks and, as time goes by, much of its architecture is replaced by fatty tissue. In old age, the thymus is reduced to a tiny, fatty rudiment. Despite this age-related involution, evidence from adoptive transfers indicates that aged thymuses retain some function.

Some of the functions of the thymus can be restored to nude or thymectomized mice by a diffusible product of the thymus. This can be demonstrated by enclosing a thymus within a chamber, the walls of which can be permeated by molecules but not by cells. Placed within the peritoneal cavity of an NTx animal, such an implant restores some thymic function even though the pores of the chamber are too small ($< 0.5\,\mu$m) to permit any traffic of cells in or out. This suggests that the early speculations about the thymus were correct; it *does* have an endocrine function. The thymus produces a number of diffusible substances which can restore cell mediated immune responses.

The hormones of the thymus have been intensely studied. Different research groups have used varied sources of the hormones and different assay methods. As a result, considerable uncertainty exists about the

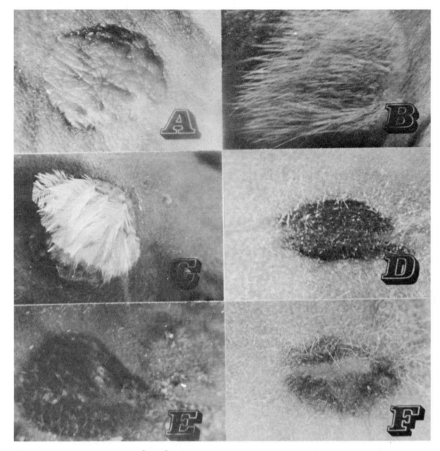

**Figure 7.7** Various grafts of xenogeneic skin maintained on nude mice. A: Human after 60 days. B: Cat at 51 days. C: Chicken at 32 days; the feathers were already present when the graft was made. D: Chameleon at 41 days. E: Fence lizard at 28 days. F: Tree frog at 40 days. [Courtesy of Dean D. Manning from D. D. Manning et al., *J. Exp. Med.* **138**:488, 1973.]

precise number and identity of the various hormones. The mixture of active molecules (they all appear to be polypeptides) is collectively known as "thymosin."

A few of these polypeptides have been extracted from calf thymuses (those that did not end up on a restaurant table as "sweetbreads"), purified and sequenced. One of these, called thymopoietin, contains 49 amino acid residues. Both thymosin and thymopoietin are able to restore certain cell-mediated functions when injected into nude or thymectomized mice.

The thymus is exceedingly sensitive to corticosteroids. An injection of cortisol leads to rapid (within hours) shrinking or involution. This is probably the mechanism of "stress involution" as well, where disease or other stress also leads to rapid shrinking of the thymus. The stress triggered release of steroids from the adrenal cortices presumably mediates the involution associated with stress. The response is so rapid that a thymus of normal size is rarely seen at autopsy. Childhood deaths under circumstances requiring an autopsy usually occur following a period of disease or other stress. At one time, the shrunken thymus seen under such circumstances was mistakenly considered to be normal. On the rare occasions when an otherwise unexplained death occurred without stress involution, a normal thymus was incorrectly considered to be pathological, and led to a diagnosis of "*status thymicolymphaticus.*"

## 7.4   The Bursa of Fabricius

This lymphoid organ is found only in birds. It is a saclike structure connected to the cloaca at the posterior end of the gut (Figure 7.8). Like the thymus, it consists of an epithelium surrounding masses of lymphoid cells. It forms at approximately the tenth day of development and reaches its maximum size 3 weeks after hatching. At 8 weeks, the bursa begins to involute.

In a series of papers published in *Poultry Science* from 1955 through 1957, Bruce Glick and his associates at Ohio State University first revealed that the bursa plays an essential role in immunity. They found that young chicks whose bursa had been removed at the time of hatching failed to manufacture antibodies when injected with bacterial antigens.

Almost a decade passed before this intriguing observation was followed up. Researchers then found that bursectomy did not suppress such cell-mediated responses as graft rejection and DTH to tuberculin. However, thymectomy (followed by x-irradiation) had the same effect in birds that it has in mammals: uniform suppression of cell-mediated immune responses but no effect on humoral responses to thymus-independent antigens or on overall levels of circulating gamma globulins. Thus the two branches of the immune system appeared, in chickens at least, to depend upon different organs. The realization that the functional duality of the immune system was reflected in a structural duality opened up lines of research that continue to be enormously productive, as we shall see.

The discovery of the function of the bursa in birds led, of course, to a

**Figure 7.8**   The central lymphoid organs of the chick. T lymphocytes mature in the thymus, B lymphocytes in the bursa of Fabricius.

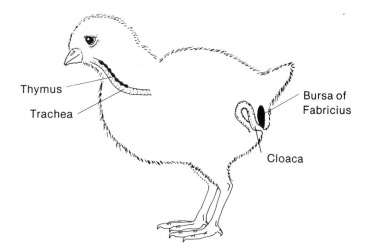

vigorous search for the equivalent organ in mammals. Many candidates were proposed, but as we shall see, the bulk of the evidence suggests that in the adult mammal, the cells responsible for antibody synthesis begin development in the bone marrow.

## 7.5 Lymph Nodes

Lymph nodes are lymph filters found at strategic locations in the lymphatic system (Figure 7.1). Each receives a flow of lymph from one or more afferent lymph vessels (Figure 7.9). The source of this lymph is the system of lymph capillaries that drains most of the tissue spaces of the body. The large pores at the origin of the lymph capillaries permit particulate matter as well as extracellular fluid to enter the capillaries. Thus foreign material that breaches the interfaces, like the skin, between the external and internal environments can be immediately picked up by the lymphatic system. Tests with isolated lymph nodes show that more than 99% of the bacteria entering a node are trapped in it.

Lymph nodes are roughly spherical or bean-shaped structures enveloped in a capsule of connective tissue. Just beneath the capsule is a phagocyte-lined meshwork, the subcapsular sinus. Lymph entering the node by the afferent lymph vessels trickles into this region and any particulate matter contained within it may be phagocytosed here.

The cortex lies just beneath the subcapsular sinus. It is densely packed with lymphocytes and macrophages organized into spherical nests of cells called **follicles.** When stimulated by antigen, the follicles become enlarged. Intense cellular proliferation occurs in the center, the **germinal center,** of the follicle. An active follicle produces clusters of dividing lymphocytes and antibody-secreting plasma cells (Figure 7.2) that extend down into the medulla of the node (Figure 7.9). Many lympho-

**Figure 7.9** Diagrammatic representation of a section of a lymph node. The paracortical area is also called the deep or diffuse cortex.

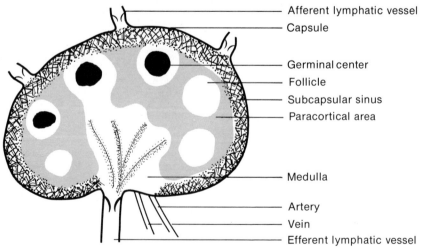

Afferent lymphatic vessel
Capsule

Germinal center
Follicle
Subcapsular sinus
Paracortical area

Medulla

Artery
Vein
Efferent lymphatic vessel

**Figure 7.10** A: Cortical area of a lymph node draining the ear of a mouse immunized with the type 3 pneumococcal polysaccharide, a thymus-independent (TI) antigen. The follicle shows intense mitotic activity, especially in the germinal center (gc), and contains plasma cells. The paracortical or thymus-dependent area (tda) shows little activity. B: Appearance of a node draining the ear of a mouse challenged (on the ear) with oxazolone, a contact sensitizer that elicits a cell-mediated, DTH reaction. The tda is packed with lymphoblasts; the follicle (or primary nodule, "pn") shows little activity and has no germinal center. C: Same experimental protocol as B except that the mouse has been neonatally thymectomized. In this case, the paracortical area (tda) failed to respond to the oxazolone treatment. [Courtesy of Drs. M. de Sousa and D. M. V. Parrott.]

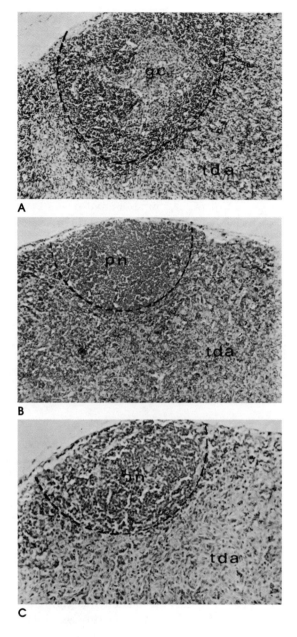

cytes and the antibodies produced by the plasma cells are released into the lymph that leaves by way of a single efferent lymphatic vessel (Figure 7.9).

Between the follicles and the medulla lie masses of lymphocytes that form the **paracortical area.** This region is also known as the *deep* or *diffuse cortex.*

The lymph nodes of a neonatally thymectomized mouse have normal follicles, but the paracortical area is severely depleted of cells. The same condition occurs in the nude mouse. For this reason, the paracortical area is called the thymus-dependent or **T-dependent** area of the node. Bursectomized birds have nodes with normal appearing paracortical

143

areas but no follicles. Therefore, this region is said to be bursa dependent or **B dependent.**

Earlier in the chapter, we examined some of the evidence linking the thymus to cell mediated immune responses as well as humoral responses to T-dependent antigens. The bursa (or bone marrow in mammals) is necessary for all antibody responses and exclusively so for responses to T-independent (TI) antigens. This functional dichotomy is beautifully illustrated in the lymph nodes. Exposed to a TI antigen like the type 3 pneumococcal polysaccharide, the lymph nodes develop an intense response in their follicles (Figure 7.10). The paracortical area reveals little cellular activity.

The center panel of Figure 7.10 shows the appearance of a lymph node in an animal treated with a skin sensitizer (oxazolone) to which it has mounted a DTH reaction. Note that in this case, the paracortical (T-dependent) area of the node is active while the nearby follicle is not.

The bottom photomicrograph shows a node taken from a neonatally thymectomized, oxazolone-treated mouse. Without its thymus, the animal fails to mount a DTH response when challenged with the sensitizing antigen. The paracortical area of the nodes draining the challenged area (the ear in this case) show no response.

## 7.6  The Spleen

The spleen serves two major functions in the body. It is largely responsible for the destruction of old and damaged red blood cells, and it is a major site for mounting immune responses. As for its immune reactivity, the spleen functions much like a lymph node *except* that the fluid it filters is blood not lymph.

The two functions of the spleen are localized in two anatomically distinct regions. Red cell processing goes on in the **red pulp.** Immune responses are generated in the **white pulp.**

Blood entering the spleen passes into a system of ever-finer arteries and arterioles that eventually deposit the blood in the red pulp. Surrounding each arteriole is a cylindrical mass of lymphoid cells, which makes up the **periarteriolar lymphoid sheath** or **PALS** (Figure 7.11). Scattered through the PALS are spherical nests of cells, the follicles. Like lymph node follicles, the follicles of the PALS are B dependent, and when an intense humoral immune response is being generated, they have germinal centers. The nonfollicular area of the PALS is T dependent and resembles the paracortical area of lymph nodes. The periarteriolar lymphoid sheaths, together with their follicles, make up the white pulp.

Blood is deposited in the red pulp along with its load of circulating cells and any antigens it may contain. Blood-borne lymphocytes, antigens, and tissue fluids move to the boundary (called the marginal zone) between the red and white pulp. This is a region of intense phagocytic activity and the juxtaposition here of antigen, antigen-trapping phagocytes, and lymphocytes sets the stage for an immune response. Lymphocytes also migrate into the PALS itself where the immune response develops. Some of

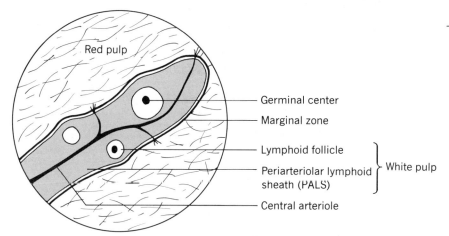

**Figure 7.11** Diagrammatic representation of a section through the spleen as it would be seen under low magnification.

the antibodies and lymphocytes produced in an immune response leave the spleen in its lymphatic drainage. Most, however, leave in the system of veins that drains blood from the red pulp.

How does the immune reactivity of the spleen differ from that of lymph nodes? Because of its role as a blood filter, the spleen plays a major role in mounting immune responses to blood-borne antigens such as bacteria that reach the circulation. The response of lymph nodes is more localized, responding only to antigens reaching them from a particular tissue. While humans can thrive without a spleen, they tend to have a particularly difficult time coping with blood-borne infections.

Small lymphocytes pack both the T-dependent and B-dependent areas of the lymph nodes (as well as of the spleen and other peripheral lymphoid tissues). Morphologically, nothing distinguishes these two populations of cells. However, a variety of functional and serological criteria does distinguish them. In the following two sections, we will examine the evidence for the existence of two distinct populations of lymphocytes: T lymphocytes dependent upon the thymus and B lymphocytes dependent upon the bursa (in birds) and upon its equivalent in mammals, the bone marrow. B lymphocytes (or simply "B cells") are the cells that develop into antibody-secreting plasma cells (Figure 7.2). Thus B cells are directly responsible for humoral immunity. T lymphocytes are responsible for all forms of cell-mediated immune responses. In addition, T cells "help" B cells respond to many kinds of antigens (Figure 7.12).

## 7.7  T Lymphocytes

Seen under the microscope (light or electron), the lymphocytes that populate the T-dependent areas of lymph nodes and spleen look just like those that reside in the B-dependent areas. However, T lymphocytes and

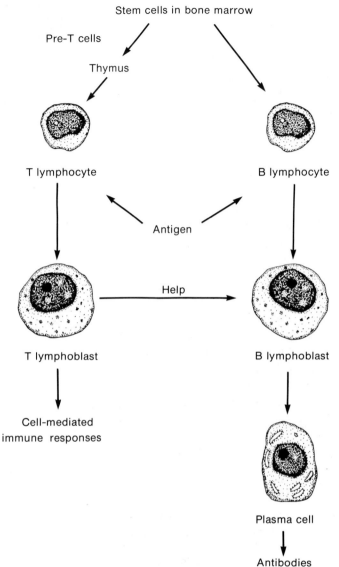

Stem cells in bone marrow

Pre-T cells

Thymus

T lymphocyte

B lymphocyte

Antigen

T lymphoblast

Help

B lymphoblast

Cell-mediated
immune responses

Plasma cell

Antibodies

**Figure 7.12** Pathways of development of the cells active in the two branches of the immune system: T cells for cell-mediated immune responses and B cells for humoral responses. A subset of antigen-stimulated T cells participate ("help") in the induction of humoral immunity to certain "thymus-dependent" (TD) antigens.

B lymphocytes express certain surface antigens and have functional properties that distinguish them. Furthermore, within each population, there are subsets of cells with their own special properties. Thus, for example, several subsets of T cells have been defined in terms of the different functional roles they play: helper, cytotoxic, suppressor, etc. Each of these subsets can also be defined in terms of a particular combination of surface antigens. These generalizations hold true for both the T lymphocytes of mice and those in humans. In fact, the more that is learned about human and mouse T cells, the more parallels are found between them. However, separate nomenclatures have developed for each, so we shall consider them separately here.

The T lymphocytes that populate the T-dependent areas of peripheral lymphoid tissue are mature, immunocompetent cells; i.e., they are capable of responding to an appropriate antigen. In mice, they all express on their surface a protein designated Thy-1 (also called theta, $\theta$). Two allelic forms of this antigen have been identified: Thy-1.1, which occurs in a few inbred strains, such as AKR, and Thy-1.2, which is found in most of the commonly used inbred strains (C57BL/10, A, BALB/c, etc.). The two alleles differ by a single amino acid residue. Because of the universal occurrence of Thy-1, treatment of a lymphocyte suspension with anti-Thy-1 antibodies and complement effectively destroys all the T cells present (Section 5.13).

Roughly two-thirds of the T lymphocytes in the spleen express a surface antigen designated L3T4. Most of the remaining T cells express two other antigens called Ly-2 and Ly-3, but no L3T4. Thus L3T4, on the one hand, and Ly-2,3 on the other, distinguish two nonoverlapping subsets of T cells in the mouse. Most of the T lymphocytes that (1) proliferate in response to antigens, (2) elicit DTH reactions ($T_D$), or (3) serve to help or amplify humoral and/or cell-mediated immune responses belong to the L3T4$^+$ subset. Most of the T cells that are cytotoxic ($T_C$) for other cells or suppress immune reactivity ($T_S$) belong to the Ly-2,3$^+$ subset. The molecules that carry the Ly-2 and Ly-3 determinants are covalently linked and one is never expressed without the other. Therefore, we shall usually designate this subset simply as Ly-2$^+$.

The L3T4$^+$ subset of T cells also expresses large amounts of the Ly-1 antigen. Most Ly-2$^+$ cells express much lower amounts of Ly-1. The difference in level of Ly-1 expression makes possible an effective method of purifying functional subsets of T cells. Treatment of a cell suspension with anti-Ly-1 destroys all those cells in the $T_H$ and $T_D$ subsets, while sparing the cells in the cytotoxic ($T_C$) and suppressor ($T_S$) subsets. Conversely, treatment with anti-Ly-2 or anti-Ly-3 and complement spares the $T_H$, $T_D$, and other L3T4$^+$ subsets.

The Ly-1 antigen was originally designated Ly$t$-1; the $t$ was included because it was thought that the antigen occurred on T cells only. However, some B cells have been found that express this antigen, so we shall use the Ly-1 designation. The Ly-2 and Ly-3 antigens have been found only on T cells, and so the designations Lyt-2 and Lyt-3 continue to be commonly used for them.

Huber and her colleagues have found that the commitment of T cells to one or the other subset appears to be irreversible. When irradiated, thymectomized mice are reconstituted with bone marrow and a suspension of T cells depleted of Ly-2$^+$ cells, the mice fail to regenerate this subset of cells. Even after 6 months, they fail to develop cytotoxic T cells ($T_C$), but their T helper function is unimpaired. Similarly, thymectomized mice reconstituted with a purified Ly-2$^+$ population fail to generate Ly-1$^+$, Ly-2$^-$ cells. These mice are able to mount a CMC response, but are unable to generate $T_H$ cells.

All the various kinds of T cells found in the peripheral lymphoid system are formed in the thymus. Their precursors, called pre-T cells, originate in the bone marrow and then migrate to the thymus (Figure 7.13). Here the cells — now called thymocytes — gradually develop immunocompetence; i.e., the ability to respond to antigen. The process of thymocyte maturation is accompanied by changes in the surface antigens they express as well as in certain other properties. For example, the immature thymocytes of many mouse strains express surface antigens called *thymus leukemia antigens* or **TL antigens.** As the name suggests, TL antigens are also expressed on leukemic cells. However, the TL antigens are probably not tumor-specific antigens as such but rather antigens associated with (as other tumor-associated antigens may well be) an early stage of cell differentiation.

Immature thymocytes also express Thy-1, Ly-1, and *both* Ly-2, 3 and L3T4. Thus at this stage we do not see the mutually exclusive T cell subpopulations (L3T4$^+$, Ly-2$^-$ and L3T4$^-$, Ly-2$^+$) characteristic of mature T cells.

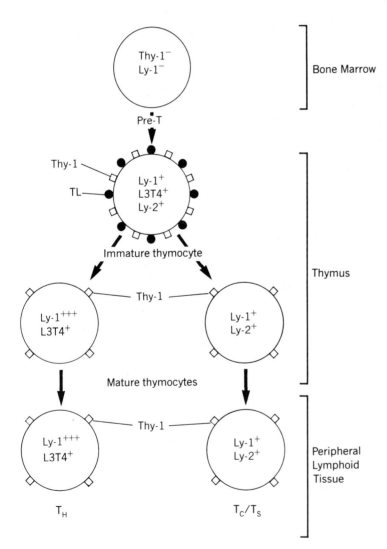

**Figure 7.13** Differentiation of T lymphocytes in mice. Immature thymocytes are localized in the cortex of the thymus; most mature thymocytes are in the medulla. Immature thymocytes are sensitive to cortisone; mature thymocytes are resistant. The Ly-3 antigen is always associated with Ly-2. The L3T4$^+$ subset "sees" antigen in association with class **II** MHC-encoded molecules; the Ly-2$^+$ subset with class I molecules.

Immature thymocytes can also be distinguished from mature T cells by their extreme sensitivity to the lethal effects of corticosteroids like cortisone. It is this effect that accounts for the rapid involution of the thymus in times of stress or corticosteroid treatment (Section 7.3).

As the differentiation of thymocytes proceeds, they become relatively resistant to the effects of corticosteroids. During this period, they also lose the TL antigen and enter one or the other pathway leading to the formation of the mature $L3T4^+$, $Ly-2^-$ and $L3T4^-$, $Ly-2^+$ subsets (Figure 7.13).

What is the nature of the pre-T cell that migrates from the bone marrow to the thymus? For technical reasons, it has been difficult to establish its properties. However, treatment of bone marrow cell suspensions with anti-Thy-1 or anti-Ly-1 does not diminish the number of pre-T cells, so we can assume that neither of these characteristic T cell markers are present on pre-T cells.

## In Humans

The differentiation of human T cells resembles that of mice in several ways. As in mice, immature human T cells can be distinguished from mature T cells by their surface antigens. And, again as in mice, mature T cells occur in discrete subsets ($T_H$, $T_C$, etc.) each of which has characteristic surface antigens. Most of these antigens are detected with monoclonal antibodies. Because monoclonal antibodies identifying the same antigen (but not necessarily the same epitope on that antigen) have been developed in different laboratories and given different designations, a confusing system of alternative nomenclatures has arisen. In an attempt to bring some order out of this chaotic situation, a new system of nomenclature for these antigens was proposed in 1984. In this system, all those monoclonal antibodies that appear to detect a particular antigen are assigned to a numbered "cluster of differentiation" (CD). Thus, for example, immature human thymocytes, which make up the bulk of the cells in the thymic cortex, express an antigen now designated CD1. They also express two other antigens designated CD4 and CD8 (Figure 7.14).

Mature human thymocytes no longer express the CD1 antigen. Furthermore, they become subdivided into two nonoverlapping subsets: one expressing CD4 but not CD8 ($CD4^+$, $CD8^-$), the other being $CD4^-$, $CD8^+$. The $CD4^+$ subset contains the T cells that proliferate most vigorously in response to antigen, and presumably the cells that elicit DTH reactions. The $CD8^+$ subset includes cytotoxic T cells ($T_C$) and suppressor cells ($T_S$). Thus the $CD4^+$ subset appears to be the counterpart of the $L3T4^+$ subset in mice. In fact, the L3T4 antigen was discovered after the corresponding human antigen and derived its designation from the earlier nomenclature (Leu 3/T4) of the human antigen. (A list of CD antigens with some of the most frequently used equivalents appears on the inside front cover of this book.) The $CD8^+$ subset appears to be the human counterpart of the $Ly-2^+$ subset in mice.

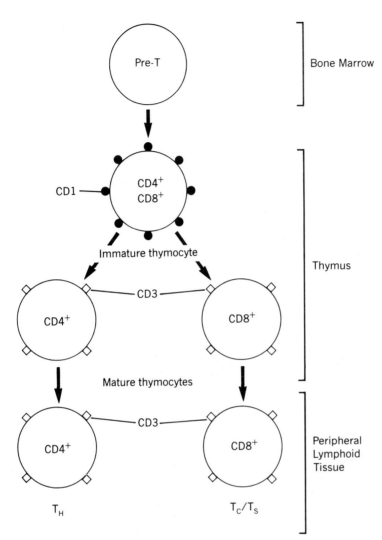

**Figure 7.14** Differentiation of T lymphocytes in humans. CD3 molecules ("T3") are associated with the T cell receptor for antigen and their appearance marks the acquisition of immunocompetence by the cell.

The mature T lymphocytes of humans also carry receptors which, fortuitously, bind to determinants on the surface of sheep red blood cells. When mixed with SRBC, each T cell binds a cluster of SRBC to its surface, forming a rosette (Figure 7.15). Such "E" (erythrocyte) rosettes not only provide a convenient way to identify and count human T cells, but also a way to separate T cells from B cells. After mixing peripheral blood lymphocytes with SRBC, the rosetted T cells can be separated from B cells by their increased density.

Both the CD4+ and CD8+ subsets of mature T cells express an antigen called CD3 (or T3). This molecule is closely associated on the surface of the cell membrane with the T cell receptor for antigen. Thus the appearance of CD3 in a maturing thymocyte marks the acquisition of immune competence by the cell: its ability to interact with and be stimulated by a particular antigen. Details about the properties of the T cell receptor for antigen are presented in Chapter 11.

**Figure 7.15** Mechanism of formation of three types of rosettes. The formation of E rosettes can be used to distinguish (and separate) human T lymphocytes from B lymphocytes. Fc receptors (FcR) and C3b receptors (C3bR) are also found on macrophages in several species. Furthermore, both lymphocytes and macrophages may express several types of Fc receptors, each specific for a different class (or subclass) of heavy chain (Fc$_\gamma$R for IgG, Fc$_\epsilon$R for IgE, etc.)

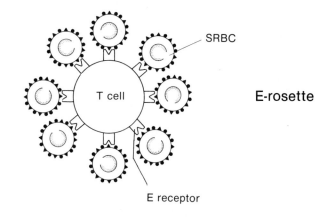

SRBC

T cell

E-rosette

E receptor

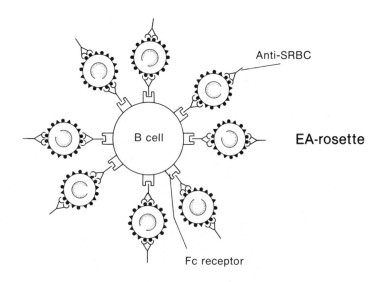

Anti-SRBC

B cell

EA-rosette

Fc receptor

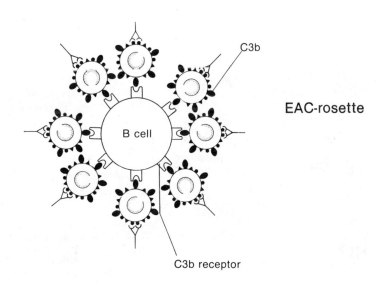

C3b

B cell

EAC-rosette

C3b receptor

## Response to Mitogens

A variety of substances have been discovered that bind to the surface of lymphocytes and, in so doing, stimulate them to undergo mitosis. Actively dividing lymphocytes, which are called lymphoblasts, are somewhat larger than resting lymphocytes (Figure 7.16). Their cytoplasm increases in volume and becomes filled with ribosomes. Their nucleus is less compact and develops nucleoli. The conversion of a resting lymphocyte into a lymphoblast is called lymphocyte transformation or blast transformation.

Several lymphocyte mitogens are **lectins.** Lectins are glycoproteins found in some plants that bind specifically to certain sugar residues on the glycoproteins of the cell surface. Phytohemagglutinin (PHA) is a

**Figure 7.16**  A: Unstimulated human lymphocytes after 48 hours in culture. B: Lymphoblasts produced after culturing human lymphocytes for the same period with the mitogen phytohemagglutinin. Note the larger cell size, larger and less compact nuclei, decreased nuclear/cytoplasmic ratio, and prominent nucleoli in the lymphoblasts. (300×) [Courtesy of Drs. Kurt H. Stenzel and A. Novogrodsky.]

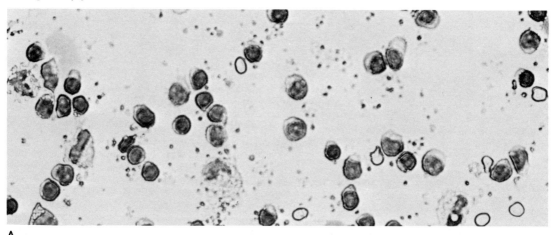

A

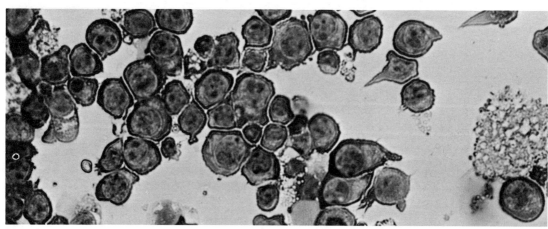

B

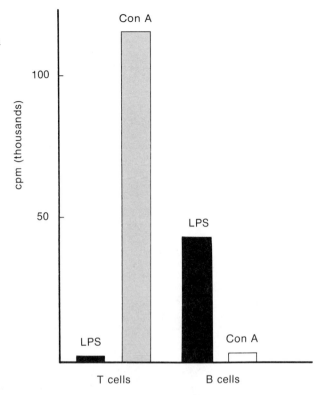

**Figure 7.17** Response of murine T lymphocytes and B lymphocytes to mitogens. Cells were cultured with the mitogen for 3 days and given tritiated thymidine during the final 12 hours of culture. LPS = lipopolysaccharide; Con A = concanavalin A.

lectin extracted from the red kidney bean, *Phaseolus vulgaris*. Although PHA binds to both B and T lymphocytes, it stimulates mitosis only in mature T cells. Concanavalin A (Con A), a lectin extracted from the jack bean *(Canavalia ensiformis)*, has a strong mitogenic effect on T cells (immature as well as mature) but not on B cells (Figure 7.17). Con A binds to glycoproteins with exposed $\alpha$-glucose and $\alpha$-mannose residues.

## 7.8 B Lymphocytes

In adult mammals, the precursors of B cells, like pre-T cells, arise in the bone marrow. Pre-B cells can be distinguished as a unique population by the presence of $\mu$ chains (the heavy chains of IgM) in their cytoplasm. Development of pre-B cells to mature B cells takes place while these cells remain within the bone marrow. When mature, B cells emigrate to the B-dependent areas of the peripheral lymphoid tissue.

The transition from pre-B to a mature B cell is marked by the appearance of membrane-bound immunoglobulin on the cell surface (Figure 7.18). At first this surface immunoglobulin (sIg) consists of monomers $(H_2L_2)$ of IgM. Later, IgD molecules appear as well. As many as $1.5 \times 10^5$ molecules of immunoglobulin (sIgM and sIgD) may occur on the surface of mature B cells. Their presence is easily revealed with fluorescent antibodies (Figure 7.19).

153

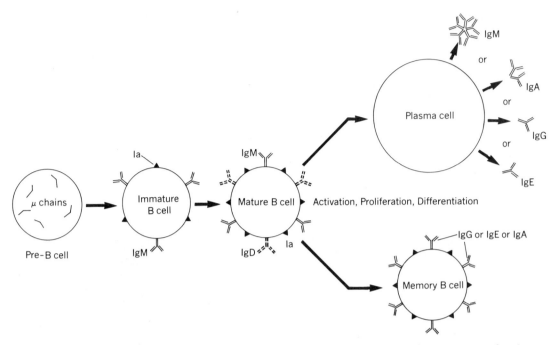

**Figure 7.18** Differentiation of B lymphocytes. Mature B cells also have surface receptors for the Fc region of IgG and for the C3b fragment of the complement system. The activation of B cells by antigen and mitogens is described in Chapter 8. Once activated, B cells develop receptors for lymphokines and monokines that stimulate proliferation (B cell growth factors — BCGFs) and differentiation (B cell differentiation factors — BCDFs). These factors are discussed in Chapter 12.

**Figure 7.19** B lymphocytes (A) and T lymphocytes (B) in a lymph node of a mouse. The B cells have been stained with a fluorescent anti-mouse immunoglobulin (thus revealing sIg); the T cells with fluorescent anti-Thy (theta) antibodies. The follicle is densely packed with B cells. B cells can also be seen around the nearby postcapillary venule (center right). Most of the T cells are in the paracortical area, although a few T cells can be seen scattered through the follicle. The latter are Ly-1$^+$ cells and presumably are helper (T$_H$) cells for B cells. These preparations were made on adjacent serial sections from the same node. [Courtesy of G. A. Gutman and I. Weissman.]

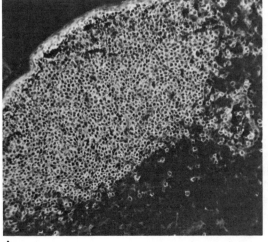

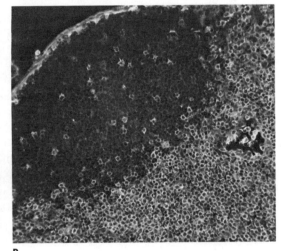

A                                B

Although the presence of an abundance of surface immunoglobulin (sIg) is the hallmark of B cells, other distinctive markers exist for them. B cells express receptors for a portion (called Fc) of IgG molecules and for the activated form (C3b) of the third component of the complement system (Section 14.2). The Fc receptor is revealed by the rosettes that B cells form with sheep red cells that have been coated with anti-SRBC antibodies of the IgG class (Figure 7.15). The C3b receptor is revealed by the rosettes formed with sheep red cells precoated with a nonlysing concentration of anti-SRBC and complement (Figure 7.15).

B lymphocytes also express Ia antigens, i.e., class II antigens encoded by the MHC. In mice, these antigens are encoded in the I-A and I-E subregions of H-2 (Figure 3.12). The Ia antigens on B cells play a role in the delivery of "help" from T cells to B cells (Figure 7.12). This role is examined in Chapter 12.

The cell walls of gram-negative bacteria such as *E. coli* contain a lipopolysaccharide (LPS) that is strongly mitogenic for a substantial fraction of the B cells in mice (but not in humans). LPS is not mitogenic for T cells in either species (Figure 7.17). Human B cells can be stimulated by pokeweed mitogen (PWM), a mixture of substances derived from pokeweed *(Phytolacca americana)*.

## 7.9  Lymphocyte Traffic

A few days after exposing cortical thymus cells to tritiated thymidine, labeled cells appear in the T-dependent areas of the peripheral lymphoid system (Figure 7.5), having been carried there by the blood. B lymphocytes migrate from bone marrow to the B-dependent areas of peripheral lymphoid tissue (Figure 7.19). In each case, the cells leave their site of origin by way of the venous blood draining the organ. Once at their destination, they stick to the endothelial cells that form the walls of the postcapillary venules; that is, the venules draining the capillaries. The lymphocytes then migrate through the wall, either by working their way between the endothelial cells or by passing directly through them. This interaction between lymphocytes and the endothelial cells of the postcapillary venules is remarkably specific. It involves a mechanism of mutual recognition ensuring that only lymphocytes will leave the circulation by this pathway.

A traffic of lymphocytes moves out of as well as into the peripheral lymphoid tissue. Both B cells and, especially, T cells migrate into the medullary sinuses of lymph nodes and pass out of the node in the efferent lymphatic vessel. The lymphatic drainage carries these cells along, and they are eventually returned to the blood at the subclavian veins (Figure 7.20). Some lymphocytes leave the spleen in its lymphatic drainage, but most exit by way of the veins draining this organ. Once in the blood, they are carried by arteries to all the tissues of the body. However, except for T cells responding to a localized antigenic stimulus elsewhere, they only leave the blood when they once again find themselves in the specialized postcapillary venules of lymphoid tissue.

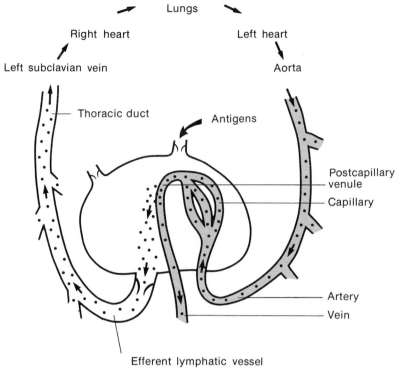

**Figure 7.20** Pathway of lymphocyte traffic. Lymphocytes leave the blood at the postcapillary venules of lymphoid tissue. They return to the blood in the lymph carried by the thoracic duct and, for the upper right quadrant of the body, a smaller lymph duct entering the right subclavian vein (see Figure 7.1).

A single lymphocyte may participate for years in this unceasing traffic between the various components and compartments of the immune system. The average life span of the circulating lymphocytes in the human is over four years. Some lymphocytes continue to circulate for 20 years or more. These figures have been established by culturing lymphocytes from patients who had received heavy doses of radiation at some precisely known time in the past. When these cells are stimulated with a mitogen and arrested at metaphase, some of them contain major chromosomal aberrations. The assumption is that the chromosomes were damaged by the earlier exposure to radiation and that the damage is so severe that these cells could never have completed a mitotic division in the interim. The discovery that some small lymphocytes may circulate through the body for decades provides a basis for the existence of immunological memory.

## 7.10 "Null" Cells

Some lymphocytes (5–10% of those in human blood) fail to reveal the characteristics of either T or B cells. Lacking either set of cell-surface markers, these lymphocytes have been called "null" cells. They are, however, associated with certain immune functions, described in Chapter 14.

## 7.11 Adherent Cells

The induction of both humoral immunity and cell-mediated immunity requires — in addition to lymphocytes — the participation of another type of cell. Attempts to generate immune responses in cell cultures have revealed this requirement. Cultures containing only lymphocytes are unresponsive, but the addition of a population of cells that adhere firmly to the bottom of the culture vessel enables the lymphocytes to respond to antigen. These adherent cells can be harvested from a variety of sources: spleen, lymph nodes, and so on. Two different categories of cells are included in the adherent cell population: *macrophages* and *dendritic cells*.

### Macrophages

Macrophages are large (10–20 $\mu$m), actively motile, phagocytic cells. They are distinguished from neutrophils (the other major group of phagocytic cell) by their unlobed nucleus and the absence of the specific granules that characterize neutrophils. Macrophages have a highly textured surface (Figure 7.21) covered with ruffles and microvilli.

Macrophages develop from the blood-borne monocytes, which are, in turn, generated in the bone marrow. Some macrophages, such as the Kupffer cells of the liver, occupy relatively fixed positions in their tissue. Others are more motile.

**Figure 7.21** Scanning electron micrograph of a macrophage (center) surrounded by several lymphocytes. [Courtesy of Drs. Jan M. Orenstein and Emma Shelton.]

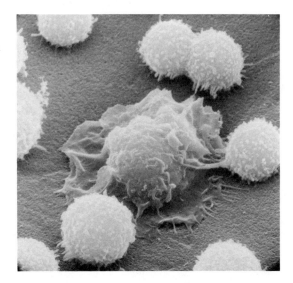

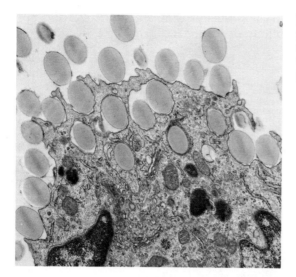

**Figure 7.22** Guinea pig macrophage ingesting polystyrene beads (14,000×). Some beads are already enclosed in vacuoles, called phagosomes, while others are in the process of being engulfed. [Courtesy of Dr. Robert J. North.]

Macrophages are highly phagocytic (Figure 7.22). They engulf foreign particles, decrepit cells and so on into phagocytic vacuoles. These fuse with lysosomes, and the contents are digested by the various hydrolases stored within lysosomes.

Phagocytosis is preceded by the binding of the particle to the surface of the macrophage. Particles coated with specific antibody ("opsonized"; see Figure 2.5) or antibody and complement adhere especially well. This is because macrophages carry surface receptors for the Fc region of IgG and receptors for the third component of complement (C3b). The Fc receptors are revealed by the rosettes that macrophages form with antibody-coated red cells (**EA**); the C3b receptors by the rosettes they form with **EAC** (Figure 7.15). Rosetting is followed by phagocytosis.

Some macrophages also express Ia antigens on their surface. This is particularly apparent with macrophages harvested from regions of intense immune activity.

Macrophages, at least $Ia^+$ macrophages, appear to be needed in order for lymphocytes to respond to antigen. This is rather puzzling because phagocytosis results in the engulfment and digestion of antigen. Perhaps macrophages do not degrade *all* the antigen to which they are exposed but retain some of it to be "presented" to lymphocytes. Certainly macrophages can often be seen in close association with lymphocytes. Although this association occurs in the absence of antigen, the binding of lymphocytes and macrophages is greatly enhanced in the presence of antigen.

### Dendritic Cells

Dendritic cells are also large, motile cells. They usually have several elongated pseudopodia. Their smooth surface also distinguishes them (Figure 7.23). Dendritic cells comprise approximately 1% of the cells in

**Figure 7.23** Two dendritic cells (lower left and upper right) from the spleen of a mouse (2200×). Compare their smooth surface with that of the two macrophages visible at the upper left. [Courtesy of Ralph M. Steinman, from R. M. Steinman et al., *J. Exp. Med.* **149**:1, 1979.]

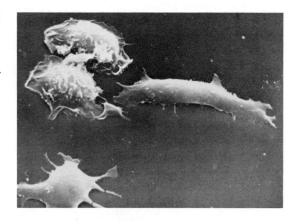

the spleen and lymph nodes. Normal skin contains a sizeable population of similar cells called *Langerhans cells.*

Dendritic cells are potent stimulators of the mixed lymphocyte reaction and of the induction of $T_C$ cells. Langerhans cells pick up antigens applied to the skin (e.g., the active ingredient of the poison ivy plant) and migrate with these into the lymph nodes draining the area where they elicit the typical DTH response of contact sensitivity (see Section 18.7). Dendritic cells are richly coated with Ia antigens. In Chapter 11, we shall examine the evidence that these play a vital role in the presentation of conventional antigen to T lymphocytes.

The role of dendritic cells in the induction of immunity has only begun to be appreciated in recent years. Because of the intimate association of dendritic cells with macrophages, it may turn out that the antigen-presenting role so often attributed to macrophages is, in fact, largely the responsibility of the dendritic cells intermixed with them. Further research should clarify this point.

## ADDITIONAL READING

1. Butcher, E. C., and I. L. Weissman, "Lymphoid Tissues and Organs," in W. E. Paul (ed.), *Fundamental Immunology,* Raven Press, New York, 1984.

2. Dialynas, D. P., et al., "Characterization of the Murine T Cell Surface Molecule, Designated L3T4, Identified by Monoclonal Antibody GK1.5: Similarity of L3T4 to the Human Leu-3/T4 Molecule," *J. Immunol.* **131**:2445, 1983.

3. Gelin, Catherine, et al., "The Heterogeneity and Functional Capacities of Human Thymocyte Subpopulations," *Proc. Natl. Acad. Sci. USA* **81**:4912, 1984.

4. Hogarth, P. M., and I. F. C. McKenzie, "Lymphocyte Antigens," in W. E. Paul (ed.), *Fundamental Immunology,* Raven Press, New York, 1984. Mostly of mice.

5. Huber, B., et al., "Independent Differentiative Pathways of Ly1 and Ly23 Subclasses of T Cells," *J. Exp. Med.* **144**:1128, 1976. (Reprinted in V. L. Sato and M. L. Gefter, *Cellular Immunology,* Addison-Wesley Publishing Co., Reading, MA, 1982.)

6. Miller, J. F. A. P., "Immunological Functions of the Thymus", *The Lancet* September 30, 1961. Describes the effects of neonatal thymectomy in mice. (Reprinted in V. L. Sato and M. L. Gefter, *Cellular Immunology*, Addison-Wesley Publishing Co., Reading, MA, 1982.)

7. Sharon, N., "Lectins," *Scientific American* **236**(6):108, June, 1977 (Offprint No. 1360).

# PART **IV**

# Immune Responsiveness

# CHAPTER 8

# The Response of B Lymphocytes to Antigen

## 8.1 The Dilemma of Antibody Diversity

By 1941 it was clear that antibodies are proteins. Although little was known about their structure, it appeared that antibody molecules, of whatever specificity, were rather similar to one another in such properties as electrophoretic mobility (hence isoelectric point), dimensions, and amino acid composition. On the other hand, the work of half a century had suggested that the capacity to synthesize antibodies of differing specificities was virtually limitless. No molecular configuration was found that could not serve as an antigenic determinant and elicit antibodies specific for it. And, as we have seen in Section 4.5, such antibodies are often capable of discriminating between subtle alterations in the structure of a determinant (refer to Figure 4.15). Thus it was believed that the humoral immune response was one of almost limitless specificity. Finally, the genetic control of protein synthesis was beginning to be glimpsed through the work of Beadle and Tatum on nutritional mutants in *Neurospora.*

All of this presented a dilemma. On the one hand, antibodies seemed to belong to a set of proteins of limited structural heterogeneity. On the other hand, on the basis of antigen-binding specificity, they seemed to belong to a set of proteins of almost inconceivable heterogeneity. But if each protein is encoded by a single gene, what accounted for such diversity?

In an effort to resolve this dilemma, Pauling suggested that antibodies are synthesized by "instruction." He proposed that globulin molecules of limited structural heterogeneity develop antibody specificity through interaction with antigen. The antigen serves as a template to establish antibody specificity. In this view, the globulin molecule is like a wad of modeling clay. Brought into contact with a particular antigenic determinant, the globulin molecule takes on a surface configuration complementary to that of the determinant (Figure 8.1). In this way, a specific binding site for antigen is created and thus a unique antibody molecule of defined specificity is synthesized.

As it turned out, the instructional theory was quite wrong. Let us examine the evidence that led to its rejection. The theory predicted that antibody-synthesizing cells must contain antigen. However, using fluorescent antibodies as probes (see Section 5.14), Coons found that no antigen could be detected in plasma cells secreting a particular antibody. How could antigen serve as a template for the synthesis of a particular antibody if the antigen was not present in the antibody synthesizing cell? Furthermore, the instructional theory fails to explain the kinetics and magnitude of the secondary response. A second dose of antigen of the same size as that given weeks or months earlier should — according to the instructional theory — produce another response just like the first one. But as we have seen (Section 2.4), the secondary response to an antigen is swifter and larger than the primary response (Figure 2.17).

Another corollary of the instructional theory is that if antibodies should be reversibly denatured ("unfolded") and then allowed to renature *in the absence of antigen,* they should fail to regain specificity. How-

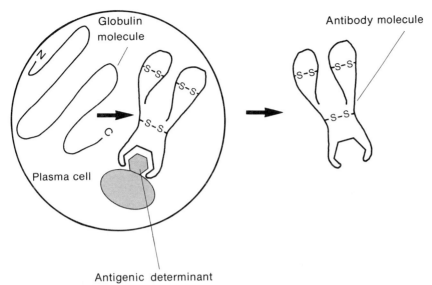

**Figure 8.1** Postulated mechanism of the synthesis of antibody molecules by "instruction."

ever, as Haber showed, the reverse was true. He denatured antibodies so that they completely lost their ability to bind antigen. Upon restoring physiological conditions of pH and salt concentration, but in the complete absence of antigen, their antigen-binding capacity was restored. In fact, this important experiment leads us far beyond the world of antibodies. The function of any protein, be it antibody, enzyme or whatever, is dependent upon its three-dimensional configuration. And its three-dimensional configuration in any given physiological environment is dependent solely upon the particular sequence of amino acids present in that protein. Thus, tertiary structure is an inevitable outcome of primary structure. The shape of a protein molecule is not impressed upon it by an outside agent; it is a reflection of the particular sequence of amino acids in that protein.

So what alternatives are there to the instructional theory? Let us now examine a theory, supported by a wealth of laboratory data, which has served as the stimulus for many productive studies in immunology. This is the theory of *clonal selection*.

## 8.2 The Theory of Clonal Selection

Several essential elements of the theory of clonal selection were proposed at the turn of the century by the pioneering immunologist Paul Ehrlich. He suggested that *prior* to exposure to antigen, the body contains cells bearing receptors able to bind that antigen. The process of binding causes the cell to manufacture more receptors of that particular specificity and, eventually, to shed these receptors into the surroundings (Figure 8.2). The shed receptors are the antibodies.

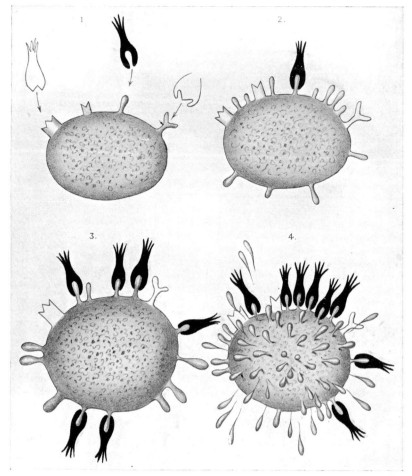

**Figure 8.2**  Clonal selection as envisaged by Paul Ehrlich at the turn of the century. The binding of antigen to a cell bearing the appropriate receptors causes an increase in the number of these receptors and their release—as antibodies—from the cell. In Ehrlich's view, each cell was multispecific, bearing receptors of many different types. The bulk of the evidence today suggests that most antigen-binding cells are monospecific with all the receptors on one cell having a single specificity. [Courtesy of The Royal Society from P. Ehrlich, *Proc. Roy. Soc.*, Series B, **66**:424, 1900.]

We owe the modern form of the theory of clonal selection to the insights of Burnet, Jerne, and Talmadge. The modern theory rests upon several postulates.

1. Every immunocompetent animal carries a heterogeneous population of cells (lymphocytes) capable of specifically binding antigen. We shall call these *antigen-binding cells* or ABCs (Figure 8.3).
2. The specificity of an ABC resides in the structure of receptor molecules present on its surface.
3. Interaction of an antigen with the receptors on an ABC stimulates it to undergo mitosis and thus to develop into a clone of cells expressing the same receptor specificity (Figure 8.3).

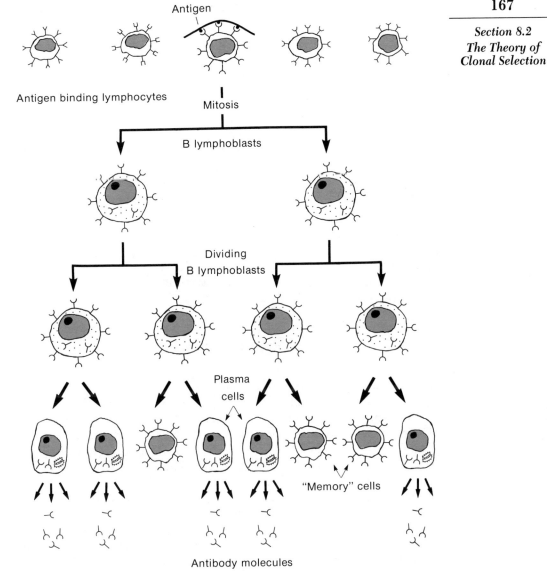

Antigen

Antigen binding lymphocytes

Mitosis

B lymphoblasts

Dividing
B lymphoblasts

Plasma
cells

"Memory" cells

Antibody molecules

Figure 8.3  Schematic representation of the clonal selection theory. Clonal selection leads to the production of antibody-secreting plasma cells *and* an enlarged pool of specific antigen-sensitive ("memory") cells. The triggering of B lymphocytes by antigen is probably a more complex process than shown here, at least for thymus-dependent (TD) antigens.

4. Among the progeny of this clone of ABCs will be plasma cells that synthesize and secrete antibody molecules of the same specificity and affinity as the receptor molecules on the ABCs that were stimulated by antigen.

Note that in sharp contrast to the instructional theory, the repertoire of ABCs in an animal is present *prior* to exposure to antigen. The theory of clonal selection states that the presence of antigen *selects* those ABCs precommitted to expressing receptors for that antigen.

While not absolutely vital to the theory, clonal selection also implies that

1. A plasma cell is a member of a clone and secretes just one kind of antibody molecule.
2. The antigen-binding cell is monospecific; it bears surface receptors of only one specificity; that is, all of its receptors for antigen are alike.

Finally, the theory holds that positive selection only occurs for clones capable of binding determinants foreign to the host. Any clones bearing receptors for self components are selected against or at least prevented from being stimulated. In this way, the ability to distinguish self from nonself is established and autoimmune responses are avoided. Let us now examine some of the evidence that has strongly supported the theory.

## 8.3 Antigen-Binding Cells (ABCs) Have Surface Receptors upon Which the Specificity of the Immune Response Depends

### Negative Selection of Antigen-Binding Cells

In 1969 Ada and Byrt reported their demonstration of (1) the existence of specific antigen-binding cells prior to exposure to the antigen and (2) the dependence of the subsequent antibody response on these cells. Their test antigen was a protein, called flagellin, extracted from the flagella of one strain of the bacterium *Salmonella adelaide* and polymerized. We will call this antigen "POL-A." They were able to label this antigen with $^{125}I$ to a very high specific activity. As a control, they used a preparation of polymerized flagellin isolated from a different strain of *Salmonella.* Let us call this antigen "POL-B."

They mixed the radioactive POL-A with a suspension of spleen cells from mice never exposed to the antigen. After washing away any unbound antigen from the cell suspension, they fixed the cells on a slide and coated them with a photographic emulsion, assuming that if any cells had bound the antigen, the radioactivity emitted from those cells would expose the emulsion. By this technique of **autoradiography,** they showed that approximately one in 5000 spleen cells had bound the antigen. They also showed that the binding was blocked if the cells were pretreated with an antimouse immunoglobulin serum. This suggested that the receptors for antigen were immunoglobulins. (The presence of immunoglobulins on the surface of B cells can be demonstrated directly with fluorescent anti-immunoglobulin antibodies — Figure 8.17.)

The specific activity of the $^{125}I$-labeled flagellin was so high that any cells binding the antigen would, after 16–20 hours, be killed by the radiation. After treating a spleen cell suspension with the radioactive POL-A, Ada and Byrt washed the free antigen away and injected the suspension into syngeneic mice whose own immune system had been

**169**

*Section 8.3
Antigen-Binding
Cells (ABCs) Have
Surface Receptors
upon Which the
Specificity of the
Immune Response
Depends*

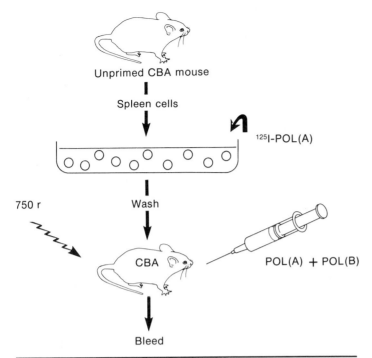

| Pretreatment of spleen cells | Anti-POL(A) antibodies | Anti-POL(B) antibodies |
|---|---|---|
| $^{125}$I-POL(A) | ± | + + + + |
| Nonradioactive POL(A) | + + + | + + + + |
| None | + + + | + + + + |

**Figure 8.4** Protocol and results of the experiment of Ada and Byrt (*Nature* **222**:1291, 1969). Destruction of those unprimed spleen cells capable of binding POL-A destroyed the capacity of the cell suspension to mount a response to POL-A upon transfer to an irradiated recipient. The ability of the cell suspension to respond to POL-B was unimpaired.

destroyed by x rays. The animals were then injected with both POL-A and POL-B (nonradioactive in each case). While these reconstituted mice were able to respond to POL-B, they were unable to produce significant amounts of antibodies to POL-A (Figure 8.4).

Variants of this experiment have since been performed in many other laboratories. The results are all comparable: an animal never before exposed to a particular antigen (i.e., "unprimed" or "virgin") possesses a low frequency (from $10^{-3}$ to $10^{-4}$) of lymphocytes capable of binding that antigen (Figure 8.5). Removal of these cells, for example, by a suicide technique, removes the animal's capacity to respond to that particular antigen.

Autoradiography of spleen cells from *antigen-primed* animals reveals a different story. After mounting a primary immune response, the frequency of ABCs for that antigen rises. Here, then, is the basis for the secondary response: an enlarged pool of ABCs.

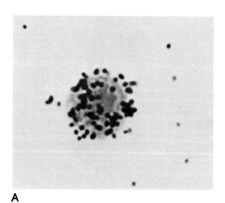

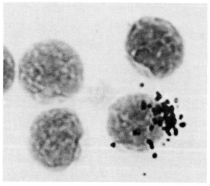

**A**                                     **B**

**Figure 8.5**  A: Autoradiograph of a lymph node cell to which molecules of tritiated POL have bound (at 0 °C). This cell was taken from an immunized mouse. B: After 15 minutes incubation at 37 °C, the radioactivity is clustered in one region because of capping of the cell's antigen-binding receptors (see Figures 8.17 and 8.18). Note the other cells that have not bound any of the radioactive antigen. Presumably they have receptors for other antigens. [Courtesy of E. Diener from E. Diener and V. H. Paetkau, *Proc. Natl. Acad. Sci. USA* 69:2364, 1972.]

### Positive Selection of Antigen-Binding Cells

Antigen suicide is a process by which specific ABCs are selected *against*. Demonstration of the specificity of the procedure depends upon showing that specific immune responsiveness has disappeared. To complete the story, it would be desirable to show selection *for* specific ABCs. One approach is to pass a cell suspension through a column packed with antigen-coated beads. Cells bearing receptors for the antigen should stick to the beads, while all other cells should pass unimpeded through the column. A number of investigators have shown that the pass-through cells are depleted of reactivity to the antigen on the beads. In other words, when these cells are used to reconstitute an irradiated animal, the animal regains the capacity to respond to all antigens except the one used to coat the beads (Figure 8.6). This is simply another example of selecting against a population of ABCs. However, it is also possible to remove the stuck cells from the beads by passing free antigen through the column. One would expect that the eluted cells would be enriched with the appropriate ABCs. Unfortunately, the process of dissociating the cells from the beads is apt to damage the cells, and most attempts to show enrichment of ABCs by this procedure have been disappointing.

Two techniques for enrichment do yield healthy cell suspensions. These are *hapten–gelatin fractionation* and the *fluorescence activated cell sorter* (FACS).

*Hapten–Gelatin Fractionation.*  A variety of haptens can be covalently coupled to gelatin. The resulting material can be used as an immunoadsorbent just like the antigen-coated beads described above. If,

**171**

*Section 8.3
Antigen-Binding
Cells (ABCs) Have
Surface Receptors
upon Which the
Specificity of the
Immune Response
Depends*

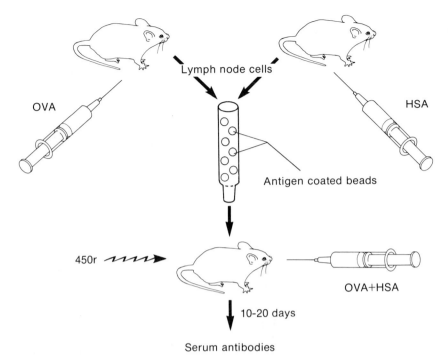

| Beads coated with | Anti-OVA | Anti-HSA |
|:---:|:---:|:---:|
| OVA | 0 | + + |
| HSA | + + | 0 |
| Not used | + + | + + + |

**Figure 8.6** Negative selection of antigen-binding cells. The presence of free antigen in the column fluid eliminates the effect presumably by occupying the receptors on the ABCs that would otherwise bind to the beads. [Based on the work of H. Wigzell and B. Anderson, *J. Exp. Med.* **129:**23, 1969.]

for example, a suspension of *normal* mouse spleen cells is spread over a layer of DNP-gelatin, a small fraction (about 0.1%) of the cells will stick to the material. The sticking occurs because of the interaction between cells containing receptors for DNP and the DNP groups on the gelatin. This binding is specific because it can be prevented by adding soluble hapten (e.g., DNP–lysine) to the mixture. The binding is also inhibited by antiserum against mouse immunoglobulins, thus indicating that the DNP receptors are immunoglobulins.

The great advantage of this system over the glass bead system is that warming the gelatin to 37°C liquefies it without harming the cells. Treatment of the resulting cell suspension with collagenase (gelatin is made from collagen) removes any residual antigen bound to the cells. These cells retain their viability and can be tested for their capacity to mount an immune response to the antigen used to select them.

Nossal and his coworkers have demonstrated that from 0.01 to 0.003% of the cells in a normal mouse spleen are ABCs for the hapten NIP (4-hydroxy-5-iodo-3-nitrophenyl acetyl) (Figure 8.7). By hapten–gelatin fractionation, they were able to produce a viable cell population

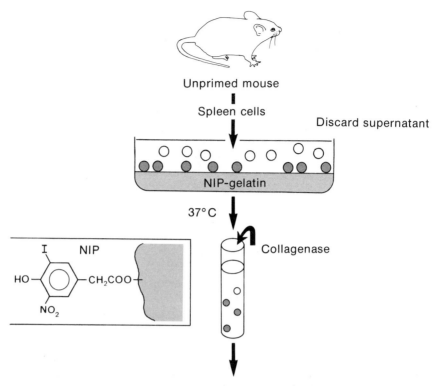

**Figure 8.7** Positive selection of NIP-binding spleen cells by hapten–gelatin fractionation. Inset: structure of NIP, (4-hydroxy-5-iodo-3-nitrophenyl) acetyl. A related hapten, NP, lacks the iodine atom. [From G. J. V. Nossal et al., "Hapten-specific B lymphocytes: Enrichment, Cloning, Receptor Analysis, and Tolerance Induction" in *Origins of Lymphocyte Diversity,* Cold Spring Harbor Symposia on Quantitative Biology, Vol. XLI, The Cold Spring Harbor Laboratory, 1977.]

in which 7% of the recovered cells were able to grow into clones of anti-NIP antibody-secreting cells (revealed by a hemolytic plaque assay). This represented roughly a 1000-fold enrichment. Here is clear evidence of clonal selection in an in vitro system. A naturally occurring population of specific ABCs has been selected *for* by exploiting the interaction between the antigen and receptors on the cell surface. From this population develop a thousand times as many anti-NIP-secreting clones as would develop from an equal number of unfractionated spleen cells.

*Fluorescence-Activated Cell Sorter (FACS).* Chapter 5 describes how fluorescent antibodies can be used to identify individual cells containing the appropriate antigen. Thanks to the cooperation of cellular immunologists and electronic engineers at Stanford University, a machine now exists that can separate cells on the basis of their fluorescence and also their size. This is the fluorescence-activated cell sorter (FACS). Briefly, it works in the following way. A cell suspension containing a subpopulation of fluorescence-labeled cells is directed into a thin stream so that all the cells pass in a single file. The stream emerges from a nozzle vibrating at 40,000 cycles per second. The vibrations break the stream up into 40,000 discrete droplets each second. Some of these droplets may contain a cell. A laser beam is directed at the stream just before it breaks up into droplets, and as each labeled cell passes through the beam, its resulting fluorescence is detected by a sensitive photocell (Figure 8.8). A second photocell detects laser light that is scattered by the cell and this provides a measure of the size of each cell. If the signals from these two detectors meet either of the two sets of criteria set for fluorescence and size, an electrical charge (+ or −) is given to the stream. The droplets retain this charge as they pass between a pair of charged metal plates. Positively charged drops are attracted to the negatively charged plate and vice versa (Figure 8.8). Uncharged droplets (those that contain no cell or contain a cell that fails to meet the desired criteria of fluorescence

**173**

*Section 8.3*
*Antigen-Binding*
*Cells (ABCs) Have*
*Surface Receptors*
*upon Which the*
*Specificity of the*
*Immune Response*
*Depends*

**Figure 8.8** The fluorescence-activated cell sorter. See text for the details of its operation.

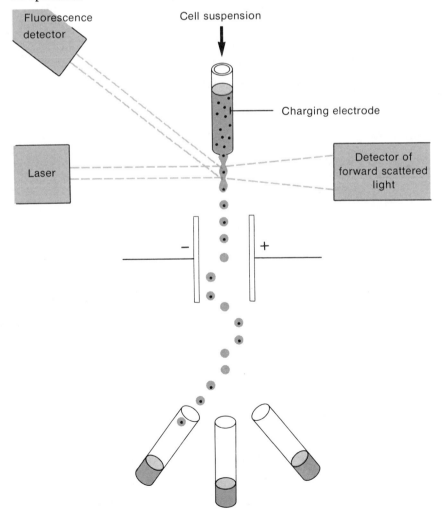

and size) pass straight into a third container and are later discarded. With this apparatus, some $18 \times 10^6$ cells can be sorted each hour. The cells are not damaged in the process of sorting. In fact, because the machine can be set to ignore the droplets containing dead cells, the percent viability of the sorted cells can be made substantially higher than that in the original suspension.

The FACS has made possible many important findings in cellular immunology. Let's look at one study, reported by Julius and Herzenberg at Stanford, that bears directly on the topic at hand.

**Figure 8.9** Adoptive transfer of DNP responsiveness by unfractionated spleen cells (right) and a population enriched with DNP-binding spleen cells by use of the fluorescence-activated cell sorter *(left)*. Each group of recipients also received an injection of helper T cells ($T_H$) from mice primed with the carrier (KLH). [Based on M. H. Julius and L. A. Herzenberg, *J. Exp. Med.* 140:904, 1974. Reprinted in V. L. Sato and M. L. Gefter, *Cellular Immunology*, Addison-Wesley Publishing Co., Inc., Reading, MA, 1982.]

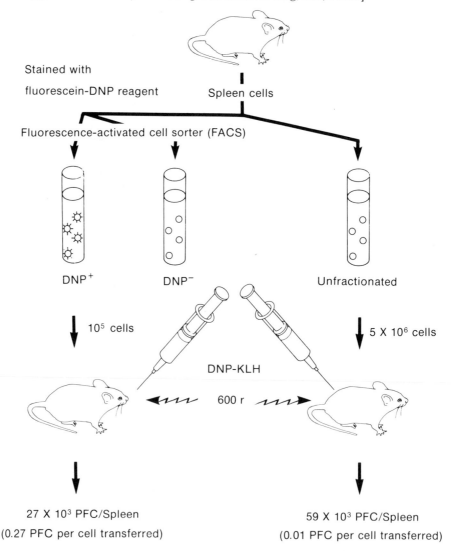

Stained with
fluorescein-DNP reagent     Spleen cells

Fluorescence-activated cell sorter (FACS)

DNP$^+$     DNP$^-$     Unfractionated

$10^5$ cells     5 $\times$ $10^6$ cells

DNP-KLH

600 r

27 $\times$ $10^3$ PFC/Spleen     59 $\times$ $10^3$ PFC/Spleen
(0.27 PFC per cell transferred)     (0.01 PFC per cell transferred)

These workers prepared a spleen cell suspension from BALB/c mice and treated the cells with a fluorescent "stain" containing DNP groups. From 1–2% of the spleen cells bound the fluorescent stain. The suspension was passed through the FACS, producing a cell suspension enriched to 91% fluorescent cells ("DNP$^+$"). Heavily irradiated (600 r) mice were given intravenous injections of either the enriched DNP$^+$ suspension or a suspension of unfractionated spleen cells (Figure 8.9). Five days later, all the animals were immunized with DNP bound to a carrier. One week after that, their spleens were assayed for anti-DNP plaque-forming cells (PFC) by the hemolytic plaque technique (Section 5.11). The results are shown in Figure 8.9. Injections of $1 \times 10^5$ DNP$^+$ cells gave approximately one-half the number of PFC as a *fifty times larger* dose ($5 \times 10^6$) of unfractionated spleen cells. In other words, the FACS had enriched the pool of anti-DNP precursors some 25-fold. These results show that it is possible to select for a population of specific antigen-binding cells (DNP–ABCs), and that such an enriched population confers—by adoptive transfer—a larger anti-DNP antibody response than does a normal population of spleen cells.

## 8.4  The Affinity of the Receptors on ABCs is the Same as That of the Antibodies Secreted by Their Progeny

The amount of antigen used to immunize an animal often has a pronounced effect on the average affinity ($K_0$, see Section 4.4) of the antibodies produced. Small doses of antigen produce a response characterized by high affinity antibodies. Large doses of antigen may elicit larger *amounts* of antibody, but these antibodies are usually of lower affinity than those elicited by smaller doses of antigen.

The concept of clonal selection provides a satisfying explanation of this phenomenon. We assume that the pool of cells capable of binding to any given antigenic determinant is heterogeneous with respect to the affinity of binding (Figure 8.10). Some cells will bear receptors capable of binding the determinant with high affinity; others will bear receptors of lower affinity. If only a small amount of antigen is presented to the pool of ABCs, then we would expect those cells with high affinity receptors to be more successful at binding antigen and being stimulated. Development of these clones should yield an antiserum containing antibodies of high affinity. Exposed to large amounts of antigen, on the other hand, all of the ABCs will be able to bind antigen, and each will develop into a clone secreting antibody of the same affinity. The pooled contributions of all of these clones will yield an antiserum with a lower $K_0$.

With the fluorescence-activated cell sorter (FACS), it is possible to examine directly the relationship between the affinity of the receptors on unprimed ABCs and the affinity of the antibodies secreted by the plasma cells derived from them. Julius and Herzenberg repeated the experiments described in the previous section using a much lower concentration of the DNP "stain." They reasoned that with a *limiting amount* of stain, only those ABCs with high affinity receptors would

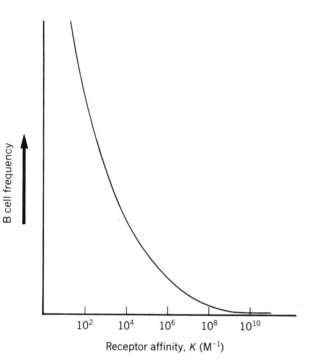

**Figure 8.10** Hypothetical distribution of receptor affinities on B cells capable of binding a particular antigenic determinant. Limiting doses of antigen would be preferentially bound by B cells carrying high affinity receptors, and the resulting antiserum would express low amounts of antibodies with a high $K_0$.

succeed in binding the stain. Once again they fractionated normal mouse spleen cells into a population that took up the stain ($DNP^+$) and one that did not ($DNP^-$). Each of these populations was injected into irradiated mice. One week after immunization with DNP–KLH, the anti-DNP response was measured by the hemolytic plaque assay. Varying concentrations of DNP–lysine were added to the assay dishes with the expectation that this reagent would inhibit the formation of plaques by competing with the DNP-coated red cells for the anti-DNP antibodies being secreted. Both groups of mice produced anti-DNP plaques. But as Figure 8.11 shows, mice that had received $DNP^+$ cells produced plaques that were much more easily inhibited by DNP–lysine than was the case for the $DNP^-$ animals. This showed that the antibodies secreted by the progeny of the $DNP^+$ cells had the *higher affinity* for the soluble ligand. Animals injected with unfractionated spleen cells produced plaques that were intermediate in the ease with which they could be inhibited. Here, then, is a direct demonstration of clonal selection: the affinity of the receptor on the ABC is directly correlated with the affinity of the antibodies secreted by the progeny of that cell.

### Affinity Maturation

The average association constant ($K_0$) of an antiserum is influenced not only by antigen dose but also by time elapsed following immunization. Eisen and Siskind demonstrated this using rabbits immunized with DNP–BGG. In the first week or two following immunization with 5 mg of the antigen, the average affinity ($K_0$) of the antibodies for DNP–L-

**Figure 8.11** Demonstration of a direct correlation between the avidity of antigen-binding cells for DNP and the affinity of the anti-DNP antibodies secreted by their progeny. [From M. H. Julius and L. A. Herzenberg, *J. Exp. Med.* **140**:904, 1974.]

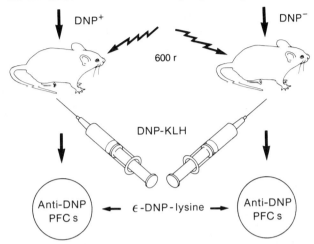

Spleen cells separated on fluorescence-activated cell sorter using limited amount of DNP stain. Only high avidity cells stained.

DNP⁺   600 r   DNP⁻

DNP-KLH

Anti-DNP PFCs ← ε-DNP-lysine → Anti-DNP PFCs

Plaques easily inhibited
∴ high-avidity cells

Plaques resistant to inhibition
∴ low-avidity cells

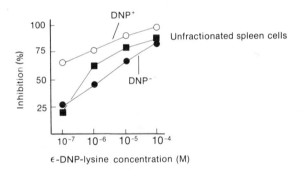

lysine was approximately $10^5\,M^{-1}$. By two months, the $K_0$ of the antibodies harvested from the same animals had risen to approximately $10^8\,M^{-1}$. This phenomenon is called affinity maturation.

How can we explain affinity maturation in terms of clonal selection? One clue is provided by Eisen and Siskind's finding that affinity maturation is most pronounced with small doses of antigen. When the antigen is first administered, we assume that many precursor cells, representing a range of affinities, will be stimulated into clonal development. If our assumption is correct that low affinity ABCs are more abundant than high affinity ABCs (Figure 8.10), we would expect their product to be dominant in the antiserum. As time goes on, antigen levels would fall as the antigen is catabolized. With antigen becoming increasingly limited, we would expect only those ABCs with high affinity receptors to be stimulated.

But this cannot be the whole story. Figure 8.12 shows affinity maturation of anti-S3 serum samples harvested at different times from a single rabbit. However, during the entire period, the rabbit was receiving weekly injections of antigen. Thus a shortage of antigen could not be driving affinity maturation in this case. However, animals immunized in this way make copious amounts of anti-S3 antibodies (Figure 2.7), enough to bind all the freshly injected antigen. Thus the serum antibodies can compete with ABCs for the available antigen. As the $K_0$ of the serum rises, only those ABCs with receptors of still higher affinity would be stimulated. If these higher affinity ABCs represent just a small part of the pool (Figure 8.10), then we would expect that the *number* of clones participating in the late stages of maturation might be smaller. And, in fact, electrophoresis of the serum of these animals often reveals what appear to be the products of a small number of clones dominating the response (Figure 2.7).

Why do the high affinity ABCs not participate in the response from the very first? Perhaps they do, but their numbers are so small that their contribution is swamped by the outpouring from cells of lower affinity. But recent evidence suggests that in some cases they are not even there early in the response!

Milstein and his co-workers (see reference 5 at the end of the chapter) have sequenced the mRNA from a series of hybridomas generated

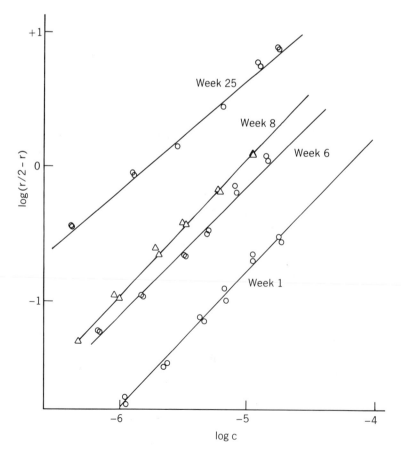

**Figure 8.12** Sips plots showing affinity maturation in the serum of a rabbit repeatedly immunized with type 3 pneumococci. The average association constant ($K_0$) of the antibodies rose from $1.6 \times 10^4 \, M^{-1}$ at week 1 to $6 \times 10^5 \, M^{-1}$ at week 25. [From J. W. Kimball, *Immunochemistry* **9**:1169, 1972.]

against the antigen 2-phenyloxazolone. They find that one week after immunization, most of the hybridomas they created express what appear to be inherited ("germline") genes for the L and H chains. By day 14, however, most of the hybridomas are expressing L and H chain genes that seem to be mutated versions of the genes used earlier in the response. For example, by day 14, mutations leading to an average of two changes in amino acid residues had occurred in the L chain genes they analyzed. What is particularly revealing for our story is that the day-14 mRNA molecules encoded antibodies with substantially higher affinity than was the case at day 7. Most of the day 7 hybridomas secreted antibodies with a $K$ around $3 \times 10^6$ $M^{-1}$. The association constants of the antibodies secreted by day-14 hybridomas were on the order of $20 \times 10^6$ $M^{-1}$. Most of the point mutations occurred in codons responsible for the hypervariable regions of the antibody molecules; i.e., the regions responsible for binding antigen (Section 9.13). These point mutations clearly generated antibody molecules with a higher affinity for the antigen. Presumably, those ABCs expressing mutated receptors better able to bind antigen were selected for clonal expansion and produced this example of affinity maturation. The role of somatic mutation in the generation of antibody diversity is explored further in Section 10.12.

**179**

*Section 8.5*
*The Receptors on Antigen-Binding Cells Have the Same Idiotype as the Antibodies Secreted by Their Progeny*

## 8.5 The Receptors on Antigen-Binding Cells Have the Same Idiotype as the Antibodies Secreted by Their Progeny

The idiotype of an antibody molecule consists of a small set of antigenic determinants associated with antibody molecules of a particular specificity and affinity. In fact, you may recall from the discussion of idiotypes in Section 2.3 that idiotypic determinants are generally located close to the antigen-binding site of the molecule.

Idiotypes are defined operationally by their interaction with anti-idiotypic sera. Anti-idiotypic sera are best raised in allotypically matched animals of the same species as the producer of the idiotype. Other species can be used, but then extensive absorptions must be carried out on the antiserum in order to remove anti-isotype and/or anti-allotype antibodies. It is also best to use a homogeneous preparation of the idiotype for immunization. Often this is not feasible because, as we have seen, even a purified preparation of, for example, anti-DNP antibodies consists of a pool of molecules having substantial diversity of affinity, electrophoretic mobility, and thus structure.

Myeloma proteins, on the other hand, are an excellent source of homogeneous immunoglobulins. Myeloma proteins are the product of a neoplastic (cancerous) clone of plasma cells. These plasma cell tumors are called *plasmacytomas*. The uncontrolled proliferation of the clone yields large amounts of a single kind of immunoglobulin molecule (Figure 4.17).

Myelomas can be induced (by intraperitoneal injections of mineral oil or similar materials) in mice of the BALB/c and NZB strains. Once in-

$$CH_3-\overset{\overset{\displaystyle CH_3}{|}}{\underset{\underset{\displaystyle CH_3}{|}}{\overset{+}{N}}}-CH_2-CH_2-\overset{\overset{\displaystyle O^-}{|}}{\underset{\underset{\displaystyle O^-}{|}}{P}}=O$$

**Figure 8.13** Phosphorylcholine (PC), a major determinant of the C polysaccharide.

duced, a given plasmacytoma can be propagated in other mice of the same strain. In this way, large amounts of the protein produced by the tumor can be harvested and studied.

The induction of a plasmacytoma appears to be a random event. Attempts to elicit myeloma proteins of a predetermined specificity have been disappointing. However, if one screens a myeloma protein against an extensive panel of antigens, it is sometimes possible to find an antigen to which the protein binds with a reasonably high affinity.

For reasons that are not entirely clear, a surprising number of myeloma proteins induced in mice precipitate with "C polysaccharide," a polysaccharide found in the walls (not the capsule) of pneumococci. These myeloma proteins also bind to phosphorylcholine (PC), a group (Figure 8.13) that contributes a major antigenic determinant to the C polysaccharide.

Two PC-binding myeloma proteins have been intensively studied. These are designated TEPC-15 and MOPC-167 (MOPC = *m*ineral *o*il *p*lasma*c*ytoma). While they share the same antigenic specificity for PC, they are different proteins. TEPC-15 binds to PC with a $K$ (not $K_0$; these are homogeneous proteins) of $2.3 \times 10^5 \text{ M}^{-1}$, while the $K$ for MOPC-167 is $1.2 \times 10^5 \text{ M}^{-1}$. Antibodies raised against the idiotypic determinants of TEPC-15 do not bind to MOPC-167 and vice versa.

When BALB/c mice are immunized with the C polysaccharide (by injecting them with "rough" pneumococci — see Section 2.1), most of the antibodies produced in the primary response express the same idiotype as TEPC-15. When spleen cells from these animals are examined in the hemolytic plaque assay, the addition of anti-TEPC-15 serum to the dishes strongly inhibits the appearance of plaques. Anti-idiotypic antibodies raised against MOPC-167 are far less inhibitory (Figure 8.14).

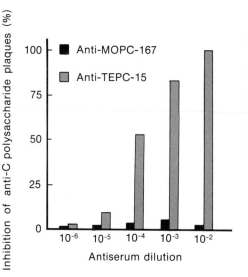

**Figure 8.14** An anti-idiotypic serum raised against the phosphorylcholine-binding myeloma protein TEPC-15 strongly inhibits the formation of plaques by the spleen cells of BALB/c mice immunized with the C polysaccharide. An anti-idiotypic serum raised against MOPC-167, another PC-binding myeloma protein, produces little or no inhibition. Thus the natural response of BALB/c mice to immunization with C polysaccharide is dominated by antibodies expressing the TEPC-15 idiotype. [From H. Cosenza and H. Köhler, *Proc. Natl. Acad. Sci. USA* **69**:2701, 1972.]

**181**

*Section 8.5*
*The Receptors on*
*Antigen-Binding*
*Cells Have the Same*
*Idiotype as the*
*Antibodies Secreted*
*by Their Progeny*

Presumably the anti-TEPC-15 antibodies bind at or close to the antigen-binding site on the antibodies being released by a majority of the plasma cells. This binding prevents the antibodies from binding to the red cells coated with C polysaccharide. Both the antigen and the anti-idiotypic antibody molecules are competing for the same unique site on the secreted antibodies.

In 1972 Cosenza and Köhler secured evidence that the PC-binding plasma cell precursors in BALB/c mice express the TEPC-15 idiotype just as the anti-PC antibodies do. They found that the injection of anti-TEPC-15 serum into a mouse had a powerful inhibitory effect on the *induction* of immunity to PC. The number of anti-PC plaque-forming cells was greatly reduced in BALB/c mice receiving 0.3 ml of anti-TEPC-15 serum one day prior to immunization with rough pneumococci. The effect was specific. (1) anti-MOPC-167 serum had no suppressive effect on the induction of anti-PC plaques, and (2) anti-TEPC-15 serum had no effect on the response to SRBC (Figure 8.15).

These results show that the receptors on the PC-binding cells in un-primed BALB/c mice carry the same idiotypic determinants as the anti-PC antibodies secreted by the progeny of these cells. Thus we see for idiotypes, as we have for specificity and affinity, that the receptors on ABCs are equivalent to the antigen-binding sites on the antibodies secreted by their progeny.

The discovery that anti-idiotypic antibodies are also antireceptor antibodies raises several fascinating possibilities. Could anti-idiotypic antibodies be used to *specifically* suppress allergic responses as they do the PC response in BALB/c mice? If this turned out to be feasible, it would represent a major breakthrough in transplantation medicine. Antisera directed against the idiotypes of receptors for the foreign histocompatibility antigens might be able to protect the graft from rejection while not interfering with other immune responses (just as anti-TEPC-15 serum had no effect on the response to SRBC). The present methods for suppressing graft rejection are general, not specific. To the extent that methods of general immunosuppression do their job, they simultaneously expose the transplant recipient to a wide variety of infections because the entire immune system is suppressed.

Considerable evidence exists that the immune system, like all physiological systems, is under homeostatic control. These controls limit the

**Figure 8.15** The ability of the mice to mount a response against phosphorylcholine (PC) was greatly suppressed by injecting them with anti-TEPC-15 serum prior to immunization with pneumococci. This suggests that most of their PC-sensitive B lymphocytes have receptors expressing the same TEPC-15 idiotype that is found on the anti-PC antibodies of these animals. [From H. Cosenza and H. Köhler, *Proc. Natl. Acad. Sci. USA* **69:**2701, 1972.]

| Mice pretreated with 0.3 ml of | Anti-PC PFC/spleen | Anti-SRBC PFC/spleen |
|---|---|---|
| Normal mouse serum | 139,000 | 164,000 |
| Anti-TEPC-15 serum | 1,300 | 106,000 |
| Anti-MOPC-167 serum | 162,000 | 247,000 |

duration and magnitude of the immune response. In Chapter 15 we examine evidence leading to the conclusion that auto-anti-idiotypic antibodies, elicited within the animal in response to its own production of idiotypic antibodies, may play an important role in suppressing further production of those antibodies.

## 8.6 Evidence That Plasma Cells Secrete Only One Kind of Antibody Molecule

One tenet of the modern theory of clonal selection is that each plasma cell is a member of a single clone of cells and secretes antibody molecules of only a single kind. If this is true, we should be able to demonstrate that a single plasma cell produces antibody molecules (1) of a single specificity, (2) of a single isotype, (3) bearing a single set of allotypic determinants, and (4) of a single idiotype. Let us examine the evidence.

### Specificity

The hemolytic plaque assay can be used to demonstrate that individual plasma cells are monospecific. One begins by immunizing an animal against *two* different antigens. The spleen cells are then plated with a mixture of target red cells: one set carrying one antigen; the second set the other. If all plasma cells are monospecific, only cloudy plaques should be seen. This is because a single plasma cell would be able to lyse only those surrounding red cells (about 50% of the total) bearing the antigen against which its antibodies are directed. To take a specific example, let us look at an experiment reported in 1979 by Couderc and his colleagues. They immunized mice against both TNP and phosphorylcholine (PC), each hapten being coupled to hemocyanin. As target cells for the hemolytic plaque assay, they used sheep red blood cells coated with PC and pigeon red cells coated with TNP. Pigeon red cells, like all bird red cells, retain their nucleus and therefore they can easily be distinguished from SRBC under the light microscope (Figure 8.16). Almost all (99%) of the plaques seen were cloudy. Around each of the PFCs, *either* the sheep cells *or* the pigeon cells were lysed. A clear plaque was occasionally seen (Figure 8.16), but when the cell at its center was subcultured, its progeny synthesized antibodies of one or the other specificity, not both. Thus we may conclude that plasma cells secrete antibody molecules of a single specificity.

### Isotype

Plasma cells usually synthesize only a single isotype at any one time. This can be demonstrated with fluorescent antibodies. By preparing fluores-

183

*Section 8.6
Evidence That
Plasma Cells
Secrete Only One
Kind of Antibody
Molecule*

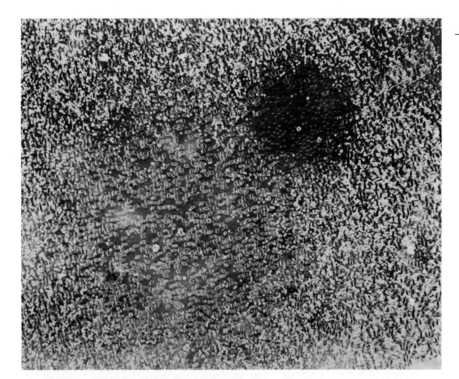

**Figure 8.16** Plaques formed by spleen cells of mice immunized simultaneously with two different antigens and plated with a mixture of sheep red blood cells (SRBC) coated with one antigen, pigeon red blood cells (PRBC) with the other. Most of the plaques were cloudy, with lysis of either the SRBC (left center) or the PRBC, although approximately 1% of the plaques were clear (upper right) with both types of indicator cells lysed. Note the spleen cell at the center of each plaque. The faint objects in the clear plaque are the nuclei remaining after lysis of the pigeon red cells. [Courtesy of Jacques Couderc from J. Couderc et al., *J. Immunol.* **123**:173, 1979.]

cein-tagged antibodies against one isotype (such as IgG) and rhodamine-tagged antibodies against a second (for example, IgA), one can look for the presence of plasma cells that are stained by both reagents. Such double-staining cells are rarely found. However, it has been observed that some normal plasma cells will, for a brief period of time, stain for both IgM and IgG molecules (of the same specificity). The evidence suggests that these cells are in the process of switching over from IgM to IgG production. However, when IgG synthesis begins, the only remaining IgM synthesis is occurring on undegraded messenger RNA molecules. This indicates that in plasma cells gene transcription, if not translation, is restricted at any time to a single isotype. The genetic mechanisms involved in isotype switching are examined in Section 10.10.

## Allotype

Fluorescent antibodies can also be used to examine the antibody allotypes expressed by individual plasma cells. In animals that are heterozygous for the expression of a particular allotype (e.g., b5 and b9, which are expressed on rabbit kappa chains — see Figure 2.15), single plasma cells stain with one or the other fluorescent stain, not both. Thus, while both b5 and b9 molecules are represented in the serum antibody pool of a heterozygous rabbit, any single plasma cell synthesizes one or the other. This phenomenon is called "allelic exclusion." It violates the usual rule that both alleles are expressed in a heterozygous cell. However, an analogous phenomenon does occur in female mammals with the alleles on the X chromosome that undergoes X inactivation in a given cell.

## Idiotype

A single plasma cell secretes antibodies expressing only a single idiotype. You will recall from the preceding section that antibodies against the TEPC-15 idiotype shut off virtually all plaque formation by BALB/c mice immunized against phosphorylcholine (PC). If a plasma cell was producing anti-PC antibodies of *both* the TEPC-15 idiotype and a *second* idiotype (e.g., MOPC-167), the molecules of the second idiotype should still be able to form a plaque.

While there are occasional exceptions, some of which can be explained by known mechanisms and some of which as yet cannot, in general we may conclude that a single plasma cell synthesizes and secretes a single kind of antibody molecule.

## 8.7   Is the Antigen-Binding Cell Monospecific?

One tenet of the theory of clonal selection is that each ABC is committed — even before it encounters antigen — to expressing on its surface a single kind of antigen receptor. In other words, each ABC is monospecific; it can interact with only one kind of antigenic determinant.

We have already examined evidence that the antigen-binding receptors on B cells are membrane bound immunoglobulin molecules. They can be visualized by staining the cell with fluorescent antibodies directed against the immunoglobulins of the species. For example, rabbit anti-mouse immunoglobulin antibodies can be coupled with fluorescein. When living mouse B cells are treated with this reagent, the surface of the cell becomes fluorescent (Figure 8.17). In the cold (4°C), the fluorescence is distributed in "patches" over the surface of the cell. However, when these cells are warmed to 37°C, the fluorescence quickly moves to one pole of the cell and forms a "cap" (Figure 8.17). In due course, the fluorescent material is taken into the cell by pinocytosis. A fresh application of the stain at this time shows that no immunoglobulin remains on the surface. (After a few hours, however, freshly synthesized immunoglobulin appears again on the surface.) If monovalent fragments

**Figure 8.17** Patching and capping of the surface immunoglobulin (sIg) on B lymphocytes. Anti-Ig Fab fragments, which are monovalent, will bind to the cell surface but do not initiate patching and capping.

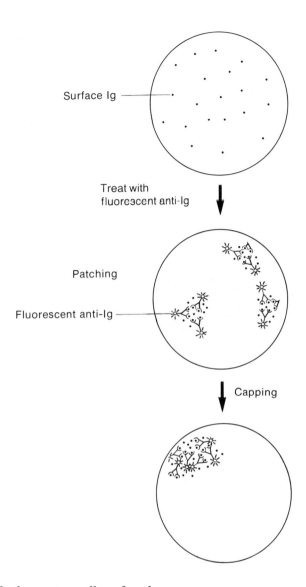

Surface Ig

Treat with fluorescent anti-Ig

Patching

Fluorescent anti-Ig

Capping

of fluorescein-coupled antibodies are used, the entire cell surface becomes diffusely stained, but neither patching nor capping follows. This suggests that the membrane receptors must be cross-linked for patching and capping to occur.

If these immunoglobulin molecules are receptors for antigen, then we might expect that a multivalent *antigen* would induce the same surface changes in the appropriate ABCs. Polymerized flagellin (POL) has many repeating determinants and is thus multivalent. Raff and his coworkers (who discovered the phenomenon of capping in 1969) have shown that approximately 0.005% of the spleen cells of an unprimed mouse bind specifically to POL. At 37°C, the receptor–POL complexes are capped. This can be shown by first treating the cells (at 4°C) with rhodamine-conjugated rabbit anti-POL antibodies (Figure 8.18). While still in the cold, the cells are then exposed to fluorescein-conjugated rabbit anti-mouse-immunoglobulin antibodies. This reagent reveals that all the immunoglobulin on the POL-binding cells has been capped at the same

**185**

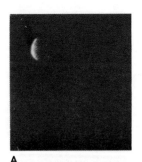

A

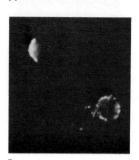

B

**Figure 8.18** Spleen cell from a mouse immunized with POL and exposed first to POL under conditions allowing capping to take place and then to rhodamine-conjugated rabbit anti-POL antibodies *and* fluorescein-conjugated rabbit antimouse immunoglobulin antibodies under noncapping conditions (i.e., at 0 °C in the presence of sodium azide). A: Rhodamine fluorescence shows that the anti-POL receptors have been capped. B: Fluorescein fluorescence shows that the immunoglobulins on the cell surface have been identically capped. Note the patchy distribution of sIg on the two cells that had not bound POL. [From M. C. Raff et al., *J. Exp. Med.* **137**:1024, 1973.]

location. Little or no staining can be seen elsewhere on the cell. On the other hand, surrounding lymphocytes that had not bound POL now are revealed by the interaction of the fluorescent stain with their uncapped immunoglobulin receptors (presumably specific for other antigenic determinants). One can, of course, argue that the POL-binding cells might have also had receptors of other specificities but that these were swept into the cap along with the POL receptors. However, B cells have a number of other types of cell surface molecules (e.g., H-2K, H-2D, and receptors for lectins) and ligands (antibodies or lectins) to any one of these cause only that type of receptor to cap.

## 8.8   The B Cell Repertoire

The theory of clonal selection tells us that B cells acquire a particular antigen specificity prior to encountering antigen. In view of the seemingly limitless number of antigens to which the immune system can respond, we are confronted with the question of how diverse are the receptor specificities expressed by the B cell population in an unprimed animal. In Section 8.3, we learned that Ada and Byrt had found approximately 1/5000 spleen cells from unprimed mice to bind their test antigen (POL). However, B cells share the spleen with other cells (e.g., T cells) so the frequency of POL-binding B cells must be on the order of 1/2500 or less. Similar studies using other antigens usually give ABC frequencies of this order of magnitude.

The counting of ABCs may not give us a reliable estimate of the diversity of the *functional* repertoire of B cells. The cells capable of binding antigen in vitro under certain conditions of concentration, etc., may represent a smaller (or larger) population than the cells capable of responding to the antigen in vivo. We can, of course, count the progeny of the cells that have responded by counting antibody-secreting cells in a hemolytic plaque assay, but without knowing how many cell divisions produced these cells, we cannot estimate the original number of precursor cells. Fortunately, this information can be secured by using the technique of **limiting dilution analysis.**

Limiting dilution analysis attempts to determine the frequency of responding cells in a cell population. It involves setting up cell cultures with graded dilutions of the cell suspension to be tested. If the quantity of cells in the suspension is so high that each culture receives several specific precursor B cells of the specificity being tested, then all the cultures will be positive. If the concentration of precursor B cells in the suspension is very low, then only rarely will a positive culture be found. Between these extremes, the response can be quantitated as a function of cell dose.

To help us understand the principle of limiting dilution analysis, let us first take, as a hypothetical example, a suspension of cells containing 1000 specific precursors in 1000 ml of tissue culture medium. The average number of precursor cells per ml, a value we shall designate $m$, is, of course, 1. Let us now dip a pipette into the suspension and withdraw a series of 1 ml samples and place these in individual culture wells. Intuitively, I think that you would not expect to get exactly 1 cell at each attempt. Sometimes you *will* get one cell, occasionally more than one, and often you will come up empty handed. The frequency for each of these outcomes follows a Poisson distribution. You can expect to withdraw 1 cell and to come up empty handed at the same frequency, 0.368 or roughly 37% of the time. The frequencies for the various outcomes are

| | |
|---|---|
| 0 | 0.368 |
| 1 | 0.368 |
| 2 | 0.184 |
| 3 | 0.061 |
| 4 | 0.014 |
| 5 | 0.003 |
| >5 | 0.002 |

While we have no way of distinguishing between culture wells that received one and those that received more precursors, we can determine the frequency of cultures receiving no precursors. We shall call this $F_0$. This value is related to the average number of precursor cells per culture $(m)$ by the expression $F_0 = e^{-m}$ where $e = 2.7183$, the base of natural logarithms. In our hypothetical example, $m = 1$ and, as we found, $F_0 = 0.368$.

Having looked at a theoretical example where we "knew" $m$ in advance, let us now turn to a practical example where we are trying to determine $m$. Solving the equation $F_0 = e^{-m}$ for $m$, we get $m = -\ln F_0$. Suppose one dilution of a cell suspension gave 10% negative cultures $(F_0 = 0.1)$, the average number of precursor B cells $(m)$ in each culture would be 2.3. If a greater dilution of the cell suspension gave 20% negative cultures, $m$ becomes 1.6. Whichever dilution of the cell suspen-

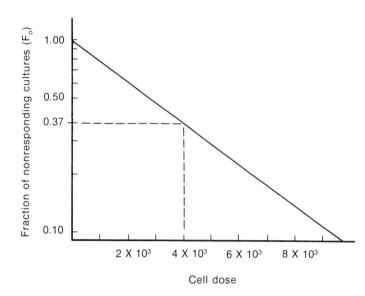

**Figure 8.19** Limiting dilution analysis. A semilogarithmic plot is made of the fraction of negative cultures as a function of the dose of cells placed in each culture. Assuming that one responding cell is sufficient to produce a positive culture, the cell dose yielding 37% negative cultures gives the frequency of cells in the population capable of responding to the antigen. In this case, a dose of $4 \times 10^3$ cells produced 37% negative cultures; thus the frequency of responding cells in the suspension is 1/4000.

sion gives 37% negative cultures, $m = 1$, and we have established the frequency of precursor cells in the suspension. For example, if 37% of the cultures established with 4000 cells per culture are negative, then the frequency of precursor cells is one in 4000. Even if none of the dilutions chosen happens to give exactly 37% negative cultures, that value can be determined by interpolation. The log of the fraction of negative cultures is plotted as a function of cell dose (Figure 8.19). If one responding cell is all that is needed to produce a positive culture, and if any other cells that participate are present in excess, then the plot should be a straight line extrapolating to one. The reciprocal of the cell dose that would yield 37% negative cultures gives the precursor frequency.

Figure 8.20 shows the results of limiting dilution analysis applied to the spleen cells of A/J mice. In this example, the spleen cells were stimulated to divide by the B-cell mitogen LPS (see Section 7.8). Each culture was tested for the presence of antibodies expressing a particular idiotype designated $CRI_A$. When A/J mice are immunized with azobenzenearsonate (ABA), most of the antibodies they produce express this idiotype. When limiting dilution analysis is applied to the spleen cells from *unprimed* A/J mice, approximately 1/300,000 cells is capable of developing into a clone secreting antibodies of the $CRI_A$ idiotype (Figure 8.20). This is, of course, a much lower frequency than Ada and Byrt (and others) have found typical of ABCs. However, only 7% of the B cells in A/J spleens respond to LPS and no more than 50% of the cells in the spleen are B cells. So as a fraction of the B cells capable of responding in this assay, the frequency turns out to be approximately 1/12,000. Limiting dilution analysis of such commonly used antigens as SRBC, TNP, and NIP yield frequencies that range from 1/10,000 down to 1/40.

What about animals primed with antigen? When A/J mice are tested after being immunized with ABA, the frequency of $CRI_A^+$ cells in their spleen rises almost 600-fold (Figure 8.20). This large increase in the frequency of precursor cells is characteristic of antigen-primed animals and provides the cellular basis for the secondary response.

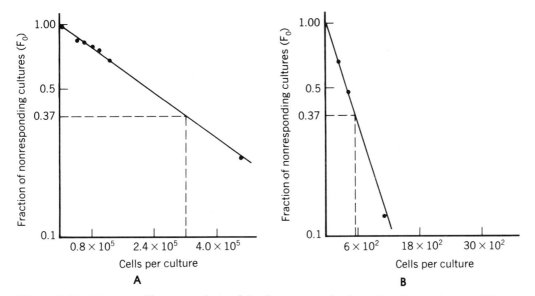

**Figure 8.20** Limiting dilution analysis of the frequency of splenic B cells in A/J mice able to develop into clones secreting antibodies of the $CRI_A$ idiotype. A: The frequency in unprimed mice is approximately 1 in 300,000. B: After immunization with azobenzenearsonate (ABA–KLH) the frequency rises to $\approx 1/500$. [From M. Slaoui et al., *J. Exp. Med.* **160**:1, 1984.]

## 8.9 Thymus-Dependent (TD) vs. Thymus-Independent (TI) Antigens

The response to most antigens (probably all in humans) requires functioning T cells. Thus nude mice (Section 7.3) or mice that have been neonatally thymectomized, irradiated, and reconstituted with bone marrow cells are unable to respond to soluble protein antigens (e.g., OVA), haptenated conjugates of these (e.g., TNP–OVA), or to particulate antigens like sheep red blood cells (SRBC). These antigens are thymus dependent (TD) because B cells cannot respond to them unless they receive "help" from T cells. Thus the response to TD antigens involves the interaction of $T_H$ and B cells. The nature of these interactions is the chief topic of Chapter 12.

Some antigens, such as the type 3 pneumococcal polysaccharide, can induce an immune response without the assistance of $T_H$ cells. Such antigens work perfectly well in mice deficient in T cells. (In fact, these animals may give a better response than normal animals do, a point that we shall examine later.)

In addition to pneumococcal polysaccharides, TI antigens include such materials as the lipopolysaccharide (LPS) from the walls of gram-negative bacteria like *E. coli* and such polymeric substances as polyvinylpyrrolidone (PVP), poly(I-C) (polyinosine-polycytosine), polymerized flagellin (POL), dextran (poly-D-glucose) as well as haptenated forms of these molecules. These substances share two properties: an orderly arrangement of repeating antigenic determinants (see Figure 2.3); and

**189**

mitogenicity. These properties have led to different models of how B cells are activated by TI antigens. In one model ("cross-linking"), a minimum number of identical, properly spaced antigenic determinants are needed to trigger the B cell. Using haptenated synthetic polymers, Dintzis et al. (see paper cited at the end of the chapter) have deduced that approximately 20 antigen receptors on the surface of the B cell must be cross-linked by an antigen molecule before the cell can respond.

Another model proposes that it is receptors for the mitogenic part of the molecule that are the key to activation. We have already seen that LPS serves as a powerful mitogen for B cells. The response to high concentrations of LPS is nonspecific or *polyclonal*. Exposure to a sufficient concentration of LPS will trigger a wide variety of antigen binding B cells to proliferate and differentiate into antibody production of a similar wide range of specificities. For this reason, the response to TI antigens depends more critically on the dose administered than is the case with thymus-dependent antigens. At low doses, TI antigens induce good antibody responses of great specificity. At high doses, however, TI antigens induce antibody production of a wide variety of specificities. Perhaps what distinguishes a TI antigen from a thymus-dependent antigen is the ability of TI antigens to interact *simultaneously* with antigen-specific receptors as well as with receptors that trigger cell proliferation. Thus the one molecule provides two signals: (1) an antigenic determinant for the antigen receptor and (2) a proliferative signal that replaces the one ordinarily provided by $T_H$ cells. At low doses, only the specific ABCs bind enough antigen — through both types of receptors — to proliferate. At higher doses, B cells of other specificities bind enough antigen through their mitogen receptors to proliferate.

There is an inbred mouse strain designated CBA/N that is unable to respond to certain TI antigens such as the type 3 pneumococcal polysaccharide and poly(I-C), while it can respond normally to other TI antigens

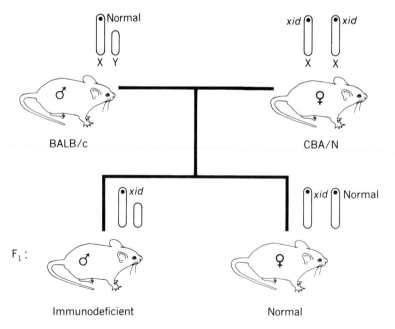

**Figure 8.21** Pattern of inheritance of X-linked immunodeficiency. Females homozygous for the *xid* gene are unable to respond to such "type 2" thymus-independent antigens as the pneumococcal polysaccharide S3. When mated to normal mice, all their male offspring, being hemizygous for the gene, are similarly immunodeficient.

such as haptenated *Brucella abortus.* This selective immunodeficiency is controlled by an X-linked recessive gene designated *xid* (X-linked immune deficiency). When homozygous CBA/N females are mated to normal males of any strain, all their male offspring ($F_1$) are immunodeficient while their daughters respond normally (Figure 8.21).

Those TI antigens that are able to induce a response in *xid* mice have been classified as type 1 TI antigens; those that cannot as type 2. This dichotomy also seems to hold for the B cells of normal neonatal mice, leading to the suggestion that B cells responsive to type 2 TI antigens represent a mature population that fails to develop in *xid* mice.

## 8.10 The Response of B Cells to Antigen

The foundation of clonal selection is a pool of antigen-binding cells representing a broad diversity of specificities. These ABCs are resting, $G_0$, B cells each of which expresses many copies of a receptor with a single antigen specificity. The construction of the particular antigen-binding site has occurred during the maturation of the B cell from its precursor (pre-B) cell. The mechanism by which a particular receptor specificity is generated is described in Chapter 10.

The antigen-binding receptors on B cells are immunoglobulin molecules. Two isotypes are generally found on virgin, mature B cells: IgM and IgD. However, on a single B cell both isotypes have the same binding specificity (and idiotype).

Why both IgM and IgD are present simultaneously is uncertain. Possibly IgM and IgD transduce different signals to the cell upon binding antigen. The heavy chain of IgM lacks the hinge region found in IgD and perhaps multivalent binding is less easily accomplished with the IgM receptor (which is present as a monomer, not the pentamer of secreted IgM).

The theory of clonal selection postulates that upon binding antigen, B cells are activated to enter the cell cycle, proliferate through a series of mitotic divisions, and then differentiate into antibody-secreting plasma cells. Because of the low number of ABCs of any particular specificity, it is difficult to study the effect of antigen binding on normal populations of B cells. Consequently, much of the analysis of the events of B cell activation, proliferation, and differentiation has been performed with B cell mitogens rather than with antigens. B cell mitogens act on a large number of B cells regardless of their antigen specificity. For mice, these polyclonal activators include anti-$\mu$ and anti-$\delta$ antibodies as well as LPS. Each of these materials can stimulate B cells to enter the cell cycle, proliferate, and ultimately differentiate in a way that seems to mimic the events that would occur following antigen binding.

### Activation

Exposure of mature, resting B cells to such mitogens as anti-$\mu$, anti-$\delta$, or LPS causes them to enter the $G_1$ phase of the cell cycle. The density of Ia

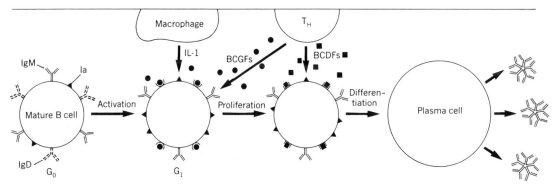

**Figure 8.22**  Response of B cells to antigen or mitogens. B cells proliferate in response to the monokine IL-1 and one or more B cell growth factors (BCGFs) secreted by $T_H$ cells. $T_H$ cells also secrete one or more B cell differentiation factors (BCDFs) which cause the proliferating cells to differentiate into plasma cells. Presumably the response of B cells to monokines and lymphokines is mediated by specific receptors for each. $T_H$ cells are also needed for B cells to be *activated* by T-dependent antigens (see Figure 12.11). The plasma cell is shown here secreting IgM, but any *one* of the other isotypes might have been chosen instead.

molecules on the cell surface increases while the IgD molecules at the surface disappear (Figure 8.22). This activated B cell now becomes, for the first time, sensitive to certain soluble factors that are able to drive it through the cell cycle. There is evidence that the monokine IL-1, secreted by macrophages, is one such factor. Activated T cells also secrete one or more lymphokines that cause activated B cells to proliferate. Because of their effect on B cell proliferation, these lymphokines are called **B cell growth factors** (BCGFs). Presumably, the ability of activated B cells to respond to BCGFs and/or IL-1 reflects in each case the new expression of specific receptors for these factors (Figure 8.22).

Recently, techniques have been developed for purifying B cells of a predetermined specificity in such a way as not to alter their physiology in the process. When purified B cells of a given specificity are exposed to the appropriate antigen, they become activated just as they do in response to mitogens. Exposed to type 1 thymus-independent (TI) antigens, they begin to proliferate vigorously. However, exposure to such thymus-*de*pendent (TD) antigens as hapten–protein conjugates does not activate B cells unless the cells also interact with $T_H$ cells specific for the same antigen (as well as for the Ia molecules on the B cells). The interaction of TD antigens with B cells is examined in Chapter 12.

### Proliferation and Differentiation

Whether in response to antigen or mitogen, activated B cells become responsive to the influence of factors (IL-1, BCGFs) that drive them into a series of mitotic divisions. Thus a B cell of a particular specificity will generate progeny of the same specificity, i.e., a clone.

In due course, some at least of the progeny of dividing B cells become responsive to one or more soluble factors that take them out of the cell

192

cycle and cause them to differentiate into plasma cells. These factors are called **B cell differentiation factors** or BCDFs. They are produced by T cells. As with the BCGFs, the acquisition of sensitivity to BCDFs is probably a function of the expression of receptors specific for the factors (Figure 8.22). To what degree B cells in T cell deficient mice are able to use other proliferation and differentiation factors and the source of such factors (the B cell itself?) remain to be determined.

The differentiation of a plasma cell from a B lymphoblast includes the formation of an elaborate rough endoplasmic reticulum and the synthesis of large amounts of one kind of immunoglobulin molecule of the same specificity as the original receptor. The secreted immunoglobulin may be IgM but, if so, the secreted molecule uses a different C terminal segment on its heavy chains and is pentameric $(H_2L_2)_5$, not monomeric like the IgM receptor. However, the secreted molecule might be IgG, or IgA, or IgE, although still of the same antigen-binding specificity as the original B cell receptor. In any case, no surface immunoglobulin (sIg) remains on the plasma cell and the plasma cell no longer expresses Ia molecules either (Figure 8.22). The mechanisms involved in switching from the synthesis of membrane-bound immunoglobulin (sIg) to secreted antibody molecules and in switching from IgM or IgD to some other isotype are examined in Chapter 10.

Certainly for thymus-dependent antigens (and perhaps to a degree for supposedly thymus-independent antigens), B cell proliferation and differentiation depend upon soluble molecules derived from macrophages and T cells. Further details of the role of cell interactions in the B cell response to thymus-dependent antigens are presented in Chapter 12.

## 8.11 Summary

The ability to make antibodies in response to an antigen depends on the preexistence of a small population of B lymphocytes which have surface receptors able to bind that antigen. The receptors are immunoglobulin molecules: IgM and IgD in animals that have never before been exposed to that antigen. All the receptors on any one B lymphocyte have identical binding sites for the antigen.

Binding of antigen to a B lymphocyte, accompanied by some additional stimulus, activates the cell to enter the cell cycle. Because the progeny of the dividing cell express the same receptor specificity, a *clone* of antigen-specific B cells develops. Proliferation of the clone is maintained by the presence of several B cell growth factors (BCGFs).

Under the influence of B cell differentiation factors (BCDFs), some B cells of the expanding clone begin to differentiate into plasma cells. These synthesize and secrete antibody molecules with the same antigen-binding site as the surface receptors on the ancestral B lymphocyte.

Other B cells of the clone revert to resting lymphocytes. These "memory" B cells express surface receptors of the original binding specificity, but they may be of other isotypes such as IgG, IgA, or IgE. The increased frequency of antigen-specific B lymphocytes after a primary response provides the basis for a larger "secondary" response to a subsequent encounter with the antigen.

The pool of B cells capable of responding to a given antigenic determinant includes cells representing a spectrum of receptor affinities for the determinant. Over the course of an immune response, clones with higher affinity receptors may come to dominate the response leading to affinity maturation: the secretion of antibodies of increased affinity for the antigen.

Most antigens are thymus dependent (TD); i.e., the ability of B lymphocytes to respond to them depends on T helper ($T_H$) lymphocytes.

## ADDITIONAL READING

1. Ada, G. L., and Pauline Byrt, "Specific Inactivation of Antigen-reactive Cells with $^{125}$I-Labelled Antigen," *Nature* **222:**1291, 1969. (Reprinted in V. L. Sato and M. L. Gefter, *Cellular Immunology,* Addison-Wesley Publishing Co., Inc., Reading, MA, 1982.)

2. Burnet, F. M., *The Clonal Selection Theory of Acquired Immunity,* Cambridge University Press, Cambridge, 1959.

3. Dintzis, R. Z., et al., "Specific Cellular Stimulation in the Primary Immune Response: Experimental Test of a Quantized Model," *Proc. Natl. Acad. Sci. USA* **79:**884, 1982. Experimental evidence that the response of B cells to a TI antigen requires that their surface receptors be cross-linked by the antigen in clusters of approximately 20.

4. Eisen, H. N., and G. W. Siskind, "Variations in Affinities of Antibodies During the Immune Response," *Biochemistry* **3:**996, 1964. Affinity maturation of the response to DNP-BGG.

5. Griffiths, G. M., et al., "Somatic Mutation and the Maturation of Immune Response to 2-Phenyl Oxazolone," *Nature* **312:**271, 1984.

6. Haber, E., "Recovery of Antigen Specificity after Denaturation and Complete Reduction of Disulfides in a Papain Fragment of Antibody," *Biochemistry* **52:**1099, 1964.

7. Julius, M. H., and L. A. Herzenberg, "Isolation of Antigen-Binding Cells From Unprimed Mice," *J. Exp. Med.* **140:**904, 1974. (Reprinted in V. L. Sato and M. L. Gefter, *Cellular Immunology,* Addison-Wesley Publishing Co., Inc., Reading, MA, 1982.)

8. Mishell, Barbara B., and S. M. Shiigi (eds.), *Selected Methods in Cellular Immunology,* W. H. Freeman, San Francisco, 1980. The principles and practice of limiting dilution analysis are presented in Chapter 5.

9. Scher, I., "The CBA/N Mouse Strain: An Experimental Model Illustrating the Influence of the X-Chromosome in Immunity," *Adv. Immunol.* **33:**1, 1982. And establishing the distinction between TI-1 and TI-2 antigens.

10. Snow, E. C., et al., "Activation of Antigen-Enriched B Cells. I. Purification and Response to Thymus-Independent Antigens," *J. Immunol.* **130:**607, 1983.

# The Immunoglobulins

## 9.1 Introduction

In this chapter, we shall explore the diversity of antibodies as revealed by serological techniques and by the techniques of protein chemistry. In the following chapter, we examine the mechanisms that generate the diversity of antibodies.

When an antiserum is subjected to electrophoresis, most of the antibody activity is associated with the slowest migrating proteins, the gamma globulins (Figures 2.7 and 2.8). However, even antibodies of a single specificity display a substantial range of electrophoretic mobility. In contrast to such serum proteins as albumin and transferrin, then, antibodies are structurally diverse. This diversity is also seen when antibody affinity is studied by equilibrium dialysis (Section 4.4). Antibodies of a single specificity synthesized in a single animal usually represent a wide spectrum of affinities. For example, an anti-DNP serum with a $K_0$ of $10^7$ $M^{-1}$ may frequently contain subsets of antibody molecules with association constants ranging from $10^5$ to $10^{10}$ $M^{-1}$.

## 9.2 Subunits of Antibodies

Such heterogeneity of charge and affinity implies a corresponding heterogeneity of structure. Nevertheless, underlying the heterogeneity of antibodies are certain uniformities that made possible some of the early insights into antibody structure. Ultracentrifugation revealed that a large portion of antibody activity in a rabbit antiserum settles with a sedimentation coefficient of just under 7S. This corresponds to a molecular weight of ~150,000. In addition, most of the antibody activity in an antiserum can be separated from other serum proteins by precipitation with high concentrations of salt, e.g., $(NH_4)_2SO_4$, or by passing the serum through an ion exchanger like DEAE–cellulose.

### The Fab and Fc Fragments

In the late 1950s, Rodney Porter and his colleagues used the methods described above to isolate the gamma globulin fraction of serum from rabbits that had been immunized with antigens such as BSA or OVA. They treated this material with the proteolytic enzyme papain. The digest was then fractionated on another ion-exchange medium, carboxymethylcellulose, which also separates molecules on the basis of electrostatic charge. Some protein, designated fraction I, passed directly through the column. Then, by gradually increasing the salt concentration of the buffer, they eluted the remaining protein from the column. The protein concentration of the fractions was monitored by absorption at 280 nm, the wavelength which tryptophan and tyrosine residues absorb most strongly.

Figure 9.1 shows the results. Almost 90% of the digested protein was recovered in three distinct fractions. The areas under the three curves were approximately equal, indicating that the fractions each contained the same amount of protein. Furthermore, each fraction sedimented at approximately 3.5S in the ultracentrifuge, indicating a molecular weight of some 50,000.

By several criteria, the material collected in fractions I and II was similar but quite distinct from the material in fraction III. Both fractions I and II retained the capacity to bind to the antigen for which the antiserum was specific. For this reason, the material in these fractions was called the fragment antigen binding or **Fab.** Although these fractions could no longer *precipitate* the antigen, their antigen-binding capacity could be demonstrated by their ability to inhibit the corresponding precipitin reaction with undigested antibody. The reason for the inability of Fab fragments to precipitate antigens is that Fab fragments are monovalent, and thus no opportunity exists for lattice formation (Section 4.1). The monovalency of Fab fragments can be demonstrated by equilibrium dialysis where $r$ approaches 1 as $r/c$ approaches zero (Section 4.4).

Fraction III differed from the other two in several ways. It was much less soluble in buffer; in fact, at pH 7 it crystallized out of solution. Because of this behavior, it was designated the **Fc** fragment (fragment crystalline). The ease with which the material in fraction III forms crystals also suggests a degree of molecular homogeneity absent in the other

**Figure 9.1** Chromatography on carboxymethylcellulose of a preparation of rabbit gamma globulin digested by papain. The protein in fraction I passed directly through the column. That in fractions II and III was eluted by gradually increasing the salt concentration of the buffer. Fractions I and II contained Fab fragments; fraction III contained Fc fragments. The yield in III was roughly one-half of the combined yields of I and II. [From R. R. Porter, *Biochem. J.* 73:119, 1959.]

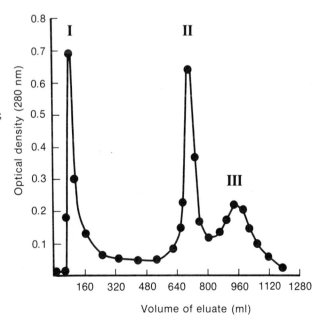

two fractions. Subsequent work, as we shall see, demonstrated this uniformity.

The Fc fragment does not inhibit antigen–antibody precipitation. It does, however, retain some of the biological properties of antibodies, such as the ability to bind complement. The Fc fragment also contains a substantial amount of carbohydrate (as hexose and hexosamine residues).

The equimolar recovery of the three fractions and their uniform molecular weight of about 50,000 suggested that the intact antibody molecule is made up of two Fab fragments and one Fc fragment. Subsequent work showed, however, that any single antibody molecule contains two *identical* Fab fragments. Thus no single antibody molecule would contain one Fab fragment from fraction I and a second from fraction II. The appearance of Fab fragments in two different fractions reflects the distribution of electrostatic charge on the Fab fragments in the entire pool of rabbit antibody molecules.

## The F(ab')₂ Fragment

Nisonoff and his associates showed that when rabbit antibodies are digested with pepsin, a single large fragment is produced along with a heterogeneous assortment of small peptides. The large fragment (MW = ~95,000) retains the same antigen-binding capacity of the intact antibody; that is, it is still bivalent and still capable of precipitating antigen. It is designated F(ab')₂.

When treated with a reagent capable of reducing disulfide bonds, the F(ab')₂ fragment is broken into two fragments, called Fab', that have the same properties as the Fab fragments produced by papain digestion. The model of antibody structure shown in Figure 9.2 is consistent with this. The molecule is constructed of two symmetrical halves linked by one or more disulfide bridges. Cleavage by pepsin occurs on the Fc side of the bridge(s); cleavage by papain on the opposite side.

The region where the two Fab and the Fc regions join is called the *hinge region.* As the name suggests, the hinge region confers a certain amount of flexibility on the molecule. One outcome of this is shown in Figure 9.3. The electron micrographs show some of the frequent molecular configurations taken by anti-DNP antibodies mixed with a hapten containing DNP groups at each end of a short chain of eight carbon

**Figure 9.2** Structural basis of the fragments produced by papain and pepsin digestion of antibodies.

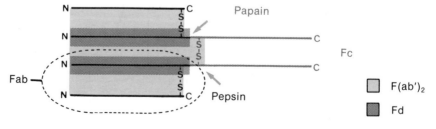

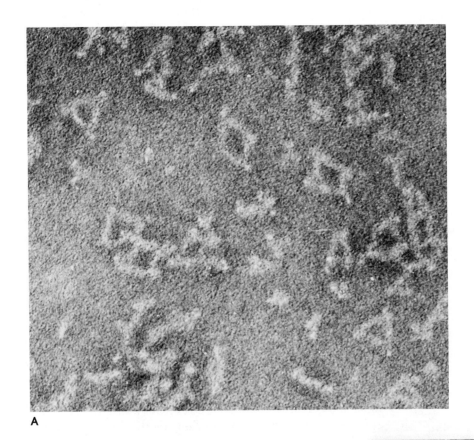

**A**

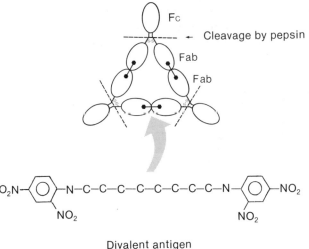

Fc

← Cleavage by pepsin

Fab

Fab

$O_2N$—⟨⟩—N—C—C—C—C—C—C—C—C—N—⟨⟩—$NO_2$

$NO_2$                    $NO_2$

Divalent antigen

**B**

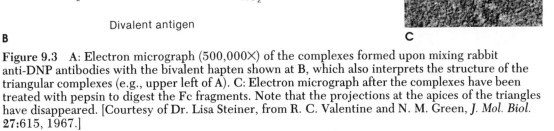

**C**

**Figure 9.3** A: Electron micrograph (500,000×) of the complexes formed upon mixing rabbit anti-DNP antibodies with the bivalent hapten shown at B, which also interprets the structure of the triangular complexes (e.g., upper left of A). C: Electron micrograph after the complexes have been treated with pepsin to digest the Fc fragments. Note that the projections at the apices of the triangles have disappeared. [Courtesy of Dr. Lisa Steiner, from R. C. Valentine and N. M. Green, *J. Mol. Biol.* **27**:615, 1967.]

atoms. Triangles and quadrangles can be seen with tails attached at each corner. The ability of these antibodies to form both triangles and quadrangles demonstrates the flexibility of the hinge region. After treating the complexes with pepsin, the triangles, quadrangles, etc., remain, but the tails are gone. The interpretation of these results is given in the figure.

### Heavy (H) and Light (L) Chains

Many proteins, insulin for example, consist of two or more polypeptide chains linked covalently by disulfide bridges established between cysteine residues in the two chains. These disulfide bridges can be broken with a reducing agent and prevented from reforming with an alkylating agent like iodoacetic acid. Porter and his colleagues found that if they combined gentle reduction of the S—S bonds with the use of an agent (e.g., acetic or propionic acid) to disrupt hydrophobic interactions, they could isolate two distinct types of polypeptide chains. Separation was achieved by gel filtration, i.e., on the basis of molecular size. The first material to leave the column consisted of chains of about 50,000 molecular weight. These were designated heavy or H chains. The chains in the second peak had a molecular weight of approximately 25,000 and were designated light or L chains (Figure 9.4). The yield of the two types of chains was approximately equimolar; i.e., the ratio of H:L was 1:1. Taken with the molecular weight data, this indicated that the intact antibody molecule is constructed from 2 H chains and 2 L chains ($H_2L_2$).

Porter then used the Ouchterlony method to examine the behavior of the chains with (1) an antiserum raised against the Fab fragment or (2) an antiserum directed against the Fc fragment. Anti-Fab serum precipitated both H and L chains; anti-Fc serum precipitated H chains only. With two chains participating in making the Fab fragment and two Fab fragments in an IgG molecule, the intact antibody molecule appeared once again to be made of four polypeptide chains: two L chains each linked to an H chain by a disulfide bridge (as well as noncovalent forces) and two H

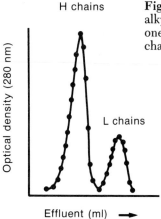

**Figure 9.4** Characteristic results of gel filtration of a reduced and alkylated preparation of gamma globulin. Although L chains represent only one-half of the protein recovered, because their size is one-half that of H chains, the yield of the two types is equimolar.

| Class | H chain | L chain | Structure | Sedimentation coefficient (S) | MW | Carbohydrate (%) | Concentration in serum (mg/ml) | Able to fix complement |
|---|---|---|---|---|---|---|---|---|
| IgG | $\gamma$ | $\kappa$ or $\lambda$ | $H_2L_2$ | 7 | 150,000 | 3 | 13 | |
| IgG1 (60–70%) | $\gamma1$ | $\kappa$ or $\lambda$ | | | | | | + |
| IgG2 (14–24%) | $\gamma2$ | $\kappa$ or $\lambda$ | | | | | | + |
| IgG3 (4–8%) | $\gamma3$ | $\kappa$ or $\lambda$ | | | | | | + |
| IgG4 (2–6%) | $\gamma4$ | $\kappa$ or $\lambda$ | | | | | | −[1] |
| IgM | $\mu$ | $\kappa$ or $\lambda$ | $(H_2L_2)_5 + J$ | 19 | 970,000 | ~12 | 0.5–2.5 | + |
| IgA | $\alpha$ | $\kappa$ or $\lambda$ | $H_2L_2$ | 7 | 160,000 | ~9 | 0.5–3 | −[1] |
| IgA1 | $\alpha1$ | $\kappa$ or $\lambda$ | $(H_2L_2)_2$ + J + SC | 11 | 405,000 | | | |
| IgA2 | $\alpha2$ | $\kappa$ or $\lambda$ | | | | | | |
| IgD | $\delta$ | $\kappa$ or $\lambda$ | $H_2L_2$ | 7 | 175,000 | ~10 | 0.03 | −[1] |
| IgE | $\epsilon$ | $\kappa$ or $\lambda$ | $H_2L_2$ | 8 | 190,000 | 12 | 0.0003 | − |

[1] Can fix complement by the alternative pathway.

**Figure 9.5** Characteristics of the human immunoglobulins.

chains linked together by one or more disulfide bridges (Figure 9.2). This four chain structure ($H_2L_2$) turned out to be the basic structure of all types of antibody molecules (Figure 9.5).

Immunization of a goat with rabbit serum produces an antiserum that will precipitate three distinct kinds of antibody molecules: IgG, IgA, and IgM (Figure 2.12). These three major isotypes or classes of antibodies are also found in humans, mice, and other mammals. In addition, mammals synthesize two other classes of antibodies: IgD and IgE, but their concentration in serum is too low to be detected by precipitation.

The five classes of antibody molecules are constructed from one or more ($H_2L_2$) monomers. What distinguishes one class from another is the nature of its heavy chain. The respective H chains are designated $\gamma$ for IgG, $\mu$ for IgM, $\alpha$ for IgA, $\delta$ for IgD, and $\epsilon$ for IgE (Figure 9.5). There are two different classes of light chains called kappa ($\kappa$) and lambda ($\lambda$). However, all classes of antibodies draw indiscriminately on a common pool of these L chains. Thus, it is the nature of the heavy chain that determines to which class (IgG, IgM, etc.) a given antibody molecule belongs.

## 9.3 The Search for Homogeneous Antibodies

In retrospect, it is remarkable that the early workers deduced as much as they did about antibody structure. They employed biochemical methods, but they did not have the luxury of working with purified preparations of a single molecular species. Thus they could not exploit some of the techniques available for the study of such homogeneous proteins as myoglobin and lysozyme. These techniques included amino acid sequence determination of polypeptide chains and x-ray crystallographic analysis of three-dimensional structure.

## Myeloma Proteins

A major advance toward the resolution of this research problem came with the growing realization that the abnormal proteins produced in certain disease states were immunoglobulins. If you look back at Figure 2.7, you will be reminded that the electrophoresis of human (or rabbit) serum usually reveals diffuse material appearing between a few sharp bands. The sharp bands represent such homogeneous proteins as albumin and transferrin. The diffuse areas represent proteins of such heterogeneity that no single molecular type can be distinguished. In most sera, the slowest migrating serum proteins, the gamma globulins, are extremely heterogeneous. In intensively immunized individuals, the concentration of gamma globulins rises but the same diffuse pattern remains. However, electrophoresis of the serum from multiple myeloma patients reveals quite a different pattern (Figure 4.17). These sera often contain a distinct band in the gamma region that may be as sharp and intense as the albumin band. These patients thus contain high concentrations of a gamma globulin that appears to be as homogeneous as albumin.

The explanation for this unusual protein is that multiple myeloma is the outcome of the malignant proliferation of a (usually) single clone of plasma cells. The unchecked proliferation of these cells produces the homogeneous gamma globulin as well as other manifestations of the disease. The latter include the colonization of a large portion of the bone marrow, leading to anemia and a shortage of the other blood cells. As the disease progresses, the interior structure of the bone itself is destroyed, causing the bones to become very brittle.

The importance of myeloma proteins here is that many of them appear to represent *one* of the possible kinds of antibody molecules that the organism can synthesize. Each such myeloma protein can be assigned to a particular immunoglobulin class — such as IgG, IgA, IgM — and many contain the $H_2L_2$ chain structure that we have established for antibodies.

A sizable fraction of multiple myeloma patients synthesize a homogeneous protein with a molecular weight of approximately 25,000. This protein appears in the serum and is also excreted in the urine. Such proteins are named **Bence-Jones proteins** after the physician who first described them in 1847. He noted their association with multiple myeloma and also reported on their unusual solubility properties. When the urine of a patient excreting a Bence-Jones protein is heated to $50-60°C$, the protein precipitates. Bringing the mixture to a boil or cooling it below $50°C$ causes the protein to redissolve. Bence-Jones proteins are important sources of information about antibody structure because they generally represent the light (L) chain — or dimers of the light chain — of the myeloma protein synthesized by the patient.

The majority of human myeloma proteins belong to the IgG class, the most abundant class of immunoglobulins in the serum. In fact, the frequency of each class of myeloma protein roughly approximates the proportion of that class of immunoglobulin in normal serum. Although some IgM myeloma proteins are found, most of the monoclonal IgM proteins found in humans are found in victims of Waldenström's macroglobulinemia, a malignant proliferation of lymphocytes.

Myeloma proteins also occur in other mammals, including mice. In fact, you have already (in Section 8.5) seen examples of myeloma proteins found in mice. There are several advantages to working with mouse myeloma proteins. One is that they can often be propagated indefinitely. The protein is the product of a clone of malignant cells (a "plasmacytoma"). If the clone has arisen in an inbred strain, it can be propagated by injecting the malignant cells into other members of the strain. Thus, while an individual mouse yields only a small amount of a myeloma protein, the opportunity to propagate the malignant clone in many mice can yield ample amounts of material for experimental work.

Plasmacytomas can be induced artificially in two inbred strains of mice, the BALB/c and the NZB. This can be done by injecting mineral oil or other polymeric materials into the peritoneal cavity. A substantial number of mice so treated develop a plasmacytoma yielding a monoclonal myeloma protein. The plasmacytomas are given various alphanumeric designations, for example, MOPC-41 represents the *mineral oil plasmacytoma* #41. Human myeloma proteins are usually designated by two or three letters derived from the name of the patient, for example, Eu, Daw, Ou.

The validity of using myeloma and Bence-Jones proteins to study antibody structure rests on the assumption that these proteins do in fact possess normal antibody structure. This is not necessarily an assumption to be made lightly. Malignant cells are abnormal cells, and their secreted product might very well be expected to be abnormal. Furthermore, antibodies are defined as antibodies by their ability to bind antigens. Are myeloma proteins able to bind antigens? One way to approach this question is to test various myeloma proteins against a large panel of antigens. From time to time, a myeloma protein that binds to a particular antigen does turn up. In a few cases, both human and mouse myeloma proteins have been found that bind particular antigens with substantial affinity. For example, the mouse myeloma protein MOPC-315 binds the hapten $\epsilon$-DNP-L-lysine with a $K$ of $1 \times 10^7 \text{ M}^{-1}$. (Note that this value is given as $K$, not $K_0$. Being homogeneous, all the molecules of MOPC-315 bind $\epsilon$-DNP-L-lysine with the same association constant.) A number of mouse myeloma proteins specific for phosphorylcholine (PC) have also been identified and have proved to be valuable experimental tools (Section 8.5).

## Monoclonal Antibodies Secreted by Hybridomas

The development by Köhler and Milstein of a technique for making B cell hybridomas has now resolved the problem of producing large amounts of homogeneous antibodies of *defined specificity*. The technique is described in Section 4.8. B cell hybridomas retain the proliferative capacity of their myeloma parent while secreting a monoclonal antibody of any desired specificity. Thus hybridomas make it possible to produce virtually unlimited amounts of a monoclonal antibody of predetermined specificity. Structural studies on these monoclonal antibodies are proceeding in many laboratories.

## 9.4   Variable (V) and Constant (C) Regions

The realization that myeloma and Bence-Jones proteins provide legitimate models of antibody structure quickly brought them under intense scrutiny. All the techniques of protein chemistry that had been so successfully applied to other homogeneous proteins were brought to bear on them.

Peptide mapping of a number of different Bence-Jones proteins soon led to an intriguing observation. In this procedure, the protein is first partially digested by an enzyme such as trypsin. In order to separate the resulting peptides, they are subjected to electrophoresis in one direction followed by chromatography run at a right angle. The resulting distribution of spots provides a map or fingerprint of the protein (Figure 9.6). When such maps were prepared for several different Bence-Jones proteins (which happened to be the kappa type), the spots fell into two categories: (1) a set of peptides that was unique to each Bence-Jones protein and (2) a set that was common to them all. The reason for this curious pattern became clear once actual amino acid sequence data became available for several Bence-Jones proteins (Figure 9.7). The se-

**Figure 9.6**   Peptide mapping ("fingerprinting"). In this example, the peptides produced by the partial digestion of the protein are separated by electrophoresis and chromatography run at right angles to each other.

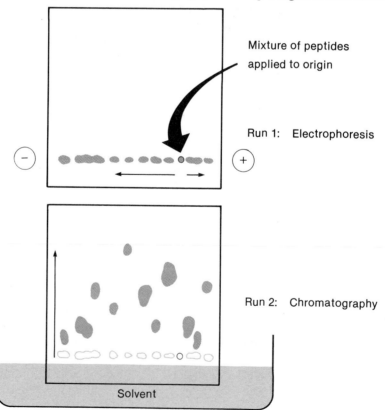

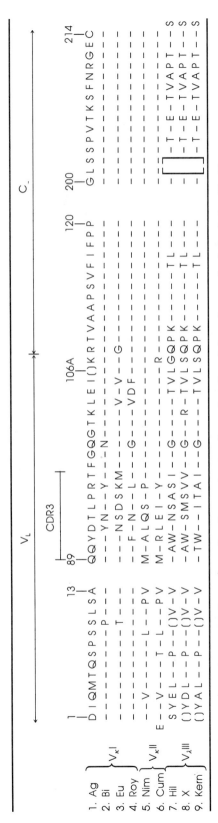

**Figure 9.7** Amino acid sequences of portions of six human kappa chains (1–6) and three human lambda chains (7–9). The single-letter code of amino acids is given inside the front cover. A dash indicates that the amino acid residue is the one located at that position in the first sequence (Ag). Gaps have been introduced in some sequences to maximize the homology of the alignment. Note (1) the uniformity of the C_L sequences for each class of light chain; (2) the consistent differences—both in V_L and C_L—between kappa and lambda chains; (3) the consistent differences in the V regions that distinguish the V_κI and V_κII subgroups; (4) the high degree of variability—even within a subgroup—of residues 89–97.

quence of amino acids in the amino terminal half of any one Bence-Jones protein was very different from that of any other. On the other hand, the carboxyl terminal halves of all the proteins (of any one class) were identical (or almost so). For this reason, the 107 or so amino acids that comprise the N terminal half of light chains are said to make up the variable (V) region of the chain; the remainder of the chain is called the *constant (C) region.*

Today, the complete amino acid sequence of over one hundred light chains is known. These include Bence-Jones proteins, light chains isolated from myeloma proteins, light chains isolated from homogeneous antibodies induced by certain bacterial vaccines, and light chains secreted by hybridomas. These light chains have come from humans, mice, rabbits, and other vertebrates. But the story remains the same. With but a few special exceptions (which we shall examine later), no two identical V regions have been identified. However, within a species, the C regions of the L chains fall into a limited number of identical sets. A similar pattern is found with heavy chains as we shall see.

## 9.5 Light Chains

### Classes of Light Chains

When a rabbit is immunized with a Bence-Jones protein from one patient, the resulting antiserum precipitates many other, but not all other, human Bence-Jones and myeloma proteins. If one then takes one of the Bence-Jones proteins with which the antiserum did *not* react, and uses *it* as an immunogen, the resulting antiserum reacts with *all* the Bence-Jones and myeloma proteins with which the first antiserum failed to react. Thus these two antisera define two distinct classes of light chains. These are called kappa ($\kappa$) and lambda ($\lambda$) after Korngold and Lipari, the investigators who established their existence. The amino acid sequences of their C regions are quite different (Figure 9.7). For example, the mouse kappa chain sequence corresponds to the lambda sequence at only 35% of the residues. That is, when the two sequences are aligned to achieve maximum homology, the same residue is found at only 35% of the positions. (However, when a mouse C-kappa sequence is compared with a *human* C-kappa sequence, the degree of homology rises to 60%.)

All the light chains present on a single antibody molecule (2 for IgG) are alike; i.e., either kappa or lambda, never both. But each individual produces both kinds of light chains and thus the pool of antibody molecules in a single person contains two subsets: $\kappa$ and $\lambda$. For example, about 60% of the IgG molecules in a human carry kappa chains, the remainder carry lambda.

Kappa and lambda light chains are also found in other species. However, their proportions in the antibody pool vary with the species. More than 95% of the antibody molecules in mice and rats carry kappa L chains. On the other hand, lambda chains are heavily favored in dogs, cats, and cows.

Examination of many C regions of human light chains reveals that even within a single class (kappa or lambda), certain limited differences are found. These appear to fall into two categories.

## Subclasses of Light Chains

Amino acid interchanges are found at positions 152 and 190 in human lambda chains. Light chains with glycine at position 152 are designated Kern$^+$; light chains with serine at position 152 are designated Kern$^-$. Light chains with lysine at position 190 are called Oz$^+$; those with Arg-190 are Oz$^-$. Three of the four possible combinations have been identified so far: Ser/Arg, Ser/Lys, and Gly/Arg. In addition, humans secrete a fourth type of lambda light chain (designated Mcg) that differs from all the others at positions 112, 114, and 163 (Figure 9.8). Although any single Bence-Jones protein shows only one of these patterns, all four are present in the pool of normal lambda chains of each individual. These differences thus establish four isotypic subclasses of lambda constant regions. Three subclasses of lambda constant regions have been found in inbred mice. These are designated $C_{\lambda 1}$, $C_{\lambda 2}$, and $C_{\lambda 3}$. Only a single isotype of kappa light chain has been identified in mice and humans.

## Allotypic Variants of Light Chains

***Human Km Allotypes.*** Another highly limited pattern of amino acid interchanges is found in the constant region of human *kappa* chains. These occur at positions 153 and 191. Again, three combinations have been identified: Val/Leu, Ala/Leu, and Ala/Val. These interchanges are designated Km1 ("kappa marker 1"), Km1,2, and Km3 respectively (Figure 9.9). (An earlier nomenclature, Inv1, Inv1,2, and Inv3, is also used for these variants.)

The Km L chain variants differ in one important respect from the Kern–Oz variants. No more than two of these three variants can be found in the serum of any *one* person. Furthermore, the pattern of Km variants in an individual is inherited as a single gene trait according to

**Figure 9.8** Human $C_\lambda$ isotypes.

| | 112 114 | | 152 | | 163 | | 190 |
|---|---|---|---|---|---|---|---|
| Kern$^-$, Oz$^-$ | Ala - Ser | ··· | **Ser** | ··· | Thr | ··· | **Arg** |
| Kern$^-$, Oz$^+$ | Ala - Ser | ··· | **Ser** | ··· | Thr | ··· | **Lys** |
| Kern$^+$, Oz$^-$ | Ala - Ser | ··· | **Gly** | ··· | Thr | ··· | **Arg** |
| Mcg | Asn - Thr | ··· | Gly | ··· | Lys | ··· | Arg |

**Figure 9.9** Human $C_\kappa$ allotypes.

| | 153 | 191 |
|---|---|---|
| Km1 | Val | Leu |
| Km1,2 | Ala | Leu |
| Km3 | Ala | Val |

Mendel's rules. Thus these three kinds of kappa chains represent a set of allotypes, not isotypes (see Section 2.3).

The gene locus is designated *Km*. Three alleles, *Km¹*, *Km¹,²*, and *Km³*, exist in the gene pool of the human population, but any one individual can inherit only two of them.

The limited amino acid interchanges characteristic of the Km allotypes are quite typical of other allelic genes. For example, the Glu/Val interchange at position 6 of the beta chain of sickle cell hemoglobin (Hb$^s$) is one of many hemoglobin mutant forms inherited as alleles.

*Rabbit Kappa Chain Allotypes.* Inherited allotypic variants are also found in rabbit light chains. Four allotypic variants of kappa chains have been identified in domestic rabbits. These are designated b4, b5, b6, and b9. The pattern of inheritance is like that of the human *Km* genes. Thus all the offspring produced by a *b4/b4* dam mated to a *b5/b5* sire will have both b4 and b5 chains in their serum.

## Complex vs. Simple Allotypes

The rabbit b allotypes differ from the human Km allotypes in one notable respect. Each b specificity is associated with a sizeable number of amino acid interchanges (Figure 9.10). Aligning rabbit C-kappa sequences shows that each b allotype differs from each of the others by up to one-third of its amino acids. In other words, the degree of homology between the C-kappa regions of any two b allotypes ranges from 65 to 80%.

Such multiple amino acid interchanges are in sharp contrast to the one or two interchanges associated with the Km allotypes. They also contrast sharply with the differences associated with other allelic genes; e.g., the single Val → Glu interchange at position 6 which distinguishes sickle cell hemoglobin from hemoglobin A. Thus although the b allotypic specificities are inherited like codominant alleles, the gene products do not resemble other examples of alleles.

In recent years, a number of laboratories have reported that rabbits occasionally express the "wrong" allotype. For example, the serum of a rabbit produced by mating a homozygous b4 animal to a homozygous b5

**Figure 9.10** Sequences of rabbit $C_\kappa$ peptides from position 139–149 for three allotypic variants. Deletions have been placed in two sequences to maximize the homology (boxed areas). Over the entire C region, the b4 and b9 chains differ by 35% of their sequence. Thus these allotypic variants are complex, not simple. [From A. D. Strosberg, *Biochem. Soc. Trans.* 4:41, 1976.]

|     | 139 |     |     |     |     |     |     |     |     | 149 |     |
|-----|-----|-----|-----|-----|-----|-----|-----|-----|-----|-----|-----|
| b4  | Tyr - Phe - | Pro | - ( ) - | Asp | - Val - Thr - | Val - Thr - Trp | - Glu |
| b6  | Tyr - Phe - | Pro | - ( ) - | Asp | - Thr - Gly - | Val - Thr - Trp | - Lys |
| b9  | Phe - Arg - | Pro | - Asp - | Asp | - Ile - Thr - | Val - Thr - Trp | - Lys |

animal would be expected to react with both anti-b4 and anti-b5 antisera. However, this rabbit on occasions may exhibit additional b specificities. Strosberg reported one of the first examples. He found that during the immune response to a bacterial vaccine, one b4b5 rabbit reacted with anti-b6 serum as well. Although the animal showed only the b4 and b5 specificities before the immunization period, during the height of the immune response, the b6 specificity appeared also, sometimes at re- markably high concentrations (several mg/ml). Unless an animal is poly- ploid or chimeric, however, it cannot express three allelic genes. The genetic mechanism by which unexpected allotypes occasionally appear is not yet understood.

## 9.6  IgG

IgG is the most abundant class of antibody in the serum of mammals (Figure 9.5). It is also the most commonly seen myeloma protein. A myeloma protein designated Eu from a human patient was the first im- munoglobulin to be completely sequenced. The work was performed by Edelman and his colleagues (Figure 9.11). The sequence of the heavy chain revealed several striking features. One is the recurring pattern of disulfide bridges that draw the chain together in four places. In each case, the disulfide bridges span a segment of the chain about 65 residues in length. Furthermore, if one examines the sequence along the constant portion of the chain, a number of amino acid residues, in addition to the cysteines, reappear in characteristic order. This can be demonstrated by dividing the $C_H$ sequences into three segments of approximately 100

**Figure 9.11**  Structure of the human IgG myeloma protein designated Eu. Note the recurring pattern of intrachain disulfide bonds that participate in drawing the chain into a series of com- pact domains. The $C_H$ region has 3 domains designated $C_H1$, $C_H2$, and $C_H3$. Various effector functions (such as fixing complement) are carried out by one or another of the $C_H$ domains. The primary structure of Eu was worked out by Edelman and his colleagues. The residue numbers are those found in this particu- lar molecule. CHO = carbohydrate residues. [From G. M. Edelman et al., *Proc. Natl. Acad. Sci. USA.* **63**:78, 1969.]

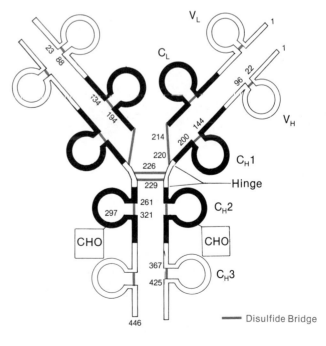

C<sub>H</sub>1 (118 → 164)
C<sub>H</sub>2 (231 → 283)
C<sub>H</sub>3 (342 → 387)

```
      A S T K G P S V F P L A P S S K S C JT S G G T A A L G C L V K D Y F P E P V T V C JS W N S C JG A L T
                                                                    S
A P E L L G G P S V F L F P P K P K D T L M I S R T P E V T C V V V D V S H E D P Q V K F N W Y V D G C JV Q
                                                                    S
      Q P R E P Q V Y T L P P S R E E C JM T K N Q V S L T C L V K G F Y P S D I A V C JE W E S N D C JG E
```

C<sub>H</sub>1 (165 → 215)
C<sub>H</sub>2 (284 → 341)
C<sub>H</sub>3 (388 → 446)

```
S G C JV H T F P A V L Q S S G L Y S L S S V V T V P S S S L G T Q C JY I C N V N H K P S N T K V L C JD K R V   — Hinge (216 → 230)
                                           S
V H N A K T K P R E Q Q T B S T Y R V V S V L T V L H Q N W L D G K E Y K C K V S N K A L P A P I C JE K T I S K A K G
                                           S
P E N Y K T T P P V L D S D G S F F L Y S K L T V D K S R W Q Q G N V F S C S V M H E A L H N H Y T Q K S L S L S P G
                                           S
```

**Figure 9.12** Amino acid sequence of the C<sub>H</sub>1, C<sub>H</sub>2, and C<sub>H</sub>3 domains of IgG Eu aligned for maximum homology. The degree of homology (about 30%) between these three segments of the C region has led to the suggestion that this portion of the chain is encoded by a gene derived by duplication and subsequent divergence of a primordial gene encoding a chain of about 100 amino acid residues. This sequence was determined by Edelman and his colleagues.

residues each and aligning the sequences to give the maximum degree of homology (Figure 9.12). It turns out that some 30% of the residues are homologous between any $C_H$ segment and the next. For this reason, these segments are called *homology units*. Thus the constant region of the gamma chain is constructed from three homology units. These are designated $C_H1$, $C_H2$, and $C_H3$. The chain of amino acid residues that makes up each homology unit is folded into a compact globular "domain." Each domain probably has a distinct function to perform for the molecule, such as fixing complement or binding to a cell receptor.

## The Hinge Region

The constant region of gamma chains contains a stretch of amino acid residues (15 in IgG Eu) between $C_H1$ and $C_H2$. This region shows no homology with any of the homology units. It is rich in proline residues and also contains the cysteines that link the two heavy chains together (Figure 9.11). This segment is called the *hinge region* because it appears to allow a certain amount of flexibility in the angle between the Fab and Fc fragments. The amino acids in the hinge region are exposed to the surrounding medium and thus are easily attacked by proteolytic enzymes. The preparation of Fab and Fc fragments by papain digestion and $F(ab')_2$ fragments by pepsin digestion involve cleavage of peptide bonds in the hinge region.

## Subclasses of IgG

Four distinct types of gamma chain are found in humans (and in mice). Nevertheless, an antiserum raised in *rabbits* to human IgG produces a single precipitin arc (like that shown in Figure 2.12) when human serum is subjected to immunoelectrophoresis. When, however, rhesus monkeys are immunized with human IgG, immunoelectrophoresis reveals three distinct precipitin arcs (Figure 9.13). Each, of course, represents a

**Figure 9.13** Demonstration of 3 of the 4 subclasses of human IgG in normal human serum. The arcs were formed with an antiserum from rhesus monkeys immunized with pooled human IgG. The antiserum was then absorbed with an IgG1 myeloma protein (upper trough) and an IgG2 myeloma protein (lower trough). A fourth subclass (IgG4) was discovered at about the same time by Grey and Kunkel. [Based on W. D. Terry and J. L. Fahey, *Science* 146:400, 1964.]

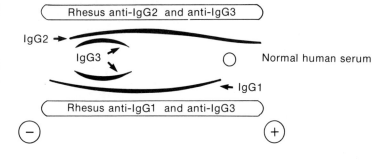

separate group of molecules. These arcs define three subclasses of IgG, today designated IgG1, IgG2, and IgG3. (Their heavy chains are called gamma-1, gamma-2, etc.) A single human myeloma protein gives a line of identity with only one of these three arcs. The occasional human IgG myeloma that does not, defines a fourth subclass, IgG4.

Every human synthesizes IgG molecules of each of the four subclasses. However, any IgG myeloma protein, being the product of a single clone of plasma cells, belongs to only one subclass. The relative proportion of each of the four IgG subclasses in normal human serum is shown in Figure 9.5. Mice also synthesize four subclasses of IgG. These are designated IgG1, IgG2a, IgG2b, and IgG3.

The reason that antiserum raised in rhesus monkeys distinguishes IgG subclasses, while rabbit antiserum does not, reflects their closer phylogenetic relationship to humans. The antigenic determinants *shared* by all IgG subclasses are foreign to rabbits and thus rabbit antiserum precipitates all these molecules identically. On the other hand, our primate relative, the rhesus monkey, sees a smaller set of IgG determinants as foreign. These are distributed discretely among the subclasses of IgG and thus rhesus antisera discriminate among these molecules.

The antigenic determinants detected by rhesus antisera are localized on the heavy chains (Figure 9.14). Ouchterlony analysis of papain digests reveals further that the determinants are confined to the Fc fragment (Figure 9.14).

Why do we describe these four antigenically different types of H chains as representing "sub" classes rather than full fledged classes? The reason is simply that the antigenic differences and the amino acid sequence differences between them are much less pronounced than those that distinguish gamma chains from the other classes of heavy chains: mu (IgM), alpha (IgA), delta (IgD), and epsilon (IgE). Overall, more than 90% of the amino acid residues in the $C_H$ regions of the four IgG subclasses are the same. This suggests a closer evolutionary relationship between subclasses than between classes; i.e., that the genes encoding the subclasses have duplicated and diverged more recently than those encoding the different classes.

Sequence studies of the four subclasses of gamma chains reveal not only characteristic sequence differences in the $C_H$ domains (which give rise to the antigenic differences) but also differences in the structure of

**Figure 9.14** The antigenic determinants that distinguish IgG2 are shown to be located in the C terminal half of the heavy chain (Fc fragment). The center wells contained an absorbed rhesus antiserum specific for gamma-2 chains. The Fab and Fc fragments were prepared from the same IgG2 myeloma used in the bottom set of wells *(right)*. HGG = pooled human gamma globulin. [After W. D. Terry and J. L. Fahey, *Science* 146:400, 1964.]

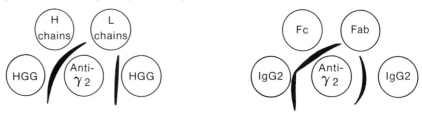

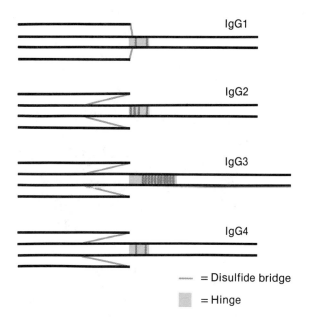

**Figure 9.15** Chain structure of the four subclasses of human IgG. Note the extra-long hinge region of IgG3 and its large number of inter-H chain disulfide bonds. The different gamma chains vary in their effector functions; for example, IgG4 is unable to fix complement by the classical pathway.

----- = Disulfide bridge

▨ = Hinge

the hinge region (Figure 9.15). For example, the hinge region of human gamma-3 chains is quite different from the others: it contains 62 amino acid residues. These include 11 cysteines which establish 11 S—S bonds between the heavy chains. The exact position of the disulfide bridges linking the H and L chains also differs among the IgG subclasses.

## The Gm Allotypes

Some two dozen allotypic variants have been found associated with human gamma chains. These were first identified serologically. Certain human antisera, such as those from victims of rheumatoid arthritis, contain antibodies that bind with gamma chains of some, but not all, other humans. The specificity identified by each type of antiserum is given a Gm number. Each Gm specificity is associated with one or the other of the four subclasses of gamma chains (Figure 9.16). These antisera make it possible to show that the particular specificities are inherited as single gene, codominant traits.

Thanks to the availability of IgG myeloma proteins, certain Gm specificities have been correlated with particular amino acid substitutions. For example, gamma-1 myeloma proteins, which have the sequence Asp-Glu-Leu at positions 356–358 (thus in $C_H3$), react with antisera that define G1m(1) ("gamma-1 marker 1"). The alternative determinant, called G1m(non-1), has Glu-Glu-Met at these positions. Chains of the gamma-1 subclass also show allotypic variation at position 214 (therefore in $C_H1$). Lys at this position establishes the allotype G1m(17); the alternative form, G1m(3), has Arg at position 214. The allotypic determinant expressed at position 214 is inherited as a unit with the one expressed at positions 356–358. Thus the vast majority of gamma-1 chains are either G1m(1)/G1m(17) or G1m(non-1)/G1m(3).

213

| Marker | Chain | Domain | Sequence |
|--------|-------|--------|----------|
| Human | | | |
| G1m(17) | $\gamma1$ | $C_H1$ | Lys-214 |
| G1m(3) | | | Arg-214 |
| | | | 356 357 358 |
| G1m(1) | $\gamma1$ | $C_H3$ | Asp-Glu-Leu |
| G1m(non-1) | | | Glu-Glu-Met |
| G2m(23) | $\gamma2$ | $C_H2$ | Not known |
| G2m(non-23) | | | |
| G3m(21) | $\gamma3$ | $C_H2$ | Tyr-296 |
| G3m(non-21) | | | Phe-296 |
| | | | 308 309 310 |
| G4m(4a) | $\gamma4$ | $C_H2$ | Val-Leu- His |
| G4m(4b) | | | Val-(   )- His |
| Rabbit | | | |
| d11 | $\gamma$ | Hinge | Met-225 |
| d12 | | | Thr-225 |
| e14 | $\gamma$ | $C_H2$ | Thr-309 |
| e15 | | | Ala-309 |

**Figure 9.16**  Structural correlates of representative heavy chain allotypes.

The G1m(non-1) sequence, Glu-Glu-Met, is found at the same position in everyone's gamma-2, gamma-3, and gamma-4 chains — even those of people who have the G1m(1), Asp-Glu-Leu, sequence on their gamma-1 chains. Thus this region is not immunogenic in G1m(non-1) people and no human antiserum exists for it. An antiserum against it can be prepared in some other animal, but such an antiserum reacts with *all* human sera irrespective of the type of gamma-1 chain they contain. Such determinants are called nonmarkers or isoalleles.

## 9.7  IgM

The concentration of IgM in the serum (0.5–2.5 mg/ml) is usually less than a tenth of that of IgG (Figure 9.5). IgM molecules sediment under ultracentrifugation at 19S, which represents a molecular weight of some 970,000. Carbohydrate residues account for approximately 12% of this.

The basic building block of IgM is a subunit that has the same $H_2L_2$ chain structure that we found for IgG. Five of these subunits are covalently linked to form the intact antibody (Figures 9.17 and 9.18). In addition, another polypeptide chain, called the joining or J chain, is covalently attached to two of the 10 H chains in the molecule.

The light chains in IgM belong to the same two classes as those for IgG; that is, the light chains in a given IgM molecule are either all kappa or all lambda. However, the structure of the H chains in IgM, called mu ($\mu$) chains, is quite different from those in IgG. The $\mu$ chain is longer than the

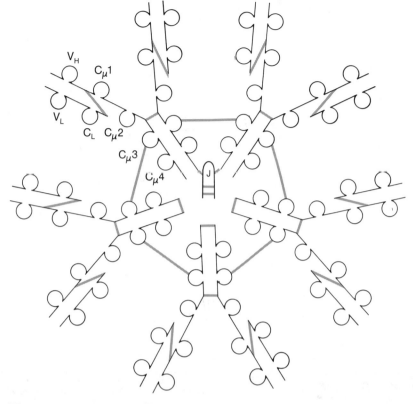

**Figure 9.17**   Structure of human IgM. The oligosaccharides are not shown.

**Figure 9.18**   Electron micrograph of a mouse IgM plasmacytoma protein (270,000×). Note the radial arrangement of 5 (usually) Y-shaped subunits (arrow). [Courtesy of R. R. Dourmashkin from R. M. Parkhouse et al., *Immunology* **18**:575, 1970.]

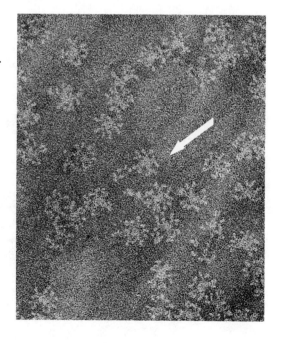

IgG ($\gamma$) heavy chain (MW = 72,000 instead of 50,000). This is because the constant region is made up of four homology units. In addition, the C terminus of the $\mu$ chain has a "tail" of 20 amino acids. The extra carbohydrate attached to the $\mu$ chain also contributes to its higher molecular weight. However, $\mu$ chains have no hinge region.

IgM serves as an antigen receptor on mature, virgin B cells (Section 8.10). This membrane-bound IgM differs from secreted IgM in two ways: (1) it is present as a monomer ($H_2L_2$), not as a pentamer, and (2) membrane-bound $\mu$ chains have a different C terminal "tail." The tail of the membrane-bound form has 46 amino acids (in the mouse). These include a long stretch of hydrophobic residues, which presumably spans the hydrophobic interior of the cell membrane. The genetic basis for this difference in their C terminals is shown in Figure 10.25.

By analogy with IgG, we would expect IgM molecules to bind haptens with a valence of 10. This can be demonstrated for certain small haptens. For other haptens, however, a valence of five or even less has been found. The reason for the lower values may be that the binding of the hapten at one site interferes with the binding of a second hapten at an adjacent site.

The binding affinity of a single site on IgM is often quite low, but this is offset by the presence of multiple sites. Thus IgM antibodies tend to be more avid than IgG molecules. By establishing multiple binding sites with a single macromolecular antigen, the antigen–antibody complex is kept intact even as one site or another momentarily dissociates.

Antigen-complexed IgM fixes complement with great efficiency. In fact, a *single* IgM molecule bound to the surface of a red cell can trigger the lysis of that cell. Recall that plasma cells secreting IgM are detected in the hemolytic plaque assay simply by adding complement, whereas IgG-producing PFCs usually can be revealed only by developing them with an anti-immunoglobulin serum (see Section 5.12).

Gentle reduction of IgM (e.g., with mercaptoethylamine) separates the five subunits ($IgM_s$) and also releases the J chain. The high avidity and hemolytic efficiency of IgM are destroyed by this treatment.

IgM is the first class of antibody to appear in the immune response to most antigens. In the case of thymus-independent (TI) antigens like DNP-POL or purified pneumococcal polysaccharide, the response usually consists exclusively of IgM antibodies.

---

## 9.8 IgA

The concentration of IgA in human serum falls approximately in the same range (0.5–3 mg/ml) as that of IgM and thus is well below that of IgG. However, IgA is the dominant immunoglobulin found in external secretions such as saliva, tears, colostrum, and the mucus-containing fluids that bathe the respiratory passages and the intestine. These locations suggest that IgA represents a first line of defense against microorganisms or other antigens that threaten to cross these interfaces between the external and internal environments.

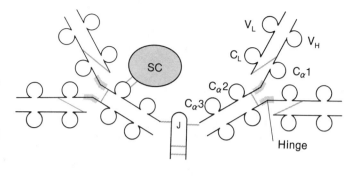

**Figure 9.19** Structure of human secretory IgA1. In IgA2 there is no S—S bridge connecting the L chain with the H chain; the two are held together by noncovalent forces only. The exact number and location of the S—S bridges linking the J chain and the secretory component (SC) to the heavy chains is still uncertain. The primary structure of human IgA1 was worked out by F. W. Putnam and his collaborators [Y-S. V. Liu et al., *Science* 139:1017, 1976.]

Most of the IgA in the *serum* is in the form of monomers containing 2H and 2L chains. The L chains are, as with the other classes of antibodies, either kappa or lambda. Again, it is the nature of the H chains, called alpha ($\alpha$) chains, that establishes the molecules as IgA. In humans, two antigenically distinct subclasses of alpha chains have been discovered. The antibody molecules synthesized from these are designated IgA1 and IgA2, respectively. (Figure 9.5). Both forms have three constant domains, a hinge region, and a "tail" at their C terminus.

Some of the IgA in the serum consists of dimers or even higher multimers of the $H_2L_2$ chain structure. The multimeric forms are linked by one or more disulfide bridges to a 15,000 dalton J chain identical to the J chain found in pentameric IgM.

IgA in secretions occurs mainly as a dimer. In addition to the J chain, each molecule of secretory IgA contains a polypeptide chain called *secretory component* (SC). Secretory component has a molecular weight of approximately 80,000. It is attached to the alpha chain by disulfide bonds and/or noncovalent forces (Figure 9.19).

IgA is synthesized in plasma cells that are especially abundant in the mucous membranes of the body. These cells synthesize and assemble an IgA dimer $(H_2L_2)_2$ linked by the J chain. These completed molecules are secreted from the plasma cell and bind to special receptors on the interior surface of epithelial cells. The IgA/receptor complex is taken into the cell by endocytosis. The receptor molecule is cleaved in two, with its N terminus remaining attached to IgA as secretory component. The complete molecule is discharged at the external face of the epithelial cell (Figure 9.20).

Secretory component is a single polypeptide containing five domains resembling those of immunoglobulins both in general structure and in sequence. Each domain is 100–105 residues in length and has an intradomain disulfide bridge spanning 60–70 residues.

Studies with such proteolytic enzymes as pepsin and trypsin reveal that secretory IgA is more resistant to degradation than serum IgA. This suggests, then, at least one function of SC. In view of the protective role that secretory IgA plays in the intestine, its resistance to digestion by the body's own proteases must be of substantial biological benefit.

Inherited (allotypic) variants are found in human alpha chains. IgA2 molecules occur in two allotypic forms designated A2m(1) and A2m(2).

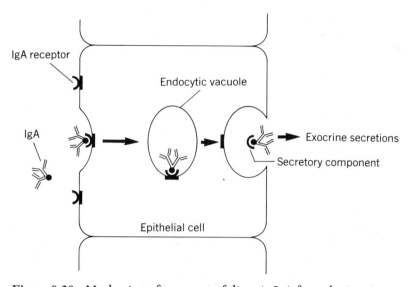

**Figure 9.20** Mechanism of transport of dimeric IgA from the interior surface to the external side of glandular epithelia. IgA molecules bind to receptors on the basal surface; the complex is internalized by endocytosis; cleavage of the receptor frees the IgA for discharge at the exterior surface. The portion of the receptor that remains attached to the IgA is called secretory component (SC). It is a single polypeptide containing 629 amino acid residues organized into five domains of 100–115 residues apiece. The domains have an intrachain S—S bond spanning 60–70 amino acids and show marked homology to each other as well as to the V domains of immunoglobulins. The transport mechanism is responsible for depositing IgA in the various exocrine secretions: saliva, milk, bile, tears, sweat, as well as in the mucus layer that protects the inner lining of the nasopharyngeal passages, intestine, and genito-urinary tract. Pentameric IgM can be transported by the same mechanism, raising the possibility that the receptor is specific for J chain, which both multimeric IgA and IgM use.

Again, remember that *all* humans synthesize both *classes* of IgA, but whether your IgA2 molecules are A2m(1)or A2m(2) or both depends on what genes you inherited from your parents.

## 9.9 IgD

IgD was originally identified as a human myeloma protein. An antiserum raised against this protein would not react with IgG, IgM or IgA molecules once its anti-L chain activity had been removed by adsorption with free light chains. The resulting antiserum defined a previously unknown type of heavy chain, designated the delta ($\delta$) chain. The availability of a specific antidelta antiserum revealed the presence of IgD in human serum. However, its concentration in the serum is very low — on the order of 0.03 mg/ml.

IgD myeloma proteins consist of 2 L chains (either kappa or lambda) each linked by a single disulfide bridge to a delta chain. In humans (but apparently not in mice) the delta chains are held together by a single disulfide bridge. Thus IgD has the same basic $H_2L_2$ chain structure of the other classes of immunoglobulins.

Although only a minor component of the serum, IgD is a major membrane immunoglobulin. During the course of B-cell differentiation, these cells synthesize and display IgD molecules as well as IgM molecules. While this appears to contradict our one cell = one immunoglobulin rule (Section 8.6), the antigen-binding sites of the two types of molecules and their light chains are identical. Only their $C_H$ regions differ. The membrane-bound IgD may serve as one of the receptors with which B cells bind antigen and are stimulated to undergo clonal proliferation.

## 9.10   IgE

The concentration of IgE in normal human serum is approximately 0.3 $\mu$g/ml, only 1/100 of the concentration of IgD and 1/40,000 that of IgG. Despite its presence in such low concentration, this class of antibody was first identified directly in human serum. This was possible because of its potent biological activity.

You may recall from Section 5.8, the demonstration by Prausnitz of the passive transfer of immediate hypersensitivity. In this procedure, serum is taken from a patient who is allergic to, for example, ragweed pollen. A small quantity of this serum is injected intradermally into a normal recipient. After several hours have elapsed, the antigen (ragweed pollen or a protein extracted from the pollen) is injected into the same site. Within minutes, a wheal and flare reaction (Figure 5.17) is observed. This is the *Prausnitz–Küstner (P-K) reaction*.

For many years, the antibodies capable of transferring a P-K reaction were called *reaginic antibodies*. Little more was known about them until the Ishizakas demonstrated that reaginic antibody activity was not inactivated by antisera specific for the H chains of IgG, IgM, IgA, or IgD myeloma proteins. However, polyvalent antiserum or antiserum directed against L chains did precipitate the active material. They thus established that reaginic antibodies belong to a fifth class of immunoglobulins: IgE.

In the ensuing years, a few IgE myeloma proteins have been discovered. The availability of this material has enabled us to learn more about the structure of IgE. Again, the molecule is composed of two L and two H chains. The L chains are of the same two types as occur in all immunoglobulins, that is, kappa or lambda. The H chains, called epsilon ($\epsilon$) chains, are unique to IgE.

The biological activity of IgE is accounted for by its property of binding to basophils and to their tissue equivalent, mast cells. The binding occurs between receptors on the mast cell and a portion of the epsilon chain localized in the Fc region. This can be shown by the ability of Fc fragments of IgE to block the sensitization of mast cells by intact, antigen specific, IgE antibodies.

The binding of IgE molecules by their Fc region leaves the two Fab arms free to bind to antigen. When they do so, the mast cell is triggered to degranulate. Its granules contain histamine, leukotrienes, and other vasoactive substances. The release of these materials increases the permeability of nearby capillaries, producing, in the skin, the characteristic wheal and flare response. Elsewhere, the interaction of antigen and IgE-sensitized mast cells leads to such allergic reactions as the severe bronchial constriction of asthma and the swollen mucous membranes of the nasal passages of the hay-fever sufferer.

Degranulation of mast cells requires the cross-linking of the receptors for IgE. Normally this occurs when antigen binds to adjacent IgE molecules (Figure 14.11). Haptens alone will not bring about degranulation. In fact, haptens specifically inhibit degranulation by intact multivalent antigens. Antibodies, but not their Fab fragments, raised against an IgE myeloma protein will also degranulate mast cells that have first been incubated with IgE or its Fc fragments. This again suggests the need for cross-linking of the mast cell receptors in order for degranulation to occur. In fact, antibodies against the Fc receptor itself will cause degranulation.

## 9.11 Light Chain Variable Regions

Although the V regions of L chains are enormously diverse, the diversity is not distributed uniformly along the chain. When large numbers of chains are compared, it is found that certain positions are, in fact, invariant. Some examples are the cysteines at positions 23 and 88, and a tryptophan at position 35.

### V Region Subgroups

Many other positions show only limited amino acid interchanges. The distribution of amino acid interchanges in this category is not random. A particular amino acid residue at one position in a given V-kappa region is often associated with a particular amino acid at other positions as well. Thus, if sequence analysis of a human V-kappa region reveals a glutamine (Q) at position 3, in all likelihood the chain will also have serine (S) at position 9, alanine (A) at 13, and a number of other predictable residues (Figure 9.7). The presence of certain invariant positions among a subset of V-kappa regions establishes the *subgroup* of that V-kappa region.

Establishing the number of different subgroups is a somewhat arbitrary process. If a chain is found that differs at only one of the residues associated with a given subgroup, should it be assigned to another subgroup? What if three chains are found sharing the same difference? Certainly the more sequence data that become available, the easier it is to recognize the existence of subgroups. Most workers presently agree that human V-kappa regions fall into four subgroups, human V-lambda into six. Only two V-lambda subgroups (which are very similar to each other) have been identified in the mouse, but the mouse has at least 26 V-kappa subgroups.

Whatever the diversity of subgroups, the sequences associated with any given V-kappa subgroup are never found with a C-lambda region and V-lambda is never associated with C-kappa. To put it another way, once you have established that you are sequencing a V-kappa region, you know that the C terminal half of the molecule will be C-kappa, not C-lambda. As we shall see later, the existence of subgroups of V-kappa and V-lambda regions must be taken into account in any theory of the genetic basis for antibody diversity.

## Hypervariable Regions

Comparison of the sequences of many light chain V regions (both kappa and lambda) reveals an especially large amount of sequence variability in three regions of the chain called *hypervariable regions* (Figure 9.21). To take an extreme example, 11 of the 20 amino acids used in the synthesis of proteins have been found at position 96 of human kappa chains.

The degree of variability anywhere along the chain can be expressed quantitatively. Elvin Kabat and his colleagues have developed an index of "variability."

$$\text{Variability} = \frac{\text{Number of different AA found at a given position}}{\text{Frequency of the most common AA at that position}}$$

where AA = amino acid. For each position along the chain, they determine the number of different amino acid residues that have been identified among all the chains with a known sequence. This value is divided by the frequency with which the most commonly found amino acid at that position occurs in the set of known chains. The quotient is designated "variability." It can vary between one and, theoretically, 400. That is, if only one amino acid has even been found at a given position (the position is invariant), its frequency is also one (e.g., found in 37/37 proteins) and

**Figure 9.21** Plot of the variability (defined in the text) of amino acid residues in human light chains (both kappa and lambda). Note the three so-called hypervariable regions. The residues in these regions participate in the formation of the antigen-binding site. For this reason, these regions of the chain are also called complementarity-determining regions (CDR). [From E. A. Kabat, T. T. Wu, and H. Bilofsky, *Sequences of Immunoglobulin Chains*, National Institutes of Health, 1979.]

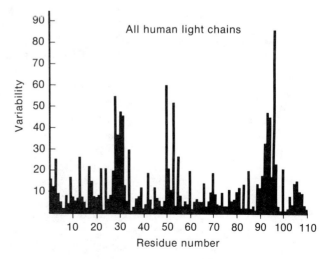

the index of variability is one. However, if all 20 amino acids have been found at that position *and in equal numbers,* the frequency of any one amino acid is 1/20 and the index of variability is 400 (20/0.05).

Figure 9.21 shows a plot of the variability found in the light chains (both kappa and lambda) of humans. Because the three hypervariable regions participate in establishing the antigen-binding specificity of an antibody, they are referred to as complementarity-*d*etermining *r*egions (CDRs). The CDRs of light chains extend from positions 24–34 (CDR1), 50–56 (CDR2), and 89–97 (CDR3). The regions in between the CDRs are called **framework regions (FR)**. The four framework regions are thus designated FR1 (1–23), FR2 (35–49), FR3 (57–88), and FR4 (98–107).

## Comparing Amino Acid Sequences

A certain amount of natural variation in length occurs among both light and heavy chains, even within a given class. Nevertheless, close inspection of several sequences reveals characteristic residues at approximately the same locations. This suggests that the length variation arises from a small number of extra amino acids added to certain chains (insertions) or deleted from certain chains (gaps). In order to establish the degree of homology between two chains, they are first aligned so that the maximum degree of overlap occurs. This often means, then, that gaps must be inserted in order to make the smaller chain align properly with the longer (Figure 9.10).

In view of these variations in length, how are we to identify particular positions in the chain? One approach is to simply number each chain sequentially from its N terminus to its C terminus. But this results in certain characteristic, often invariant, residues bearing a different number in each chain. A second approach is to number a prototype chain, often the first to be sequenced, and then to add whatever insertions or gaps appear to be needed to other chains to achieve maximum homology with the prototype. Where amino acids must be added, letters are used for the extras. For example, the third hypervariable region of many light chains contains extra amino acid residues between position 97 and the invariant Phe that occupies position 98 (the start of FR4). These additional residues are thus designated 97A, 97B, etc. In cases where a segment of chain is shorter than the prototype, the missing positions are simply indicated by gaps.

Unfortunately, several competing prototype sequences have appeared in the literature. This has caused considerable confusion, especially with respect to heavy chain sequences. In this book, we shall use either (1) the actual residue number of the chain being discussed or (2) when comparisons between different chains are being made, the numbering scheme adopted by Kabat, Wu, and Bilofsky. These workers have compiled a register of all the immunoglobulin sequence data available and have numbered the sequences according to a uniform scheme. By adhering to their numbering system, we shall be able to describe and compare immunoglobulin sequences in a uniform, useful way.

The primary structure of $V_H$ regions resembles that of $V_L$ regions in several respects. As in light chains, the term variable should not suggest that the entire region (usually 118–124 residues in length) is uniformly variable. Certain positions are invariant. These include the cysteines at positions 22 and 92 that establish an intrachain disulfide bridge. Other invariant residues include a Pro at position 14, a Gly at 26, and the tryptophan residues at positions 36 and 47.

Other positions show a low degree of variability when one is comparing all known $V_H$ sequences. However, a predictable pattern of invariant residues is found among some, but not all, $V_H$ regions. These patterns establish the subgroups of the region. Human $V_H$ regions fall into four distinct subgroups, mouse $V_H$ regions into seven. These subgroups represent isotypic, not allotypic differences. In other words, every human (and every mouse) synthesizes $V_H$ regions representing each of the subgroups.

Figure 9.22 shows a plot of the variability found in all human $V_H$ regions for which sequence data are available. As in $V_L$ regions, three regions of hypervariability are clearly seen. In the next three sections, we shall examine the evidence that these three regions participate in creating the binding site for the antigenic determinant. For this reason, we shall again refer to these three regions as complementarity-determining regions (CDR). The CDRs of $V_H$ regions occupy positions 31–35 (CDR1), 50–65 (CDR2), and 95–102 (CDR3) (Figure 9.23). However, this does not mean that CDR1 always contains five residues, CDR2 has 16, and CDR3 has 8. The length of a CDR is itself quite variable. Additional amino acid residues (35A, 35B) are frequently inserted between position 35 and the invariant Trp at position 36. Similarly, positions 52 in CDR2 and 100 in CDR3 are often followed by insertions (52A, 100A, 100B, etc.).

The regions flanking the CDRs are called (as in L chains) the framework (FR) regions. For $V_H$ regions, these are FR1 (1–30), FR2 (36–49),

**Figure 9.22**  Plot of the sequence variability found among all the known human $V_H$ regions. Three regions of hypervariability are evident. As in light chains, these regions of the molecule participate in forming the antigen-binding site. [From E. A. Kabat, T. T. Wu, and H. Bilofsky, *Sequences of Immunoglobulin Chains*, National Institutes of Health, 1979.]

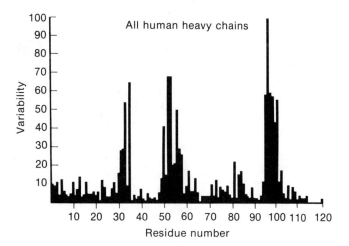

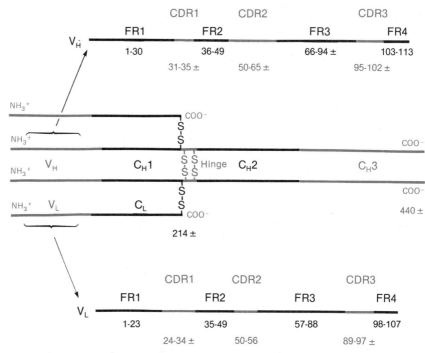

**Figure 9.23** Distribution of framework regions (FR) and complementarity-determining regions (CDR) in the $V_L$ and $V_H$ regions of a human IgG1 molecule. The numbering is that of Kabat, Wu, and Bilofsky and applies to all kinds of H and L chains.

FR3 (66–94), and FR4 (103–113) (Figure 9.23). Many mouse and some human FR3 regions have extra residues (88A, 88B, and so on) between positions 88 and 89.

## 9.13 The Location of the Antigen-Binding Site

Antibody molecules have two quite different sets of properties. On the one hand, the antibodies in an individual animal represent a broad spectrum of specificities. On the other hand, antibodies, regardless of specificity, share certain properties. For example, most are able to bind complement components. IgE molecules, whatever their specificity, bind to receptors on mast cells.

Thus we are faced with both a high degree of variability in function and certain shared functions. As we have seen, the primary structure of antibodies reveals a similar dichotomy. We might expect, then, that V regions would be involved in antigen binding while C regions would be involved in such shared properties as complement fixation and mast-cell binding. Put another way, antibody molecules have (1) a recognition function, reflected in specificity of binding to an antigenic determinant, and (2) effector functions, reflected in the biological activities that they trigger. In this section, we shall examine some of the evidence linking the recognition function to V regions.

**Figure 9.24** DNP binding activity of recombined heavy and light chains purified from rabbit anti-DNP antibodies or normal rabbit serum. The heavy chains play the dominant role in this (and many other) cases. [Based on E. Haber and F. F. Richards, *Proc. Roy. Soc., Series B* **166**:176, 1966.]

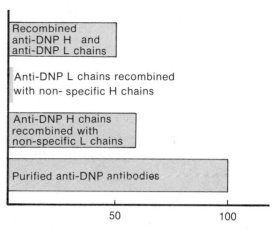

Recombined anti-DNP H and anti-DNP L chains

Anti-DNP L chains recombined with non-specific H chains

Anti-DNP H chains recombined with non-specific L chains

Purified anti-DNP antibodies

50          100

Percent DNP-binding relative to purified antibodies

The work of Porter showed that antigen binding occurs in the Fab fragments. Each Fab is constructed from a light chain ($V_L + C_L$) and a portion ($V_H + C_H1$) of a heavy chain. Two questions follow from this.

1. Do both chains participate in antigen binding?
2. Is antigen binding localized in the V region, the C region, or both?

Porter's procedures for isolating heavy and light chains provide the material with which to answer the first question. Isolated L chains (when returned to physiological conditions of pH, etc.) retain little or none of the antigen-binding capacity of the antibodies from which they are derived. In the few instances where isolated L chains have been shown to retain specific binding, the affinity has been extremely low ($10^2$ M$^{-1}$ or less). Isolated H chains, on the other hand, frequently retain the capacity to bind to the appropriate antigen. However, the affinity of the binding site of an isolated H chain is usually much less than that of the intact antibody molecule.

When isolated H and L chains are allowed to recombine under physiological conditions, much of the antigen-binding capacity of the original antibodies is regained (Figure 9.24). Furthermore, when antigen-specific H chains are allowed to recombine with nonspecific L chains (isolated from preimmune serum), the binding affinity may still be appreciable. (Figure 9.24). However, antigen-specific light-chains combined with nonspecific H chains show little or no antigen binding. These and many other results indicate that the heavy chain usually plays the dominant, but not exclusive, role in antigen binding. Only a few cases have been found where the L chain plays the dominant role.

## 9.14 Affinity Labels

We could localize the antigen-binding site of an antibody molecule if, once within the site, the antigen remained there. Then we could separate the chains to see if either or both were bound to the antigen. Peptides

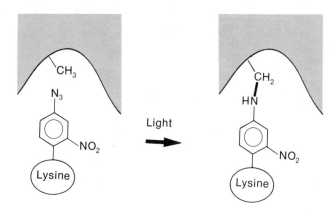

**Figure 9.25** Affinity labeling. Once the hapten is bound noncovalently within the site of the anti-DNP antibody, activation of the azide (N$_3$) group causes it to form a covalent bond with a nearby amino acid residue. Then the antibody chains can be separated and analyzed to pinpoint the location of the affinity label.

could be prepared and sequence analysis performed to see exactly which amino acids participated in the construction of the site. However, the binding of an antigenic determinant occurs through noncovalent forces (Section 4.3), and the treatment necessary to separate L and H chains, for example, would cause the antigen to dissociate quickly from the binding site.

The solution to this dilemma is to prepare a hapten which, once within its site, can establish a covalent bond with amino acids in or near the site. Such a reagent is called an *affinity-labeling reagent.* Figure 9.25 shows the structure of one such reagent. The molecule is essentially ε-DNP-lysine in which one of the NO$_2$ groups has been replaced by the azide (N$_3$) group. This change does not interfere seriously with the ability of anti-DNP antibodies to bind the hapten. The azide group is inert in the dark. It absorbs light strongly, however, and becomes highly reactive as it does so.

The procedure is to first allow the antibodies to bind to the hapten in the dark. Once the hapten is snug within its site, the hapten–antibody complex is exposed to the light. The now activated azide group will establish a covalent bond with any amino acid side chain located nearby.

In affinity labeling, we must establish that the binding is specific. Preincubation of the antibodies with unmodified hapten should block the binding of the affinity label. Conversely, affinity-labeled antibodies should lose the capacity to bind the unmodified hapten. Nonspecific immunoglobulin should not be labeled by the reagent.

The results of a number of affinity-labeling studies are quite consistent. The label is sometimes bound by the light chain but more often by the heavy chain. Heavy chains are favored over light chains by ratios that range from 2:1 to 8:1, depending upon the particular antibody population being studied.

Because of the heterogeneous nature of most antisera, it is difficult to pinpoint the particular amino acid residue to which the affinity label has bound. The use of antigen-binding myeloma proteins circumvents this difficulty. MOPC-315 is a mouse myeloma protein that binds several DNP-containing haptens, in some cases with substantial affinity. Figures 9.26 and 9.27 show the results of a series of experiments using a set of related affinity-labeling reagents. In one of these, N-bromoacetyl-N-DNP-ethylenediamine (''BADE''), the DNP group is located at one end

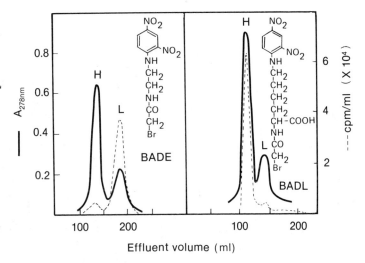

**Figure 9.26** Fractionation by gel filtration of protein (solid lines) and radioactivity (dashed lines) of the dissociated H and L chains of MOPC-315 after affinity labeling with $^{14}$C-BADE *(left)* and $^{14}$C-BADL *(right)*. BADE labeled the L chains almost exclusively while BADL labeled the H chains. [From J. Haimovich, D. Givol, and H. N. Eisen, *Proc. Natl. Acad. Sci. USA* **67**:1656, 1970.]

of the molecule, the reactive bromoacetyl group at the other. When MOPC-315 binds this reagent in its active site, the covalent bond is almost exclusively formed with the light chain. In fact, the bond is formed with the tyrosine residue at position 32. This residue, you may recall, is in the first complementarity-determining region (CDR1). A second reagent, called BADL (*N*-bromoacetyl-*N*-DNP-lysine), binds almost exclusively to the heavy chain. The distance between the DNP group and the bromoacetyl group is five angstroms greater in BADL than in BADE. The covalent bond formed with BADL occurs with the side group of lysine at position 52 in CDR2 of $V_H$. Reagents in which the

**Figure 9.27** Electrophoretic patterns of affinity-labeled MOPC-315 under conditions that normally separate the H and L chains. The bifunctional reagent "DIBAB" cross-links some of the H and L chains. The position of the extra band formed with DIBAB corresponds to a molecule with the molecular weight (72,000) expected of 1H + 1L chain. [Based on D. Givol et al., *Biochemistry* **10**:3461, 1971.]

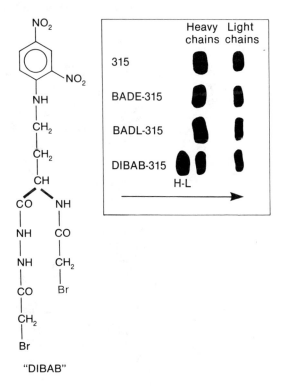

spacing between the DNP and the bromoacetyl groups is intermediate between that of BADE and BADL label one or the other chain without marked preference.

The synthesis of a DNP reagent with *two* bromoacetyl groups—one located with respect to the DNP as in BADE, the other as in BADL—provides the capstone of this story. With this reagent, *both* chains are covalently bound to the reagent and thus to each other. Now any attempt to separate the H and L chains by the usual methods fails (Figure 9.27).

Workers in many laboratories have devised and used affinity labeling reagents. Whatever the specificity involved, the affinity label is almost always bound to a residue in or near a hypervariable region. This provides strong justification for calling these hypervariable regions *complementarity-determining regions (CDR)*. However, the CDRs of both H and L chains occur at widely separated portions of the chain. Are the CDRs in the intact, folded molecule close enough to each other to participate in the building of a binding site? A direct answer to this question requires that the three-dimensional structure of the variable regions be determined. And, for this, one must turn to x-ray analysis of crystals.

## 9.15 The Three-Dimensional Structure of Immunoglobulins

The formation of crystals involves the orderly assembly of identical subunits. A number of homogeneous proteins, such as myoglobin, can form crystals, and the x-ray analysis of these reveals their three-dimensional structure. But antibody populations are normally far too heterogeneous to permit crystal formation. However, a few myeloma proteins, myeloma Fab fragments, and several V-region dimers (Bence-Jones proteins) have been crystallized. Let us examine the results gained from the x-ray crystallographic analysis of

1. The Fab′ fragment of a human IgG1 myeloma from a patient designated New and
2. The Fab fragment of McPC-603, a mouse IgA myeloma.

X-ray analysis reveals in each case a molecule with the overall dimensions of $80 \times 50 \times 40$ Å. The molecules are divided into two compact globular regions: one made up of $V_L$ and $V_H$; the other made up of the $C_L$ and $C_H1$ domains (Figure 9.28). The portions of the L and H chains connecting the two globular regions are elongated and exposed to their surroundings. This region is called the "switch" region and, like the hinge region, it is easily attacked by proteolytic enzymes.

The two domains that make up each globular region are close together (Figure 9.28) and interact with each other through hydrophobic residues that face each other. The $C_L$ and $C_H1$ domains are more tightly pressed together than are the $V_L$ and $V_H$ regions.

The peptide chain within a domain is folded back and forth on itself. Multiple hydrogen bonds link parallel segments forming two pieces of beta-pleated sheet, a classic example of secondary structure. Nine paral-

**229**

*Section 9.15*
*The*
*Three-Dimensional*
*Structure of*
*Immunoglobulins*

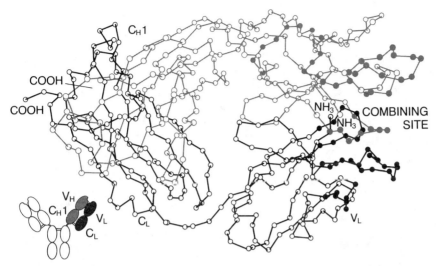

**Figure 9.28** Tertiary structure of the Fab fragment of McPC-603. Note how the L and H chains are exposed to solvent between their respective V and C domains. This region is known as the switch region. The combining site of the molecule—which binds phosphorylcholine—is at the right. [From J. D. Capra and A. B. Edmundson, "The Antibody Combining Site," Copyright © 1977 by *Scientific American, Inc.* All rights reserved.]

lel (or, better, "antiparallel") stretches exist in each V region; 7 in each C domain (Figure 9.29).

The ends of each straight segment are connected by sharp bends. The flexibility imparted by glycine residues is often exploited to make these bends. Many of the invariant glycines are located here.

Each pair of cysteines that forms one of the four intrachain disulfide bridges in the Fab fragment are, as you would expect, located within a few angstroms of each other. These are $23 \rightarrow 88$ for $V_L$, $134 \rightarrow 194$ for $C_L$, $22 \rightarrow 92$ for $V_H$, and $142 \rightarrow 208$ for $C_H1$ (using the Kabat–Wu numbering).

The three-dimensional structure of Fab' New also provides a structural basis for understanding the Kern–Oz isotypic variants and the Km allotypic variants described in Section 9.5. The light chain of Fab' New carries Ser at position 152 (Kern⁻) and Lys at position 190 (Oz⁺). Both of these residues are located at the *surface* of $C_L$ and thus are accessible to form antigenic determinants (Figure 9.29).

Although the L chain of Fab' New is lambda and thus does not exhibit Km variants, we can deduce from its structure the serological basis for these kappa chain allotypes. The Km allotypes are dictated by the residues at positions 153 and 191 in kappa chains. To discriminate the Km1,2 allotype (Ala-153/Leu-191) from Km1 (Val-153/Leu-191) and Km3 (Ala-153/Val-191), the anti-Km1,2 antibodies must recognize *both* residues simultaneously. In other words, both residues must make up a *single* antigenic determinant (Figure 9.30). Assuming that the tertiary structure of human kappa chains resembles that of lambda chains, these two residues are only about eight angstroms (Å) apart, a distance easily encompassed by an antigen-binding site (Section 4.2).

The hypervariable regions of both $V_L$ and $V_H$ are clustered close to

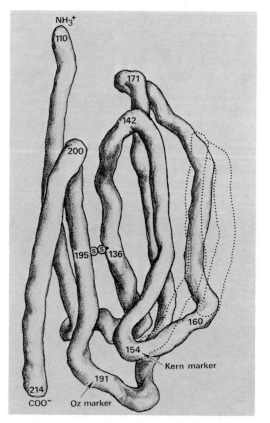

**Figure 9.29** Folding of the polypeptide chain characteristic of $C_L$ and $C_H1$ regions (solid lines). Seven antiparallel segments of the chain are hydrogen-bonded to form two pieces of $\beta$-pleated sheet. The dotted lines represent the two additional stretches of chain found in $V_L$ and $V_H$ regions. Residues marked 136, 154, 191, and 195 correspond to 134, 152, 190, and 194 in the Kabat–Wu system. [Courtesy of R. J. Poljak from R. J. Poljak et al., *Proc. Natl. Acad. Sci. USA* **70**:3305, 1973.]

each other near the tip of the V domain. Here they are exposed to their surroundings and are ideally situated to interact with an antigenic determinant. The hypervariable regions form a cavity or depression. In Fab' New, this cavity is 15 Å long, 6 Å wide and 6 Å deep. It is bounded at one end by part (Gly-25 to His-31) of CDR1 of the L chain. The other end is bounded by the sequence Asn-31 to Tyr-33 of CDR1 and Tyr-50 to Asp-58 of CDR2 of the H chain. The sides of the depression are flanked by Ser-90 to Arg-96 of CDR3 of the L chain and Asn-95 to Cys-100 of CDR3 of the heavy chain.

The organization of the complementarity-determining regions in McPC-603 (Figure 9.28 and 9.31) is similar in many respects to that of Fab' New. In this case, however, the CDRs form the walls of a consider-

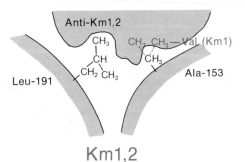

**Figure 9.30** To discriminate the Km1,2 allotype (Ala-153/Leu-191) from Km1 (Val-153/Leu-191) and Km3 (Ala-153/Val-191), the anti-Km1,2 antibody molecule must recognize both residues simultaneously. The presence of Val-153 on Km1 molecules prevents the antibody from binding to Leu-191.

**231**

*Section 9.15*
*The*
*Three-Dimensional*
*Structure of*
*Immunoglobulins*

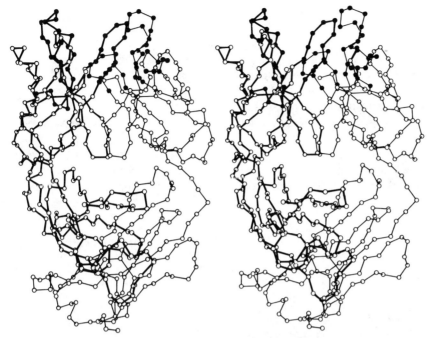

**Figure 9.31** Stereoscopic representation of the Fab fragment of McPC-603. The heavy chain is represented by the thicker line. The V regions — and thus the antigen-binding site — are at the top. The alpha carbons of the amino acid residues in the hypervariable regions are shown as solid circles. If a stereo viewer is not available, you may be able to fuse the images by erecting a stiff paper or cardboard between the views so that the left eye sees only the left-hand image, the right eye the right-hand image. It helps to have both sides illuminated evenly and 12–18 inches away from your eyes. [From D. R. Davies and H. Metzger, "Structural Basis of Antibody Function" in *Ann. Rev. Immunol.* **1**:87, 1983.]

ably larger and deeper cavity: 20 Å long, 15 Å wide, and 12 Å deep. Curiously, the second hypervariable region of the L chain plays no part in forming the cleft of either Fab' New or Fab McPC-603. In the case of Fab' New, there is a deletion of residues 55–61 of the light chain, which removes two residues of the second hypervariable region (55 and 56) and displaces the remaining residues away from the site. In McPC-603, there is a six-residue insertion in CDR1 of the light chain, which causes it to block the second hypervariable region from access to the site. The lack of participation of the second hypervariable region of the light chains of these two proteins is probably not representative of all antibodies. Sequence analysis and affinity labeling suggest that the second hypervariable region of light chains plays an important role in building the antigen-binding site of many antibodies.

Although Fab' New and Fab McPC-603 are both derived from myeloma proteins, they each have antibody activity. Fab' New binds several haptens with appreciable affinity. The best of these is a derivative of vitamin K (called vitamin $K_1OH$), which is bound with an affinity of $1.7 \times 10^5$ M$^{-1}$. The Fab of McPC-603 binds phosphorylcholine (PC) with an affinity of $1.6 \times 10^5$ M$^{-1}$.

In both cases, it has been possible to analyze the x-ray diffraction patterns of these fragments with and without the hapten present. In each case, the hapten lies within the site formed by the complementarity-determining regions. Vitamin $K_1OH$ almost entirely fills the binding site of Fab' New. Phosphorylcholine, on the other hand, occupies only a portion of the binding site of McPC-603. This may reflect that the antibody is directed against an antigenic determinant of which PC is only a part. Or possibly this molecule has more than one specificity; i.e., perhaps it can bind PC in one portion of its site or some other determinant elsewhere in the site.

The orientation of phosphorylcholine within the binding site reveals several opportunities for noncovalent interactions between it and amino acid side chains in the site (Figure 9.32). Two of the oxygen atoms on the

**Figure 9.32**   Schematic representation of the binding of phosphorylcholine to the binding site of McPC-603. In addition to the complementarity of shape, there are several opportunities for electrostatic interactions and hydrogen bonding (dashed lines) to nearby amino acid residues. Most of the contact residues are located in the complementarity-determining regions of the heavy chain ("—H"). Asn-90 and Trp-104a are residues 95 and 100a, respectively in the Kabat–Wu system and thus within CDR3. [From J. D. Capra and A. B. Edmundson, "The Antibody Combining Site," Copyright © 1977 by *Scientific American, Inc.* All rights reserved.]

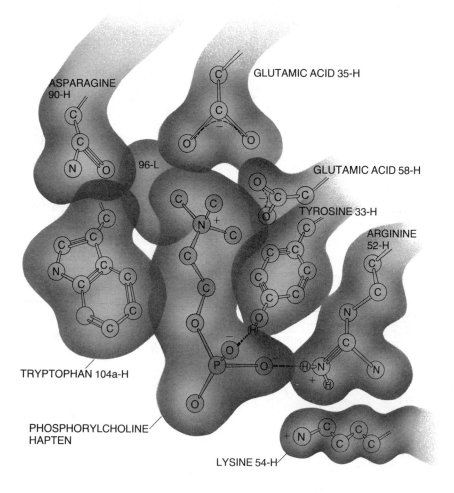

phosphate group of PC are positioned so that they can form hydrogen bonds with the side chains of Tyr-33 and Arg-52 of CDR1 and CDR2 of the heavy chain. The positively charged terminal amino group on Lys-54 in the H chain is also close to the negatively charged phosphate group. Phosphorylcholine carries a positively charged nitrogen atom at the other end of the molecule (Figure 9.32). This is positioned close to the negatively charged carboxyl group of Glu-35 and of Glu-58 of the H chain. The central portion of the PC molecule is occupied by a short chain of carbon atoms. This hydrophobic region makes close contact with the hydrophobic benzene ring of Trp-104a in CDR3 of the heavy chain. Note that all of these residues (called "contact" residues) are on the heavy chain. The only part of the $V_L$ region that seems to contribute to the PC-binding portion of the site are some of the residues in CDR3, especially Leu-96. This confirms the dominant role that the heavy chain plays in the binding activity of so many antibodies (Figure 9.24).

You may argue that knowing the three-dimensional structure of two Fab fragments hardly permits us to generalize about the whole universe of antibody molecules. On the other hand, the marked similarities between these human and mouse proteins and the conservation of structure in the framework regions suggests that these two molecules do indeed reveal the basic mechanism on which antibody specificity depends.

## ADDITIONAL READING

1. Davies, D. R., and H. Metzger, "Structural Basis of Antibody Function," *Ann. Rev. Immunol.* **1**:87, 1983.

2. Ishizaka, K., and T. Ishizaka, "Studies on Immunoglobulin E: The Impact of a Sojourn with Professor Dan H. Campbell at Cal Tech," *Immunochemistry* **12**:527, 1975. A brief review of the elucidation of the properties of IgE by the key players in the story.

3. Kabat, E. A., et al., *Sequences of Proteins of Immunological Interest,* National Institutes of Health, Bethesda, MD, 1983.

4. Kohler, G., and C. Milstein, "Continuous Cultures of Fused Cells Secreting Antibody of Predetermined Specificity," *Nature* **256**:495, 1975. (Reprinted in V. L. Sato and M. L. Gefter, *Cellular Immunology,* Addison-Wesley Publishing Co., Reading, MA, 1982.)

5. Koshland, Marian E., "Structure and Function of the J Chain," *Adv. Immunol.* **20**:41, 1975.

6. Nisonoff, A., J. E. Hopper, and Susan B. Spring, *The Antibody Molecule,* Academic Press, New York, 1975. A monograph on the structures and properties of the immunoglobulins.

7. Padlan, E. A., et al., "Structural Basis for the Specificity of Phosphorylcholine-Binding Immunoglobulins," *Immunochemistry* **13**:945, 1976. On the Fab of McPC-603.

8. Poljak, R. J., "X-Ray Diffraction Studies of Immunoglobulins," *Adv. Immunol.* **21**:1, 1975. On Fab' New.

9. Solari, R., and J.-P. Kraehenbuhl, "The Biosynthesis of Secretory Component and Its Role in the Transepithelial Transport of IgA Dimer," *Immunology Today* 6:17, 1985.

10. Strosberg, A. D., et al., "A Rabbit with the Allotypic Phenotype: a1a2a3 b4b5b6," *J. Immunol.* 113:1313, 1974. The first report of the occasional non-allelic behavior of complex allotypes.

# CHAPTER 10

# The Genetic Basis of Antibody Diversity

## 10.1 Introduction

Antibodies are proteins, and proteins are synthesized following the instructions encoded in genes. Thus the antibody repertoire of an animal must represent the expression of genetic information encoded in its DNA. So far, so good. The problem comes when we compare the extraordinary diversity of antibodies with the rather limited diversity of the other proteins of the body. Insulin, beta-galactosidase, clotting factor VIII, and many other proteins exist within the individual as one or two molecular species. They represent the product transcribed and translated from, usually, a single gene locus. Diploid organisms having inherited two of every (autosomal) gene locus can express at most two allelic forms of these proteins.

No one knows how many different kinds of antibody molecules a single human or mouse can synthesize. Some workers estimate that the mammalian genome carries the information for as many as $10^7$ different kinds of antibody molecules. Others set the figure lower. But even if we can synthesize only $10^6$ different antibody molecules, we are confronted with a genetic situation far different from that involved in the production of other proteins of the body.

The instructional theory of antibody synthesis, described in Section 8.1, was one of the early attempts to resolve the dilemma. This theory postulates that an immunoglobulin molecule acquires its antigen-binding specificity by being synthesized in contact with antigen, which acts as a template (Figure 8.1). Thus the instructional theory does not demand a large number of immunoglobulin genes. However, we have already examined the evidence (in Section 8.1) that disproves the theory. The specificity of an antibody is dictated by its three-dimensional structure, and its three-dimensional structure is dictated by its primary structure, i.e., its sequence of amino acids. We must assume that its sequence of amino acids is dictated, as it is for all other proteins, by the sequence of coding nucleotides in DNA.

As soon as it was realized that the diversity of antibodies is dictated by the genes, immunologists began to assemble into two schools of thought. On the one hand, there were those who saw no reason to postulate special genetic mechanisms for the production of antibodies. If we can make $10^6$ different kinds of antibodies, then we must have inherited $10^6$ different kinds of genes for doing the job. This view became called the "strict germline theory."

A second school of thought could not accept the possibility of such inherited genetic diversity. Its proponents wondered how an organism could afford to devote so much of its genome to antibody genes. In particular, what selective forces would have enabled a species to retain, through countless past generations, the genes for antibodies directed against such recent laboratory products as DNP, (T,G)-A-L, etc. The extreme view of this camp was that the germline carries only one or a few pairs of genes for antibody synthesis. As the individual animal goes through its life, however, these few genes are repeatedly mutated, giving rise in the B cells to the required diversity of antibody molecules. This is the "somatic mutation" view of antibody diversity (Figure 10.1).

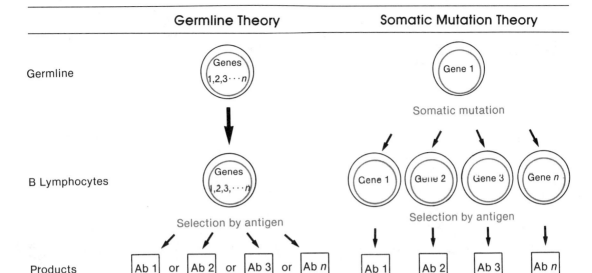

**Figure 10.1** The germline and somatic mutation models for creating antibody diversity. In the germline model, each B lymphocyte carries the genes for every possible antibody specificity. These genes have arisen during the evolutionary history of the species. In the somatic mutation model, a germline gene is repeatedly altered by mutation during the life of the individual. In both models, a single B lymphocyte expresses only a single antibody gene. Thus both models accommodate the theory of clonal selection.

As we shall see shortly, the extreme views of each camp soon became untenable. The somatic mutation people had to accept a steadily increasing number of germline genes. The strict germline people had to accept fewer genes than the number of different kinds of antibody molecules. Gradually, a middle position has developed. The view from this middle position is that there is a sizeable, but not enormous, number of genetic elements, genes or "minigenes," inherited in the germline. During the lifetime of a single organism, these genetic elements are reshuffled in varying combinations and, as a result, give rise to the abundant diversity of antibodies. What shall we call this view? If you are retreating from the strict germline camp, you call it the *recombinational germline theory*. If you are retreating from the somatic mutation camp, you call the process *somatic recombination*. In any case, the evidence is now overwhelming that somatic point mutations give rise to additional diversity superimposed on this recombinational mechanism.

## 10.2 Separate Genes Encode Heavy and Light Chains

Each antibody molecule (IgG, IgM, etc.) is made up of two or more sets of H-L chain pairs ($H_2L_2$). (We shall ignore the J chain of IgM and IgA as well as the secretory component of IgA.) Does a single gene encode both the H and the L chains? The answer is no; the two chains are encoded separately. However, this is by no means self-evident. The insulin mole-

237

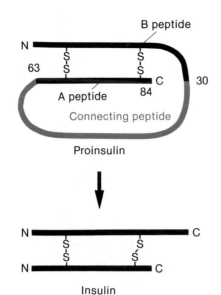

**Figure 10.2** The two chains of insulin are formed from the product — proinsulin — of a single gene. Removal of the connecting peptide occurs in the Golgi apparatus of the cell. The heavy and light chains of antibodies, in contrast, are *not* formed from a single precursor (or gene).

cule also consists of two polypeptide chains linked by disulfide bridges. Nevertheless, the insulin molecule is encoded by a single gene. The mRNA transcript of this gene encodes a single polypeptide, "proinsulin." The removal of a peptide from this molecule creates the double chain insulin molecule (Figure 10.2).

The technique of somatic cell hybridization has shown quite clearly that — in contrast to the situation with insulin — separate genes encode the L and H chains of antibody molecules and that these genes are, in fact, on separate chromosomes. The fusion of cultured Chinese hamster cells with mouse cells gives rise to cell lines that carry the full complement of Chinese hamster chromosomes but only a partial set of mouse chromosomes. The particular mouse chromosomes present varies from one cell line to the next. The DNA of each cell line can be tested for the presence of heavy or light chain genes. The purified mRNA from myeloma cells can serve as the template for the synthesis, by reverse transcriptase, of complementary DNA (cDNA) molecules. The cDNA can be radiolabeled and used as a molecular probe to search for the homologous (complementary) DNA sequences. The procedure is first to extract the DNA from a given cell line. The DNA is then partially digested by an enzyme, called a *restriction endonuclease,* that cleaves the double helix only where a particular pattern of nucleotides occurs. The pattern recognized by a particular restriction endonuclease usually occurs so infrequently that the DNA molecule is only cut at a few widely separated locations. The resulting DNA fragments are then separated into discrete bands by electrophoresis and denatured to form single-stranded molecules (ssDNA). Without altering their positions, the separated bands of ssDNA are transferred to a nitrocellulose filter and exposed to the radiolabeled cDNA. The procedure, called "gel blotting," was developed by E. M. Southern and the finished product is often called a "Southern blot." If the cDNA probe detects complementary DNA sequences, it will bind to them. The presence of the probe in a particular band is revealed by autoradiography (Figure 10.3).

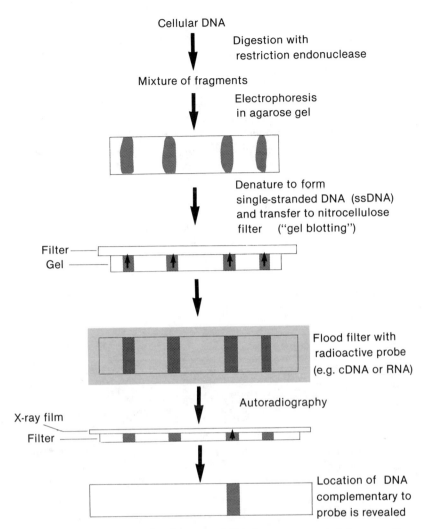

**Figure 10.3** Procedure for detecting DNA fragments containing a particular sequence. This procedure, called gel blotting, was developed by E. M. Southern (*J. Mol. Biol.* **98**:503, 1975).

Using radiolabeled cDNA corresponding to the $C_H2$ and $C_H3$ regions of the mouse gamma-2b chain, the probe binds to the DNA of only those cell lines that contain chromosome 12 of the mouse. However, cDNA corresponding to mouse kappa light chains binds to the DNA of somatic cell hybrids containing mouse chromosome 6, and cDNA for mouse lambda light chains binds only to those hybrids containing chromosome 16. Clearly, then, the light and heavy chains of mouse antibodies are encoded by separate, unlinked genes. This is consistent with the results of breeding studies in the rabbit, which show that the allotypic markers on kappa light chains (the "b" allotypes), lambda light chains (the "c" allotypes), and heavy chains (e.g., the d/e allotypes) are inherited independently.

The separate genetic control of H and L chains raises the possibility that antibody diversity could arise from the random combination of the two types of chain. This would reduce the amount of DNA needed to provide for antibody diversity. Thus only $10^3$ L chains assorting randomly with $10^3$ H chains would give rise to $10^6$ different kinds of antibody molecules while using only $2 \times 10^3$ genes. But is there evidence that any L chain can pair with any H chain?

The interaction between H and L chains involves both a disulfide bridge and extensive hydrophobic interactions between amino acid residues on the adjacent chains. Even in the otherwise highly variable V region, the residues involved in $V_H - V_L$ contact show very low variability. This suggests, then, that a wide variety of $V_H$ and $V_L$ regions should be able to pair successfully with each other.

The technique of somatic cell hybridization can also be used to fuse myeloma cells with normal plasma cells (see Section 4.8). The resulting hybrids, called *hybridomas,* retain the "immortality" of the myeloma parent and, often, synthesize both the myeloma protein and the antibody that was being synthesized by the plasma cell parent. In addition, these cells can also synthesize hybrid molecules consisting of the myeloma H chains and the antibody L chains or vice versa. This is additional evidence that H and L chains can assort randomly.

## 10.3 Separate Genes Encode the V and C Regions

As soon as accumulating sequence data clearly distinguished between the V and C regions of L and H chains, the idea was suggested (by Dreyer and Bennett) that the two regions might be encoded by separate genes (that is, two genes = one polypeptide). A number of lines of evidence provide overwhelming support for this view. Let us examine one line here. More direct evidence will appear later in the chapter.

It is now apparent that many more V regions than C regions are encoded in the germline. The existence of multiple genes for V regions is suggested by the many V region subgroups. Multiple V subgroups cannot be explained by somatic mutation within a single region of DNA. Each V subgroup ($V_H III$, $V_{\kappa 21}$, etc.) is identified by a particular set of invariant amino acid residues found chiefly in the first framework region (FR1). Every myeloma protein can be assigned to one or another of the subgroups characteristic of the species. If these molecules had been produced by the somatic mutation of a single gene, it would require that the same pattern of multiple point mutations occur in each individual member of the species. This is highly improbable. Instead, we must postulate that each V region subgroup is encoded by a separate germline gene.

On the other hand, subclasses of C regions are very rare. In the mouse, for example, the V regions of kappa chains fall into at least 26 different subgroups while only one kind of C-kappa region is found. One could argue that the germline gene for each V-kappa subgroup begins by encoding its subgroup-specific sequence and ends by encoding the same C terminal sequence as all the other V-kappa genes. However, the technique of hybridization kinetics, which is described in Section 10.11, does not support this redundant model. Hybridization of a probe for the mouse C-kappa sequence reveals only one copy of $C_\kappa$ DNA in the haploid genome. We conclude, then, that the V regions and C regions of antibody chains are encoded by separate genes and that a larger set of V region genes must share a limited number of C region genes.

Although V and C regions are encoded by separate genes, these genes are located on the same chromosome. Complementary DNA (cDNA) specific for *either* $V_\kappa$ or $C_\kappa$ DNA each bind to the DNA of somatic cell hybrids containing mouse chromosome 6. Probes for DNA encoding either $V_\lambda$ or $C_\lambda$ both bind to the DNA in somatic cell hybrids containing chromosome 16. As for heavy chains, we have seen that somatic cell hybridization shows that the DNA encoding the constant regions of mouse heavy chains is located on chromosome 12. The linked inheritance of idiotypes and allotypes suggests that $V_H$ genes are located on the same chromosome. Idiotypic determinants are located in V regions. The inheritance of a $V_H$ idiotype is closely linked to that of $C_H$ allotypes. For example, C57BL/6 mice respond to immunization with the haptenic group (4-hydroxy-3-nitrophenyl)acetyl ("NP"—see Figure 8.7) by producing antibodies expressing a particular idiotype designated $NP^b$. The anti-NP antibodies produced by CBA mice do not express the $NP^b$ idiotype. The $C_H$ regions of C57BL/6 mice contain allotypic markers different from those expressed on the $C_H$ regions of CBA mice. When (C57BL/6 × CBA)$F_1$ hybrids are backcrossed to the CBA strain, one-half of the offspring express the $NP^b$ idiotype **and,** almost always, the C57BL/6 $C_H$ allotype (Figure 10.4). The $NP^b$-negative offspring express the CBA $C_H$ allotype. This is a classic demonstration of linkage and tells us that the gene controlling the $V_H$ region is located close to the gene

**Figure 10.4** Concurrent inheritance of idiotype and allotype. The distinctive idiotypic and allotypic heavy chain markers of these two mouse strains are almost always inherited together. This indicates that the genes controlling them ($V_H$ and $C_H$, respectively) are closely linked on the chromosome. If the $V_H$ and $C_H$ genes were on separate chromosomes (or far apart on the same chromosome), the backcross progeny would include recombinants (e.g., allotype b, $NP^b$-negative) as well as the parental combinations.

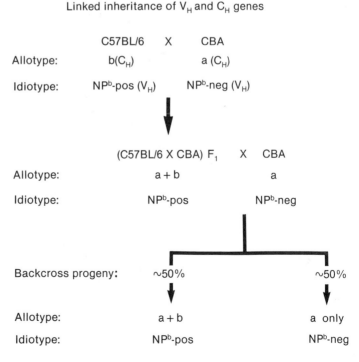

controlling the $C_H$ region. (However, the occasional appearance of recombinants proves once again that two distinct loci are involved.)

Chapter 9 examines protein sequence data showing that $V_\kappa$ regions are always associated with $C_\kappa$ and $V_\lambda$ regions with $C_\lambda$ regions. This suggests that only V and C genes on the same chromosome can be expressed in a single chain. This limitation extends to the members of a pair of homologous chromosomes. Each individual inherits a set of heavy chain genes on one chromosome (e.g., number 14 in humans) from one parent and a second set of heavy chain genes on the homologous chromosome received from the other parent. However, the expression of a pair of V and C genes is *"cis"*; i.e., each heavy chain contains either a $V_H$ and $C_H$ region inherited from one parent or a pair inherited from the other parent (Figure 10.5). Thus, when a homozygous rabbit expressing the $V_H$ allotype a2 and the $C_H$ allotype d12 is mated with a homozygous a3d11 rabbit, their offspring produce only two kinds of antibody molecules: a2d12 and a3d11. (Small amounts of a2d11 and/or a3d12 are sometimes seen, but this is probably not a case of *trans* synthesis — see the discussion of complex allotypes in Section 9.5).

Although our doubly heterozygous rabbit has both a2d12 and a3d11 molecules in its serum, a single one of its plasma cells secretes only one kind or the other. This is the phenomenon of *allelic exclusion* (see Section 8.6). The mechanism by which the V and C genes on only one of the two homologues gets expressed is uncertain but under intense study (see Section 10.8).

As long as their genes are on the same homologue, any $V_H$ region can become associated with any one of the $C_H$ regions. Evidence for this is the occurrence of each of the several $V_H$ subgroups ($V_H$I, $V_H$II, etc. — see Section 9.12) in antibodies of all the heavy chain classes. Thus $V_H$ subgroups behave differently from the $V_L$ subgroups. Each of the V-kappa subgroups is found associated only with C-kappa regions. Similarly, each V-lambda subgroup is found only with C-lambda regions. Any $V_H$ sub-

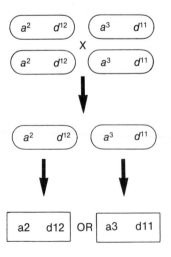

**Figure 10.5** The antibodies synthesized by a rabbit heterozygous for both *a* ($V_H$) and *d* ($C_H$) allotypes express only the combinations that were found in the parents. The product of a V gene on one chromosome cannot be paired with the product of a C gene on the homologous chromosome. Furthermore, a single plasma cell secretes only one of the two parental combinations (allelic exclusion).

Antibodies EITHER | a2  d12 | OR | a3  d11

No recombinant molecules

∴ cis translation only

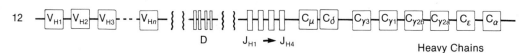

**Figure 10.6** Organization of the genetic elements encoding the kappa, lambda, and heavy chains of mice. The gaps indicate large amounts of intervening DNA. The $J_{\lambda4}$-$C_{\lambda4}$ cluster appears to be nonfunctional. In humans, the kappa, lambda, and heavy chain gene clusters are located on chromosomes 2, 22, and 14, respectively.

'group, in contrast, may be associated with *any* of the classes or subclasses of heavy chains. In other words, the V regions of mu, epsilon, alpha-1, alpha-2, as well as all four subclasses of gamma chains, draw from a single set of $V_H$ regions.

Idiotypes provide additional evidence. A given idiotype is often expressed on antibodies of more than one heavy chain class. Thus the serum of a C57BL/6 mouse immunized with NP may contain anti-NP antibodies of several classes (IgM, IgG1, and so on) all bearing the NP[b] idiotype.

All of this information leads to the following conclusions.

1. Both heavy and light chains are encoded by separate genes for the V and C regions.
2. The V and C genes for kappa, lambda, and heavy chains are located on different chromosomes (Figure 10.6).
3. Only V and C genes on the same chromosome can be expressed in a single heavy or light chain.
4. More V region genes than C region genes exist on a chromosome (except for $\lambda$ genes in inbred mice).
5. A given $V_H$ gene can become associated with any one of the $C_H$ genes.

## 10.4  V–C Joining Takes Place in the DNA

A cell could assemble two distinct gene products into a single polypeptide chain by three possible mechanisms.

1. Each gene (V and C) could be transcribed and translated separately into separate peptides which would then be linked together to form the completed chain.

2. Each gene could be transcribed separately, but the resulting RNA molecules could be joined and translated as a single unit into the complete polypeptide.
3. The DNA of the V and C genes could first be joined and then transcribed as a unit into a single RNA molecule (the primary transcript).

Let us now examine evidence showing that the first mechanism does not occur, but that the third mechanism does. (The possibility that the second mechanism may occur in certain B cells simultaneously expressing two H chain isotypes has not been ruled out—Section 10.8.)

### Each Polypeptide Chain Is Synthesized in One Piece

Polypeptide synthesis proceeds from the N terminus to the C terminus as the RNA codons are read by ribosomes traveling in the 5′ to 3′ direction on the mRNA molecule. If radioactive amino acids are supplied to a protein-synthesizing system (such as reticulocytes synthesizing hemoglobin), they will immediately begin to be incorporated into the growing polypeptide chains. Chains that were nearly complete at the time of

**Figure 10.7** Pulse labeling with radioactive amino acids shows that polypeptide synthesis proceeds from the N terminal to the C terminal. After a brief exposure (pulse) to radioactive amino acids (roughly 0.5–5 min depending on conditions), the completed chains are partially digested and the radioactivity of the resulting peptides measured and plotted. The graph is characteristic not only of such polypeptides as the alpha and beta chains of hemoglobin but of the H and L chains of antibodies as well.

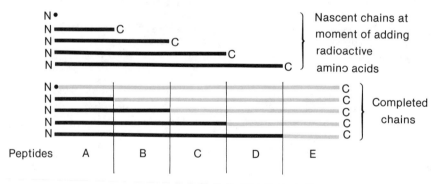

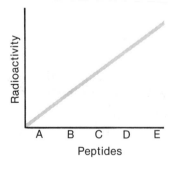

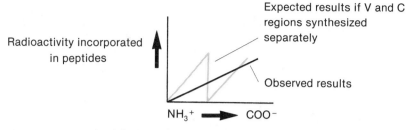

Figure 10.8   Pulse labeling of plasma cells reveals that for both the H and the L chains, the entire chain is synthesized in one piece even though its V and C regions are encoded by separate genes.

addition will have radioactive residues only near the C terminal end. Chains that were half-complete when the radioactive amino acids were added will, when completed, be nonradioactive in the N terminal half, radioactive in the C terminal half. Chains that were just beginning to be synthesized will be entirely radioactive. If after a brief interval the protein is digested into small peptides and these are separated by chromatography, the amount of radioactivity in each peptide sample should increase with the proximity of that peptide to the C terminal end of the original chain. One finds this during the synthesis of the alpha and beta chains of hemoglobin (Figure 10.7). This also occurs during the synthesis of both the L and the H chains of immunoglobulins. If the V and C regions had been synthesized on separate ribosomes, then the plot of radioactivity versus peptide position would yield a saw tooth curve (Figure 10.8). However, this is not found, and we conclude that V – C joining must occur at a stage prior to the synthesis of the chain.

## Each Polypeptide Chain Is Synthesized From a Single mRNA Molecule

Eukaryotic messenger RNA (mRNA) molecules characteristically include regions at each end that are not translated. These are the 5′ untranslated region (5′UT) and the 3′UT plus the poly-A "tail" (Figure 10.9). If V regions and C regions were translated from separate messengers, then we would expect that the quantity of nucleotide fragments derived from, for example, the 3′UT region would be twice that of the quantity of oligonucleotides derived from either the V or C region. But as Milstein and his coworkers have shown, the concentration of 3′UT oligonucleotides in purified light chain mRNA is equimolar with that of both V and C region nucleotides. In fact, only a single 3′UT sequence is found, which in itself would be highly unlikely if two different messengers were involved. In addition, these workers isolated an oligonucleotide with a sequence encoding four amino acids that span the V – C junction (105 – 108).

Let us, then, turn to the third model: that V genes and C genes are first joined at the DNA level and then are transcribed as a single unit into a single primary transcript that is processed to yield a single mRNA molecule.

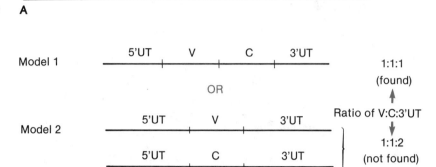

**A**

**B**

**Figure 10.9** A: Structure of a messenger RNA (mRNA) molecule. B: If V and C are translated from separate mRNA molecules (model 2), then the molar ratio of V : C : 3'UT fragments should be 1 : 1 : 2. In fact, the ratio is 1 : 1 : 1 indicating that the entire chain is translated from a single mRNA molecule (model 1). [Based on C. Milstein et al., "Sequence Analysis of Immunoglobulin Light Chain Messenger RNA," *Nature* **252:**354, 1974.]

## V and C Genes Are Rearranged During Differentiation

In 1976 Hozumi and Tonegawa presented striking evidence that V–C joining occurs at the level of DNA. They searched for the presence of a particular V gene and a particular C gene in extracted DNA. The DNA was taken from two sources.

1. The cells of the MOPC-321 BALB/c myeloma (these cells secrete homogeneous kappa chains and are considered to be fully differentiated).
2. The cells of a 13-day BALB/c embryo. These cells were assumed to contain DNA as it is organized in the germline.

In order to search for specific DNA sequences, they used radiolabeled mRNA purified from the MOPC-321 tumor cells. They prepared a sample containing the entire mRNA molecule and also a sample consisting of the 3' half of the mRNA. Because translation proceeds 5' to 3', this half molecule contained the sequence coding for the C region of the light chain.

The DNA samples were digested with a restriction endonuclease, called BamHI, produced by the bacterium *Bacillus amyloliquefaciens*. This enzyme cleaves DNA only at sites containing the sequence

$$
\begin{array}{c}
\downarrow \\
5'\ G\ G\ A\ T\ C\ C\ 3' \\
3'\ C\ C\ T\ A\ G\ G\ 5' \\
\uparrow
\end{array}
$$

Each strand of the double helix is cut between the two guanines. Inasmuch as this particular sequence occurs rarely, the enzyme cleaves cellular DNA into a few relatively large fragments. These fragments can be separated by size by means of electrophoresis. The electrophoretic medium (generally an agarose gel) is then cut into even-sized pieces and the DNA is extracted from each piece. Portions of each DNA sample are incubated with the mRNA probes. Because the DNA is denatured (single stranded), mRNA molecules can bind to it if they can find the appropriate complementary stretches for Watson–Crick base pairing.

When the whole mRNA probe was used with embryo DNA, it bound to two different populations of DNA molecules: one population with a MW of $6 \times 10^6$ and the other with a MW of $3.9 \times 10^6$ (Figure 10.10). However, the 3'-half mRNA probe bound only to the six million DNA fragment. These results suggested that the large fragment contained the C gene (it hybridized with both probes) and the small fragment contained the V gene (it hybridized only with the mRNA containing V region sequences).

When the experiment was repeated with tumor-cell DNA, the pattern was quite different. Each mRNA probe hybridized with the *same* fraction of DNA, a fraction containing molecules with a MW of $2.4 \times 10^6$ (Figure 10.10). Evidently, at some time between embryonic development and

**Figure 10.10** Demonstration that the location of V and C genes changes during differentiation. In the embryo, the V and C genes (for the $\kappa$ chain of MOPC-321) are found on separate fragments of DNA (I and II). In the differentiated antibody-secreting cell, the V and C genes are located on a single DNA fragment (III) smaller than either embryo fragment. [From N. Hozumi and S. Tonegawa, *Proc. Natl. Acad. Sci USA* **73**:3628, 1976. Reprinted in V. L. Sato, and M. L. Gefter, *Cellular Immunology*, Addison-Wesley Publishing Co., Inc., Reading, MA, 1982.]

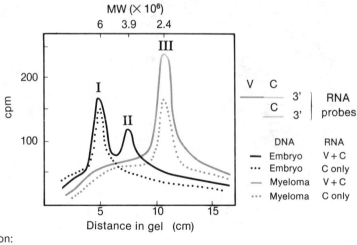

Interpretation:

the differentiation of the plasmacytoma cell, the V gene and C gene became relocated in the DNA. In the embryo, they are located so far apart that even though the C region (about 330 nucleotides) is embedded in a stretch of DNA some 18,000 nucleotides long and the V region (also about 330 nucleotides) is embedded in a fragment 12,000 nucleotides in length, at least one enzyme cleavage site occurs between these two long pieces. In the plasma cells, on the other hand, the V and C genes are both present in a single fragment smaller than either of the embryo fragments.

There is one puzzling feature of these results. Only a single pattern of rearranged DNA is seen in the plasmacytoma. What about the second chromosome 6 (the other one carrying kappa genes)? Did it undergo precisely the same rearrangement? Probably not. The subsequent analysis of many plasmacytomas has revealed three types of pattern: (1) a single rearranged gene (as here in MOPC-321) with the second gene having been lost (a deletion) perhaps as a result of an abortive rearrangement of its chromosome, (2) both the rearranged gene and a gene remaining in the embryonic configuration (Figure 10.11 shows an example), and (3) two rearranged genes, one expressed and the other aberrantly rearranged and unable to encode a complete chain. This pattern is particularly common with heavy chain genes.

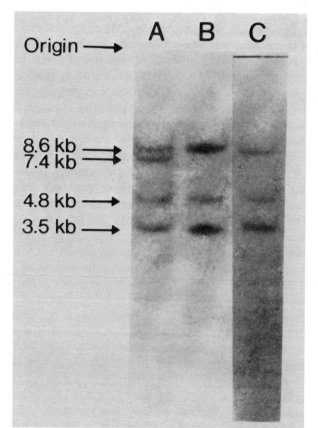

**Figure 10.11** Gel blotting analysis of the DNA fragments carrying $\lambda$ genes in the cells of a BALB/c embryo (B), H2020, a plasmacytoma, which produces $\lambda 1$ chains (A), and MOPC-321, which synthesizes kappa chains (C). The DNA fragments were hybridized with radioactive cDNA from H2020. A fragment containing the $C_{\lambda 1}$ gene (8.6 kb) and fragments containing the $V_{\lambda 1}$ and $V_{\lambda 2}$ genes (4.8 and 3.5 kb) are found in the embryo DNA as well as in both the $\lambda$-secreting (A) and $\kappa$-secreting (C) plasmacytoma DNA. However, the $\lambda$-secreting plasmacytoma (A) also shows an additional fragment (7.4 kb) that contains both the V and C genes. The embryonic, nonrearranged pattern often coexists with the differentiated pattern in differentiated cells. Presumably the embryonic pattern persists in the No. 16 chromosome that is not being expressed. The close homology of $V_{\lambda 1}$ and $V_{\lambda 2}$ accounts for them both binding to the $V_{\lambda 1}$ probe. [From C. Brack et al., *Cell* **15**:1, 1978 (© M.I.T.).]

In 1978, Tonegawa and his colleagues reported the nucleotide sequence of a gene coding for the V region of a lambda chain. The gene was taken from the DNA of a 12-day-old mouse embryo and thus represented a germline gene. This remarkable achievement required the use of three technological innovations.

1. The use of several restriction endonucleases, each of which cleaves DNA at a unique site established by a particular sequence of nucleotides.
2. The use of recombinant DNA technology. This made it possible to duplicate the isolated gene millions of times (i.e., to "clone" it) and thus to provide enough material for sequence analysis.
3. Techniques for establishing the linear order of nucleotides in DNA.

### Recombinant DNA Techniques

In order to clone a segment of DNA, it must be inserted into a type of DNA, like bacteriophage DNA, that can be replicated in a bacterium. The accepting DNA is called the "vector." Tonegawa and his colleagues chose as their vector bacteriophage lambda ($\lambda$), whose host is *E. coli*. Many restriction endonucleases cleave double-stranded DNA in an off-set fashion (see Section 10.4). The result is that a short segment of single-stranded DNA extends out at each end of the double-stranded molecule. By treating both the bacteriophage DNA and the mouse DNA with the same restriction endonuclease, the same type of "sticky" ends are produced. The sticky ends of the mouse DNA fragments can base pair with those of the bacteriophage DNA fragments forming "recombinant" molecules of bacteriophage DNA carrying a segment of mouse DNA. If the recombinant DNA has regained the infectivity of the bacteriophage DNA, it can be replicated in enormous numbers by its host.

The digestion of the total genomic DNA of a mouse yields an extremely diverse mixture of fragments. Somewhere in that heterogeneous collection is the gene, or a fragment of the gene, that interests you. The next step in locating this needle in a haystack is to expose the mixture of mouse DNA fragments to a sufficiently large number of vector DNA molecules so that each mouse fragment can anneal to one (Figure 10.12). Then this heterogeneous collection of mouse–vector DNA molecules is mixed with living host cells *(E. coli)* and the mixture plated in a petri dish of agar. All of the bacterial cells begin growth. However, those that have been infected by the bacteriophage are soon lysed and release progeny bacteriophage. These infect nearby *E. coli* cells, and the process is repeated. After 24 hours or so, the petri dish contains a "lawn" of uninfected *E. coli* cells dotted with circular clear zones, the plaques, each of which represents a center of bacteriophage infection. Each plaque contains many copies of the vector–mouse DNA complexes. By gently

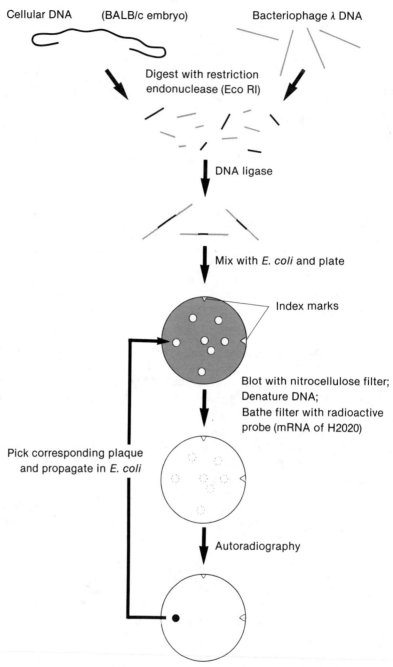

Cellular DNA     (BALB/c embryo)

Bacteriophage λ DNA

Digest with restriction
endonuclease (Eco RI)

DNA ligase

Mix with *E. coli* and plate

Index marks

Blot with nitrocellulose filter;
Denature DNA;
Bathe filter with radioactive
probe (mRNA of H2020)

Pick corresponding plaque
and propagate in *E. coli*

Autoradiography

**Figure 10.12**   Cloning a gene for a lambda chain of BALB/c antibodies.
Embryo DNA and the DNA of bacteriophage λ were each digested with
EcoRI forming complementary sticky ends in all the resulting fragments.
The fragments were allowed to reanneal at random and then were
sealed covalently with DNA ligase. Those recombinant molecules that
regained infectivity produced plaques in the lawn of *E. coli* cells.
Radioactive mRNA from H2020, a λ1 secreting plasmacytoma, was used
to identify plaques producing complementary DNA. Once identified,
the DNA can be propagated indefinitely. In this particular example,
the cellular DNA had been enriched for Vλ DNA prior to cloning.
[S. Tonegawa et al., *Proc. Natl. Acad. Sci. USA* **74**:3518, 1977.]

pressing a nitrocellulose filter against the surface of the agar, the DNA in each plaque is transferred to the filter. The DNA is then denatured, to form single strands, and the filter is bathed with a solution containing a radioactive DNA or RNA molecule complementary to the mouse DNA that you are looking for. Where the probe encounters such DNA, it binds by Watson–Crick base pairing, and the radioactivity acquired by that plaque identifies it.

By screening some 4000 plaques, Tonegawa was able to isolate a recombinant bacteriophage that contained 4800 base pairs of mouse DNA including a sequence homologous to the V region half (see Section 10.3) of the mRNA of the λl myeloma protein H2020. (Do not confuse the term lambda for light chains with the same name for the bacteriophage.) Propagation of the recombinant bacteriophage yielded 5 mg of DNA for sequence analysis.

## Sequencing DNA

Maxam and Gilbert at Harvard University developed the technique of DNA sequencing used in this study. It involves the use of inorganic

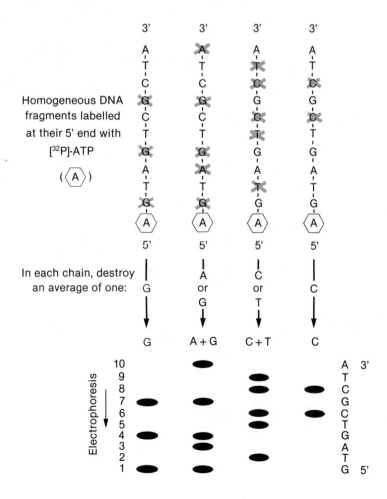

**Figure 10.13** The "chemical" method of sequencing DNA. [A. M. Maxam and W. Gilbert, *Proc. Natl. Acad. Sci. USA* **74:**560, 1977.]

reagents to cleave single-stranded DNA (ssDNA) by destroying particular nucleotides in the chain. The procedure is illustrated in Figure 10.13. Fragments of DNA are labeled at one end (5′ or 3′) with radioactive ATP and separated into single strands. This material is then divided into four portions. Each portion is subjected to chemical attack specific for G, A+G, C, and C+T, respectively. The strength of the reaction is carefully controlled so that most of the strands get cut only once. Each mixture is then subjected to electrophoresis, which separates the fragments by size. Single nucleotides travel the farthest, dinucleotides come next, trinucleotides follow the dinucleotides, etc. A photographic emulsion is exposed to the electrophoretogram for autoradiography, and each position containing the radiolabel is revealed. By comparing the respective electrophoretograms, the nucleotide sequence can be read directly (Figure 10.14). The positions containing A are determined by the positions that contain A+G fragments but not the G-only fragments. Similarly, the positions containing C+T fragments, but not C-only, establish the presence of T.

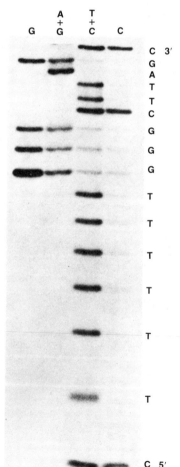

**Figure 10.14** Autoradiograph of a sequencing gel. The fragments in each lane were produced by chemical attack on the bases indicated at the top. The original DNA fragment was labeled at its 5′ end, and the migration of the cleavage products was from top to bottom. Thus the sequence of the original fragment is 5′ CTTTTTTGGGCTTAGC 3′. [Courtesy of Dr. David Dressler.]

The precise sequence of nucleotides was established for a stretch of DNA containing 750 base pairs (Figure 10.15). In some regions, both the anticoding ($5' \rightarrow 3'$) and the coding ($3' \rightarrow 5'$) strands were sequenced independently. In other regions, the sequence for one strand was derived from the sequence determined for the other.

The DNA begins with a stretch of 81 base pairs which do not code for any known protein. This is followed by the codon ATG for Met, the first amino acid in the hydrophobic signal peptide or "leader" that is found at the N terminus of all newly synthesized antibody chains (both heavy and light) but which is removed before the chain is secreted. The DNA sequence continues for 42 more base pairs, which establish the codons corresponding exactly to the known sequence of amino acids (from $-19$ to $-5$) in the signal peptide of the light chain found in the myeloma

**Figure 10.15** DNA sequence of the embryonic $V_{\lambda 2}$ gene of the BALB/c mouse. The amino acids specified by the coding portions (exons) of the sequence are listed above the DNA sequence. This sequence of amino acid residues corresponds to the established sequence of the $\lambda 2$ chain of MOPC-315 except for the residues at positions 38, 55, and 94–96 (the residues present at those positions in MOPC-315 are shown in boxes). Note that 4 of the 5 shifts occur in the complementarity-determining regions (the numbering is for this particular chain and does not match Kabat–Wu numbering precisely). Probably the 5 changes seen in MOPC-315 reflect somatic mutations in the germline gene shown here. The signal peptide ($-19$ to $-1$) enables the newly synthesized light chain to enter the endoplasmic reticulum after which the signal peptide is cleaved away. [From S. Tonegawa et al., *Proc. Natl. Acad. Sci. USA* 75:1485, 1978. Reprinted in V. L. Sato and M. L. Gefter, *Cellular Immunology*, Addison-Wesley Publishing Co., Inc., Reading, MA, 1982.]

```
              -19                                                        -5
              Met Ala Trp Thr Ser Leu Ile Leu Ser Leu Leu Ala Leu Cys Ser

5'...81bp...ATGGCCTGGACTTCACTTATACTCTCTCTCCTGGCTCTCTGCTCAGGTCAGCAGCCTTTC
                                                      └─────────────────────→

TACACTGCAGTGGGTATGCAACAATACACATCTTGTCTCTGATTTGCTACTGATGACTGGATTTCTTACCTGTTTGCA
←──────────────────── Intron (93bp) ─────────────
 -4            1                      10                                 20
 Gly Ala Ser Ser Gln Ala Val Val Thr Gln Glu Ser Ala Leu Thr Thr Ser Pro Gly Gly Thr Val Ile Leu Thr Cys

GGAGCCAGTTCCCAGGCTGTTGTGACTCAGGAATCTGCACTCACCACATCACCTGGTGGAACAGTCATACTCACTTGT

                          30                           │Ile│  40
Arg Ser Ser Thr Gly Ala Val Thr Thr Ser Asn Tyr Ala Asn Trp Val Gln Glu Lys Pro Asp His Leu Phe Thr Gly
└────────────── CDR1 ────────────────┘
CGCTCAAGTACTGGGGCTGTTACAACTAGTAACTATGCCAACTGGGTTCAAGAAAAACCAGATCATTTATTCACTGGT

  50               │Asp│        60                              70
Leu Ile Gly Gly Thr Ser Asn Arg Ala Pro Gly Val Pro Val Arg Phe Ser Gly Ser Leu Ile Gly Asp Lys Ala Ala
            └──────── CDR2 ────────┘
CTAATAGGTGGTACCAGCAACCGAGCTCCAGGTGTTCCTGTCAGATTCTCAGGCTCCCTGATTGGAGACAAGGCTGCC

    80                            90                │Phe│Arg│Asn│  98
Leu Thr Ile Thr Gly Ala Gln Thr Glu Asp Asp Ala Met Tyr Phe Cys Ala Leu Trp Tyr Ser Thr His Phe
                                                   └──────── CDR3 ────────┘
CTCACCATCACAGGGGCACAGACTGAGGATGATGCAATGTATTTCTGTGCTCTATGGTACAGCACCCATTTCCACAAT

GACATGTGTAGATGGGGAAGTAGAACAAGAACA...162bp...3'
```

protein MOPC-315. [The light chains of MOPC-315 belong to the $\lambda2$ class, but the $V_{\lambda1}$ and $V_{\lambda2}$ genes are so similar that the H2020 probe ($V_{\lambda1}$) had "fished out" a $V_{\lambda2}$ gene.] Then come 93 base pairs that do not match any known protein sequence. Then the codons begin again to correspond to the final four amino acids of the light chain signal peptide. This is followed without interruption by a stretch of 294 base pairs, the codons of which correspond almost exactly with the known N terminal 98 amino acids of the $\lambda2$ light chain of MOPC-315. There are only five places where the amino acid specified by the DNA differs from that found in the MOPC-315 light chain. Four of the discrepancies (positions 55 and 94–96) are located in CDRs.

Two possible explanations exist for these discrepancies. Perhaps the MOPC-315 cells are expressing a germline $V_\lambda$ gene different from the one isolated from the embryonic DNA. Alternatively, the MOPC-315 gene may be the end result of several point mutations in the embryo (germline) $V_{\lambda2}$ gene that occurred during the differentiation of the MOPC-315 cells. In Section 10.12, we shall examine evidence strongly supporting the second alternative.

Following the codon for Phe at position 98, the DNA sequence continues for 201 base pairs. This would be enough to encode the remainder of the V region and a substantial part of the C region as well. However, the amino acids specified by these bases do *not* correspond to any of the sequences found in this region of mouse lambda light chains. Thus this fragment of DNA does not encode the *entire* V region.

The noncoding DNA (93 base pairs) that "splits" the DNA encoding the signal peptide is called an *intervening sequence* or *intron*. Such sequences have been found in many other eukaryotic genes, such as the ovalbumin gene, but are not found in prokaryotic genes. The existence of genes split by intervening sequences tells us that a processing step must occur in eukaryotes between DNA transcription in the nucleus and mRNA translation in the cytoplasm. It has been known for some time that the RNA molecules produced in the nucleus are much larger than the mRNA molecules attached to ribosomes in the cytoplasm. One reason is that the primary transcripts of DNA contain intervening sequences. These must be removed and the cut ends of the coding sequences spliced together to produce the mature mRNA molecule (Figure 10.16).

DNA encoding the remaining portion of a $V_\lambda$ region soon turned up on another cloned fragment of BALB/c embryo DNA. But this fragment was isolated by using a *C region* probe. The DNA fragment contained four distinct regions (Figure 10.17).

1. A noncoding section at the start.
2. A stretch of 39 base pairs that encode the remainder (residues 99–111) of the V region (of a $V_{\lambda1}$ gene in this case).
3. An intron containing 1250 base pairs.
4. A sequence of 138 base pairs that encode the first 46 amino acids of the C region.

Earlier in the chapter, we examined some of the evidence that the V and C genes became rearranged during the course of the differentiation of a plasma cell. We found that in the embryo a given V gene and C gene are very far apart. In the B cell, they are closer together (Figure 10.10).

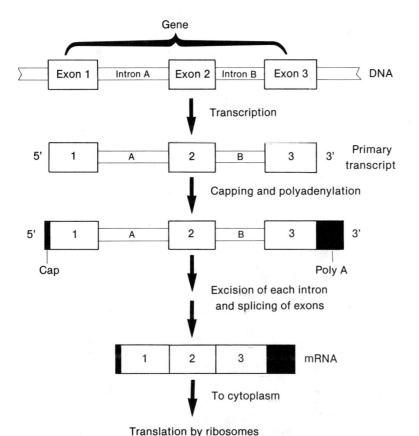

**Figure 10.16** Organization of a split gene (top), the RNA molecule transcribed from it, and the processing of this primary transcript to form a mature messenger RNA (mRNA) molecule. In addition to its "cap" and "tail," a mRNA molecule may contain regions (5'UT, 3'UT) at each end that are not translated (see Figure 10.9).

However, these results call for a reassessment. While *most* of the V gene is located far away from the C gene in embryonic DNA, the nucleotides coding for the last 13 amino acids of the V region are quite close to the C gene.

Tonegawa and his co-workers were able to pinpoint the nature of V–C joining event. They cloned and sequenced a DNA fragment encoding the entire light chain ($\lambda$1) of the H2020 *myeloma* as well as the embryonic $V_{\lambda 1}$ gene. They found that except for two base changes, the DNA sequence of the myeloma gene corresponded exactly with the embryonic $V_{\lambda 1}$ gene sequence from the signal peptide up to the end of the codon for His-97. Then without interruption, the sequence shifted to the 39 base pairs found in the fragment isolated with the C region probe. The myeloma DNA continued on with the same 1250 base pair intron followed by the 138 base pairs encoding the first portion of the $C_{\lambda 1}$ region (Figure 10.17). Thus the joining event that occurred during the differentiation of the H2020 plasmacytoma occurred at the *start* of the DNA that follows the nucleotides coding for position 97 and the *end* of the DNA preceding the nucleotides encoding position 98. The stretch of 39 base pairs that joins the DNA containing the C gene to the DNA containing the V gene

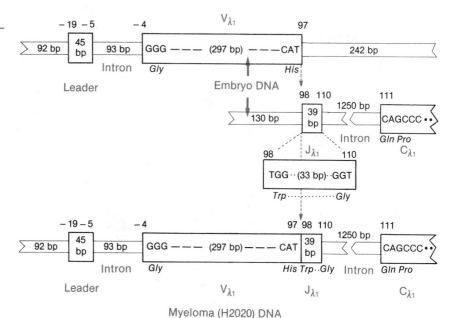

Myeloma (H2020) DNA

**Figure 10.17** Assembly of the gene segments encoding a λ1 light chain. The
$V_{\lambda 1}$ sequence in the myeloma DNA corresponds precisely to the amino acid
sequence of the λ1 chains of H2020. It differs at two bases from the $V_{\lambda 1}$
sequence in *embryo* DNA. Presumably the expressed gene in the myeloma is
the product of two point mutations that occurred in the embryonic $V_{\lambda 1}$ gene.
The new codons created by each of these base changes alter two amino acid
residues (both in CDR1). The DNA following the embryonic $V_{\lambda 1}$ segment and
the DNA preceding $J_{\lambda 1}$ contain recognition sites that appear to be required for
the proper splicing of the two segments (see Figure 10.19). [Based on O.
Bernard et al., *Cell* **15**:1133, 1978.]

segment is called the joining or J gene segment. (Don't confuse this J
gene with the gene that encodes the J *chains* that link subunits of IgA and
IgM.)

## The Organization of Kappa Genes

Most (>95%) of the antibodies synthesized by mice carry kappa, not
lambda chains. Many kappa myeloma proteins have been sequenced and
these are far more varied than lambda chains. Some 26 $V_\kappa$ subgroups
have been identified as compared with only the 2 $V_\lambda$ subgroups.

Although the kappa system is more varied than the lambda, there are a
number of similarities between the two. Again, split gene segments encode a signal peptide and the first 95 amino acids of the V region. In the
embryo, these gene segments are located far away from the DNA that
encodes the C region. The DNA encoding the $C_\kappa$ region (there is only one
$C_\kappa$ gene) is preceded by an intron of approximately 2500 base pairs. This
long intron is, in turn, preceded by five J regions, each separated from
the next by a small intron of 246–310 base pairs (Figure 10.18). The
amino acids encoded by all but the middle of these J regions correspond

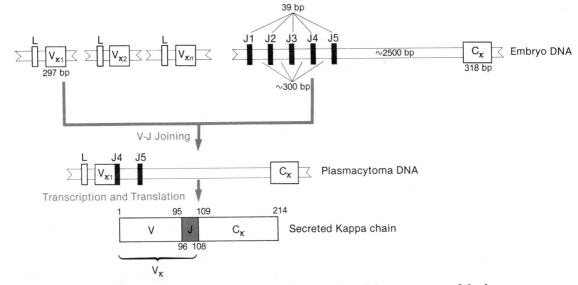

**Figure 10.18** Organization in the germline, in a plasma cell, and the expression of the kappa gene segments in the mouse. The amino acid sequence specified by the J3 segment has not been found in any kappa chains probably because the J3 gene segment is preceded by a defective recognition signal. L = signal peptide.

precisely with those found in one or another of a number of kappa-secreting myelomas. In 28 out of 36 myeloma proteins studied, positions 96–108 correspond to either J1, J2, J4, or J5. This arrangement of four J regions with many different V regions suggests that any single J region can be associated with any V region. Should these short stretches of nucleotides be called genes? minigenes? gene segments? Whatever we call them, the important point is that the light chains are encoded by three separate genetic elements: V, J, and C.

In the course of the differentiation of a plasma cell, the V gene segment becomes joined directly to one J gene segment. In the first example sequenced, a V gene segment had joined J1 in the plasmacytoma cells. J1 was then followed by

1. the other 4 J gene segments separated by the small introns,
2. the large intron (2500 base pairs), and
3. the C gene.

If joining had occurred between V and, say, J4, it would have resulted in the removal of the other three J regions as well as of their small introns (Figure 10.18).

---

## 10.6  V–J Joining

Careful examination of the DNA that follows each of the $V_\kappa$ genes that have been sequenced and of the DNA immediately preceding the four active $J_\kappa$ gene segments reveals some striking similarities. Every $V_\kappa$ is followed by

1. an identical sequence of seven bases (5′ CACAGTG 3′). This heptamer is followed by
2. a "spacer" of 11 or 12 bases which differ markedly from gene to gene. This is followed by
3. the nonamer 5′ ACAAAAACC 3′ which, with an occasional single base change, is found with all $V_\kappa$ gene segments.

The $J_\kappa$ gene segments are *preceded* by a similar pattern.

1. the nonamer 5′ GGTTTTTGT 3′,
2. a spacer of 23 or 24 bases,
3. the heptamer 5′ CACTGTG 3′.

Note that the base sequences of both the nonamer and heptamer preceding the $J_\kappa$ gene segment are *inverted complements* of the corresponding sequences following the $V_\kappa$ gene segment. In other words, the 5′ → 3′ sequence of one matches — by the rules of base pairing — the 3′ → 5′ sequence of the other. The regularities of these arrangements have led to the suggestion that these regions serve as a "recognition signal" for joining the $V_\kappa$ gene segment with one or another $J_\kappa$ gene segment. It is perhaps significant that the lengths of the spacers correspond to one (11–12) or two (23–24) turns of the DNA helix.

The same recognition signals follow $V_\lambda$ genes (see Figure 10.15) and precede the $J_{\lambda 1}$ gene segment, but in this case, the spacer in the $V_\lambda$ recognition signal is a "two turn" spacer (23 bases); that for $J_\lambda$ is "one turn" (Figure 10.19). Several models have been proposed as to how these recognition signals might serve to bring about V–J joining. Two of these are shown in Figure 10.20. Each assumes that the fusion of V and J results in the "looping out" and loss of all the intervening DNA, including all the V gene segments and J gene segments that had been located between the rearranged segments.

Each of the kappa J gene segments encodes two residues of the third complementarity determining region (CDR3). The first of these, position 96 (Kabat–Wu numbering), can be Trp, Tyr, Phe, or Leu depending on whether J1, J2, J4, or J5 is used. Here, then, is one mechanism which

**Figure 10.19** Recognition signals found in the DNA following (3′ side) and preceding (5′ side) representative V and J gene segments (and on both sides of a D segment). Bases that differ from the "consensus" sequence are underlined. Note that a "one-turn" spacer (11-12 bp) is always paired with a two-turn (23 bp) spacer even in heavy chain DNA where a D gene segment is spliced between $V_H$ and $J_H$. The exact length of the spacer varies by one or two bases in different recognition signals.

|  | Heptamer | | Nonamer | Nonamer | | Heptamer |  |
|---|---|---|---|---|---|---|---|
| $V_{\kappa 21C}$ | —CACAGTG - - | [11 bp] - - | ACAAAAACC | GGTTTTTGT - - - - | [23 bp] - - - - | CACTGTG | $J_{\kappa 1}$ |
| $V_{\lambda 1}$ | —CACAATG - - | [23 bp] - - | TCAAGAACA | GTTTTTGC - - - | [12 bp] - - - - | CACAGTG | $J_{\lambda 1}$ |
| $V_{H141}$ | —CACAGTG - - | [23 bp] - - | ACAAATACC | GGTTTTTGT - - — | [23 bp] - - - - | TAGTGTG | $J_{H2}$ |
| Consensus: | CACAGTG | | ACAAAAACC | GGTTTTTGT | | CACTGTG | |

GATTTTTGT - - [12 bp] - - TACTGTG — D — CACAGTG - - [12 bp] - - ACAAAAACC

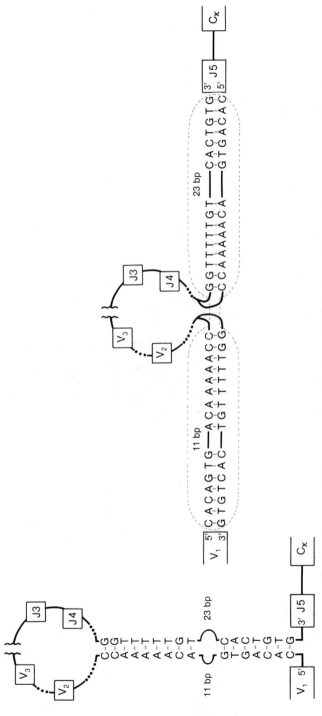

**Figure 10.20** Two models to explain how recognition signals might be used to splice a V gene segment with a J gene segment. The stem model (left) assumes that base pairing switches from interstrand to intrastrand at the recognition signals. In the second model, each strand remains paired with the opposite strand, and a joining protein binds simultaneously to the two recognition signals drawing together the ends to be spliced. In each model, the intervening gene segments are looped out and lost from the DNA being expressed. The stem model is described in E. E. Max et al. (cited at the end of the chapter); the joining protein model in P. Early et al. (*Cell* 19:981, 1980).

259

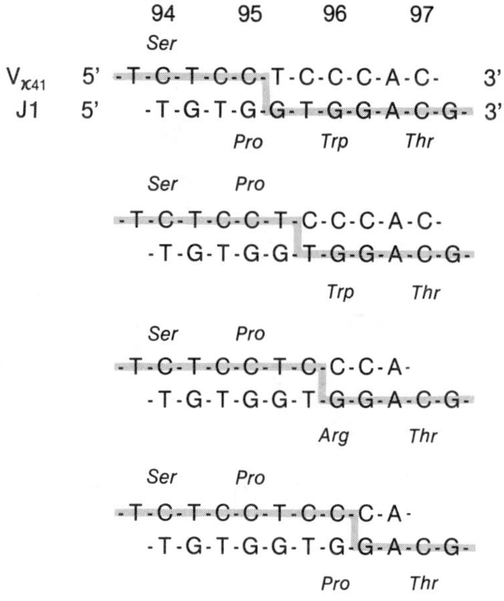

Figure 10.21 Changed amino acid sequences in CDR3 that would be created by shifts in the point of splicing of $V_{\kappa 41}$ with J1. Myeloma proteins with Arg-96 and Pro-96 are known, although no germline $J_\kappa$ gene encodes these residues. [Based on E. E. Max et al., *Proc. Natl. Acad. Sci. USA* **76**:3450, 1979.]

can diversify the antigen-binding site. (Position 97 appears to be an invariant Thr in all BALB/c chains.) However, position 96 in some BALB/c kappa chains is a Pro; in others, an Arg. Is there any mechanism (other than somatic mutation) to account for these residues?

One possible way to introduce additional diversity at the V–J junction is to vary slightly the exact point at which breakage of the coding segments from their introns and subsequent fusion occurs. Figure 10.21 shows four possible points of fusion between a $V_\kappa$ gene and the J1 gene. In every case, the resulting codon would encode Pro at position 95. However, position 96 might be a Trp or Arg or Pro. And, in fact, a BALB/c myeloma protein with Arg-96 and one with Pro-96 have been sequenced. Both of these proteins use the J1 gene (or possibly J2 in the second case).

In a similar fashion, variations in the exact point of fusion between a $V_\kappa$ gene and J2, J4, and J5 (J3 appears to be nonfunctional—probably because of a defect in its recognition signal) can give rise to different amino acids at position 96. Some of these have already been identified in myeloma proteins; we might well predict that those that have not simply await the working out of additional V-kappa sequences.

## 10.7 Heavy Chain Genes

The same techniques that proved so successful in establishing the organization of light chain genes have also been applied to heavy chain genes. In most respects, the organization and behavior of heavy chain genes resembles that of light chain genes. $V_H$ and $C_H$ genes, like $V_L$ and $C_L$ genes, become rearranged during the course of B cell differentiation. This can be shown by comparing the DNA fragments containing the V and C genes from undifferentiated and differentiated cells. Embryo DNA presumably carries the $V_H$ and $C_H$ genes in their undifferentiated (germline) pattern. DNA extracted from a plasmacytoma is assumed to carry the genes in the differentiated pattern of mature B cells. The sizes of the fragments in each case can be revealed by *gel blotting analysis* (similar to that shown in Figure 10.3).

Gel blotting analysis shows that the fragments containing heavy chain gene sequences produced by digesting plasmacytoma DNA are not the same size as those produced by the digestion of embryo DNA. This is evidence that a rearrangement of heavy chain DNA as well as of light chain DNA occurs during differentiation.

In most (~90%) plasmacytomas, the heavy chain DNA on both copies of chromosome 12 has been rearranged. However, only one of the rearrangements is functional; i.e., allows the formation of a complete, normal heavy chain. The other may have such defects as a missing DNA segment or an out of phase reading frame. Perhaps the rearrangement process is highly error prone, and most B cells that succeed in becoming plasmacytomas do so following the second attempt at rearrangement. How many B cells fail at both attempts and never make a mu chain at all is unknown. Such cells would, of course, not be able to express sIg and thus would not be subject to clonal selection.

Although there are many similarities between the two, the organization of heavy chain genes differs from that of light chain genes in three important respects.

1. The V regions of heavy chains are usually encoded by three, not two, separate segments of DNA: V, D, and J.
2. $C_H$ genes, unlike $C_\kappa$ and $C_\lambda$ genes, are split. Each of the $C_H$ domains of heavy chains (and the hinge region in gamma, alpha, and delta chains) is encoded by a separate coding segment (exon). These are arranged in the same order ($5' \rightarrow 3'$) as the domains they encode ($C_H1 \rightarrow C_H2 \rightarrow$ etc.).
3. The $C_H$ genes for all classes of immunoglobulins are located in a cluster on the same chromosome. A single $V_H$ gene can become associated with any one of these. A single $V_H$ gene can be associated with $C_\mu$ and $C_\delta$ genes at the same time. However, the same $V_H$ can later switch to another $C_H$ gene ($C_{\gamma1}$, $C_\epsilon$, $C_\alpha$, etc.).

Let us now examine each of these three special features of heavy chain genes in each of the following three sections.

## 10.8  The Assembly of $V_H$ Region Genes

The cloning and sequencing of fragments of heavy chain DNA, both from mouse embryos and plasmactyomas, has revealed the following.

1. The V region of most heavy chains is encoded by three separate gene segments: $V_H$, D, and $J_H$.
2. The $V_H$ gene segment, like its light chain counterparts, consists of

two coding sections (exons) separated by an intron. The first coding section encodes the first 15 amino acids ($-19 \rightarrow -5$) of the signal peptide. The next exon completes the signal peptide and goes on to encode the $V_H$ region through to the end of the third framework region (FR3), which is residue 94 in the Kabat–Wu system (Figure 10.22). In embryonic DNA, coding stops at this point.

3. There are four $J_H$ gene segments in the mouse. These are located in a cluster approximately 8000 base pairs upstream (i.e., on the 5' side) of the $C_\mu$ gene.

4. Like the J gene segments of kappa chains, any $J_H$ appears able to join with any $V_H$ gene segment.

5. The J gene segments encode part of CDR3 and all of FR4 (Figure 10.22).

6. Most myelomas contain a number of amino acid residues in CDR3 that cannot be encoded by nucleotides in the $V_H$ and $J_H$ gene segments. At least some of these amino acids are encoded by one or another of a dozen (in the mouse) independent gene segments called diversity or **D gene segments.**

7. D gene segments vary in length, encoding anywhere from two to 14 amino acids in the third complementarity determining region (CDR3) (Figure 10.22).

8. The nonamer–heptamer sequences at the 3' end of embryonic $V_H$ gene segments are separated by some 23 nucleotides (approxi-

**Figure 10.22** A: Coding relationships between $V_H$ gene segments and the $V_H$ polypeptide (Kabat–Wu numbering). B: Representative myeloma sequences showing the contribution of D and $J_H$ gene segments to the third complementarity-determining region (CDR3). The single letter code for amino acids is shown on the inside front cover. A dash indicates that the residue is the same as the one above it in the first sequence. The first base of the codons specifying the underlined residues is located in the D segment. So far as is known, a given $V_H$ segment can be associated with any one of 4 $J_H$ segments and any D segment. In addition, variation in the exact point of splicing between $V_H$ and D, and D and $J_H$, probably adds, subtracts, or changes codons as well. [From H. Sakano et al., *Nature* 286:676, 1980.]

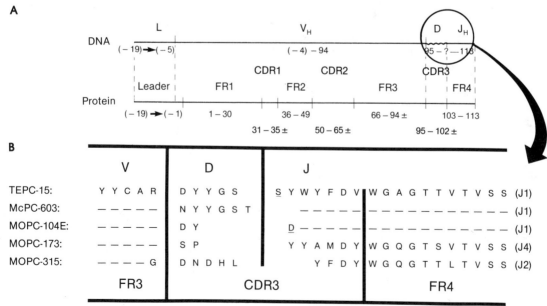

mately two turns of the double helix) as are the sequences on the 5′ side of the $J_H$ gene segments. This is not the pattern we found for $V_\lambda - J_\lambda$ and $V_\kappa - J_\kappa$ gene segments, where a two turn spacer is matched in each case with a one turn spacer (Figure 10.19). The patterns flanking V and J in the heavy chain system led to the prediction that when isolated (unrearranged) D segments were found and sequenced, they would be flanked on *both* sides by the recognition sequences separated by one turn spacers. This has turned out to be the case in both humans and mice (Fig. 10.19).

9. As with light chain genes, the exact point at which the 5′ end of the $J_H$ gene segment becomes connected to the 3′ end of the D segment (and the 5′ end of D becomes joined to the 3′ end of $V_H$) is variable. This variability causes codons to be added, deleted, and even creates new codons when the splice point occurs within codons. These cause changes in the length and sequence of amino acids in CDR3. Chapter 9 examines evidence implicating CDR3 as playing a major part in establishing the antigen-binding specificity of the complete antibody molecule.

10. The DNA of assembled heavy chain genes often contains a few nucleotides on either side of D that do not match any known embryonic gene segments. Perhaps these nucleotides have been inserted (without regard to template specificity) at the time of splicing D to $J_H$ and $V_H$. If so, these so-called N (for nucleotide) **regions** would yield still greater opportunities for diversity in CDR3 but at the price of increasing the risk of shifting the codon reading frame and causing a nonfunctional gene to be produced.

11. The exact number of D gene segments and their location in embryonic DNA is uncertain. Five have been identified in humans; over a dozen in mice. In each species, the D gene segments are arranged in orderly, tandemly repeated arrays. By analogy with the sequential (5′ → 3′) order of gene segments we have already noted (a pattern which appears again in heavy chain gene switching — see Section 10.10), we would expect the D gene segments to be located downstream of the V segments and upstream of the $J_H$ gene cluster (Figure 10.6). One D gene segment has been found upstream from the $J_{H1}$ gene segment in mouse embryo DNA.

12. The random assortment of different germline V gene segments with one of several different D segments and any one of four $J_H$ gene segments provides considerable opportunity for the creation of antibody diversity. The creation of diversity is further enhanced by (a) variations in the exact splice points at which D joins $J_H$ and, probably, $V_H$ joins D and (b) the incorporation of N regions at one or both sides of D.

## Allelic Exclusion

A developing B cell has six chromosomes from which to draw the genetic information to encode a complete antibody molecule. In the mouse, these are two each of chromosome 12 (H chain genes), chromosome 6 (kappa chain genes), and chromosome 16 (lambda chain genes). But as we have seen (Section 8.6) only one chromosome 12 is used for H chain synthesis (allelic exclusion). Furthermore, the light chains synthesized in a given B cell show isotypic exclusion as well as allotypic (allelic) exclusion. In other words, the cell uses either kappa or lambda chains and, whichever is chosen, only one of the encoding chromosomes. For other autosomal genes, both the maternal and paternal copies are expressed in a given cell. What, then, could be the mechanism which excludes one allele in antibody-producing cells?

An examination of the pattern of genetic rearrangements in B cells provides a clue. As we have noted, most (~90%) mouse plasmacytomas have undergone rearrangements on both copies of chromosome 12. One of these is expressed, the other is defective in some way (e.g., $D_H$ joined with $J_H$ but lacking a $V_H$, or an extra nucleotide destroying the correct reading frame). This high frequency of abortive rearrangements suggests that the gene joining process may be quite prone to error. Perhaps a cell on the path to becoming a pre-B cell rearranges one chromosome 12 and, if it is done incorrectly, turns to the other. Perhaps many cells fail with both.

To become a mature B cell, the cell must also correctly rearrange a set of L chain gene segments in order to provide a light chain for its completed antigen receptor. This may be a somewhat easier task. Only one-

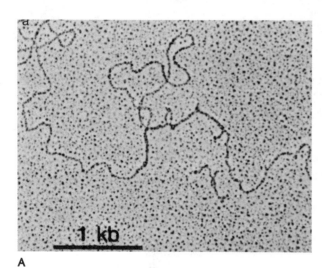

A

**Figure 10.23** A: Electron micrograph of a mRNA–DNA hybrid molecule formed by mixing purified mRNA from MOPC-141 with single-stranded DNA cloned from the same tumor. The bar indicates the length equivalent to 1000 bases. B: Interpretation of the structure. The solid line represents the DNA; the dotted line the mRNA. The loops represent the introns ($I_A$, $I_B$, etc.) that separate the exons ($E_1$, $E_2$, etc.) encoding the domains of the constant region (see Figure 10.24). The unhybridized portion of the mRNA is probably the poly-A tail at the 3′ end of mRNA. [From R. Maki et al., *Proc. Natl. Acad. Sci. USA* 77:2138, 1980.]

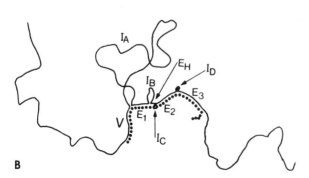

B

third to one-half of B cells synthesizing kappa chains show either a deletion or an abortive rearrangement of the unexpressed kappa allele. The remainder have their unexpressed kappa gene segments in the germline configuration suggesting that these cells succeeded at the first attempt. Curiously, both sets of lambda genes are in the germline configuration in these cells. However, cells synthesizing lambda chains usually contain abortive rearrangements and/or deletions of *both* their sets of kappa-encoding DNA. All this leads to the notion that once a pre-B cell has succeeded in making a heavy chain, it tries to make its light chain using kappa gene segments. If this fails for both kappa chromosomes, it turns to lambda gene segments as a last resort.

The process of allelic exclusion is probably regulated. The successful production of an antibody chain, H or L, appears to turn off further attempts to rearrange gene segments to make that chain. One striking piece of evidence to support this view comes from the deliberate introduction of a fully assembled $\kappa$ chain gene into the germline of mice (by injecting eggs with the gene). When these mice grow up, some of their B cells express the introduced gene. The remarkable aspect of this feat of genetic engineering for our story is that all of the animal's own complement of L chain genes remain in their germline configuration in these cells. It looks therefore as though the successful production of an L chain by the introduced gene prevents any rearrangements of the animal's own L chain gene segments. There is also evidence that B cells expressing an introduced, completely assembled H chain gene fail to rearrange their own H chain gene segments.

## 10.9 The Structure of $C_H$ Genes

Light chains have only a single C domain. Heavy chains have three (gamma and alpha) or four (mu and epsilon). In addition, gamma and alpha chains have a hinge region between $C_H1$ and $C_H2$. Considerable evidence suggests that the DNA sequences that encode each of these domains (as well as the hinge region in gamma—but not in alpha—chains) are separated from one another by intervening sequences. One way in which this has been shown is by preparing hybrid molecules consisting of a single strand of DNA encoding a $C_H$ region and the corresponding mRNA. Because of their sequence complementarity, a mRNA molecule can hybridize with the coding strand of the corresponding DNA molecule. When such hybrid molecules are examined by electron microscopy, a series of loops are seen. Figure 10.23 shows four loops ($I_A$, $I_B$, $I_C$, $I_D$) formed when a mRNA molecule from the cells of an IgG2b-secreting plasmacytoma is allowed to hybridize with the homologous single-stranded DNA cloned from the same tumor. The loops are flanked by five regions (V, $E_1$, $E_H$, $E_2$, $E_3$) where the two strands have hybridized. That no mRNA sequence corresponds to the loops of DNA indicates that they represent introns. Thus the DNA encoding the C region of this gamma-2b chain is split into four exons separated by three introns (Figure 10.24). The number and size of the hybridized segments suggest that

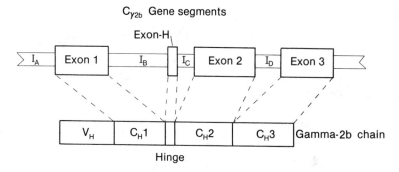

**Figure 10.24** Organization of the introns and exons in a mouse $C_\gamma$ gene segment and their relationship to the $C_H$ domains of the chain. The introns are labeled to correspond to those identified in Figure 10.23.

each corresponds to a single domain of the heavy chain. $E_1$ would encode $C_H1$, $E_H$ the hinge; $E_2$ and $E_3$ would encode $C_H2$ and $C_H3$ respectively.

This interpretation has been verified by actual sequence analysis in some cases. At each point in the DNA where the codons begin to correspond to the known sequence of amino acids in the $C_H$ region, that point marks the start of one of the domains. For example, DNA sequence data have revealed that the intron–exon margins correspond precisely to the margins of the four domains found in mu chains (Figure 10.25).

**Figure 10.25** Genetic basis for the membrane-bound and the secreted heavy chains of IgM. The alternative C terminal regions are encoded by different exons, both of which are included in the primary transcript. Alternative patterns of excision and splicing produce the mRNA molecules for each version of the chain. A similar situation is found for IgD and the other classes as well. $\mu_s$ = heavy chain of secreted IgM. $\mu_m$ = heavy chain of IgM bound at the membrane surface of B lymphocytes. 3'UT = 3' untranslated region. The poly-A tail of the mRNA molecules is not shown. [Based on P. Early et al., *Cell* **20**:313, 1980.]

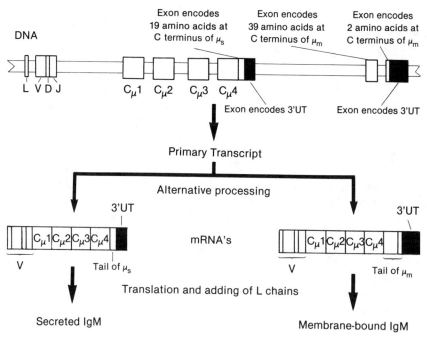

The $C_\mu 4$ domain of secreted mu chains is followed by a "tail" of 20 amino acids. The DNA that encodes this region is contiguous with the DNA encoding $C_\mu 4$ (Figure 10.25). This stretch of nucleotides is followed immediately by the nucleotides encoding the 3' untranslated tail (3' UT) of the mRNA molecule. As is the case for all the genes, the entire DNA region is transcribed into RNA. Then the regions represented by the intervening sequences are removed from the RNA to form the mature mRNA molecule. The 3' UT is retained in mature mRNA but is not translated into protein.

Early in their development, B cells display large numbers of IgM molecules on their surface. The C terminus of these membrane-bound molecules differs from that of secreted IgM molecules. Instead of the "tail" of 20 amino acids that follows the $C_\mu 4$ domain of secreted IgM, there is a longer tail of 41 amino acids. Many of these are hydrophobic and probably help anchor the molecule in the cell membrane. DNA sequencing has shown that the exon encoding the tail of the membrane-bound molecule (along with its 3' UT) is located downstream from the exon encoding $C_\mu 4$ and the tail of the secreted form of the molecule. The primary transcript of these gene segments contains *both* regions. Two different types of RNA processing then produce two different mRNAs and these, in turn, are translated into the two forms of IgM (Figure 10.25).

The $C_H$ exon clusters of each of the other classes of H chain also contain separate exons for the secreted and membrane-bound versions of the molecule. While virgin B cells seem to express only IgM and IgD at their surface, memory B cells express one or another of the other heavy chain classes as integral membrane proteins (Figure 7.18).

## 10.10  Heavy Chain Gene Switching

In Section 10.3, we examined some of the evidence that all the $C_H$ genes are located on the same chromosome and that any $V_H$ gene can become associated with any $C_H$ gene. Considerable evidence exists that a particular $V_H$ gene may become associated with more than one $C_H$ gene. The evidence comes from both the analysis of the gene products, antibody molecules, and the analysis of the genes themselves. Let us first examine the evidence at the protein level.

### Different $C_H$ Regions May Share the Same $V_H$ Region

Early in their differentiation, B cells express both IgM and IgD on their surface. This appears to violate our one cell = one immunoglobulin rule (see Section 8.6). But the violation is more apparent than real. The evidence suggests that the V region of these two classes of immunoglobulin are identical. Let us examine some of this evidence.

The lymphocytes of victims of chronic lymphocytic leukemia (CLL) may display both IgM and IgD molecules on their surface. Often the IgM is also *secreted* and appears in the serum as a homogeneous (monoclonal) product like those of multiple myeloma and Waldenström's macroglobulinemia. The IgM can be isolated and used to produce an anti-idiotypic antiserum; i.e., an antiserum specific for V region determinants. When the leukemic cells are treated with the anti-idiotypic antiserum, both the surface IgM and the surface IgD molecules are capped (see Section 8.7). This indicates, then, that the IgD molecules carry the same V region as the IgM molecules. The fact that a cell can synthesize two kinds of immunoglobulins bearing the same V region but different C regions, strongly supports the idea that these regions are under separate gene control.

In an earlier discussion of the monospecificity of antigen-binding cells (Section 8.7), we noted that one *antigen* caps all the immunoglobulin molecules on the cell surface. If the antigen-binding cell has two kinds of immunoglobulin on its surface (e.g., IgM and IgD), then this result suggests that the two kinds share the same antigenic specificity. In other words, here again is evidence of two kinds of molecules encoded by identical V genes but different C genes.

In 1976 Goding and Layton reported a direct demonstration of this. They used gelatin conjugated with NIP-POL to secure a spleen cell population enriched in NIP-POL specific cells. When exposed to soluble NIP–POL, these cells bound the antigen and capped it. By the use of fluorescent antisera, these workers were able to show that the caps contained both IgM and IgD molecules and that neither IgM nor IgD was present elsewhere on the cell surface.

The preceding experiments deal with cells that simultaneously express two classes of membrane-bound immunoglobulin. Cells can also switch from the synthesis of one class to the synthesis of another. Using the B-cell mitogen LPS, it is possible to stimulate isolated spleen cells to undergo several rounds of mitosis. The resulting clone of daughter cells can then be examined individually for the class of H chain they are synthesizing. In most cases, the class expressed by the mother cell will be expressed by all her progeny. In a substantial number of cases, however, mother cells synthesizing mu chains (IgM) produce progeny synthesizing gamma chains (IgG) as well as mu chains (Figure 10.26) or, in a few cases, gamma chains exclusively. Evidently during clonal development, some cells switched on a previously unexpressed $C_H$ gene. This experiment does not, however, tell us anything about the expression of V region genes during clonal development because the antigen-binding specificity of these immunoglobulins is unknown.

However, with a modification of the hemolytic plaque assay, it can be demonstrated that an IgM → IgG switch sometimes occurs during the development of a clone and that no change in specificity accompanies this switch. The procedure involves isolating a single IgM plaque-forming cell (which lyses SRBC "directly", i.e., simply with the addition of complement) and to stimulate it to proliferate. The daughter cells are then tested in the hemolytic plaque assay for either IgM production or IgG production (the latter by the use of anti-IgG and complement — see Section 5.12). Approximately 40% of the IgM PFCs that are cloned

**Figure 10.26** Evidence of class switching within a single clone of mouse B cells. A single mother cell and 10 of her progeny have been stained (with fluorescent antibodies) for $\mu$ chains (left) and $\gamma$ chains (right). The mother cell shows surface IgM. The daughter cells show IgM in their cytoplasm and, in some cases, IgG as well. [Courtesy of Dr. Matthias Wabl, from M. R. Wabl et al., *Science* 199:1078, 1978.]

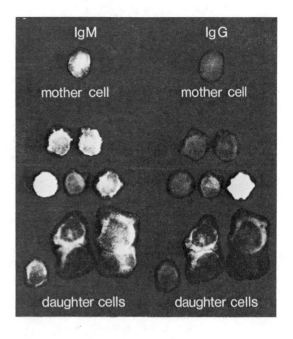

produce daughter cells that lyse SRBC with IgG. Thus a single cell synthesizing anti-SRBC antibodies of the IgM class can give rise to daughter cells secreting IgG antibodies of the same specificity. Because the specificity is unchanged, we assume that the cell has continued to express the same V region genes while it has switched from the expression of $C_\mu$ to $C_\gamma$ genes.

*Biclonal Myelomas.* Electrophoresis of the serum of most victims of multiple myeloma shows the myeloma protein as a single band (Figure 4.17). On rare occasions, however, human myeloma patients have displayed *two* discrete bands. In one of the first cases to be identified, one of the bands was an IgM protein, the other was IgG2. Careful analysis revealed that the *light* chains in the two proteins were identical in their V as well as their C regions. Furthermore, the $V_H$ regions on each protein were the same. Thus the only difference between the two proteins was that the heavy chain of one contained a $C_\mu$ region, the other was $C_{\gamma 2}$. The most reasonable interpretation for this finding was that one or more daughter cells of the original malignant clone of IgM producers had switched from expressing the $C_\mu$ gene to expressing the $C_{\gamma 2}$ gene. The expression of the $V_H$, $V_L$, and $C_L$ genes remained unchanged. Other patients with biclonal myelomas (e.g., IgM with IgA and IgG2 with IgA) have been identified. In each of these cases, the light chains as well as the $V_H$ regions on the two proteins appeared to be identical.

These data show that the product of a single $V_H$ gene can become associated with the product of different $C_H$ genes during the course of the differentiation of a B cell. We might well predict that these changes would be the outcome of changes in the association of the genes themselves. This turns out to be the case.

269

# The C$_H$ Gene Cluster

The rearrangement that occurs in *light* chain DNA during B cell differentiation appears to be a single event. The situation for heavy chains is more complex. The DNA extracted from IgM myeloma cells contains not only C$_\mu$ genes but also the other C$_H$ genes in the cluster (Figure 10.6). The presence of each of these genes can be revealed by hybridization with a radiolabeled cDNA probe for those gene sequences. However, when the DNA from an *IgA*-secreting myeloma is tested with these probes, the intervening C$_H$ sequences are either missing entirely or present in reduced amounts (perhaps on the number 12 chromosome that is not being expressed in this cell). These results and others like them lead to several important conclusions.

1. During B cell differentiation, certain C$_H$ genes become lost.
2. This could be expected if the process of V$_H$–C$_H$ joining occurred with the loss of all the intervening DNA.
3. The earliest antibody detected in B cells is IgM. The evidence above suggests that these cells still retain all the remaining C$_H$ genes.
4. As differentiation proceeds, the B cell switches from the expression of one C$_H$ gene (e.g., mu) to the expression of another (e.g., $\gamma$1). The light chain gene and the V$_H$ gene remain the same.
5. The evidence above also suggests that this later stage of differentiation occurs by another gene rearrangement.
6. These later rearrangements occur with the loss of all the C$_H$ genes "upstream" from the one currently expressed.
7. This suggests that the conversion of an IgM-secreting cell to an IgG- or IgA-secreting cell is irreversible.
8. The analysis of the number of gene copies remaining in various myeloma cells and the cloning of large fragments of mouse embryo DNA containing overlapping sequences in the C$_H$ gene cluster has made it possible to establish the linear order of C$_H$ genes on the chromosome. The order is C$_\mu$, C$_\delta$, C$_{\gamma3}$, C$_{\gamma1}$, C$_{\gamma2b}$, C$_{\gamma2a}$, C$_\epsilon$, and C$_\alpha$ (Figure 10.6).

The V$_H$ gene expressed in the IgA myeloma designated McPC-603 has been sequenced and provides powerful evidence of C$_H$ gene switching. We have already noted that the J$_H$ gene segments are linked to the C$_\mu$ gene in the germline with 8000 bases of intron separating them. The DNA fragment containing the V$_H$ gene of McPC-603 includes a germline J$_H$ sequence plus a stretch of noncoding nucleotides extending toward C$_\mu$. However, the C gene being transcribed in this myeloma is the C$_\alpha$ gene, not the C$_\mu$ gene. This shows that two distinct DNA rearrangements have occurred during the differentiation of the McPC-603 cells. The first rearrangement brought the V$_H$, D, and J$_H$–C$_\mu$ gene segments together. Presumably, the cell at this stage of its differentiation synthesized a phosphorylcholine-binding IgM antibody (and probably IgD as well). Later the intron downstream from J$_H$ became separated from the C$_\mu$ gene and became attached to the intron upstream from another C$_H$ gene. Perhaps this second C$_H$ gene was the C$_\alpha$ gene and the differentiation of McPC-603 was complete (Figure 10.27). Or perhaps one or more inter-

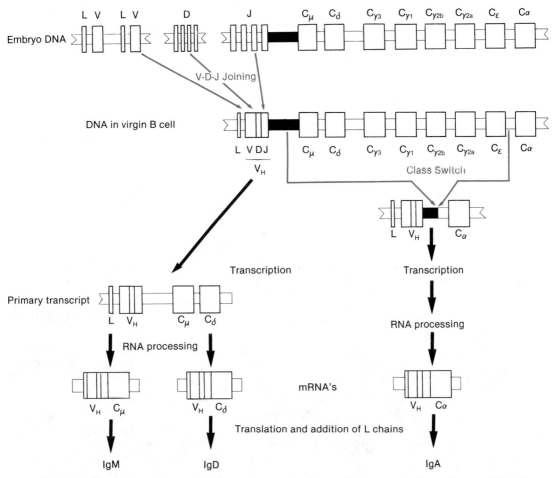

**Figure 10.27** One gene rearrangement (V–D–J joining) is sufficient to produce the $\mu$ and $\delta$ chains of IgM and IgD. However, a second rearrangement—called class switching—is needed to produce $\alpha$ (or $\gamma$) chains. Part of the intron (shaded) between the $J_H$ gene segment and the $C_\mu$ gene is still present between $J_H$ and $C_\alpha$. Similar evidence of a two-step rearrangement has been found in the genes of cells secreting $\gamma$ chains. The introns flanking the various $C_H$ genes appear to contain sequences that serve as switching signals analogous to the recognition signals that guide V–D–J joining. The introns that split the $C_H$ genes are not included in this figure.

mediate switches occurred, linking the $V_H$–D–$J_H$ complex for a time to first one, then another, of the $C_\gamma$ genes before the final switch to $C_\alpha$ took place.

## Switch (S) Regions

Class switching involves a rearrangement of an assembled $V_H DJ_H$ gene from its initial position just upstream of $C_\mu$ to a position upstream of one of the other $C_H$ genes (Figure 10.27). The switch occurs within the introns separating the $C_H$ genes. Naturally, these introns have been examined for the presence of a specific sequence that might mediate the recombination. All of the introns (except between $C_\mu$ and $C_\delta$) turn out to

**271**

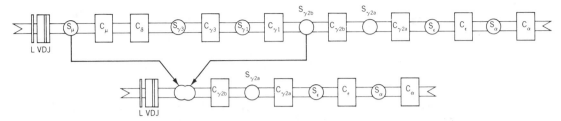

**Figure 10.28** Location of the switch (S) regions in the heavy chain gene cluster of mice (top) and the DNA rearrangement causing the cell to switch from IgM to IgG2b synthesis. The transcription enhancer, which is located between J and $S_\mu$, is shown in Figure 20.4.

have a region containing many tandem repeated pentamers. These regions are called S regions (Figure 10.28). There does not seem to be a class-specific sequence for each S region nor, for that matter, does recombination always occur at a given spot within an S region. The length of the S regions vary from 1000 to 10,000 base pairs. Curiously, there is a correlation between the abundance of each class of antibody in the serum and the length of the S region of its $C_H$ gene. In the mouse, for example, the S region for the gamma-1 chain (IgG1) is ten times longer than that for the epsilon chain (IgE).

There is no S region between the $C_\mu$ and $C_\delta$ genes (Figure 10.28). These genes are much closer to each other than are the other $C_H$ genes in the cluster. In fact, they are closer to each other than $J_H$ is to $C_\mu$. We have seen that IgD is expressed along with IgM early in the differentiation of B cells. However, the transitory appearance of IgD is preceded by and followed by the production of IgM alone. This violates our rule of the irreversibility of the $C_H$ gene switch. In this case, however, both the $C_\mu$ and $C_\delta$ genes are transcribed (along with $V_H DJ_H$) as a single unit. RNA processing can then produce both $VC_\mu$ and $VC_\delta$ mRNA molecules.

There have been reports of class switching occurring in B cells without the loss of the intervening $C_H$ genes. Perhaps in these cases, the new $V - C_H$ combination is produced by alternative RNA processing of a single transcript in much the same way that both IgM and IgD are. However, a primary transcript able to generate, for example, alpha chains without the loss of the $C_\mu$ gene and other intervening genes would have to be huge — some 180,000 bases long. Whatever the mechanism, some workers feel that all class switching *begins* with the alternative processing of a multigene primary transcript. Only as the B cell differentiates into a plasma cell and becomes committed to the new isotype does physical switching of the $V_H DJ_H$ gene occur (possibly as a result of signals from "helper" T cells).

## The Transcription Enhancer

The process of $V_H - D - J_H$ joining not only assembles a complete H chain gene, but also turns on its efficient transcription by the B cell. Activation of transcription depends on a stretch of DNA located between the $J_H$

cluster and $S_\mu$, the switch region upstream of the $C_\mu$ exon cluster (Figure 20.4). Enhancers stimulate transcription from promoters which must be on the same chromosome but can be some distance away (up to a few thousand bases) from the enhancer. Each $V_H$ gene segment appears to have its own promoter, but until gene rearrangement occurs, these are too far away to be influenced by the heavy chain gene enhancer.

The action of the enhancer is tissue specific. Rearranged H chain genes are transcribed efficiently only in B cells. B cells contain a factor, probably a protein, that binds to the enhancer and in so doing enables it to do its job.

Because of its position upstream (5′) to $S_\mu$, the H chain enhancer is retained after class switching (Figure 10.28). This makes possible efficient production of the new class of heavy chain. A transcription enhancer has also been found upstream of the $C_\kappa$ gene segment.

## 10.11  Counting Genes

Throughout this chapter we have examined evidence for a sizable number of immunoglobulin genes or gene segments carried in the germline. Some of this has been done by actual DNA sequence data (e.g., the five distinct J-kappa segments), but most stems from amino acid sequence data. The occurrence within the catalog of myeloma proteins of a set of V regions that are similar or identical (especially in their framework regions) to each other but quite different from other myeloma proteins establishes a subgroup. On the assumption that no two mice (or humans) could have undergone the same pattern of mutations leading to two identical or closely similar myeloma proteins, we postulate that two proteins assigned to the same subgroup have been derived from the same germline gene. The very fact that mouse myeloma proteins of the $V_H III$ subgroup resemble human $V_H III$ myelomas more closely than they do mouse $V_H I$ myeloma proteins strongly supports this argument.

But within most subgroups, a number of different myeloma sequences are known. Some of these differ in one or two framework residues, but most of the differences occur in the complementarity-determining regions (CDRs). Regions of DNA that encode CDRs are already present in the germline in the V, D, and J gene segments. So we are still left with the question of whether there is a separate germline gene segment for each of the known sequences or whether somatic point mutation gives rise to diversity superimposed on germline sequences.

One way to approach this question is to attempt to count the number of copies of a given subgroup gene present in the genome of the organism. If the number of genes in a subgroup is smaller than the number of myeloma proteins in that subgroup, then we conclude that somatic mutation has contributed to antibody diversity. Two methods for attacking this question have been used. Both use a radiolabeled probe carrying the nucleotide sequence of the gene in question to search for similar sequences in cellular DNA.

# Hybridization Kinetics

Two types of probes can be used in order to search for specific DNA sequences: a mRNA complementary to the sequence in question or a cDNA prepared from such a messenger. The principle of hybridization kinetics is the same for each.

In either case, the probe is radiolabeled and mixed with an excess of DNA fragments extracted from cells such as myeloma cells or liver cells (the latter presumably carrying immunoglobulin genes in the germline number and arrangement). Therefore, the reaction vessel contains (1) multiple copies of a probe, carrying a unique sequence of nucleotides corresponding to a gene or gene fragment, surrounded by (2) an incredibly diverse collection of DNA fragments carrying nucleotide sequences representing the entire gene content of the organism. When and if a probe molecule collides with a DNA fragment with which it can base pair over most of its length, a duplex is formed. This duplex can be separated from the surrounding single-stranded molecules and its presence detected by its radioactivity.

Given a pool of DNA fragments from a single source (e.g., mouse liver), the ability of the probe molecules to find complementary molecules will depend upon the initial concentration $(C_0)$ of the probe and the time $(t)$ available to search. The concentration is usually expressed as moles/liter and the time in seconds. Their product, $C_0t$, is designated the "Cot" value.

Figure 10.29 shows typical examples of the type of results seen. At low values of Cot, most of the probe molecules remain unhybridized. At high values of Cot, the probe molecules approach a maximum value of hybridization. These values usually span several orders of magnitude so that the log of Cot is plotted.

The shape of the hybridization curve is roughly sigmoid, with hybridization occurring most rapidly in the middle part of the curve. The Cot value at the point when the probe molecules have achieved 50% of their maximum hybridization can usually be read with considerable precision. This is known as the $Cot_{1/2}$ value.

The Cot curves for the genes encoding the alpha and beta chains of hemoglobin and the genes encoding the 18S RNA subunit of ribosomes

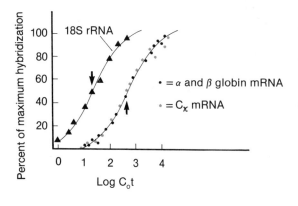

**Figure 10.29**  Hybridization kinetics of mouse 18S rRNA, globin mRNA, and $C_\kappa$ mRNA with DNA extracted from mouse liver cells. The $C_0t1/2$ values are indicated with arrows. The value for $C_\kappa$ mRNA indicates that only a few copies of the $C_\kappa$ gene are present in mouse cells. [From S. Tonegawa et al., *Proc. Natl. Acad. Sci. USA* **73**:203, 1976.]

(both in mice) are shown in Figure 10.29. A radiolabeled purified globin mRNA was used as the probe in the first case; purified rRNA in the second. The $Cot_{1/2}$ values are indicated with arrows. The mouse genome is thought to contain approximately 200 rRNA genes; there are probably no more than four globin genes.

Using standards such as these, one can establish $Cot_{1/2}$ values for immunoglobulin genes. A number of laboratories have pursued such studies. While the values reported have varied between laboratories, the variations have been remarkably small. In general, probes specific for a particular C gene (e.g., $C_\kappa$) give $Cot_{1/2}$ values that indicate only one or two copies (probably one in the case of $C_\kappa$) of the gene in the (haploid) genome (Figure 10.29). This is certainly all the sequence data demand and provides strong support for the concept that any of a multiple set of V genes can be associated with a single C gene (Section 10.3). So the problem of antibody diversity is really one of V region diversity.

There are many (26 or more) $V_\kappa$ subgroups in the mouse. In order to derive useful information from Cot data, the extent to which any $V_\kappa$ probe can cross-hybridize with different subgroups must be established. Considerable hybridization data have been accumulated with probes for the $V_{\kappa21}$ subgroup. The $V_{\kappa21}$ subgroup is the most complex of all the $V_\kappa$ subgroups. There are a large number of $V_{\kappa21}$ myeloma sequences known and many of these fall into recognizable subsets. For this reason, the $V_{\kappa21}$ subgroup should probably be subdivided into at least six sub-subgroups ($V_{\kappa21A}$, $V_{\kappa21B}$, $V_{\kappa21C}$, etc.). The degree of sequence homology between the subsets of $V_{\kappa21}$ ranges upward from 80%. However, the degree of homology between the differently numbered $V_\kappa$ subgroups (e.g., $V_{\kappa21}$ versus $V_{\kappa19}$) is only about 50%. Hybridization studies indicate that any $V_{\kappa21}$ probe will hybridize extensively with any and all $V_{\kappa21}$ genes. However, a $V_{\kappa21}$ probe will be unlikely to hybridize with $V_\kappa$ genes of other numbered subgroups. Using a $V_{\kappa21C}$ mRNA probe, Tonegawa arrived at a value of two to three germline $V_{\kappa21}$ genes. As we shall see in the following section, this value is probably a little low. But even if there are six $V_{\kappa21}$ genes in the genome (one for each of the lettered sub-subgroups), this number is too small to produce — without somatic modification — all the $V_{\kappa21}$ protein sequences known.

## Counting Genes by Gel Blotting

The gel blotting procedure lends itself admirably to establishing the minimum number of copies of a gene in the genome. Let us assume that a sample of mouse liver DNA contains six closely similar $V_\kappa$ genes located at various places on chromosome number six. Let us further assume that these six genes are flanked by DNA sequences that differ for each gene. Digestion of the DNA with a restriction endonuclease will produce a complex mixture of DNA fragments of different sizes. These are subjected to electrophoresis (Figure 10.30). Any fragments homologous to a radiolabeled probe will bind that probe and can be visualized by autoradiography. The number of bands that appear thus establish the *minimum* number of different copies of the gene sequence being probed. (Two

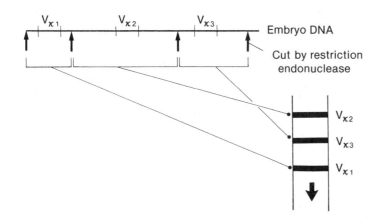

**Figure 10.30** Counting genes by gel blotting. The number of bands produced gives a minimum estimate because (1) two V genes might be present in a single fragment and (2) two or more V genes might be flanked by identically positioned enzyme cleavage sites.

copies of the gene might be present in a single fragment. Or, if two copies of the gene were each flanked by DNA containing enzyme-cleavage sites spaced exactly alike, then each would be present in a fragment of identical size and they would migrate as a single band during electrophoresis.) Using this technique Tonegawa's colleagues showed that a digest of BALB/c embryo DNA produced six different fragments that hybridized to a cDNA probe prepared from the mRNA of the MOPC-321 myeloma. The light chains of MOPC-321 belong to the $V_{\kappa 21}$ subgroup. Therefore the mouse carries at least six different $V_{\kappa 21}$ genes in its germline. Taken with the earlier evidence that (1) there are six well-defined $V_{\kappa 21}$ sub-sub-groups (A, B, C, D, E, and F) and (2) any $V_{\kappa 21}$ probe will cross-hybridize extensively with the genes for all the sub-subgroups ($V_{\kappa 21A}$, $V_{\kappa 21B}$, etc.), we are led to the tempting conclusion that each $V_{\kappa 21}$ sub-subgroup is encoded by a single germline gene. However, some 33 myeloma proteins have been assigned to the $V_{\kappa 21}$ subgroup. If six germline genes produce 33 different gene products, we must look for a means of somatically diversifying the germline genes. And, in fact, within a sub-subgroup (e.g., $V_{\kappa 21C}$), the differences observed are (a) primarily confined to the CDRs and (b) can be accounted for by single base changes; i.e., they appear to be examples of point mutations.

Some 26 distinct subgroups of $V_{\kappa}$ regions have been identified in the mouse. If each subgroup is represented by, say, five different germline genes, that would provide 130 different inherited $V_{\kappa}$ genes. As for humans, gel blotting suggests that we have fewer than 50 germline $V_{\kappa}$ genes.

The germline pool of $V_{\lambda}$ gene segments is quite limited in mice. As we have seen (Section 10.5), the BALB/c mouse inherits only two $V_{\lambda}$ gene segments. Not surprisingly, only a small ($\sim$5%) fraction of mouse antibodies carry lambda chains. The proportion of lambda-carrying antibodies in humans is higher ($\sim$40%), and gel blotting predicts that the number of $V_{\lambda}$ gene segments in the human genome is on the order of two dozen.

Gel blotting has also been used to estimate the size of the pool of $V_{H}$ gene segments. Complementary DNA (cDNA) probes specific for a particular $V_{H}$ subgroup may reveal anywhere from 1 to 30 bands depending on the subgroup analyzed. Seven $V_{H}$ subgroups have been identified in mice, four in humans. Taking a value of 20 for each subgroup, this gives a rough estimate of 140 germline $V_H$ gene segments in the mouse, 80 in humans.

**277**

*Section 10.12*
*Further Evidence*
*for Somatic Muta-*
*tions in V Genes*

## 10.12 Further Evidence for Somatic Mutations in V Genes

Only 5% or so of the antibodies synthesized by mice carry lambda light chains. Myelomas with lambda chains are correspondingly rare. Nevertheless, the amino acid sequences of the V regions of over 20 myeloma light chains of the $\lambda 1$ family have been studied and compared. Over half of these are identical. Remembering that each of these myelomas arose in a different mouse, this suggests that each of the identical sequences was the expression of a single germline gene. Each of the other chains differed from the "germline" sequence at one to three amino acid residues, and *no two of these variant chains were alike.* In almost every case, the variant amino acid residue could have been encoded by a single base change. Furthermore, almost all of the amino acid replacements in the variant chains were found in the three complementarity-determining regions (CDRs). If each of the variant chains was the product of another germline gene, one would have expected to find some duplicates. Although indirect, this evidence strongly favors the existence of somatic point mutations in the generation of antibody diversity.

As we noted in Section 10.5, Tonegawa's group actually sequenced the V gene of the light chain of H2020, a myeloma with $\lambda 1$ light chains, and compared it with the sequence of the embryonic $V_{\lambda 1}$ gene. The myeloma gene was identical to the embryonic gene except for two bases. Each of these base changes produced the appropriate codon for the two amino acids that distinguish the H2020 light chain from the commonly occurring "germline" $\lambda 1$ protein sequence (Figure 10.17). This provides direct evidence for the occurrence of point mutations in the generation of antibody diversity.

Comparison of myeloma $V_\kappa$ genes with embryonic $V_\kappa$ genes have turned up some cases where the sequences were identical and some where one or more point mutations seem to have occurred in the germline sequence during the differentiation of the myeloma cells.

A similar story is emerging for $V_H$ genes. Bothwell and his colleagues made hybridomas (see Section 4.8) of C57BL/6 spleen cells producing anti-NP antibodies carrying the NP[b] idiotype (see Section 10.3). One hybridoma was derived from the spleen cells of a mouse mounting a primary response to the antigen, and this hybridoma secreted IgM anti-NP antibodies. A second hybridoma was derived from a mouse that was giving a secondary response to the antigen, and this hybridoma secreted IgG2a anti-NP antibodies.

Complementary DNA (cDNA) was prepared for the heavy chains of each of these hybridomas, cloned and sequenced. The genes differed by 10 base pairs in their $V_H$ gene segment. Their D segments were very different, and their J gene segments ($J_{H2}$) were the same.

The sequence differences between the two $V_H$ gene segments resulted in eight codon differences. One of these was "silent" (encoded the same amino acid). The other seven encoded different amino acids. Three of these were located in CDR2; one in CDR1; the rest in framework regions.

These workers used the cDNA of the IgG2a $V_H$ to isolate a number of similar "germline" genes from C57BL/6 embryo DNA. Seven of these were sequenced. One turned out to be identical to the $V_H$ of the IgM hybridoma sequence and more closely related than any of the others to the $V_H$ of the IgG2a gene as well. Thus they concluded that (1) the $V_H$ gene segment expressed in the IgM-secreting hybridoma was the germline gene, and (2) the $V_H$ gene segment in the IgG2a-secreting hybridoma had been derived by repeated point mutations from the germline gene.

Hood and his colleagues at Caltech have found a similar situation in the TEPC-15 system. They sequenced a germline gene (cloned from BALB/c sperm) that encodes the $V_H$ of the TEPC-15 myeloma (as well as nine other phosphorylcholine (PC)-binding myeloma and hybridoma immunoglobulins that have identical $V_H$ regions). Another nine PC-binding immunoglobulins differ from the TEPC-15 sequence at from one to eight residues each. Presumably these variants were produced by mutation of the TEPC-15 gene because no other germline gene was found that could have encoded them. All of the variants were either IgG or IgA. Without exception, the IgM molecules carried the sequence encoded in the germline gene.

It has been known for a long time that the affinity of IgM antibodies does not increase with the passage of time, but that the affinity of IgG antibodies does (Section 8.4). Perhaps mu chains are assembled with germline genes and the introduction of point mutations occurs with heavy chain switching. This would provide a mechanism by which the affinity of IgG antibodies could be increased during the course of the immune response. In any case, other laboratories have shown that the V regions of IgG antibodies of a single specificity are considerably more diverse than those of IgM antibodies of the same specificity.

We have seen that the random assortment of V and J gene segments (V, D, and J in heavy chains), coupled with minor variations in the exact point at which the gene segments join each other, creates many opportunities for the somatic generation of variability in CDR3. But what of CDR1 and CDR2? The evidence presented here of point mutations clustered in the regions of V gene DNA encoding these CDRs provides a somatic mechanism for introducing the variability that we know from protein sequences is so characteristic of these regions (see Figure 9.22).

Perhaps the best place to look for evidence of somatic point mutation in $V_H$ and $V_\kappa$ genes is in their J gene segments because we know how many there are in the germline (4 $J_H$ and 5 $J_\kappa$) and what the germline sequence is for each (Figure 10.22). When the amino acid sequences of the J regions (e.g., $J_{H2}$) expressed in different myeloma proteins are compared with the sequence encoded by the germline $J_H$ gene, it turns out that

1. some are identical to the germline sequence;
2. some show alterations corresponding to slight variations in the point where D and J meet; and

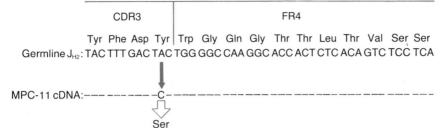

Figure 10.31 Somatic mutation in the $J_{H2}$ gene segment encoding the heavy chain of MPC-11. Both the germline $J_{H2}$ gene segment and the cDNA sequence of MPC-11 have been sequenced. The single base difference between the two accounts for the presence of Ser instead of Tyr at the end of CDR3 in the heavy chain of the myeloma protein. The base change occurs too far into $J_{H2}$ to be explained by splicing effects at the D–J junction. [Based on D. Givol et al., *Nature* **292**:426, 1981.]

3. a few reveal an amino acid substitution in the *middle* of the J region.

For example, the heavy chain of MPC-11 uses the $J_{H2}$ gene segment. However, there is a base alteration (A → C) in the myeloma $J_{H2}$ gene segment that changes the codon for the final amino acid in CDR3 from Tyr to Ser (Figure 10.31). A point mutation occurring in the germline $J_{H2}$ gene best explains this.

## 10.13  Summary

Where does the great debate stand now? Who was right about the mechanism that generates antibody diversity? The answer appears to be: everyone (partly) and no one (entirely). Let us summarize.

1. There are many genes inherited in the germline that encode antibodies with diverse antigen-binding sites — fewer than the germline proponents had predicted, but more than the defenders of somatic mutation had predicted. In the mouse, there are around 150 $V_H$ genes, a similar number of $V_\kappa$ genes, two $V_\lambda$ genes, as well as four $J_H$, four functional $J_\kappa$, and three functional $J_\lambda$ gene segments and a dozen or so D gene segments.
2. Germline V and J gene segments can be assorted in any combination. This is true for both light chains and heavy chains. In addition, heavy chains also have a D region, which is encoded by a separate gene segment carried in the germline. So the proponents of the recombinational germline (or somatic recombination) theories are substantially vindicated.
3. The site of nucleotide joining between V and J and, in heavy chains, between V and D and between D and J provides additional opportunities for sequence variability. In each of these cases, the nucleotide interchanges, additions or deletions in the assembled gene are located in CDR3 at the V–D and D–J boundaries (V–J for light chains).
4. The sporadic appearance of nucleotides in myeloma genes, which

cannot be found in what appear to be the corresponding germline genes, provides a strong argument for the occurrence of somatic mutations in V genes during the development of the B cells in a single animal.

5. There is combinatorial association of H and L chains; i.e., a given H chain can be associated with one or another of many different L chains. How important a factor this is in the generation of binding site diversity is still uncertain. In some cases, several different L chains can occur with the same $V_H$ region without altering the antigen specificity of the complete molecule. In other cases, however, substituting a different L chain with a given H chain creates a new antigen-binding specificity.

In any case, the mechanisms examined here — when taken together — are more than sufficient to account for the extraordinary range of antibody diversity.

## ADDITIONAL READING

1. Bentley, D. L., "Most κ Immunoglobulin mRNA in Human Lymphocytes Is Homologous to a Small Family of Germ-line V Genes," *Nature* **307**:77, 1984. Gel blotting yields an estimate of ≤50 germline $V_\kappa$ genes in humans.

2. Crews, S., et al., "A Single $V_H$ Gene Segment Encodes the Immune Response to Phosphorylcholine: Somatic Mutation Is Correlated with the Class of Antibody," *Cell* **25**:59, 1981. Evidence that the germline $V_H$ gene segment that encodes all PC-binding IgM antibodies (and TEPC-15) is somatically mutated in some PC-binding myelomas and hybridomas of the IgG and IgA classes.

3. Davis, M. M., et al., "An Immunoglobulin Heavy-Chain Gene Is Formed by at Least Two Recombinational Events," *Nature* **283**:733, 1980. (Reprinted in V. L. Sato and M. L. Gefter, *Cellular Immunology*, Addison-Wesley Publishing Co., Inc., Reading, MA, 1982.) Discusses the evidence for the alpha chain of McPC-603.

4. Dreyer, W. J., and J. C. Bennett, "The Molecular Basis of Antibody Formation: A Paradox," *Proc. Natl. Acad. Sci. USA* **54**:864, 1965.

5. Ephrussi, Ann, et al., "B Lineage-Specific Interactions of an Immunoglobulin Enhancer with Cellular Factors in Vivo," *Science* **227**:134, 1985.

6. Gillies, S. D, et al., "A Tissue-Specific Transcription Enhancer Element Is Located in the Major Intron of a Rearranged Immunoglobulin Heavy Chain Gene," *Cell* **33**:717, 1983.

7. Goding, J. W., and Judith E. Layton, "Antigen-Induced Co-capping of IgM and IgD-like Receptors on Murine B Cells," *J. Exp. Med.* **144**:852, 1976.

8. Honjo, T., "Immunoglobulin Genes," *Ann. Rev. Immunol.* **1**:499, 1983.

9. Leder, P., "The Generation of Antibody Diversity," *Scientific American* **246**(5):102, May, 1982 (Offprint No. 1518). The story in a nutshell.

10. Liu, C.-P., et al., "Mapping of Heavy Chain Genes for Mouse Immunoglobulins M and D," *Science* **209**:1348, 1980. (Reprinted in V. L. Sato and M. L.

Gefter, *Cellular Immunology*, Addison-Wesley Publishing Co., Inc., Reading, MA, 1982.) How alternative processing of one primary transcript could produce both IgM and IgD in a single B cell.

11. Max, E. E., J. G. Seidman, and P. Leder, "Sequences of Five Potential Recombination Sites Encoded Close to an Immunoglobulin Constant Region Gene," *Proc. Natl. Acad. Sci. USA* **76**:3450, 1979. (Reprinted in V. L. Sato and M. L. Gefter, *Cellular Immunology*, Addison-Wesley Publishing Co., Inc., Reading, MA, 1982.) Includes a description of the stem model of V-J joining.

12. Ritchie, K. A., et al., "Allelic Exclusion and Control of Endogenous Immunoglobulin Gene Rearrangement in κ Transgenic Mice," *Nature* **312**:517, 1984.

13. Rogers, J., et al., "Two mRNAs with Different 3′ Ends Encode Membrane-Bound and Secreted Forms of Immunoglobulin μ Chains," *Cell* **20**:303, 1980.

14. Schilling, J., et al., "Amino Acid Sequence of Homogeneous Antibodies to Dextran and DNA Rearrangements in Heavy-Chain V-Region Gene Segments," *Nature* **283**:35, 1980. (Reprinted in V. L. Sato and M. L. Gefter, *Cellular Immunology*, Addison-Wesley Publishing Co., Inc., Reading, MA, 1982.) Evidence of D segments at the protein level.

15. Swan, D., et al., "Chromosomal Assignment of the Mouse Light Chain Genes," *Proc. Natl. Acad. Sci. USA* **76**:2735, 1979. How somatic cell hybrids can be used to determine the chromosomal location of genes.

16. Tonegawa, S., "Somatic Generation of Antibody Diversity," *Nature* **302**:575, 1983. Includes a model for the production of N regions.

# The Response of T Lymphocytes to Antigen

## 11.1 Most T Cells Respond Only to Cell-Bound Antigens

In Chapter 8, we examined some of the experiments that showed that the response of B cells to a particular antigen is limited to a subset of cells capable of binding that antigen on their surface. This work, which placed the theory of clonal selection on a solid foundation, was quickly followed by attempts to find analogous phenomena with T cells. It quickly became clear, however, that T cells do *not* respond to antigen in the same fashion that B cells do. In contrast to B cells, most T cells do not bind *soluble* antigen on their surface. Therefore, attempts to count antigen-specific T

282

**Figure 11.1** T cells respond to antigen only in the presence of antigen-presenting cells (APCs). Both the T cells (a clone designated DO-11.10) and the APCs (dendritic cells) were H-$2^{k/d}$. The T cells are specific for OVA *associated with* I-A$^d$. Adding anti-I-A$^d$ antibodies to the cultures blocked the response; anti-I-A$^k$ had no effect. The magnitude of the T-cell response is measured by their production of IL-2 (Section 6.2). The cells of the DO-11.10 clone also respond to H-$2^b$ alone and to certain, but not all, other bird egg albumins. (From G. H. Sunshine et al., *J. Exp. Med.* **158:**1745, 1983.)

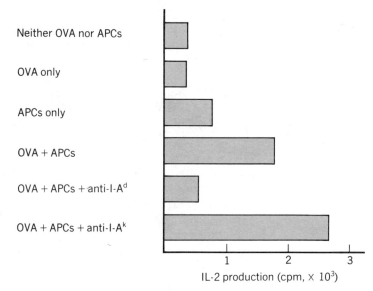

Neither OVA nor APCs

OVA only

APCs only

OVA + APCs

OVA + APCs + anti-I-A$^d$

OVA + APCs + anti-I-A$^k$

1    2    3

IL-2 production (cpm, $\times$ 10$^3$)

cells by exposure to radiolabeled antigen followed by autoradiography (as Ada and Byrt did for B cells — Section 8.3) do not succeed. Unable to *bind* soluble antigen, you would predict that T cells are unable to be activated by soluble antigen and this is the case. Figure 11.1 provides a demonstration of this using a clone of T cells specific for chicken egg ovalbumin (cOVA). One of the earliest events that occurs when T cells become activated (by antigens or mitogens) is the secretion of IL-2 (Section 6.2). However, when these OVA-specific T cells are cultured with *soluble* OVA, they secrete no more IL-2 than they do in the absence of antigen. But if they are cultured with syngeneic dendritic cells along with OVA, there is a substantial increase in the production of IL-2 (Figure 11.1). In other experiments (not shown in the figure), dendritic cells that had been *pre*cultured with OVA and then washed before mixing them with the T cells, could still provide a potent stimulus. Furthermore, the antigen-pulsed dendritic cells and the antigen-specific T cells actually bind specifically to each other.

## 11.2 Conventional and Histocompatibility Antigens

The antigens to which T lymphocytes are capable of responding appear to fall into two categories. On the one hand, T cells respond to the same sorts of conventional antigens that B cells do. These include proteins (e.g., OVA, KLH), and haptens (e.g., DNP) coupled to some type of carrier molecule. Like B cells, each T cell seems to express a single antigen specificity. Furthermore, the frequency of T cells specific for a particular conventional antigen, as a fraction of the total pool of T cells, is of the same order of magnitude as for B cells.

The *specificity* of T cells is also comparable to that of B cells. In other words, the ability of antigen-primed T cells to distinguish between the priming antigen and related structures is similar to that of antibodies. Figure 11.2 illustrates this using T cells harvested from a guinea pig primed with DNP coupled to mycobacteria as the carrier. The T cells proliferate vigorously when cultured with DNP coupled to OVA, an unrelated carrier. Because they do not respond to OVA itself, the response is specific for the hapten. *Antibodies* raised in an animal primed to DNP on one carrier will also bind to DNP presented on an unrelated carrier. These T cells also respond to TNP–OVA and, as we have seen (Figure 1.3), DNP and TNP are cross-reactive for antibodies as well.

There are, however, some subtle differences between the response of T cells and B cells to antigenic determinants. T cells seem to be less dependent than B cells on the three-dimensional structure of protein antigens. Primed to a protein antigen in its native configuration, T cells may also be able to respond to the denatured antigen or even to small peptides derived from the antigen. Antibodies raised against the native protein usually bind well only to determinants that preserve the configuration they had on the native antigen. One possible reason for this difference between T cells and B cells (antibodies) is that T cells may not *be* primed by native antigen but instead be primed by some form of "processed" antigen (i.e., denatured antigen or antigen fragments) displayed for them by antigen-presenting cells (APCs).

T lymphocytes also respond to histocompatibility antigens, especially to those encoded in the major histocompatibility complex. Mouse T cells that express L3T4, large amounts of Ly-1, and no Ly-2 respond vigorously to foreign class II (I region encoded) antigens. This is well illustrated by the mixed lymphocyte reaction (Figure 6.5). T cells that are Ly-2$^+$, on the other hand, respond most vigorously to class I histocompatibility antigens (encoded in the K and D regions). This can be demonstrated by the cell-mediated cytotoxicity (CMC) assay (Figure 6.6). The CMC assay can also be adapted to measure T cell responsiveness to *conventional* antigens present on the target cell surface, but in this case the conventional antigen must be expressed *along with* a class I antigen.

The T cell response to histocompatibility antigens differs from that to conventional antigens in a remarkable way. Whereas the frequency of T cells capable of responding to a particular conventional antigen is on the

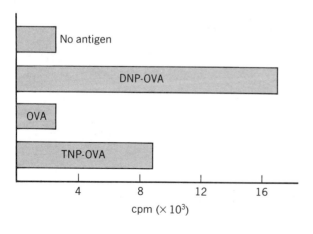

Figure 11.2 Proliferative response of DNP-primed T cells to in vitro culture with various antigens. The T cells were harvested from guinea pigs immunized with DNP coupled to mycobacteria. The proliferative response is measured by the uptake of tritiated thymidine. (cpm = counts per minute). [Based on C. A. Janeway, Jr., in *Contemporary Topics in Immunobiology* 9:171–203, Plenum Press, 1980.]

order of one in several thousand, the frequency of T cells capable of responding to a particular foreign MHC-encoded antigen (e.g., class II) has been estimated at from 0.5 to 10%. These figures are so high that they cast into serious question the validity of clonal selection in the response to these antigens. If one in every ten T cells responds to a single foreign H-2 haplotype (e.g., H-2$^b$), and if, as seems likely, as many as 100 H-2 haplotypes occur in mice, it seems to force us to conclude that any one T cell can respond to more than one histocompatibility antigen. If the figure is closer to 1 in 100, each T cell might be monospecific for a single H-2 haplotype, but what T cells would be left to respond to other kinds of antigens, for example, minor histocompatibility antigens and conventional antigens?

Peavy and Pierce have nonetheless provided strong evidence that the response of T cells to alloantigens *is* clonal. In a manner analogous to that of Ada and Byrt (see Section 8.3), they have shown that the suicide of a population of splenic T cells capable of responding to one H-2 haplotype (H-2$^b$) does not destroy the ability of the same population of cells to respond to a second foreign H-2 haplotype (H-2$^d$). They set up one way, mixed lymphocyte cultures using H-2$^b$ cells as stimulators and H-2$^q$ cells as responders. Thirty-six hours later, they added tritiated thymidine. Its specific activity was sufficiently high that any cell incorporating it in the process of DNA synthesis would be killed. After removal of excess $^3$H-TdR, a second set of stimulator cells (H-2$^d$) was added. Five days later, portions of the cells were assayed separately for CMC against $^{51}$Cr-labeled H-2$^b$ and H-2$^d$ cells, respectively. As Figure 11.3 shows, the cells were not active against H-2$^b$ but were strongly active against H-2$^d$. These results suggest, at least for this pair of H-2 haplotypes, that neither the responding nor the effector cells are multispecific. Later in the chapter

**Figure 11.3** Demonstration that the T cells responsive to one set of histocompatibility antigens (H-2$^b$) represent a separate population from those responsive to a second set (H-2$^d$). These data suggest that T cells are clonally restricted to a particular antigen just as B cells are. [From D. L. Peavy and C. W. Pierce, *J. Immunol.* 115:1521, 1975.]

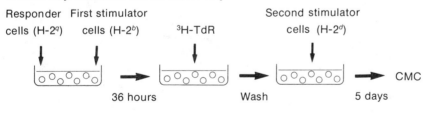

| Responder cells | First stimulator cells | Suicide pulse | Second stimulator cells | Specific $^{51}$Cr release (%) H-2$^b$ targets | Specific $^{51}$Cr release (%) H-2$^d$ targets |
|---|---|---|---|---|---|
| H-2$^q$ | H-2$^b$ | + | H-2$^d$ | 9 | **55** |
| H-2$^q$ | H-2$^b$ | None | None | 93 | 15 |
| H-2$^q$ | None | + | H-2$^d$ | 12 | 62 |

we shall examine possible explanations for the massive commitment to alloantigens by T cells that nonetheless appear to be monospecific.

## 11.3  Associative Recognition by T Cells

Perhaps the major feature that distinguishes the response of T cells to conventional antigen from that of B cells is the T cell requirement for associative recognition. In order to respond to a conventional antigen, the T cell must "see" that antigen associated with an antigen encoded by the major histocompatibility complex. An instructive example is presented in Section 3.7. You may recall that delayed-type hypersensitivity can be adoptively transferred by an infusion of T cells ($T_D$) from an immune donor to an unprimed recipient. That is, an injection of the same antigen into the recipient will elicit a DTH reaction even though the recipient has never encountered the antigen before. However, as Miller and his colleagues have shown, there is the further requirement that the donor and the recipient must express the same I region encoded ("Ia") antigens. In this case, either identity of the $A_\alpha A_\beta$ or $E_\alpha E_\beta$ genes appears to be sufficient. If donor and recipient have different I region genes, there is no response even though the transferred T cells are exposed to the priming antigen. This makes good sense if we assume that the T cells were primed to a particular combination of conventional antigen and Ia antigen in the donor and these cells can only respond to the same combination "presented" by the APCs (e.g., dendritic cells) of the recipient.

Figure 11.4 shows an in vitro experiment that also demonstrates MHC restriction; in this case the ability of antigen-primed T lymphocytes to *proliferate* in response to spleen cells precultured with the antigen (DNP–OVA). The spleen cell population is exposed to both the antigen and to mitomycin C. Treatment with mitomycin C ensures that none of the cells in the spleen population will contribute to the proliferative response in the culture.

When the donor of the antigen-presenting cells and the donor of the T cells are syngeneic, a vigorous proliferative response occurs (Figure 11.4). However, when the antigen is presented by cells having the same background genes but a different H-2 haplotype, very little antigen-specific stimulation occurs. (We must specify "antigen specific" because allogeneic cells trigger a proliferative response to MHC antigens alone — the MLR — and the data must be corrected for this portion of the response.) The experiment reveals two important points about the recognition of antigen by T cells.

1. It tells us that something other than simple recognition of DNP–OVA is involved. If T cells primed to DNP–OVA needed only to encounter DNP–OVA again in order to respond, they should be able to respond to DNP–OVA presented on any cell surface. But this is not the case.
2. The crucial factor in determining whether an antigen-presenting cell can stimulate a T cell specific for that antigen is to be found in its MHC. The fact that the phenomenon of associative recognition is tied

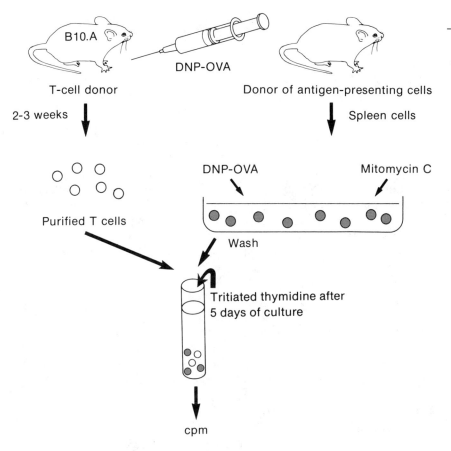

| T-cell donor | Donor of antigen-presenting cells | H-2 region identity | Percent of syngeneic response |
|---|---|---|---|
| B10.A | B10.A | Complete (syngeneic) | 100 |
| B10.A | B10 | None (allogeneic) | 9 |
| B10.A | B10.A(5R) | $E_\alpha \rightarrow D$ | 14 |
| B10.A | B10.A(4R) | $K \rightarrow E_\beta$ | 127 |
| B10.A | A.TL | $A_\alpha \rightarrow D$ | 94 |

**Figure 11.4** Antigen-primed T cells proliferate in culture only when they once again encounter the antigen on the surface of cells expressing the same $A_\alpha A_\beta$ (line 4) or $E_\alpha E_\beta$ (line 5) molecules as before. (Based on A. Yano et al., *J. Exp. Med.* **146:**828, 1977.)

to the MHC has led to these responses as being described as "MHC restricted."

By using recombinant congenic strains, these workers were able to pinpoint the region of the MHC that restricts the response. Once again, it was the I region that was crucial. If the antigen-presenting cells have either the same $A_\alpha A_\beta$ (fourth row) or the same $E_\alpha E_\beta$ (fifth row) molecules as the T cell donor, vigorous proliferation occurs.

## 11.4 The Activity of $T_C$ Cells Is Restricted by the Class I MHC Antigens of Their Targets

Immunization with alloantigens or with conventional antigens associated with cell surfaces can elicit the formation of cytotoxic T cells. As its name suggests, the cytotoxic T cell or $T_C$ cell is a cell that destroys other cells. $T_C$ cells are immune cells in the fullest sense: only those cells expressing the immunizing antigens can serve as susceptible targets. The activity of $T_C$ cells is assayed in an in vitro assay: cell-mediated cytotoxicity (CMC). The principles of the assay are described in Section 6.6.

Lymphoblasts are the target cells most commonly used in CMC assays. These can serve as targets if they carry the appropriate MHC antigens on their surface, perhaps alone (an allogeneic response) or together with some non-MHC antigen, producing MHC restriction. The non-MHC antigens that can serve as part of the target "seen" by T cells include (1) minor histocompatibility antigens, (2) foreign proteins like KLH and OVA, (3) haptens (such as TNP) coupled to cell-surface components, (4) certain antigens expressed on tumor cells, and (5) antigens expressed on the surface of cells infected by viruses. Let us examine the phenomenon of MHC restriction as illustrated by the response of $T_C$ cells to virus-infected cells. In fact, the earliest demonstration of MHC restriction was made with virus-specific $T_C$ cells. The demonstration arose, as so many crucial scientific advances have, from a chance observation.

Lymphocytic choriomeningitis virus (LCMV) causes a serious, sometimes fatal, disease in mice (and humans). Moderate doses of the virus, when injected intraperitoneally, cause a disease from which the animal may recover. If the virus is injected within the cerebrum, however, the progress of the infection is rapid and fatal. At the height of the disease, the spleen of the infected animal contains a large population of $T_C$ cells that are specific for virus-infected cells. Their presence can be demonstrated by culturing spleen cells from the infected animals with $^{51}$Cr-labeled virus-infected cells from another animal of the same inbred strain (Figure 11.5). The response is virus specific; that is, these Tc cells do not lyse uninfected, syngeneic target cells nor target cells infected with some other virus.

In response to reports that certain mouse strains are less susceptible to LCMV than others, Zinkernagel and his colleagues attempted to see if this was reflected in the relative efficiency of their $T_C$ cells. They tried culturing LCMV-specific $T_C$ cells of one strain with LCMV-infected target cells from another strain. Much to their surprise, the amount of lysis produced was no greater than with uninfected targets. For example, $T_C$ cells from virus-infected BALB/c mice were unable to lyse virus-infected target cells from C3H mice. The success or failure of the interaction between $T_C$ cells and targets turned out to depend on their respective H-2 regions. Thus $T_C$ cells from CBA mice can lyse infected C3H targets because both strains carry the H-2$^k$ haplotype. $T_C$ cells of the congenic strain C3H.SW cannot lyse C3H target cells. The C3H.SW strain differs from C3H only in the H-2 region; it carries the H-2$^b$ haplotype on the C3H background. By using various recombinant strains as a source of $T_C$ cells, the crucial genes within H-2 can be identified. Infected C3H tar-

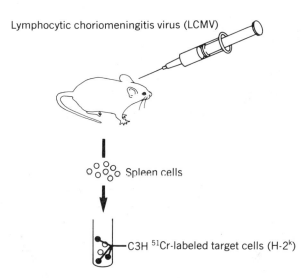

289

*Section 11.4*
*The Activity of $T_C$*
*Cells Is Restricted*
*by the Class I MHC*
*Antigens of Their*
*Targets*

| Immune spleen cells | | $^{51}$Cr release (%) | | |
|---|---|---|---|---|
| Strain | Haplotype | Infected targets | Uninfected targets | Interpretation |
| C3H | kkkkkk | **78** | 25 | Syngeneic combination— works |
| BALB/c | dddddd | 18 | 17 | Allogeneic combination— does not work |
| CBA | kkkkkk | **86** | 21 | Other H-2$^k$ strains work |
| C3H.SW | bbbbbb | 31 | 22 | Same background; different H-2—does not work |
| A.TL | sskkkd | 18 | 18 | Identity at loci between H-2K and H-2D insufficient |
| B10.A | kkkkkd | **73** | 17 | Identity at H-2K only—works |
| C3H.OH | dddddk | **57** | 22 | Identity at H-2D only—works |
| (CBA × C57BL) | H-2$^{k/b}$ | **56** | 17 | F$_1$ cells work, if they share one haplotype with targets |

**Figure 11.5** Cytotoxic T cells induced in a virus-infected H-2$^k$ mouse can only lyse virus-infected target cells that express the same H-2K$^k$ and/or H-2D$^k$ antigens. The loci for each haplotype are given in the order K, A$_\beta$, A$_\alpha$, E$_\beta$, E$_\alpha$, and D. [Based on R. M. Zinkernagel and P. C. Doherty, *Nature* **248**:701, 1974; P. C. Doherty and R. M. Zinkernagel, *J. Exp. Med.* **141**:502, 1975; and R. J. Blanden et al., *Nature* **254**:269, 1975.]

gets are not lysed by A.TL $T_C$ cells even though the strains are identical at all H-2 loci except K and D (and A$_\alpha$). However, identity at *either* H-2K *or* H-2D permits efficient lysis as seen by the success of $T_C$ cells from B10.A (identical at H-2K) and C3H.OH (identical at H-2D) mice against C3H targets (Figure 11.5). $T_C$ cells from hybrid mice can lyse targets with which they share at least one H-2 haplotype.

Thus the activity of $T_C$ cells, like several other T cells, is restricted by the MHC. However, the restriction on $T_C$ cells is imposed by the class I molecules of the MHC whereas we have seen that the MHC restriction displayed by $T_D$ cells and proliferating T cells is imposed by class II molecules. (Although the *cytolytic* activity of $T_C$ cells is usually restricted by only K or D, the *induction* of $T_C$ cells, because it requires $T_H$ cells, is restricted by the I region as well—Section 13.3.)

## 290

*Chapter 11*
*The Response of T*
*Lymphocytes to*
*Antigen*

### 11.5 Testing Models of T-Cell Recognition

A variety of hypotheses have been developed to account for the remarkable biological phenomenon of associative recognition. But most of these are simply variants of one or the other of two distinctly different models: (1) the two-receptor hypothesis and (2) the single-receptor hypothesis.

The **two-receptor hypothesis** postulates that a T cell recognizes conventional antigen and MHC antigen through separate receptors borne on its surface (Figure 11.6). Associative recognition would require that the T cell be able to bind both types of determinant, each to its own receptor. What the T cell sees as self could either be established by its own genotype or be learned during its differentiation. If what is self *is* learned, the process of acquiring its final specificity could occur in two steps: a step, presumably early in its differentiation, when the T cell precursor is selected for its ability to recognize self MHC and a later step when it is selected for clonal expansion by the presence of conventional antigen (see Section 13.6, Thymic Education).

The **single-receptor hypothesis** postulates that T cells employ a single type of antigen receptor that binds to a determinant constructed from both the conventional antigen and the MHC-encoded antigen. This hypothetical Ag/MHC complex has been called a *neoantigen* and a determinant on such a neoantigen is called a *compound antigenic determinant* (CAD—Figure 11.6). In this model, the T cell is selected for clonal expansion at the time of antigen presentation.

A *clone* of T cells with two different MHC-restricted antigen specificities would be the ideal tool for testing the alternative hypotheses for associative recognition. In 1981, two research groups reported success at this. In each case, their results supported a one-receptor rather than a two-receptor model. The approach in each laboratory was to develop clones of T cells that were reactive with an antigen (X) restricted by one H-2 antigen (CAD = X + H′) and simultaneously reactive with a second

**Figure 11.6** Alternative models of associative recognition.

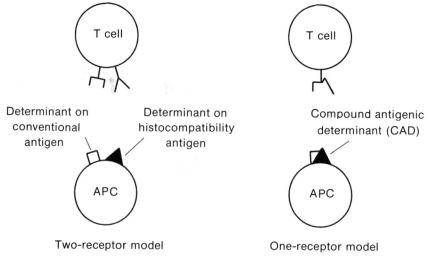

antigen (Y) restricted by a different H-2 (CAD = Y + H″). If MHC restriction involves separate receptors for the H-2 antigen and the conventional antigen, then these cells should not only lyse both X + H′ and Y + H″ targets but X + H″ and Y + H′ as well. On the other hand, if MHC restriction involves a single kind of receptor for a compound antigenic determinant (CAD), then only X + H′ and Y + H″ targets should be lysed. Both groups found the latter to be the case.

Kappler, Marrack, and their colleagues used the technique of somatic cell hybridization to fuse B10.A (H-2ᵃ) lymph node cells specific for OVA with B10.M (H-2ᶠ) lymph node cells specific for KLH. By limiting dilution (see Section 8.8), they cloned and subcloned cells from successful fusions. The various clones and subclones were then cultured with the four combinations of the conventional antigens (OVA and KLH) and antigen presenting spleen cells of the two restricting haplotypes (H-2ᵃ and H-2ᶠ). A high proportion of the clones continued to respond to both OVA presented by H-2ᵃ cells and to KLH presented by H-2ᶠ cells. But not a single clone responded to OVA presented by H-2ᶠ cells or to KLH presented by H-2ᵃ cells (Figure 11.7).

**Figure 11.7** Clones of T cells simultaneously specific for OVA restricted by H-2ᵃ and KLH restricted by H-2ᶠ do not respond to OVA presented by H-2ᶠ nor to KLH presented by H-2ᵃ. These results are incompatible with the two-receptor model of associative recognition. [Based on J. W. Kappler et al., *J. Exp. Med.* **153**:1198, 1981.]

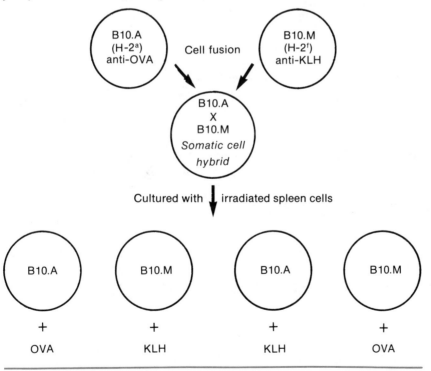

The activity of $T_C$ cells against *minor* histocompatibility antigens is also restricted by the MHC. Hünig and Bevan at MIT used clones of $F_1$ hybrid $T_C$ cells that were *simultaneously* specific for

1. one minor histocompatibility antigen ("X") restricted by H-2D$^d$ (CAD = X + D) and
2. a second minor histocompatibility antigen ("Y") restricted by H-2K$^d$ (CAD = Y + K).

These clones lysed both X + D and Y + K targets but were unable to lyse X + K or Y + D targets. If two separate receptors were involved in associative recognition, then all four kinds of targets should have been lysed.

A major drawback of the concept of the compound antigenic determinant is that it is difficult to envisage the molecular basis for such a structure. No such compound molecules have been isolated and they may not exist. However, the mobility of molecules of antigen (Ag) and MHC molecules in the plane of the cell surface membrane probably allows for transient associations between the two. At the instant of their association, they could then be bound by a single receptor structure able to encompass portions of each with sufficient affinity.

Recent evidence, which we shall examine later in this chapter (Section 11.8), reinforces the conclusion that T cells bear a single receptor for Ag/MHC. But before we examine this evidence, let us turn to some of the attempts that have been made to characterize the T cell receptor by serological methods; i.e., by using antibodies directed against it.

## 11.6 Serological Analysis of the T Cell Antigen Receptor

In Chapter 8, we saw that the antigen receptor on B cells is an immunoglobulin molecule. To summarize: (1) antisera or monoclonal antibodies raised against immunoglobulins, especially IgM and IgD, bind to the surface of B cells. This can be revealed by tagging the antibody molecules with a fluorescent label (see Figure 8.17). (2) The pretreatment of B cells with anti-immunoglobulin molecules prevents the B cells from binding antigen.

What about T cells? Despite many attempts, it has not been possible to show that antibodies directed against C region determinants on immunoglobulins (i.e., anti-isotype antibodies such as anti-$\mu$ or anti-$\delta$) are able to bind to T cells or interfere with their response to antigen. On the other hand, many experimenters have reported that antibodies directed against *idiotypic* determinants on antibody molecules *do* react with structures on the surface of T cells and do alter (interfere with or, sometimes, enhance) the response of those T cells to antigen. Because idiotypic determinants are confined to V regions (usually on the heavy chain but often requiring the presence of the L chain as well), these findings have led to the suggestion that the same V region gene segments that encode the V regions of antibodies are used to encode the antigen-binding portion of the T-cell antigen receptor.

One of the earliest demonstrations that anti-idiotypic antibodies could

interfere with T cell mediated responses in a specific fashion was reported by McKearn and his colleagues in 1974. They used rats as their
experimental animals: two inbred strains, Lewis (LEW) and Brown Norway (BN), as well as their $F_1$ hybrids (LEW × BN). Their experimental
procedures are shown in Figure 11.8. Lewis rats injected with BN-
tumor cells develop antibodies against the BN histocompatibility antigens. When these anti-BN antibodies ("Ab1") are injected into $F_1$ animals, they elicit the production of anti-antibodies ("Ab2"). We should
expect these anti-antibodies to have the properties of anti-idiotypic anti-

**Figure 11.8** Suppression of a graft versus host reaction in a rat synthesizing anti-idiotypic antibodies.
Although the anti-idiotypic antibodies (Ab2) were elicited by antibodies (Ab1), they suppress the
activity of T cells. This suggests that they are antireceptor antibodies and that T cell receptors
express determinants similar to those of antibodies of the same specificity. [Based on T. J. McKearn,
*Science* 183:94, 1974.]

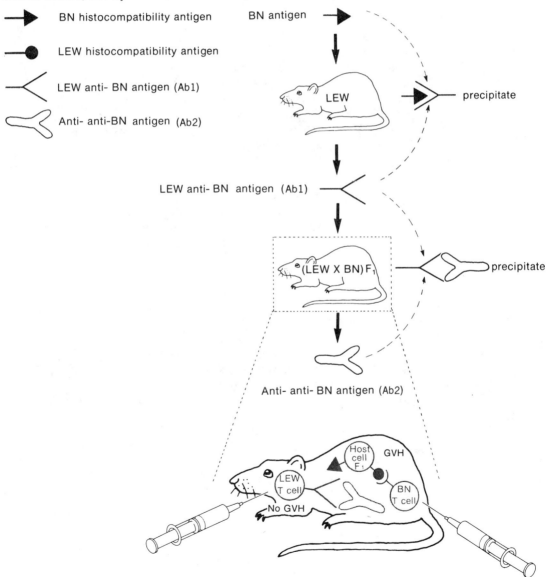

bodies because all isotypic and any allotypic determinants on the anti-BN antibodies would be present on the immunoglobulins of the $F_1$ animals and thus not be immunogenic.

The classic way of assaying for graft vs. host reactivity is to inject parental type T cells into an $F_1$ recipient (see Section 6.4). When either Lewis or Brown Norway lymphocytes are injected into a lymph node of an $F_1$ recipient, a localized swelling occurs as a result of a GVHR. Lewis lymphocytes trigger a GVHR in response to the BN histocompatibility antigens of the recipient; BN lymphocytes respond to the Lewis histocompatibility antigens. However, only BN lymphocytes are able to elicit a GVHR in hybrids that have been immunized earlier with the Lewis anti-BN antibodies (Figure 11.8). The injection of Lewis lymphocytes has no effect. This suggests that the anti-idiotypic antibodies circulating in these animals interact in some suppressive way with receptor structures on those Lewis T cells that would otherwise recognize BN histocompatibility antigens. These receptors must share some of the idiotypic determinants that are associated with the antigen-binding site of Lewis anti-BN antibodies.

Later, these workers reported that prolonged and intense immunization of Lewis rats with BN histocompatibility antigens *spontaneously* elicits a population of antibodies having the same properties as the anti-idiotypic antibodies produced in the $F_1$ animals. This serum factor appears at the time when the idiotypic antibodies (anti-BN) disappear. In Ouchterlony plates, the line of precipitate between anti-BN serum and the anti-id antibodies in the $F_1$ serum produces a reaction of identity with the precipitate formed with antibodies produced spontaneously in the hyperimmunized Lewis rats (Figure 11.9). This suggests that the blocking of a cell-mediated immune response by anti-idiotypic antibodies may not simply be a laboratory curiosity but may well reflect a normal homeostatic response in the intact animal.

These experiments, along with many others showing that anti-idiotypic antibodies can react specifically with T cells, led to the suggestion that the T cell antigen receptor is encoded by V gene segments drawn from the same pool as that used by B cells to make antibodies. However, the failure of anti-isotype sera to react with T cells suggested that any C region genes ("$C_T$") used by T cells were quite distinct from those used by B cells.

But if T cells borrow immunoglobulin V gene segments ($V_H$, D, $J_H$) to associate with their own $C_T$ segment, then we would expect to find evidence — as we do for B cells — for a rearrangement of the DNA en-

**Figure 11.9** Reaction of identity between the anti-idiotypic antibodies induced in $F_1$ rats (following the protocol shown in Figure 11.8) and those induced in Lewis rats following hyperimmunization with BN histocompatibility antigens. [Based on T. J. McKearn et al., *J. Immunol.* 113:1876, 1974.]

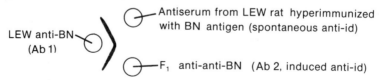

coding these regions. Thus a probe for a V region gene segment, such as $J_H$, should show a difference between its organization in embryonic DNA and in the DNA of differentiated T cells. A variety of T cell clones have been examined for this purpose. In some cases no rearrangement is seen. In other cases, there is evidence of a DNA rearrangement (e.g., of a $J_H$ segment) but the rearranged product appears to be nonfunctional. Furthermore, all attempts to detect $V_H$-specific mRNA in T cells have failed, although such efforts succeed for B cell clones.

What is needed to finally resolve the question is to isolate and study directly the T cell antigen receptor and the gene(s) that encode it. Rapid progress is being made at both of these tasks. Let us first examine the evidence at the protein level; then at the level of DNA.

## 11.7 Biochemical Analysis of the T Cell Antigen Receptor

By 1983, workers in several laboratories had succeeded in isolating from T cells a cell-surface protein that had the properties to be expected of a T cell antigen receptor. The approach taken in most cases was to immunize mice with a T cell clone (of mouse origin in some cases; human in others) and then to develop hybridomas from their spleen cells (Figure 4.18). The hybridomas were screened for those secreting a monoclonal antibody able to bind to the surface of, and/or interfere with the activity of, the T cell clone used for immunization *but not to other T cell clones.* Such clone-specific monoclonal antibodies appeared to recognize an idiotypic determinant on a set of cell-surface molecules unique to the immunizing clone; the most likely candidate for such a molecule would be the unique antigen receptor expressed by that clone.

For example, Marrack, Kappler, and their colleagues developed a B cell hybridoma that secreted monoclonal antibodies against a cOVA/H-$2^d$ specific T cell hybridoma ("DO-11.10," described in Figure 11.1), which was derived from a BALB/c mouse immunized with cOVA. These monoclonal antibodies bound to the surface of the T cell clone and also interfered with the ability of the clone to respond (by making IL-2) to cOVA (and certain other bird egg albumins) presented by H-$2^d$ cells (Figure 11.10). In order to determine the specificity of this monoclonal antibody; i.e., if it were anti-idiotypic or not, it was tested to see if it interfered with antigen (cOVA) recognition by 397 other T cell clones also derived from BALB/c mice immunized with OVA. All but one of the clones tested proved *not* to be inhibited by the anti-DO-11.10 antibodies. This remarkable example of specificity for the immunizing clone suggested that the monoclonal antibodies were recognizing a determinant unique to that clone. The one cell-surface structure that we would expect to distinguish this clone from other such clones would be its receptor for antigen. As for the one new positive clone, this one — and only this one — turned out to have precisely the same specificity as the original (DO-11.10) clone. Its pattern of response to other egg albumins was identical to that of DO-11.10. No other clone tested (over 200 of

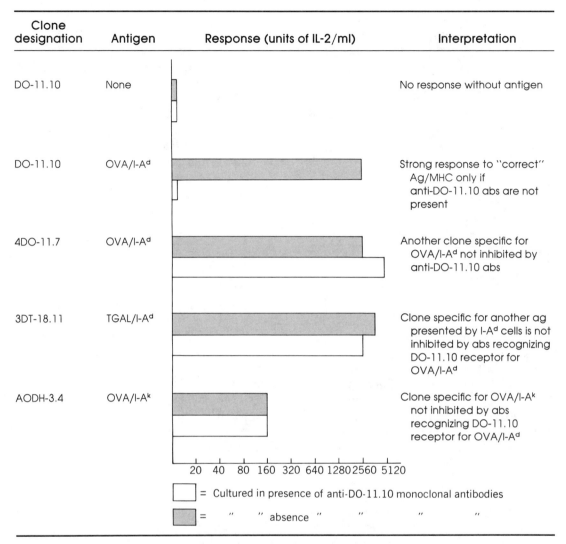

| Clone designation | Antigen | Response (units of IL-2/ml) | Interpretation |
|---|---|---|---|
| DO-11.10 | None | | No response without antigen |
| DO-11.10 | OVA/I-A$^d$ | | Strong response to "correct" Ag/MHC only if anti-DO-11.10 abs are not present |
| 4DO-11.7 | OVA/I-A$^d$ | | Another clone specific for OVA/I-A$^d$ not inhibited by anti-DO-11.10 abs |
| 3DT-18.11 | TGAL/I-A$^d$ | | Clone specific for another ag presented by I-A$^d$ cells is not inhibited by abs recognizing DO-11.10 receptor for OVA/I-A$^d$ |
| AODH-3.4 | OVA/I-A$^k$ | | Clone specific for OVA/I-A$^k$ not inhibited by abs recognizing DO-11.10 receptor for OVA/I-A$^d$ |

20 40 80 160 320 640 1280 2560 5120

☐ = Cultured in presence of anti-DO-11.10 monoclonal antibodies

▨ = " " absence " " " "

**Figure 11.10** Response of several T-cell hybridomas to antigen in the absence or presence of monoclonal antibodies elicited by clone DO-11.10. [Based on K. Haskins et al., *J. Exp. Med.* **157**:1149, 1983.]

them) showed this specificity pattern. Thus two independently derived clones (out of several hundred) that proved to respond precisely in the same way to antigens were also inhibited by the same monoclonal antibody.

Note also that the monoclonal antibody has no inhibitory effect on T cell clones that are specific for some other conventional antigen associated with H-2$^d$ nor for the same conventional antigen (cOVA) associated with H-2$^k$. Because this monoclonal antibody represents a homogeneous population of molecules having a single kind of epitope-binding site, the fact that the antibody interferes with recognition of only one particular Ag/MHC combination suggests that Ag/MHC recognition by T cells is mediated by a single receptor.

In addition to their property of binding to the cells of a particular clone, such monoclonal antibodies can also be used to isolate the cell-surface molecules — the supposed T cell antigen receptor — for further characterization.

Several laboratories have succeeded in isolating and characterizing the T cell antigen receptor. The procedure is to prepare a lysate of a T cell clone and to expose this lysate to the monoclonal antibodies specific for that clone. In each case, this precipitates a glycoprotein with a molecular mass of 80–90 thousand daltons (80–90 kd). Under reducing conditions, a disulfide bond is broken yielding two different polypeptide chains (40–50 kd each). One chain, the more acidic (pI ~5) of the two is designated the $\alpha$ chain. The other, which is more basic (pI ~7), is called the $\beta$ chain (Figure 11.11).

While the clone-specific monoclonal antibodies bind well to the cells of the clone which elicited them, they do not bind to other clones of T cells. In view of the low frequency of T cells of one particular antigen specificity, we would expect that very few cells in the T cell population of a normal, unprimed animal would be bound by these antibodies, and that is the case. However, by immunizing animals of another species (e.g., rabbit or rat) with the precipitated T cell receptor molecules, it has been

**Figure 11.11** Proposed structure of the T cell antigen receptor. The oligosaccharides are not shown. The exact positions of the cysteines thought to establish disulfide bridges vary slightly from chain to chain. In humans, the $\alpha$ and $\beta$ chains are closely associated with other integral membrane polypeptides that make up the CD3 ("T3") complex. However, CD3 is invariant and probably does not contribute to the specificity of binding.

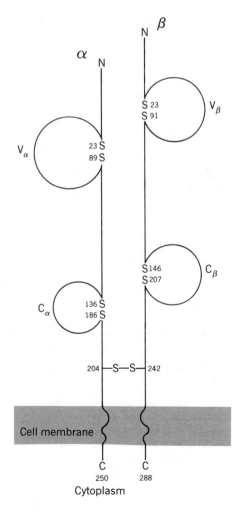

possible to produce antisera that recognize determinants *shared* by T cell receptors of many different antigen specificities. In contrast to the clone-specific antibodies, these anti-"framework" antisera bind to a variety of different T cell clones (as well as to a significant fraction of the T cell pool). Thus these antisera can be used to isolate antigen receptor molecules from a variety of T cell clones and even from normal populations of T cells. When fingerprint analysis (see Section 9.4) is performed on the digests of receptor material from several different T cell *clones,* a pattern of some common and some unique peptides is revealed. This suggests that, just as is the case for immunoglobulins, the polypeptides that make up the T cell antigen receptor have a constant region and a variable region (Figure 11.11).

## 11.8   T Cell Receptor Genes

A plasma cell is a terminally differentiated B cell largely occupied with the synthesis and secretion of large amounts of a single kind of antibody molecule (several thousand copies each second). Accordingly, the messenger RNAs encoding antibody H and L chains represent a sizeable fraction of the total mRNA pool in a plasma cell. This made practical the early work of preparing complementary DNA (cDNA) probes for isolating antibody genes. The T cell, in contrast, needs only to maintain a slow renewal of the antigen receptors anchored in its cell membrane and presumably the mRNA for this limited purpose represents only a small fraction of the many kinds of mRNA being used by the cell at one time. Among these kinds would be mRNAs for other integral membrane proteins such as Thy-1, class I antigens, receptors for hormones, and many others.

How, then, does one isolate the mRNA for the antigen receptor from all the other mRNAs in the T cell? On the assumption that B cells express most (98% or so) of the same genes that T cells do — but *not* the gene(s) for the T cell receptor — the mRNAs from B cells should hybridize with most of the cDNA prepared from a T cell clone. Removing the hybridized sequences should leave only that cDNA representing T cell specific functions (Figure 11.12). The odds of including the cDNA for the T cell receptor are improved by preparing the T cell cDNA from polysomes (rather than free cytoplasmic ribosomes) as the T cell receptor — like other integral membrane proteins — should be synthesized on polysomes. Several groups of investigators have succeeded in using this approach to develop clones of T cell specific cDNA from mouse T cell clones. You would expect that some of these clones would encode T cell specific proteins unrelated to the antigen receptor and, in fact, among the first cDNA clones isolated were some that encoded the characteristic mouse T cell marker Thy-1. However, a few cDNA clones revealed the same type of behavior that we noted with immunoglobulin cDNA clones (Figure 10.11), i.e., evidence of DNA rearrangements during T cell differentiation. When these clones were used to probe — by Southern blotting — the DNA of embryonic cells or of nonlymphoid cells (e.g., liver cells) or even of B cell clones, they yielded the same pattern of

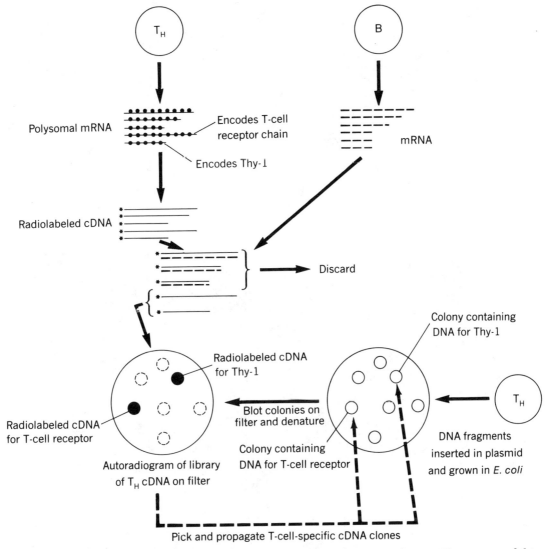

**Figure 11.12** Strategy for isolating T-cell-specific cDNA by subtractive cloning. The success of this approach can be improved by also using a subtractive step before inserting the $T_H$-cell DNA fragments into plasmids.

restriction fragments in every case. However, Southern blots of the DNA harvested from the T cell clone that provided the cDNA probe produced a different pattern of fragments. On the assumption that the DNA encoding the antigen receptor of T cells undergoes rearrangements analogous to those described in Chapter 10 for the H and L chain genes in B cells, such clones were chosen for further study.

In due course, it became apparent that some cDNA clones were detecting one set of rearranged genes—later determined to encode the $\beta$ chains of the T cell receptor; some a second set (encoding the $\alpha$ chains). Several cDNA clones were chosen for sequencing.

The results of sequencing a number of cDNA clones revealed that the T cell receptor genes encode $\beta$ chains of some 290 amino acid residues,

**299**

```
        ┌──── V_T ────┐ ≀≀≀ D_T ≀≀≀ ≀≀≀ J_T ≀≀≀        ┌──── C_T ────┐
         ┌─S—S─┐                                              ┌─S—S─┐

1. Human β (YT35)        LKIQPSEPRDSAVYFCASSFSTCSANYGYTFGSGT   PSEAEISHTQKATLVCLATGFFPDHVELSWW
2. Human β (HPB–MLT)     ---RT-RG---L------QGRETGY--P--        --------------------Y---------
3. Mouse β (86T1)        --H-SAVD-E-------HGQGVSGNTLY--E-S      --K---ANK---------R-----------
4. Mouse β (2B4)         -E--S--AG---L--L---LNW  SQDTQY--P--   --K---ANK---------R-----------
5. Human α (HPB–MLT)     FT-TA-QVV---------LDS  SASKII-----    AVYQLRDSKSSDDKS---F-D-DSQTNVSQSK
6. Mouse α (pHDS58)      --RKASVHWS----V-GFA  SALT  ------     AVYQLKDPRSQDSTL--F-D-DSQINVPKTM
7. Mouse α (TT11)        --H-RD-Q--S----L--L--VTLYGG  SGNKLI--T--  AVYQLKDPRSQDSTL--F-D-DSQINVPKTM

8. IgL chain consensus   -T-SGL-AE-A-T-Y-QQWN-SP   W--G--     -PSS-ELQ-G------IND-Y-GD-T-VA-
9. IgH chain consensus   -QMNSLRAE-T---Y--RDYYGY-  DVW-Q--    C-RSLPTSGSTVA-G--VK-Y--EP-TVVT-

         ├──FR3──┤ ├──────CDR3──────┤ ├─FR4─┤              C
```

Figure 11.13  Amino acid sequences of corresponding portions of several $\beta$ and $\alpha$ chains from T cells. The V region sequences flank the second cysteine (position ~90), which presumably participates in forming the intrachain disulfide bridge of the V domain. Similarly, the $C_T$ sequences flank the first Cys (position ~140) thought to form the intrachain S–S bond of the C domain. The most frequently observed residues of the corresponding portions of immunoglobulin light and heavy chains are shown for comparison. Sequences 1, 2, and 5 are from human leukemia cell lines; 4 and 7 from mouse $T_H$ clones. Sequence 6 is from a mouse $T_C$ clone. The amino acid sequences are those predicted from the nucleotide sequences of the cloned DNA. The single-letter code of amino acids is given on the inside front cover. A dash indicates that the amino acid residue is the one located at that position in the first sequence (YT35). Note: (1) The variability in the V regions, although some positions are highly conserved. (2) The uniformity of the $C_T$ sequences for each class of chain. The homology between human and mouse chains of one class is higher than that between the $\alpha$ and $\beta$ chains of the same species. Sequences 1 and 2 and sequences 3 and 4 use different $C_T$ genes ($C_\beta1$ and $C_\beta2$, respectively) but in the mouse these are identical over the region shown here. (3) The modest homology with the corresponding portions of immunoglobulins, especially light chains. (4) Gaps have been introduced in some sequences to increase the homology of the alignment. These tend to fall in the D regions and the larger ones (in 2 and 5) may represent chains in which a D region was not used. (5) The exact boundaries between $V_T$ and $D_T$ and between $D_T$ and $J_T$ are uncertain. (6) Sequence 6 is from a clone of $T_C$ cells; 7 from a clone of $T_H$ cells. The identity of their $C_T$ regions suggests that the choice of one or the other $C_T$ gene is not correlated with cell function.

and $\alpha$ chains of ~250 residues (Figure 11.11). Each chain contains a stretch of hydrophobic amino acids near its C terminal where the molecule probably passes through the cell membrane. This is followed by a short stretch of hydrophilic amino acid residues that extend into the cytoplasm of the cell. The predicted molecular weight of these chains is ~15 kd less than that of the chains isolated from T cell lysates. The difference is presumably accounted for by the carbohydrate covalently attached to these glycoproteins.

Although the DNA sequences themselves showed very little homology to the DNA sequences that encode antibodies, the deduced translation of these DNA sequences into amino acid sequences revealed several antibody-like features (Figure 11.13).

1. A comparison of several chains verifies that there is an N terminal variable (V) domain and a C terminal constant (C) domain (Figure 11.13). These domains are of approximately the same size as the corresponding domains of an immunoglobulin chain.
2. Two pairs of cysteine residues, spaced about the same distance apart that they are in immunoglobulin domains, are able to establish a pair of intrachain disulfide bonds.
3. A third cysteine in the C domain could form the *inter*chain linkage already demonstrated by biochemical studies of the protein.
4. The homology between the $\beta$ and $\alpha$ chains is no greater than that between either chain and immunoglobulin chains.
5. The $\beta$ and $\alpha$ chains of the mouse T cell receptor show a high degree of homology with the $\beta$ chains and $\alpha$ chains of the human.

When these cDNAs are used to probe for and isolate corresponding sequences in embryonic DNA (or DNA in somatic cells like liver cells), the sequences encoding the $\beta$ chains are found to be dispersed in four different clusters of gene segments: $V_\beta$, $D_\beta$, $J_\beta$, and $C_\beta$ (Figure 11.14). The $J_\beta$ gene segments and $C_\beta$ gene segments are organized in two tandem clusters (a feature reminiscent of lambda J–C gene segments—Figure 10.6). During its differentiation, the T cell rearranges these separate stretches of DNA so that the $V_\beta$, $D_\beta$, and $J_\beta$ regions become directly juxtaposed (Figure 11.14).

Sequencing of the DNA flanking the $V_\beta$ gene segments (3' side) $J_\beta$ (5' side), and $D_\beta$ (both sides) reveals heptamer-spacer-nonamer sequences similar to those that flank the equivalent immunoglobulin gene segments. However, in contrast to $J_H$ and $D_H$, $J_\beta$ is *preceded* by a 12-nucleotide spacer and $D_\beta$ is flanked on the 3' side by a 23-nucleotide spacer (Figure 11.15). Thus without violating the 12-23 rule (Section 10.6), this would permit direct $V_\beta$–$J_\beta$ joining (which has been observed) as well as the joining of two or more $D_\beta$ gene segments in the assembled V region gene.

Despite their remarkable similarities to antibody genes, it is not yet certain to what degree these T cell genes use the various mechanisms that contribute to antibody diversity. Combinatorial diversity of $V_\beta$, $D_\beta$ and $J_\beta$ segments occurs, but the size of the $V_\beta$ gene pool appears to be much smaller than those of immunoglobulin V genes. Furthermore, comparison of the sequences of expressed $V_\beta$ genes with their germline counterparts suggests that somatic mutation has little or no role to play in the

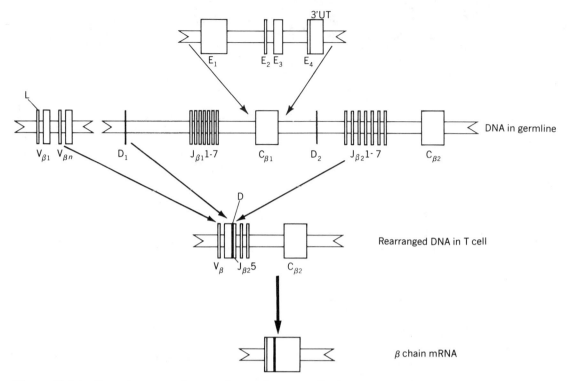

**Figure 11.14** Organization in the germline and in a T cell of the exons encoding the $\beta$ chain of the T cell antigen receptor. The size and sequence of the exons of $C_{\beta2}$ are quite similar to those of $C_{\beta1}$ (top). The use of one or the other $C_\beta$ cluster does not seem to be correlated with the type of T cell ($T_H$ or $T_C$) in which the chain is expressed. One of the $J_\beta$ gene segments in each cluster is nonfunctional (a pseudogene). Although the number of $V_\beta$ genes appears to be limited ($\sim 20$), the potential for diversity is increased by the ability of T cells (like B cells) to vary the exact point at which the gene segments are joined (junctional diversity) and to add extra nucleotides on either side of D segments (N-region diversity — see Section 10.8).

generation of T cell diversity. The relative contribution of these mechanisms to $\alpha$ chain diversity also remains to be established.

In any case, it is now clear that the genes encoding the T cell receptor are assembled from a distinct set of gene segments that are significantly different from Ig gene segments in sequence, in the details of their organization, and even in their location. Although the human $\alpha$ chain genes are located on chromosome 14, which also carries the genes encoding antibody H chains, the $\beta$ chain genes are on chromosome 7, which

**Figure 11.15** Comparison of recognition signals flanking the gene segments that are assembled to make a $V_H$ gene (top) and a $V_\beta$ gene of the T cell receptor (bottom). Note that the pattern of T gene segments would permit — without violating the "12/23" rule — direct $V_\beta$–$J_\beta$ joining as well as the use of two or more $D_\beta$ gene segments. The $\alpha$ chain gene segments use the same pattern of recognition signals.

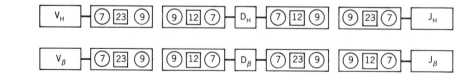

does not carry any antibody genes. In the mouse, the $\beta$ chain genes are on chromosome 6, along with the genes encoding antibody $\kappa$ chains, but the $\alpha$ chain genes are on chromosome 14, which has no antibody genes.

How does the T cell receptor construct its binding site for Ag/MHC? The immunoglobulin-like domain structure of the $\beta$ and $\alpha$ chains raises the possibility that their V regions interact by noncovalent forces to build a single binding site just as $V_H$ and $V_L$ domains do. Note, however, that each B cell receptor for antigen (e.g., sIgM) carries *two* (identical) binding sites (Fab), whereas the T cell receptor appears to carry only one. Furthermore, both chains of the T cell receptor are anchored in the cell membrane, while only the H chain is similarly anchored on B cells. More sequence data will be needed to establish the size and distribution of any hypervariable regions in the $\beta$ and $\alpha$ chains which might contribute to the specificity of binding. Whether and how the structure created by the $\beta$ and $\alpha$ chains of the T cell receptor can explain associative recognition remains to be determined.

How are we to account for the many demonstrations that antibodies elicited by antibody idiotypes are so often able to interact with T cells of the same antigenic specificity? Two possibilities (which are not mutually exclusive) come to mind. Considering the degree of amino acid sequence similarity between antibody V regions and the V regions of the T cell receptor chains, we might well expect to find a short string of amino acid residues common to each and to both of which a subset of anti-idiotypic antibodies would bind. But further, we would expect that a binding site on an antibody capable of binding, for example, the DNP group and a site on the T cell receptor capable of binding DNP would—at least in one area of each—have similar surfaces complementary to DNP. An antiserum raised against the anti-DNP antibody should contain a subset of anti-idiotypic antibodies that are specific for this site, and we would expect these to bind to the similar region of the T cell receptor. Such anti-idiotypic antibodies have been described (by Jerne) as the "internal image" of the antigen because they presumably mimic the spatial features of the antigen, in this case, the DNP group. Chapter 15 examines this concept in greater depth as part of the whole question of interacting "networks" in the immune system.

## 11.9 Why Are T Cells So Alloreactive?

The T cell clones described above use a unique antigen receptor that appears at very low frequency in the T cell pool. But the T cell pool responds to a single foreign determinant encoded on an MHC molecule by enlisting the services of up to 10% of its members. How can we reconcile these findings?

At least two possibilities have been suggested. A compound antigenic determinant (Ag/MHC) consisting of conventional antigen (Ag) associated with a self-histocompatibility antigen (MHC) is probably present on the surface of an antigen-presenting cell at a relatively low density.

Such a sparsely distributed Ag/MHC determinant would only be bound by T cells with receptors of high affinity for it. We would assume that the cells with such high affinity receptors would represent only a tiny fraction of the total pool of T cells. On the other hand, an antigen-presenting cell might have 100,000 copies of a particular class I antigen or class II MHC antigen displayed on its surface. Such a high density of identical molecules in the plane of the cell membrane would favor the binding of T cells with low affinity receptors as well as those with high. Thus the rare T cell capable of binding, for example, cOVA/H-$2^d$ with high affinity might — along with T cells of many other Ag/MHC specificities — be able to bind a foreign MHC antigen, e.g., H-$2K^b$, with low affinity.

There is abundant evidence that T cell clones specific for a particular Ag/MHC can also respond to allogeneic MHC alone. For example, the DO-11.10 clone described earlier in the chapter, which is specific for cOVA/H-$2^d$, also responds to allogeneic cells from C57BL mice (H-$2^b$) without any OVA present. Conversely, T cell clones selected for alloreactivity will sometimes be able to respond to a conventional antigen presented by syngeneic APCs.

There is a second possibility (which does not exclude the first). It may turn out that there is *no* fundamental difference between the MHC-restricted response to conventional antigen (Ag/self-MHC) and the response to foreign MHC antigens. There are many other types of molecules displayed at the surface of a cell like a dendritic cell. These would include such things as receptors for the Fc fragment of IgG, receptors for components of the complement system, receptors for insulin and other hormones, and probably many more. If these molecules *also* associate with self-MHC molecules in the cell membrane, then all T cells that are potentially capable of reacting against the combination would have to be eliminated in order to avoid an autoimmune response. This would have to be done during the early development of the immune system. But associated in the cell membrane with a *foreign* class I or class II antigen, each of these normally "self" molecules would now be associated with that foreign MHC molecule, forming a wide variety of new Ag/MHC antigens. This wide variety would engage the activities of many T cell clones yielding a massive response of the T cell pool.

In 1980, Sherman reported the results of experiments which revealed that the response of a mouse to a foreign H-2 antigen is, in fact, made up of the contributions of T cells of a wide variety of slightly different specificities. She examined the cytotoxic T cells ($T_C$) generated by culturing B10.D2 cells *(dddddd)* with irradiated B10.A(5R) stimulator cells *(bbbbkd)*. Most $T_C$ cells "see" class I molecules, and the only class I difference between these cells is at H-2K (Figure 11.16).

Using limiting dilution analysis (Section 8.8), Sherman found that the frequency of $T_C$ cell precursors ("$T_C$-P") in the spleen was 1/12,000. Assuming that 3% of the cells in the spleen are Ly-$2^+$ $T_C$-P, this yields a frequency of 1/360 — not as high as 10% but still far higher than the frequencies encountered for T cells specific for conventional antigens. Cultures were established with 2500 spleen cells, giving an average of 0.2 $T_C$-P per culture and thus making it likely that any positive culture would have been started by a single cell and represent a true clone.

| | H-2 haplotype | | | | | | |
|---|---|---|---|---|---|---|---|
| Strain | K | $A_\beta$ | $A_\alpha$ | $E_\beta$ | $E_\alpha$ | D | Function |
| B10.D2 | *d* | *d* | *d* | *d* | *d* | *d* | Responding cells |
| B10.A(5R) | *b* | *b* | *b* | *b* | *k* | *d* | Stimulator cells |
| Mutant strains | *b*(1) | *b* | *b* | *b* | *b* | *b* | Target cells |
| D2.GD | *d* | *d* | *d* | *d/b* | *b* | *b* | Negative control |
| C57BL/6 | *b* | *b* | *b* | *b* | *b* | *b* | Positive control |

(1) = mutation in H-2K$^b$.

**Figure 11.16** Haplotypes of the mouse strains used in the Sherman study. [*J. Exp. Med.* **151**:1386, 1980.]

Responding clones (43 of them) were transferred to fresh culture medium and stimulated with IL-2 until enough cells had been produced by mitosis to test for cytotoxicity against a panel of target cells. Along with the proper controls, the target cell panel was made up of cells derived from seven strains of mice containing mutations at H-2K$^b$. Such mutations are first recognized by the rejection of skin grafts between what had been, prior to the mutation, syngeneic animals. These mutations are expressed as a loss or a gain (or both) of antigenic determinants on the H-2K$^b$ molecule.

The results of testing revealed that by no means were all the $T_C$ clones the same. While they all lysed nonmutant H-2$^b$ target cells, each clone would lyse only certain mutant targets (Figure 11.17). Of the 128 ($2^7$) possible combinations of lysis and nonlysis of the seven kinds of mutant targets, 23 were observed among the 43 clones tested. Eight patterns were produced by two or more different clones; the remainder (15) appeared only once.

These results show that the response to even a single H-2 antigen represents a substantial range of specificities. If the results shown here (23 different specificities among only 43 clones tested) represent a random sampling of the total anti-H-2K$^b$ repertoire, probably more than twice that many specificities are available in the entire anti-H-2K$^b$ repertoire.

As we have seen, Sherman found 1 $T_C$-P for H-2K$^b$ in 12,000 spleen cells. Although as few as 3% of spleen cells may be Ly-2$^+$ cells, the possibility of there being, say, 50 different specificities available suggests that the frequency of $T_C$-P for any *single* antigenic specificity associated with H-2K is about 1/18,000 (12,000 × 0.03 × 50). Now we are looking at numbers that make clonal selection plausible for T cells responding to alloantigens as well as to those responding to conventional antigens. What had appeared to be very high levels (0.5–10%) of precommitment of $T_C$-P to a single H-2 haplotype may reflect instead the complexity of the antigens involved, i.e., the number of different antigenic determinants associated with each. But unless the H-2K molecule behaves very differently from conventional protein antigens, it is highly unlikely that it alone expresses 50 or more different antigenic determinants. More likely, each of these clones of $T_C$ cells is responding to a

| Pattern | No. of clones | Target cells[1] | | | | | | | |
|---|---|---|---|---|---|---|---|---|---|
| | | H-2K$^b$ | bm8 | bm1 | bm3 | bm4 | bm9 | bm10 | bm11 |
| 1 | 7 | + | + | + | + | + | + | + | + |
| 2 | 1 | + | + | + | + | − | + | + | + |
| 3 | 2 | + | + | + | + | − | + | − | + |
| 4 | 1 | + | + | − | − | + | + | − | + |
| 5 | 1 | + | + | − | − | + | − | + | − |
| 6 | 2 | + | − | + | + | + | + | + | + |
| 7 | 1 | + | − | + | − | + | + | − | − |
| 8 | 1 | + | − | − | − | + | + | + | − |
| 9 | 1 | + | − | − | − | + | + | − | + |
| 10 | 3 | + | − | − | − | + | − | + | − |
| 11 | 1 | + | − | − | + | + | + | + | + |
| 12 | 1 | + | − | − | + | + | + | − | − |
| 13 | 1 | + | + | − | − | − | + | + | − |
| 14 | 1 | + | + | − | − | − | + | − | + |
| 15 | 1 | + | + | − | + | − | + | + | + |
| 16 | 2 | + | + | − | + | − | − | − | + |
| 17 | 1 | + | − | + | − | − | + | − | + |
| 18 | 8 | + | − | − | − | − | + | − | − |
| 19 | 1 | + | − | − | − | − | − | + | − |
| 20 | 2 | + | − | − | − | − | − | − | − |
| 21 | 2 | + | − | − | + | − | + | + | + |
| 22 | 1 | + | − | − | + | − | + | − | − |
| 23 | 1 | + | − | − | + | − | − | − | + |
| | 43 | | | | | | | | |

[1] For mutant target cells, + = 60% or more of lysis of unmutated H-2K$^b$ targets; − = 25% or less of lysis of unmutated H-2K$^b$ targets.

**Figure 11.17**  Patterns of antigen specificity of 43 clones of anti-H-2K$^b$ T$_C$ cells tested against a panel of mutant H-2K$^b$ target cells. The heterogeneity shown suggests that the response to a single alloantigen involves T cells of a substantial number (~50) of different specificities. [From L. Sherman, *J. Exp. Med.* **151**:1386, 1980.]

neoantigen: a combination of an unknown molecule (X) associated with the allogeneic H-2K molecule. The X molecule need not be foreign; in fact, these two congenic strains of mice share all their background genes so we would expect their other cell surface molecules (e.g., the Fc$_\gamma$ receptor) to be identical. However, the combination of a shared X with a foreign H-2K molecule would produce a foreign neoantigen. If this view is correct, it means that the response to allogeneic cells obeys the same rules of associative recognition as the response to conventional antigens presented on syngeneic cells.

While further work is needed to determine the precise nature of the antigenic determinants recognized by T cells, Sherman's results have brought CMI responses to alloantigens within the scope of clonal selection. There is no longer any need to believe that a single T cell is multispecific in the sense of being able to respond to several different alloantigens.

Most of the T cells of the normal, unprimed animal are small, nondividing lymphocytes circulating through the T-dependent tissues of the body. The evidence suggests that even in the unprimed animal, each of these cells has already rearranged the genes for its antigen receptor and is expressing a single kind of receptor specific for Ag/MHC. So the foundation has been laid — perhaps very early in the life of the animal — for the clonal selection by foreign Ag/MIIC of thc T lymphocytes precommitted to it. As we have seen earlier in the chapter, clonal selection must begin with the "presentation" of Ag/MHC by an antigen-presenting cell like a dendritic cell. This is only the start of the story, however. In order for the resting $(G_0)$ T cell to be activated, it must receive a second signal. This is the monokine IL-1, which can be secreted by the APC itself (Figure 11.18). Once stimulated by both the appropriate antigen and IL-1, the T cell enters the cell cycle at $G_1$. The cell's metabolism increases. One manifestation of this is a sharply increased rate of protein synthesis. The $G_1$ T cell begins to synthesize and secrete IL-2. It also synthesizes its own receptors for IL-2. An activated T cell may anchor 5000–15,000 of these glycoproteins on the exterior surface of its cell membrane. The IL-2 receptors bind IL-2 with high affinity $(K > 10^{11} \text{ M}^{-1})$. This binding is absolutely necessary if the cell is to continue through the cell cycle. The binding of IL-2 first triggers DNA synthesis (S phase) and then the cell passes through $G_2$ and undergoes mitosis. In this way, a clone of antigen-specific T cells is produced.

Although IL-2 itself acts nonspecifically in promoting T cell proliferation, only those T cells expressing receptors for IL-2 are capable of

**Figure 11.18**  The response of T cells to antigen. The resting T cell is activated by (1) binding antigen and (2) the influence of IL-1. The T cell is able to bind a conventional antigen such as TNP only when (1) it is presented on the surface of an antigen-presenting cell (APC) and (2) it is presented in association with an MHC-encoded antigen. Once activated, the T cell expresses surface receptors for IL-2 and begins to secrete IL-2. This leads to its proliferation into a clone of T cells of the same specificity.

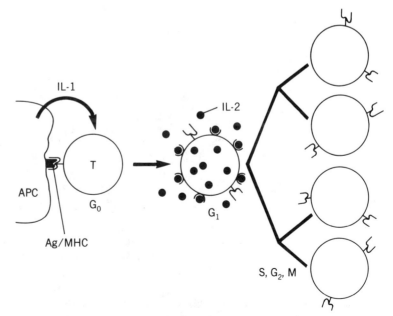

responding to it. Because only antigen-activated cells express these receptors, the proliferative response ends up being highly specific for antigen.

And it continues to be so. The daughter cells produced by mitosis do not express IL-2 receptors so they, too, must interact with the appropriate APCs if clonal proliferation is to continue. At any time that antigen should disappear, the cells of the responding clones soon lose their IL-2 receptors and once more become quiescent $G_0$ (memory?) cells.

Figure 11.18 suggests that a *single* activated T cell synthesizes IL-2 and the receptors which enable it to respond to IL-2. Although this seems to be the case, there is a good deal of evidence that a particular subset of T cells, e.g., $T_C$ cells, can be helped by the IL-2 secreted by T cells of other subsets (e.g., $T_H$) responding to the same antigenic stimulus. Thus the response of T cells to antigen seems to involve the same sort of cell–cell interactions that we have seen take place in humoral immunity. The cell interactions characteristic of cell-mediated immune responses are examined in Chapters 13 and 15.

## 11.11  Summary

All cell-mediated and most humoral immune responses require T lymphocytes. The pool of T lymphocytes consists of cells representing a wide range of antigen specificities. The antigen specificity of T lymphocytes, like that of B lymphocytes, is generated prior to encountering antigen. And, like B cells, the T cells specific for a given antigenic determinant represent a small fraction of the total repertoire.

The response of T lymphocytes to antigen differs from that of B cells in several respects.

1. T cells can bind and respond only to antigens present on a cell surface. Such antigens include foreign histocompatibility antigens as well as conventional antigens.
2. In the case of conventional antigens, the T cells can respond to the antigen only when it is associated with a particular histocompatibility antigen.
3. Murine L3T4+ and human CD4+ T cells respond to conventional antigens associated with class II histocompatibility antigens. Murine Ly-2+ and human CD8+ T cells respond to conventional antigens associated with class I histocompatibility antigens.
4. Those T cells that are able to bind a particular Ag/MHC and which receive a second stimulus, probably IL-1, enter the cell cycle. Activated $(G_1)$ T cells express surface receptors for IL-2 and also secrete IL-2. The interaction of IL-2 with its receptors causes the cell to divide and thus to develop into a clone of T cells.
5. A secondary T cell response can be elicited only when the T cell encounters the same combination of conventional antigen and histocompatibility antigen (Ag/MHC) to which the precursors of its clone responded ("MHC restriction").

6. It now seems likely that the dual specificity of T cells for Ag/MHC is mediated by a single type of receptor.
7. This receptor is constructed from two S—S linked polypeptides attached to the cell membrane.
8. As is the case for the immunoglobulin receptors of B cells, the T cell receptor is encoded by several gene segments (V, D, J, and C), which are rearranged during T cell differentiation (but prior to exposure to antigen).
9. Although the organization, behavior, and even sequence of T cell receptor gene segments resemble those of immunoglobulins, they are encoded separately and the two families of gene segments are not shared by B and T cells.

## ADDITIONAL READING

1. Bevan, M. J., "Killer Cells Reactive to Altered-Self Antigens Can Also Be Alloreactive," *Proc. Natl. Acad. Sci. USA* 74:2094, 1977. (Reprinted in V. L. Sato and M. L. Gefter, *Cellular Immunology*, Addison-Wesley Publishing Co., Inc., Reading, MA, 1982.)

2. Buchmeier, M. J., et al., "The Virology and Immunobiology of Lymphocytic Choriomeningitis Virus Infection," *Adv. Immunol.* 30:275, 1980.

3. Gascoigne, N. R. J., et al., "Genomic Organization and Sequence of T-Cell Receptor $\beta$-Chain Constant- and Joining-Region Genes," *Nature* 310:387, 1984. The two $J_\beta$–$C_\beta$ clusters in the mouse.

4. Haskins, Kathryn, et al., "The Major Histocompatibility Complex-Restricted Antigen Receptor on T Cells," *Ann. Rev. Immunol.* 2:51, 1984.

5. Hedrick, S. M., et al., "Isolation of cDNA Clones Encoding T-Cell-Specific Membrane-Associated Proteins," *Nature* 308:149, 1984. How subtractive cloning was used to isolate cDNA for a mouse $\beta$ chain.

6. Hunig, T., and M. J. Bevan, "Specificity of T-Cell Clones Illustrates Altered Self Hypothesis," *Nature* 294:460, 1981. Strong support for the single-receptor model of associative recognition.

7. Jones, Nancy, et al., "Partial Primary Structure of the Alpha and Beta Chains of Human T-Cell Receptors," *Science* 227:311, 1985. Includes the complete sequence of the HPB–MLT $\beta$ chain.

8. Kavaler, J., et al., "Localization of a T-Cell Receptor Diversity-Region Element," *Nature* 310:421, 1984. Includes the heptamer-nonamer recognition signals flanking the $V_\beta$, $D_\beta$, and $J_\beta$ gene segments.

9. Kronenberg, M., et al., "Three T Cell Hybridomas Do Not Contain Detectable Heavy Chain Variable Gene Transcripts," *J. Exp. Med.* 158:210, 1983. Evidence against the idea that the antigen specificity of T cells depends on the same pool of $V_H$ genes that B cells use for antibody synthesis.

10. Marrack, Philippa, et al., "The Major Histocompatibility Complex-Restricted Antigen Receptor on T Cells. IV. An Antiidiotypic Antibody Predicts Both Antigen and I-Specificity," *J. Exp. Med.* 158:1635, 1983. The monoclonal

antibody specific for DO-11.10 reacts with only one other cOVA/H-2$^d$ specific hybridoma (out of 397 tested).

11. McIntyre, B. W., and J. P. Allison, "The Mouse T Cell Receptor: Structural Heterogeneity of Molecules of Normal T Cells Defined by Xenoantiserum," *Cell* 34:739, 1983. Variable and constant regions of T cell receptors revealed by "antiframework" antibodies.

12. Siu, G., et al., "The Human T Cell Receptor Is Encoded by Variable, Diversity, and Joining Gene Segments That Rearrange to Generate a Complete V Gene," *Cell* 37:393, 1984.

13. Smith, K. A., "Interleukin 2," *Ann. Rev. Immunol.* 2:319, 1984.

# CHAPTER 12

# Cellular Interactions in Humoral Immunity

## 12.1   The Role of Adherent Cells

A primary immune response can be induced entirely in vitro. In the 1960s, Mishell and Dutton introduced a culture system in which all the events from antigen exposure to antibody production could take place. If sheep red blood cells (SRBC) are added to a culture containing spleen cells, specific antibody secreting cells can be detected after a few days by the hemolytic plaque assay. The number of plaque-forming cells (PFCs) rises to a peak at the fourth or fifth day and then declines (just as it does in vivo).

An unfractionated spleen cell population consists of lymphocytes (both B and T) and adherent cells, chiefly macrophages. The advantage of the in vitro system is that these cell populations can be purified and cultured in various combinations in order to determine the contribution of each.

In 1967 Mosier showed that the heterogeneous cell population of the spleen could be fractionated into a macrophage-rich population and a lymphocyte-rich population. He did this by exploiting the property of macrophages to adhere to plastic while lymphocytes do not. After cul-

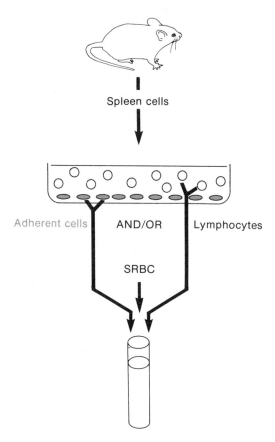

Spleen cells

Adherent cells    AND/OR    Lymphocytes

SRBC

**Figure 12.1** A primary in vitro response to sheep red blood cells (SRBC) requires the participation of adherent cells (mostly macrophages) as well as lymphocytes. The macrophages engulf SRBC by phagocytosis. Adherent cells incubated for 30 min with SRBC and then washed before mixing them with lymphocytes give an equally good response. [Based on D. E. Mosier, *Science* **158:**1573, 1967.]

|  | Anti-SRBC PFC per $10^6$ cultured cells |
|---|---|
| Normal spleen cells | 170 |
| Adherent cells only | 0 |
| Lymphocytes only | 0 |
| Adherent cells plus lymphocytes | 125 |

turing spleen cells in plastic dishes for 30 minutes, most of the macrophages adhere to the surface of the dish while most of the lymphocytes remain in the supernatant and can be poured off.

Mosier found that neither purified lymphocytes nor purified adherent cells could mount a primary anti-SRBC response when cultured alone with SRBC. Mixed together, however, the combined adherent cell–lymphocyte population produced almost as many PFCs as an unfractionated spleen cell population (Figure 12.1).

When particulate antigens are added to cultures containing macrophages, the antigens are quickly engulfed by phagocytosis. Even most soluble antigens, especially if they are somewhat aggregated, are taken up by macrophages. What is puzzling about this is that once ingested, the antigens are rapidly degraded. The phagocytic vacuoles fuse with lysosomes, and their contents are quickly digested by the proteases and other degradative enzymes contained within the lysosomes. Thus we might not expect that any antigenic determinants would remain intact to stimulate antigen-binding cell (ABCs).

As it turns out, however, not all of the antigen ingested by macrophages *is* degraded. Some of it is retained in an immunogenic form that appears to be localized on the surface membrane of the macrophage. In fact, this membrane-localized antigen is far more potent at stimulating an immune response than is free antigen (Figure 12.2). However, its effectiveness is destroyed if the membrane is treated with proteolytic en-

**Figure 12.2** Effect of soluble antigen and macrophage-bound antigen on the in vitro secondary response to DNP. Each culture was established with $12 \times 10^6$ spleen cells (which include macrophages), harvested from mice primed 4 months earlier to DNP–KLH, to which $5 \times 10^5$ macrophages and/or soluble antigen were added as indicated. Antigen-treated macrophages were incubated with antigen for 30 min and then washed thoroughly before being placed in culture. The number of IgG plaque-forming cells (PFC) was determined 4 days later. [Adapted from D. H. Katz and E. R. Unanue, *J. Exp. Med.* **137:**967, 1973.]

| Added to spleen cell culture | Anti-DNP PFC/Culture | Interpretation |
|---|---|---|
| 1. No macrophages; no antigen | 53 | No secondary response without antigen |
| 2. No macrophages; 1 µg/ml soluble DNP–KLH | 825 | Secondary response to soluble antigen |
| 3. Normal macrophages; no antigen | 53 | Untreated macrophages have no effect without antigen |
| 4. Normal macrophages; 1 µg/ml soluble DNP–KLH | 1756 | Macrophages and soluble antigen give good secondary response |
| 5. DNP–KLH-treated macrophages; no free antigen | 2234 | Antigen bound earlier to macrophages gives a good secondary response |
| 6. DNP–BGG-treated macrophages; no free antigen | 50 | Response is carrier specific |

zymes to remove the antigen or with antibodies directed against the antigen. In the latter case, the antibodies presumably mask the antigen so that it cannot be "seen" by the appropriate antigen-binding lymphocytes.

---

## 12.2 T Helper Cells

Chapter 7 presents evidence of a fundamental division in the immune system: humoral immune responses are mediated by B lymphocytes; cell mediated immune responses by T lymphocytes (see Figure 7.12). We would expect, then, that neonatally thymectomized mice or nude mice —both lacking mature T cells—would be unable to mount cell-mediated immune responses, and this is true. We *might* also expect these mice to mount normal humoral responses because their B cells are perfectly normal. But the situation is not so simple.

Neonatally thymectomized mice and nude mice *are* able to mount excellent humoral responses to certain kinds of antigens. These include the purified pneumococcal polysaccharides, polymerized flagellin (POL), and haptens coupled to these substances, for example, DNP-POL. For this reason, such antigens are called thymus independent (TI). On the other hand, these thymus-less mice cannot respond normally to foreign proteins like OVA and PPD nor to foreign particulate antigens like SRBC. Therefore these types of antigens are described as **thymus dependent**. The discussion in this chapter is exclusively concerned with thymus-dependent antigens. Some of the special features of TI antigens are examined in Section 8.9.

The reason that many antigens are thymus dependent is that the humoral response to those antigens requires a synergistic cooperation between B cells and T cells. Claman and his collaborators first clearly demonstrated this in 1966. They used heavily irradiated mice to test the activity of various syngeneic cell populations in the response to sheep red blood cells. Their experimental design is shown in Figure 12.3.

They found that neither thymus cells nor bone marrow cells could, by themselves, mediate a response to the antigen. When mixed together, however, the irradiated recipients responded well to the antigen. Spleen cells, which we now realize contain both B and T cells, also restored the ability of irradiated recipients to respond to SRBC (Figure 12.3).

If it takes both B cells and T cells to mount a humoral response to certain antigens, what is the role played by each? One approach to this question is to reconstitute irradiated mice with bone marrow cells and thymus cells that can be distinguished from each other. If, for example, we were to reconstitute an irradiated mouse with a suspension of bone marrow cells of one H-2 haplotype (say H-$2^b$) and thymus cells of another (H-$2^k$), we could see which haplotype was expressed on the antibody-secreting cells that appear a few days later. But when this experiment is done, no response at all occurs. The procedure that works for syngeneic cells does not work for allogeneic cells. On the other hand, if the bone marrow and thymus cells are only *semi-allogeneic*, they are able to coop-

**Figure 12.3** An in vivo humoral response to sheep red blood cells (SRBC) requires the participation of both thymus cells (a source of T lymphocytes) and bone marrow cells (a source of B lymphocytes). A suspension of spleen cells alone is effective because the spleen contains both B cells and T cells. [From H. N. Claman et al., *Proc. Soc. Exp. Biol. & Med.* **122**:1167, 1966.]

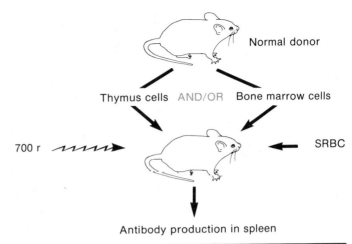

Antibody production in spleen

|  | Percent of spleen fragments with antibody activity |
|---|---|
| Thymus cells alone | 12 |
| Bone marrow cells alone | 2 |
| Thymus AND bone marrow cells | 71 |
| Spleen cells | 66 |
| None | 7 |

erate successfully. Semi-allogeneic cells share one but not both of the sets of MHC alleles (haplotypes) that a heterozygous mouse possesses. Thus the cells of a (CBA $\times$ C57BL)F$_1$ mouse (H-2$^{k/b}$) are semi-allogeneic to either CBA (H-2$^k$) or C57BL (H-2$^b$) cells.

By using the Claman reconstitution procedure with semi-allogeneic cells, Mitchell and Miller were able to show that antibody-secreting cells are derived from B cells, not T cells. They used CBA (H-2$^k$) mice that, as adults, had been thymectomized, irradiated, and reconstituted with injections of syngeneic bone marrow. Lacking a thymus, these animals were unable to generate any new T cells of their own. Two weeks later, the mice were injected with semi-allogeneic T cells and antigen (SRBC). The T cells were collected from the lymph in the thoracic duct of (CBA $\times$ C57BL)F$_1$ mice. Five days later, the spleen cells were harvested from the recipient mice and incubated with anti-H-2 serum (normal serum in the case of the controls). Then the cells were assayed for anti-SRBC plaque-forming cells (PFCs) in the hemolytic plaque assay. When treated with anti-CBA serum (anti-H-2$^k$), a drastic reduction (95–97%) occurred in the number of plaque-forming cells. In itself, this tells us little because both the bone marrow (B) cells (CBA) and the thoracic duct (T) cells (F$_1$) express the H-2$^k$ haplotype. However, treating the spleen cell suspension with anti-C57BL serum (anti-H-2$^b$), had little or no effect on the PFC response (Figure 12.4). This result shows that the antibody-secreting cells express only the H-2$^k$ haplotype. They must not have been derived from the injected thoracic duct (T) cells.

If T cells are required for the anti-SRBC response but do not secrete the anti-SRBC antibodies, what is their function? They must assist in the

**315**

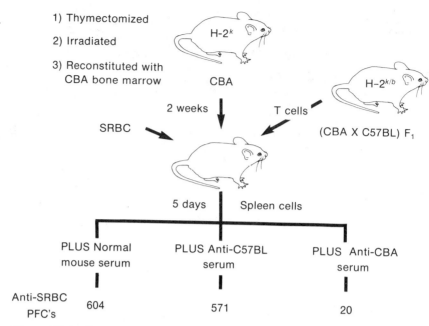

**Figure 12.4** Demonstration that antibody-secreting cells are derived from B lymphocytes, not T lymphocytes. Only the T cells expressed the H-2$^b$ antigens and treatment with anti-H-2$^b$ serum (anti-C57BL) had no inhibitory effect on plaque formation. (In separate experiments, the potency of the anti-C57BL (H-2$^b$) serum was shown by its ability to inhibit PFC production by both H-2$^b$ and H-2$^{k/b}$ spleen cells. [From G. F. Mitchell and J. F. A. P. Miller, *J. Exp. Med.* **128**:821, 1968.]

response in some way and, for this reason, we call these cells *T helper* (T$_H$) *cells*.

## 12.3  T$_H$ Cells Recognize Carrier Determinants

Anti-DNP antibodies bind to DNP attached to any carrier (see Section 4.5 for examples). However, the *induction* of a *secondary* antibody response to DNP (or any other hapten) normally requires that the animal be challenged with the same hapten–carrier complex that was used to induce the primary response (Figure 12.5). For example, an animal primed to DNP–BSA will simply produce another primary anti-DNP response when challenged with DNP–OVA. This phenomenon was discovered by Ovary and Benacerraf and called by them the *carrier effect*.

Priming an animal to a hapten and a carrier can be done separately. If an animal is immunized with a hapten coupled to one carrier (such as DNP–BSA) and then is independently immunized with another protein (e.g., OVA), the hapten coupled to the second protein (DNP–OVA) will now elicit a vigorous secondary response to DNP (Figure 12.5).

Each of these two phenomena can be adoptively transferred by the injection of the appropriate cells into irradiated, syngeneic recipients

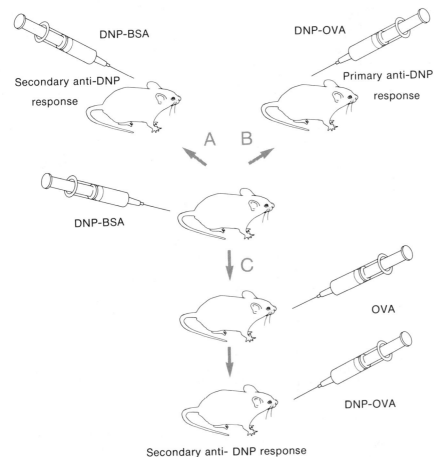

**Figure 12.5** The carrier effect. A secondary response to hapten (DNP) requires that it be presented on a carrier to which the animal has also been primed.

(Figure 12.6). For example, the irradiated recipients of spleen cells from animals primed with NIP – OVA will mount a secondary response to NIP if *either* they are injected with NIP coupled to the same carrier (OVA, experiment 1, Figure 12.6), *or* they are injected with NIP on a different carrier (e.g., BSA) *and* at the same time receive an injection of spleen cells from an animal primed with BSA (experiment #3).

This adoptive transfer system provided the means with which to examine the nature of the cells reacting with hapten and those reacting with the carrier. The procedure, devised by Raff, involves treating the spleen cell suspensions with anti-Thy-1 (anti-theta) serum and complement. Because only the T cells carry the Thy-1 antigen, we would expect this treatment to destroy T cells but not B cells. In each experiment, the irradiated animals were reconstituted with two separate cell populations given at the same time: one from an animal primed to the hapten on one carrier (H-C.1); the second from an animal primed to a second carrier (C.2) (Figure 12.7). In one experiment, cells from the donor primed to the hapten – carrier conjugate (H-C.1) were treated with anti-Thy-1 and complement before transfer to the irradiated recipients. The cells

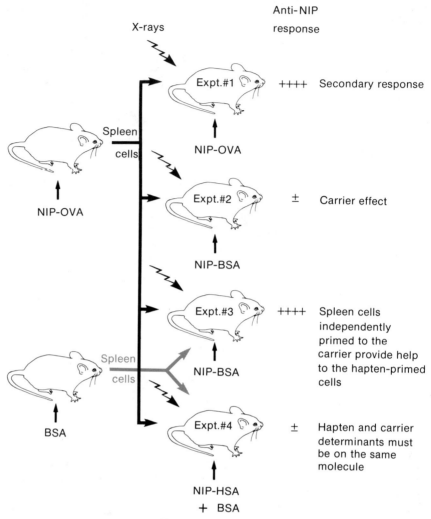

**Figure 12.6** Adoptive transfer of the carrier effect. HSA = horse serum albumin. [Based on N. A. Mitchison, *Eur. J. Immunol.* 1:18, 1971.]

primed to the second carrier (C.2) were untreated. In this case, the recipients were able to mount a vigorous antihapten response when challenged with the hapten coupled to the second carrier (H-C.2) (Figure 12.7). However, if only the carrier-primed (C.2) cells were treated with anti-Thy-1 and complement, the animal made a poor response when challenged with H-C.2. The conclusion is clear. The cells that interact with the carrier are T cells; the cells that react with the hapten are the B cells. And, as Mitchell and Miller showed, these B cells go on to produce antihapten antibodies.

Treatment of a carrier-primed spleen cell population with anti-Ly-1 serum and complement also destroys the ability of the cells to collaborate in a secondary antihapten response. However, treatment with anti-Ly-2 does not damage the cells. Thus we conclude that $T_H$ cells in the humoral response belong to that subpopulation of T cells that bear large amounts

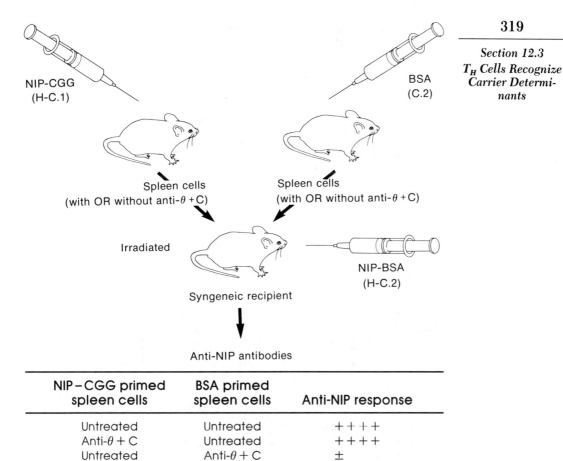

| NIP–CGG primed spleen cells | BSA primed spleen cells | Anti-NIP response |
|---|---|---|
| Untreated | Untreated | + + + + |
| Anti-$\theta$ + C | Untreated | + + + + |
| Untreated | Anti-$\theta$ + C | ± |

**Figure 12.7** Demonstration that the carrier primed helper cells in a secondary humoral response are T lymphocytes. Treatment with normal mouse serum and complement had no effect on either cell population. CGG = chicken gamma globulin. [From M. C. Raff, *Nature* **226**:1257, 1970. Reprinted in V. L. Sato and M. L. Gefter, *Cellular Immunology*. Addison-Wesley Publishing Co., Inc., Reading, MA, 1982.]

**Figure 12.8** Model of cooperative interaction between $T_H$ and B cells in the response to a thymus-dependent antigen. Any determinant on the antigen can serve as a hapten determinant (for B cells) while any other determinant can serve as a carrier determinant for $T_H$ cells. The process of binding to antigen is actually more complex than shown here. For example, antigen-presenting cells like macrophages must be present and the $T_H$ cell also binds to MHC-encoded determinants on these cells (see Section 12.4).

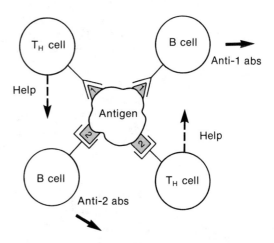

of Ly-1 antigen but no Ly-2 antigen on their surface. These cells also express the L3T4 antigen (Section 7.7).

Emphasis on this hapten–carrier system should not lead you to think that some structural feature distinguishes hapten determinants from carrier determinants. Any determinant on a T-dependent antigen might serve either as a hapten determinant or as a carrier determinant (Figure 12.8). One B cell responding to any determinant on the molecule can receive help from a T cell responding to any *other* determinant on the molecule. And, in fact, the animals described above made antibody responses to other determinants as well as to DNP. However, the *assay* was only measuring anti-DNP production.

## 12.4 The Secondary Response to Thymus-Dependent Antigens Is Restricted by the MHC

T cells respond to conventional antigens only when they are associated with antigens encoded by the major histocompatibility complex (MHC). Furthermore, T cells primed to a conventional antigen associated with one particular MHC-encoded antigen (e.g., Ia) will later be able to respond only if they once again encounter the conventional antigen associated with the same histocompatibility antigen. These facts are reviewed extensively in Chapter 11 (see, e.g., Sections 11.3 and 11.4). This phenomenon of associative recognition occurs during the interaction between $T_H$ cells and cells (e.g., macrophages and/or dendritic cells) that "present" antigen to them and also during the interaction between certain subsets of $T_H$ cells and B cells.

### The Interaction Between $T_H$ Cells and Macrophages Is Restricted by the MHC

This phenomenon was demonstrated in an elegant series of experiments reported by Erb and Feldmann in 1975. Their experimental protocol consisted of a sequential culture system. In the first culture, they mixed (1) purified T cells from CBA mice, (2) the antigen KLH (the carrier), and (3) the macrophages to be tested. After four days in culture, precise numbers of cells were removed and placed in a second culture with (1) unprimed CBA cells from which T cells (but not macrophages) had been removed and (2) antigen (TNP–KLH or, in one case, DNP–POL). Four days later, the antihapten response was measured in a hemolytic plaque assay using DNP-coated sheep red cells. (Antibodies elicited by TNP show a high degree of cross-reactivity with DNP.)

The first experiment in Figure 12.9 shows that culturing T cells with the carrier (KLH) and syngeneic macrophages produces a population of carrier-primed helper cells. These enable the B cells in the second culture to respond to hapten on the same carrier. If macrophages are not included in the first culture, few if any $T_H$ cells are produced (experiment

| First culture | Second culture | | |
|---|---|---|---|
| ⎡CBA T cells (*kkkkkk*)⎤<br>⎣  + KLH  ⎦<br> + macrophages<br>as shown | ⎡CBA B cells⎤<br>⎣ (*kkkkkk*) ⎦<br> + cells from first culture<br> + antigen as shown | Anti-DNP<br>PFC/Culture | Interpretation |
| 1. CBA (*kkkkkk*) | TNP–KLH | 377 | $T_H$ cells induced by syngeneic macrophages |
| 2. No macrophages | TNP–KLH | 63 | Poor primary response to TD antigen in absence of macrophage-induced $T_H$ cells |
| 3. (No first culture) | DNP–POL | 436 | Primary response to TI antigen in absence of $T_H$ cells |
| 4. C57BL/10 (*bbbbbb*) ("B10") | TNP–KLH | 70 | $T_H$ cells able to help CBA B cells not induced by allogeneic macrophages |
| 5. B10.BR (*kkkkkk*) | TNP–KLH | 327 | Identity at H-2 allows effective induction even though background Is different |
| 6. A.TL (*skkkkd*) | TNP–KLH | 327 | Identity at K/D not needed |
| 7. B10.A(4R) (*kkkkbb*) | TNP–KLH | 263 | Identity at $A_\beta A_\alpha$ works |

**Figure 12.9**  Effect of the H-2 region expressed on macrophages on the induction of T helper cells able to assist CBA B cells. First culture = CBA spleen cells depleted of macrophages (by giving them iron particles and then removing them with a magnet) and cultured with KLH and $5 \times 10^5$ test macrophages (depleted of T cells by anti-theta plus C) as indicated. Second culture = unprimed CBA spleen cells depleted of T cells (but still containing macrophages) and cultured for 4 days with antigen (as indicated) and no (expt. 3) or $3 \times 10^5$ $T_H$ cells produced in the first culture. [Adapted from P. Erb and M. Feldmann, *J. Exp. Med.* **142**:460, 1975.]

2). However, helper cells are not needed if the hapten is supplied to the second culture coupled to polymerized flagellin (POL). DNP–POL is a T-independent antigen, able to induce anti-DNP antibodies in neonatally thymectomized or nude mice.

When CBA T cells are cultured with antigen and *allogeneic* (C57BL/10) macrophages, they are unable to provide help to the second culture CBA cells. One interpretation of this finding is that $T_H$ cells cannot be primed with antigen unless it is presented to them by macrophages having the same histocompatibility antigens. A second interpretation (and the one I favor) is that $T_H$ cells are, in fact, induced by the *combination* of carrier (KLH) and C57BL/10 ("B10") histocompatibility antigens. When placed in the second culture, however, they are unable to provide help because, although the same carrier is present, it is seen in the context of a new set (CBA) of histocompatibility antigens. In a normal animal, of course, all the cells would share the same histocompatibility antigens.

By using congenic mouse strains, Erb and Feldmann were able to show that this phenomenon is dependent upon the nature of the H-2 region. Macrophages from the B10.BR strain are able to induce $T_H$ cells that can help B cells from the CBA strain. The B10.BR strain carries the same H-2 haplotype as CBA although on quite a different background (the C57BL/10 strain).

With the use of H-2 recombinants, these workers were able to identify the I region of H-2 as the one controlling the response. Macrophages from the recombinant strain B10.A(4R) *(kkkkbb)* enabled CBA helpers to be generated as did macrophages from the A.TL strain *(sskkkd)* (Figure 12.9). Taken together, these findings show that as long as the antigen-presenting cells in the second culture have the same $A_\alpha A_\beta$ or $E_\alpha E_\beta$ Ia antigens as the macrophages used in the first culture, they can provide help for the B cells.

## Some Interactions Between $T_H$ Cells and B Cells Are Restricted by the MHC

The induction of a humoral immune response to a thymus-dependent antigen requires the interaction of three types of cells: antigen-presenting cells (such as macrophages), $T_H$ cells, and B cells. Successful interaction between $T_H$ cells and macrophages is restricted by the MHC; in mice, the I region. What about the interaction between $T_H$ cells and B cells?

Several groups of investigators have found that successful $T_H$-B collaboration in mice requires that the $T_H$ cells recognize a particular Ia antigen expressed by the B cells. In other words, the delivery of T help is restricted by I-encoded antigens expressed by the B cells. Figure 12.10 demonstrates the effect of adding $T_H$ cells to a culture containing B cells and a thymus-dependent antigen (PC–OVA, which is phosphorylcholine coupled to the carrier ovalbumin). The $T_H$ cells are members of a clone of Ly-1$^+$ T cells derived from a mouse immunized with OVA. The B cell response is measured after five days in culture by their ability to form plaques with PC-coupled red cells in the hemolytic plaque assay. In the absence of $T_H$ cells, few anti-PC secreting cells are formed. With the addition of $T_H$ cells, however, a striking response is observed. Note that when the B cells are cultured with a T-*independent* (TI) form of the antigen (PC coupled to the bacterium *Brucella abortus*), a substantial response is seen whether or not $T_H$ cells are present.

With this system, these workers were able to establish that $T_H$ cells of a particular H-2 haplotype could deliver help only to B cells of the same haplotype. For example, $T_H$ cells derived from BALB/c mice (H-2$^d$) could help only BALB/c or other H-2$^d$ B cells. The critical region of H-2 turned out, as you would have expected, to be the I region. Furthermore,

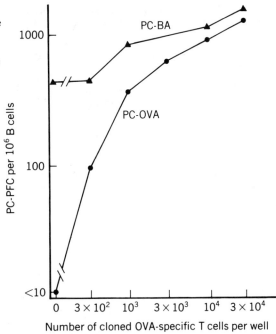

**Figure 12.10** The response of B cells to a thymus-dependent antigen (PC-OVA) requires the presence of OVA-specific $T_H$ cells (●). The response to the same hapten coupled to *Brucella abortus* (PC-BA) is T independent (▲). The ability of the $T_H$ cells to provide help is restricted by the MHC. $T_H$ cells generated in an animal with one set of class II antigens can help only B cells that express the same class II antigen(s). [From K. Bottomly et al., *J. Exp. Med.* **158**:265, 1983.]

monoclonal antibodies against I-A$^d$-encoded determinants block the ability of H-2$^d$ $T_H$ cells to give help to H-2$^d$ B cells but anti-I-A$^b$ antibodies have no such effect.

It is clear from these results that successful $T_H$-B interactions in this system are restricted by the MHC and, more particularly, by antigens encoded in the I region (A$_\alpha$A$_\beta$ and/or E$_\alpha$E$_\beta$). Many find this satisfying. First, it extends the principle we have been developing that T cells recognize antigen in association with MHC antigens. Second, it provides a function for the rich coat of Ia antigens characteristic of activated B cells and of such (other) antigen-presenting cells as dendritic cells and macrophages.

## 12.5   The Antigen/Ia Bridge Model of $T_H$-B Collaboration

In order for a secondary response to occur, both the hapten and the carrier to which the B cells and T cells have been respectively primed must *normally* be present on the *same* molecule. If, for example, the animal is reconstituted with two spleen cell populations, one primed to H-C.1 and the other to C.2, it will respond, as we have seen, to an injection of H-C.1 *or* H-C.2 (Figure 12.6). However, it will not normally respond to a *mixture* of C.2 and the hapten conjugated to a third carrier. H-C.3 (experiment 4, Figure 12.6). One might have expected that T cells encountering the carrier to which they had been primed would have been able to help the B cells respond to the hapten even though it was presented on a new carrier (C.3). We shall use the expression *linked*

323

*recognition* to describe the interaction between $T_H$ cells and B cells each primed to a determinant presented on the same molecule.

The delivery of help in the system described in the previous section (Figure 12.10) requires not only a proper MHC match but also linked recognition. The OVA-specific $T_H$ cells can help the PC-specific B cells only when PC and OVA are part of the same molecule. When these cells are cultured with a *mixture* of OVA and PC–KLH, for example, no collaborative response occurs.

The requirement for linked recognition immediately suggests a mechanism by which $T_H$ cells deliver help to B cells. This model proposes that the antigen serves as a bridge physically linking the $T_H$ cell and the B cell together (Figure 12.11). The finding that linked recognition is also MHC restricted suggests further that the "bridge" is formed by both the conventional antigen and an Ia antigen. The binding of the $T_H$ cell to the B cells could be accomplished by separate receptors — one for a carrier determinant and one for Ia. If, on the other hand, the $T_H$ cell interaction is mediated by a single antigen receptor (as seems likely — Section 11.8), then this receptor probably binds a compound antigenic determinant made up of portions of antigen and MHC (Figure 12.11). In either case, the antigen/Ia bridge model of $T_H$-B collaboration really adds B cells to the list (along with dendritic cells and some macrophages) of antigen-

**Figure 12.11**  Model of T cell help for B cells provided by linked recognition (left) and by bystander cells (right). A single receptor is postulated for the $T_H$ cells to account for their associative recognition of a carrier determinant on the antigen with a class II (Ia) histocompatibility antigen. "APC" at the top of the figure represents an antigen-presenting cell such as a dendritic cell. Antigen uptake by these cells is nonspecific. They can induce the appropriate $T_H$ cells after taking up hapten–carrier conjugates (as shown here) or carrier alone. In linked recognition, the B cell is also an APC. Antigen uptake by B cells is specific; only those B cells with immunoglobulin receptors for epitopes (hapten) on the intact antigen can bind it preparatory to presenting carrier determinants (and Ia) to $T_H$ cells. The B cell growth and differentiation factors are not antigen specific.

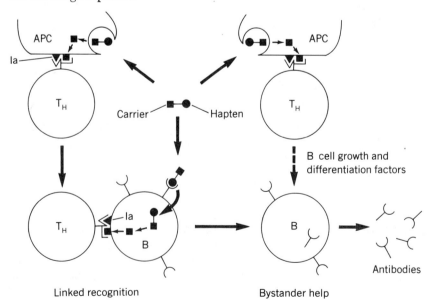

Linked recognition                    Bystander help

presenting cells (APCs) for $T_H$ cells. In contrast to macrophages and dendritic cells, however, antigen presentation by B cells is limited to those clones specific for that antigen. This is because only those B cells expressing the appropriate immunoglobulin receptor (e.g., sIgM) can bind the antigen.

The binding of antigen to a B cell by means of its immunoglobulin receptor for a "hapten" determinant on the antigen appears to be a separate event which precedes presentation of a carrier determinant (in association with Ia) to $T_H$ cells. Section 8.7 describes the evidence that antigen bound to immunoglobulin is swept into a "cap" on the cell surface and then taken into the cell by endocytosis. Lanzavecchia has shown that anything that interferes with this process blocks the ability of B cells to react later with $T_H$ cells. In due course, fragments ("carrier") of the antigen are returned to the cell surface and now, in association with Ia, they can stimulate $T_H$ cells. Linked recognition occurs because $T_H$ cells specific for determinants on, say, carrier "1" (C.1) can be presented these determinants only by those hapten-specific B cells that have taken up the H-C.1 conjugate.

Steinman and his colleagues have been able to provide striking visual and functional evidence of the cellular interactions that occur between antigen-presenting cells (they use dendritic cells), B cells, and $T_H$ cells. They have found that when spleen cells are cultured with an antigen, tight clusters of cells develop (Figure 12.12). These clusters contain dendritic cells, $T_H$ cells, and B cells. The process of clustering can be separated into two phases: an early phase (days 0–2) during which only the dendritic cells and $T_H$ cells need be present to form clusters; and a later phase (days 2–5) when antigen-primed B cells enter the cluster and differentiate into antibody-*secreting* cells. The B cells can only join the dendritic cell/$T_H$ cell cluster if they have the same Ia antigens as the dendritic cells.

Once the second phase has begun, the $T_H$ cells in the culture can be

**Figure 12.12** Phase contrast micrograph (750×) of spleen cells after two days in culture. Four dendritic cells (with the surface projections) can be seen clustered with the lymphocytes. [Courtesy of Ralph M. Steinman from K. Inaba et al., *J. Exp. Med.* **160**:858, 1984.]

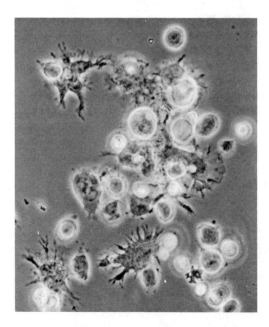

destroyed (by anti-Thy-1 and/or anti-Ly-1 and complement). Even in the absence of $T_H$ cells, however, the B cells can continue along the path to antibody-secreting cells *if* the B cells are supplied with certain soluble factors released by activated T cells. Beyond a certain point, then, completion of B cell development becomes independent of antigen-specific, MHC-restricted T cell help. We shall use the expression "bystander" help for the help given to B cells that requires neither linked recognition nor, as it turns out, I region identity between the $T_H$ and B cells.

## 12.6 Bystander Help for B Cells

The intitial activation of B cells using hapten–carrier conjugates seems always to require linked recognition. However, it is sometimes possible to demonstrate a *secondary* B cell response in the absence of any opportunity of linked recognition. In these cases, the previously-primed B cells seem to have acquired the capacity to respond to bystander help.

### Bystander Help in Vitro

Schimple, Wecker, and their colleagues have demonstrated that B cells and T cells, both primed to DNP–KLH (H-C.1), can collaborate in a secondary anti-DNP response when cultured together in the presence of KLH (C.1) *and* DNP-BGG (H-C.2) (Figure 12.13). In this situation, there is no opportunity for the KLH-specific $T_H$ cells to bind to the DNP-specific B cells. However, the interaction of carrier-primed T cells with carrier alone enables them to render bystander help. Presumably the B cells become susceptible to bystander help following their first exposure to antigen.

### Bystander Help in Vivo

Workers in a number of laboratories have also been able to demonstrate bystander help in vivo. Katz and his collaborators, for example, reconstituted heavily irradiated mice with *two* separate populations of syngeneic spleen cells. One population had been primed to DNP conjugated to a protein extracted from the nematode *Ascaris suum* (DNP–Asc). The second had been primed to the carrier (Asc) alone. When challenged four days later with Asc *and* DNP–*KLH*, a weak but significant anti-DNP response occurred although the DNP was presented on a new carrier. The positive control of DNP–Asc gave an excellent response, while the negative control of DNP–KLH alone gave a very poor response.

Thus it is clear that the interaction of carrier primed T cells with carrier alone can, at least in some circumstances, result in the delivery of help to B cells responding to a hapten conjugated to a different carrier. If a $T_H$ cell can provide help without the opportunity for antigen bridging to the

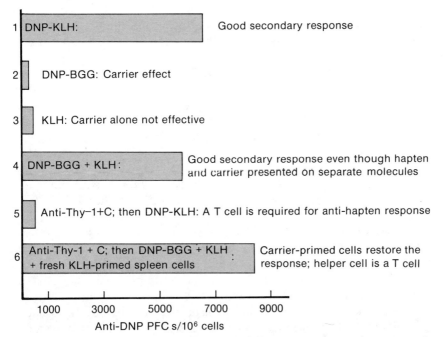

Figure 12.13  Overcoming the carrier effect in vitro. Each culture contained $5 \times 10^6$ spleen cells (thus with both B and T cells present) harvested from mice primed several weeks earlier with DNP–KLH. In experiments 5 and 6, the spleen cells were treated with anti-Thy-1 and complement (C), washed, and then cultured with antigen (5) or with antigen plus spleen cells previously primed with KLH (6). Only plaques produced by IgG were counted. [Adapted from Th. Hünig et al., *J. Exp. Med.* 145:1216, 1977.]

B cell, perhaps help in these cases is delivered by soluble factors of some sort.

## 12.7  Nonspecific Helper Factors

A number of laboratories have found evidence of helper factors that enable B cells to respond to T-dependent antigens in the absence of $T_H$ *cells.* Often these factors are nonspecific in their action; i.e., they can help B cells of any antigen specificity. Although they can *replace* $T_H$ cells, the factors are nonetheless the products of T cells which have been activated by some stimulus. Thus these factors qualify as lymphokines (Section 3.2).

### B Cell Growth Factors (BCGFs)

In a preparation of lymphocytes (from the spleen for example), the frequency of B cells specific for any particular antigen is quite low (Section 8.8). This makes it difficult to study the events that take place when a B cell binds the antigen for which it is specific. Fortunately, there are a number of agents that can activate a large proportion of B cells in a nonspecific fashion. These include mitogens like LPS (in mice — Section 7.8) and also antibodies directed against IgM and IgD. Chapter 8 presents the evidence that sIgM and sIgD serve as the antigen receptors on the surface of mature B cells. Presumably, the binding of anti-IgM (or anti-IgD) antibodies to these receptors mimics the signal that antigen binding would provide.

At relatively high concentrations, anti-IgM antibodies are mitogenic for a large proportion of B cells. In other words, the B cells are stimulated to begin mitosis. The response is polyclonal: the responding B cells probably represent most of the antigen-binding specificities available in the animal. At lower concentrations, however, anti-IgM antibodies alone cannot trigger mitosis. They must work synergistically with some other factor or factors in order to drive resting $(G_0)$ B cells to divide by mitosis. This is shown in Figure 12.14. Even at a dose of 50 $\mu$g/ml of anti-IgM, there is practically no proliferation of B cells (measured by the uptake of tritiated thymidine in S phase). However, the addition of the supernatant fluid harvested from a culture of activated T cells permits vigorous proliferation to take place. Although the cells proliferate well, they are unable to differentiate into antibody-*secreting* cells. Lymphokines that promote B cell proliferation without differentiation are called B cell growth factors (BCGFs). In addition to the factor studied by Howard and her associates (Figure 12.14), there is considerable evidence that IL-2, a well-known product of activated T cells (Section 6.2), acts as a BCGF. The macrophage product interleukin 1 (IL-1) also seems to be a BCGF.

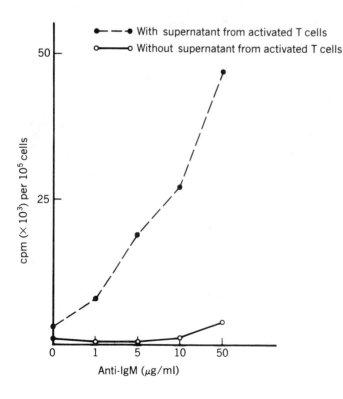

Figure 12.14 The proliferation of mitogen-activated B cells requires lymphokines secreted by activated T cells. These lymphokines are called B cell growth factors (BCGFs). The B cells were activated by treating them with anti-IgM antibodies. B cell proliferation was measured by their incorporation of tritiated thymidine. [From Maureen Howard et al., *J. Exp. Med.* **155**:914, 1982.]

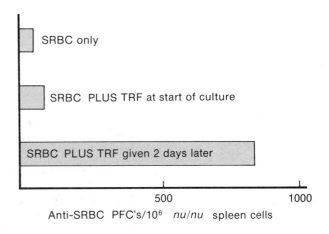

**Figure 12.15** Establishment of a primary response to sheep red blood cells (SRBC) in cultures of spleen cells from nude mice by a late-acting T-cell replacing factor (TRF). Spleen cells from nude mice ordinarily cannot respond to this T-dependent antigen. The TRF preparation consisted of the supernatant of a culture containing DNP–KLH and spleen cells from mice previously immunized with the same antigen. [From Th. Hünig et al., *J. Exp. Med.* **145**:1228, 1977.]

## B Cell Differentiation Factors (BCDFs)

In the previous section, we saw that it is sometimes possible to demonstrate a T helper effect even in the absence of linked recognition between $T_H$ and B cells. In the example shown in Figure 12.13, $T_H$ cells primed to one carrier were able to help hapten-primed B cells respond to the hapten presented on a different carrier. The help in this case can be delivered just as well by the supernatant fluid of a culture containing the $T_H$ cells and the carrier. This factor, which was called "T cell replacing factor" or TRF by its discoverers, is one of a number of T cell factors (lymphokines) that enable antigen-stimulated B cells to differentiate into antibody-secreting plasma cells. Thus this TRF is one of a number of B cell differentiation factors (BCDFs). The activity of TRF and other BCDFs is not antigen specific. Although produced by T cells responding to DNP–KLH, it enables B cells to respond to SRBC, an unrelated antigen (Figure 12.15).

When the amount of TRF is limiting, its effect is seen only when TRF is added two days after the cells are cultured with SRBC (Figure 12.15). Presumably the first two days are taken up with the process of antigen activation of resting B cells and their clonal proliferation. Only then do the proliferating cells become competent to respond to any BCDFs present. Probably the acquisition of competence is mediated by the appearance of receptors for BCDFs on the cell surface.

Evidence is accumulating for the existence of isotype-specific BCDFs. Thus a factor designated $BCDF_\mu$ induces proliferating B cells to secrete IgM while a different factor, $BCDF_\gamma$, induces them to become IgG-secreting cells.

## 12.8 Antigen-Specific Helper Factors

From time to time, reports appear of T cell replacing factors that are antigen specific in their action; that is, factors that replace $T_H$ cells in the response to one particular antigen only. These antigen-specific factors

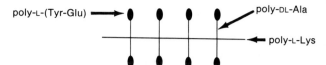

**Figure 12.16** Schematic representation of the synthetic antigen (T, G)-A-L. The side chains of this polymer are attached to the ε-amino groups of the lysine residues.

differ from the factors described in the previous section not only in their antigen specificity but in other properties as well. They all bind to the antigen for which they give help. A number of reports indicate that these factors express idiotypic determinants similar to the idiotypes expressed by antibodies of the same specificity. In a number of cases, the action of these factors is MHC restricted: they can give help only to B cells expressing the correct Ia antigens. In many cases, these factors also seem themselves to express Ia antigens.

Precise characterization of these antigen-specific factors has been difficult because of the small amounts produced. However, hybridoma technology (Section 4.8) may solve this problem. For example, Eshhar *et al.* have created a *T cell* hybridoma that secretes a helper factor specific for the synthetic antigen (T,G)-A-L (Figure 12.16). Their factor enhances the in vivo response of B cells to (T,G)-A-L (Figure 12.17) and expresses idiotypic determinants characteristic of antibodies directed against (T,G)-A-L. The factor is also associated with a polypeptide that is bound by anti-Ia antibodies. In other words, the active factor seems to express Ia antigens.

Most of the properties of antigen-specific helper factors are consistent with these factors simply being the solubilized T cell receptor(s) for antigen and Ia (Figure 12.11). Chapter 11 examines the nature of the T cell receptor for antigen; its Ag/MHC specificity, and the reasons why we might expect these receptors to express determinants similar to those of antibodies of the same specificity. Why these helper factors, which often

**Figure 12.17** Evidence for an antigen-specific helper factor. A factor secreted by a T cell hybridoma is able to substitute for $T_H$ cells in enabling primed B cells to mount a secondary response to (T,G)-A-L. The antigen specificity of the factor was shown by its inability to help B cells respond to an unrelated antigen (OVA). The factor was bound by (T,G)-A-L and also by an immunoadsorbent carrying anti-$V_H$ antibodies. The hybridoma was made by fusing (T,G)-A-L-primed T cells with mouse tumor cells (see Section 4.7). [From Z. Eshhar et al., *Nature* **286**:270, 1980.]

| Treatment[1] | Anti-(T,G)-A-L[2] antibodies (cpm) |
|---|---|
| (T,G)-A-L-primed spleen cells (B + T) | 12,000 |
| (T,G)-A-L-primed B cells only | 1,900 |
| (T,G)-A-L-primed B cells plus factor[3] | 4,200 |
| (T,G)-A-L-primed B cells plus purified factor[4] | 15,000 |

[1] Mice were irradiated (750 rad) and injected with 10 μg (T,G)-A-L and the mixtures indicated.
[2] Measured by radioimmunoassay of serum 12–14 days after treatment.
[3] Supernatant of hybridoma culture.
[4] Purified with a (T,G)-A-L-coupled immunoadsorbent.

must *recognize* a particular Ia antigen in order to work, should also *express* Ia antigens remains to be determined

## 12.9 Immune Response (Ir) Genes

Antigens that induce a humoral response in certain members of a species may fail to do so in other members. As so frequently happens in scientific work, this discovery was made in the course of experiments having quite a different goal. In an effort to reduce the heterogeneity of the antibodies produced during an immune response, Benacerraf and his coworkers tried immunizing animals with synthetic antigens of simple structure. One of these was DNP–PLL, a linear polymer of L-lysine with DNP groups coupled to the epsilon amino groups. They found that while DNP–PLL was a perfectly satisfactory antigen in some guinea pigs, other animals failed to respond to it. Breeding studies showed that the ability to respond was inherited as a dominant, single-gene trait. Thus, when strain 2 guinea pigs (responders) are mated to strain 13 guinea pigs (nonresponders), all of the $F_1$ offspring are responders. Backcrossing these $F_1$ animals with the nonresponder (strain 13) parents gives 50% responders and 50% nonresponders, the classic Mendelian ratio for a trait controlled by a single gene locus (Figure 12.18). The gene was called the PLL gene. It is an example of an *immune response* (Ir) *gene*.

A similar phenomenon was discovered in mice by McDevitt and his associates. They also used synthetic antigens. These workers found that the ability of an inbred mouse strain to respond well to (T,G)-A-L (Figure 12.16) was a function of its H-2 haplotype. Thus all strains with the H-$2^b$ haplotype (e.g., C57BL/10 and the congenic BALB.B10) are responders whereas all strains carrying H-$2^k$ (such as CBA, C3H, and AKR) are low or nonresponders (Figure 12.19).

The availability of recombinant inbred strains made it possible to map the location of the Ir gene for (T,G)-A-L. It turned out to be located between the K and S loci of H-2, and this region was designated *I*.

Figure 12.18 Inheritance of the response of inbred guinea pigs to DNP–PLL. Strain 2 animals are responders; strain 13 nonresponders.

| | | Strain 2 (RR) | | |
|---|---|---|---|---|
| | | R | R | |
| Strain 13 (rr) | r | Rr | Rr | } 100% responders |
| | r | Rr | Rr | |

| | | Strain 13 (rr) | | |
|---|---|---|---|---|
| | | r | r | |
| (2 × 13)F$_1$ (Rr) | R | Rr | Rr | 50% responders |
| | r | rr | rr | 50% nonresponders |

| Haplotype | Representative strains | Antigen | | | | |
|---|---|---|---|---|---|---|
| | | (T,G)-A-L | (Phe,G)-A-L | GLPhe | OVA | BGG |
| H-2$^b$ | C57BL/10, BALB.B10 | + | + | − | + | − |
| H-2$^d$ | BALB/c, DBA/2 | ± | + | + | + | − |
| H-2$^k$ | CBA, C3H, AKR | − | + | − | − | + |
| H-2$^a$ | A, B10.A | − | + | − | − | + |

Figure 12.19   Representative examples of immune responsiveness among various inbred mouse strains. + = responder to the antigen.

As research proceeded, the humoral response of mice to a number of other antigens turned out to be under Ir gene control. Mapping studies placed all of these genes in the I region but not always at precisely the same spot. In this way, the I region began to be divided into subregions. Some Ir genes map exclusively to the I-A subregion; but other immune responses are dependent on one gene mapping to I-A and a second to I-E.

### How Do Ir Genes Work?

The failure to make anti-DNP antibodies in response to DNP–PLL is not caused by a lack of B cells capable of responding to DNP. When DNP is coupled to some other carrier the animal can respond to, such as OVA, a normal anti-DNP response follows. So the defect in nonresponder animals involves the carrier portion of the antigen and thus involves $T_H$ cells. In fact, if the DNP–PLL complex is itself treated as a hapten by coupling it to an immunogenic carrier (OVA), nonresponders are now able to synthesize antibodies against it. Thus Ir gene defects seem to involve the ability of $T_H$ cells to respond to particular carrier determinants. In certain cases, this failure is caused by the presence of a population of suppressor T ($T_S$) cells. (The properties of $T_S$ cells are examined in Chapter 15.) In other cases, which we shall examine here, the failure of $T_H$ cells to respond to certain antigens is caused by their failure to interact success-fully with macrophages that "present" the antigen to them. Strain 13 guinea pigs do not respond to DNP–GL (DNP coupled to the synthetic polymer of L-Glu, L-Lys). Strain 2 guinea pigs do not respond to GT, a synthetic polymer of L-Glu and L-Tyr. However, the $(2 \times 13)F_1$ T cells produced by mating these strains respond (by proliferation in culture) to *either* antigen so long as $F_1$ macrophages are present in the culture (Figure 12.20). They also respond to antigen stimulated, *parental*-type macrophages but only when the macrophages are from the strain that is a responder for that antigen. Thus, strain 2 macrophages exposed to DNP–GL or strain 13 macrophages exposed to GT are able to stimulate proliferation of $F_1$ lymphocytes that have previously been primed to both of these antigens. However, the doubly primed $F_1$ T cells respond very poorly to strain 13 macrophages exposed to DNP–GL and also to strain 2 macrophages exposed to GT (Figure 12.20). (At first glance you might feel that mixing responder or nonresponder macrophages with

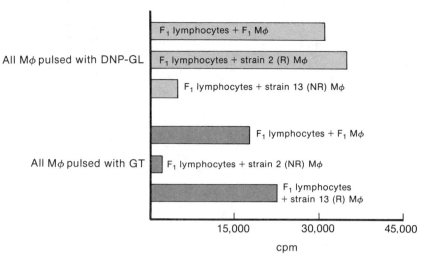

**Figure 12.20** Proliferative response (measured by the uptake of tritiated thymidine) of lymphocytes from $(2 \times 13)F_1$ guinea pigs to antigen-pulsed macrophages. Antigen-pulsed macrophages have been exposed to the antigen and then washed thoroughly before being added to the cultures. All the $F_1$ lymphocytes were harvested from guinea pigs primed to both DNP–GL and GT. $M\phi$ = macrophages. [From E. M. Shevach and A. S. Rosenthal, *J. Exp. Med.* **138**:1213, 1973.]

parental-type responder or nonresponder T cells would have been a more straightforward approach. But, of course, mixing T cells of one parental strain with macrophages of the other would have produced a vigorous MLR. The proliferative response to allogeneic histocompatibility antigens would have masked any effect contributed by the soluble antigens under study.)

What accounts for the failure of $F_1$ T cells to respond to antigen presented on nonresponder macrophages? One possibility is that macrophages from nonresponder animals are unable to "present" the antigen to T cells in an immunogenic form, that is, that the fault lies with the macrophages. A second possibility is that the fault lies with the T cells. Perhaps nonresponder strains have a gap in their T cell repertoire such that they cannot produce T cells with receptors for the complex antigenic determinant (CAD — see Section 11.5) constructed from the conventional antigen (DNP–GL or GT) *and* some portion of one of their own histocompatibility antigens (Figure 12.21). This second interpretation is supported by the evidence of Ishii et al. that responder T cells, which have been *depleted* of all alloreactive cells, are able to respond to an antigen (X) presented to them by allogeneic *non*responder macrophages. This indicates that macrophages from nonresponder strains are able to present antigen in an immunogenic form to responder T cells.

When different congenic H-2 recombinant mouse strains are immunized with each other's lymphoid cells, they produce antibodies directed against antigenic determinants encoded by H-2 genes that distinguish them. When this is done with mice that differ solely in their I region loci, the antisera that are produced define the so-called Ia or class II antigens. The genes encoding these map to the I-A and I-E subregions (Section

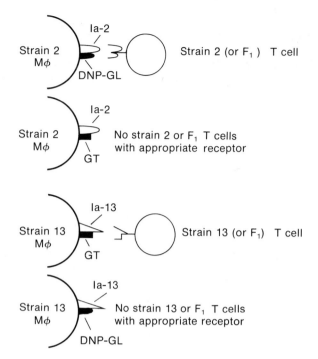

Figure 12.21 One interpretation of the results presented in Figure 12.20. According to this view, strain 2 (and $F_1$) guinea pigs lack T cells capable of recognizing the compound antigenic determinant made up of GT and a strain 2 ("self") Ia antigen. Strain 13 (and $F_1$) guinea pigs lack T cells capable of recognizing DNP–GL associated with a strain 13 Ia antigen. $F_1$ T cells can respond to either antigen presented by $F_1$ macrophages (see Figure 12.20). The importance of the Ia antigen is shown by the ability of anti-Ia-2 serum to block $F_1$ T cells from responding to DNP–GL and anti-Ia-13 serum to block them from responding to GT.

3.6). These Ia antigens are present on the surface of B cells and also on the surface of those adherent cells that take up and "present" antigen to lymphocytes.

Antisera defining their respective Ia antigens can also be raised by the reciprocal immunization of strain 2 and strain 13 guinea pigs. Anti-2 serum interferes with the response of $F_1$ T cells to DNP–GL on $F_1$ macrophages; anti-13 serum has no effect. Conversely, anti-13 serum interferes with the stimulation of $F_1$ T cells cultured with $F_1$ macrophages and GT, while having no effect on the response to DNP–GL.

The masking of the Ia antigen by antibodies (no complement was added, so no lysis occurred) prevents primed T cells from recognizing that antigen. So once again we find that T cells need to "see" something more than the conventional antigen alone (Figure 12.21).

## The Response to Some Antigens Requires Two Ir Genes

C57BL/10 mice (H-2$^b$) are unable to respond to the synthetic polymer made up of L-Glu, L-Lys, and L-Phe (GLPhe). The congenic strain B10.A, which carries the H-2$^a$ haplotype, is also a nonresponder. However, the $F_1$ hybrids produced by mating these two strains are fully responsive to GLPhe. Evidently the Ir gene defect in each can be overcome by a gene product of the other. This is because the response to GLPhe requires a responder allele at *both* I-A and I-E. The B10.A(5R) strain is a congenic recombinant strain derived from H-2$^b$ and H-2$^a$ parents and carrying a crossover within the H-2 region. It carries the alleles *(bbbb)* from the H-2$^b$ parent at the left end of its H-2 region and the alleles of the H-2$^a$

| Strain | K | I | | | | D | Responder to GLPhe |
| | | $A_\beta$ | $A_\alpha$ | $E_\beta$ | $E_\alpha$ | | |
|---|---|---|---|---|---|---|---|
| C57BL/10 (H-2$^b$) | b | b | b | b | ⓑ$^{(1)}$ | b | No |
| B10.A (H-2$^a$) | k | k | k | ⓚ | k | d | No |
| (C57BL/10 × B10.A)F$_1$ | b/k | b/k | b/k | b/k | b/k | b/d | Yes |
| B10.A(5R) | b | b | b | b | k | d | Yes |

$^{(1)}$ ○ = nonresponder allele.

**Figure 12.22** Gene complementation in the response to the synthetic polymer GLPhe (L-Glu, L-Lys, L-Phe).

parent *(kd)* at the right end (Figure 12.22). These animals respond to GLPhe. The reason for this appears to be that the response to GLPhe requires an Ia antigen constructed from a $\beta$ chain encoded in the I-A subregion and an $\alpha$ chain encoded by I-E (Figure 12.23). So the C57BL/10 (H-2$^b$) mouse is a nonresponder because it is unable to synthesize the appropriate $\alpha$ chain at I-E. The B10.A mouse is a nonresponder because it cannot synthesize the appropriate $\beta$ chain at I-A. A hybrid of the two (H-2$^{b/a}$) or a recombinant *(bbbbkd)* is able to produce both the correct $\alpha$ chain and the correct $\beta$ chain and thus can respond to the antigen. Just how the $\alpha$ and $\beta$ chains of the Ia antigens interact with a conventional antigen to facilitate or prevent antigen recognition by T cells is still unknown.

## 12.10 Immunoglobulin-Specific T$_H$ Cells

In addition to carrier-specific T$_H$ cells, immunization may elicit immunoglobulin-specific T$_H$ cells. These are T cells that give help to B cells committed to the synthesis of a particular kind of immunoglobulin molecule. For example, *feeding* antigen (SRBC) to mice induces in the Peyer's patches of the intestine a population of T$_H$ cells that preferentially helps B cells committed to producing anti-SRBC antibodies of the IgA class. These IgA-specific T$_H$ cells have surface receptors (Fc$_\alpha$R) for the constant region of IgA, which are demonstrated by the formation of rosettes with IgA-coated RBCs (Section 7.8). T$_H$ cells that preferentially help B

**Figure 12.23** Genetic control of the Ia antigen associated with the Ir gene loci controlling responsiveness to GLPhe (see Figure 12.22). The other two loci shown in the I-A subregion encode an $\alpha$ and $\beta$ chain that function in the immune response to other antigens.

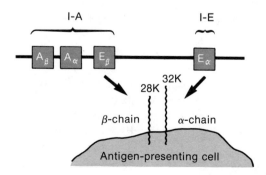

cells committed to the synthesis of IgE have also been discovered. They, too, bear Fc receptors, in this case for the constant region of IgE.

It makes good biological sense that the immune system be able to direct its response in favor of antibodies with particular effector properties. IgA is the dominant class of antibody in secretions and is structurally adapted to its role in protecting body surfaces (see Section 9.8). Thus it is appropriate that antigen in the intestine favors the production of IgA antibodies.

There is also evidence for allotype-specific and idiotype-specific $T_H$ cells. The biological significance and the mechanism of action of these types of immunoglobulin-specific $T_H$ cells are unknown. One possible mechanism of idiotype-specific T help is presented in Section 15.6 as part of an examination of the role of T cells in regulating immune responses.

## 12.11 Summary

The humoral immune response to most antigens depends on the interaction of three kinds of cells: B lymphocytes, T lymphocytes, and antigen-presenting cells (APCs). Resting ($G_0$) B lymphocytes can be activated by the antigenic determinant ("hapten") for which they bear the appropriate receptor if they receive help from a T helper cell specific for a second determinant ("carrier") on the same antigen. The $T_H$ cell is induced by interacting with an antigen-presenting cell (e.g., macrophage and/or dendritic cell) bearing a combination of the antigen and an Ia molecule for which the $T_H$ cell carries the appropriate receptor. The $T_H$ cell is able to give help to only those B cells that present it with the same carrier determinant and the same Ia molecule (MHC restriction). The $T_H$-B collaboration requires that the carrier determinant to which the $T_H$ cell responds and the haptenic determinant to which the B cell responds be present on the same molecule (linked recognition). The terms "carrier" and "hapten" are defined operationally: they refer simply to the determinants to which the T and B cells respond, respectively, without implying any particular structural features.

The continued interaction of $T_H$ cells with antigen-presenting cells causes the $T_H$ cells to release factors that can drive antigen-activated B cells first to proliferate (B cell growth factors—BCGFs) and then to differentiate into antibody-secreting plasma cells (B cell differentiation factors—BCDFs). BCGFs and BCDFs act nonspecifically, they stimulate proliferation and differentiation in activated B cells of any antigen specificity. There is also some evidence for *antigen-specific* $T_H$ factors; these have some of the properties to be expected of a secreted form of the T cell receptor for antigen.

Animals of a particular inbred strain may fail to respond to certain antigens. The immune response (Ir) genes responsible map to the same region of the major histocompatibility complex as the structural genes for Ia (class II) antigens. One explanation for this selective genetic unresponsiveness in a particular inbred strain is that the animal has no $T_H$ cells

In addition to antigen-specific $T_H$ cells, there is evidence for immunoglobulin-specific $T_H$ cells, which help only those B cells expressing a particular immunoglobulin isotype, or allotype, or idiotype.

## ADDITIONAL READING

1. Asano, Y., et al., "Role of the Major Histocompatibility Complex in T Cell Activation of B Cell Subpopulations. A Single Monoclonal T Helper Cell Population Activates Different B Cell Subpopulations by Distinct Pathways," *J. Exp. Med.* **156**:350, 1982. A single clone of KLH-specific $T_H$ cells is able to provide bystander help as well as help by linked recognition (Figure 12.11).

2. Azar, Y., et al., "In Vivo Activity of Affinity Purified Helper Factor from Antigen Specific Helper Clone," *J. Immunol.* **134**:1717, 1985. An OVA-specific $T_H$ clone secretes an OVA-specific helper factor that appears to be a soluble version of the $T_H$ surface antigen receptor.

3. Benacerraf, B., "Role of MHC Gene Products in Immune Regulation," *Science* **212**:1229, 1981. His Nobel Lecture, which provides a succinct review of Ir genes.

4. Claman, H. N., et al., "Thymus-Marrow Cell Combination. Synergism in Antibody Production," *Proc. Soc. Exp. Biol. & Med.* **122**:1167, 1966. (Reprinted in V. L. Sato and M. L. Gefter, *Cellular Immunology*, Addison-Wesley Publishing Co., Inc., Reading, MA, 1982.)

5. Ishii, N., et al., "Responder T Cells Depleted of Alloreactive Cells React to Antigen Presented on Allogeneic Macrophages from Nonresponder Strains," *J. Exp. Med.* **154**:978, 1981.

6. Kiyono, H., et al., "Isotype-Specificity of Helper T Cell Clones: $Fc\alpha$ Receptors Regulate T and B Cell Collaboration for IgA Responses," *J. Immunol.* **133**:1087, 1984.

7. Lanzavecchia, A., "Antigen-Specific Interaction Between T and B Cells," *Nature* **314**:537, 1985. Demonstrates that B cells bind antigen with their immunoglobulin receptor and then process the antigen intracellularly before presenting fragments of it to $T_H$ cells. The fragments ("carrier") are associated at the cell surface with Ia antigens but probably not with immunoglobulin.

8. Mitchell, G. F., and J. F. A. P. Miller, "Cell to Cell Interaction in the Immune Response: II. The Source of Hemolysin-Forming Cells in Irradiated Mice Given Bone Marrow and Thymus or Thoracic Duct Lymphocytes," *J. Exp. Med.* **128**:821, 1968. (Reprinted in V. L. Sato and M. L. Gefter, *Cellular Immunology*, Addison-Wesley Publishing Co., Inc., Reading, MA, 1982.)

9. Mitchison, N. A., "The Carrier Effect in the Secondary Response to Hapten-Protein Conjugates. II. Cellular Cooperation," *Eur. J. Immunol.* **1**:18, 1971. (Reprinted in V. L. Sato and M. L. Gefter, *Cellular Immunology*, Addison-Wesley Publishing Co., Inc., Reading, MA, 1982.)

10. Nakagawa, T., et al., "Effect of Recombinant IL 2 and $\gamma$-IFN on Proliferation

and Differentiation of Human B Cells," *J. Immunol.* **134**:959, 1985. IL-2 acts as a BCGF and γ-IFN as a BCDF.

11. Nepom, J. T., B. Benacerraf, and R. N. Germain, "Analysis of Ir Gene Function Using Monoclonal Antibodies. Independent Regulation of GAT and GLPhe T Cell Responses by I-A and I-E Subregion Products on a Single Accessory Cell Population," *J. Immunol.* **127**:31, 1981.

12. Raff, M. C., "Role of Thymus-Derived Lymphocytes in the Secondary Humoral Immune Response in Mice," *Nature,* **226**:1257, 1970. (Reprinted in V. L. Sato and M. L. Gefter, *Cellular Immunology,* Addison-Wesley Publishing Co., Inc., Reading, MA, 1982.)

13. Snow, E. C., et al., "Activation of Antigen-Enriched B Cells. II. Role of Linked Recognition in B Cell Proliferation to Thymus-Dependent Antigens," *J. Immunol.* **130**:614, 1983.

14. Zubler, R. H., et al., "Activated B Cells Express Receptors for, and Proliferate in Response to, Pure Interleukin 2," *J. Exp. Med.* **160**:1170, 1984. Recombinant human IL-2 acts as a BCGF for mouse B cells.

# CHAPTER 13

# Cellular Interactions in Cell Mediated Immunity

## 13.1 Introduction

It is likely that all cell-mediated immune responses involve the participation of two or more different kinds of cells. At least one kind is a T lymphocyte because all cell-mediated immune responses are strictly thymus dependent. Neither nude mice nor neonatally thymectomized animals can exhibit delayed-type hypersensitivity, allograft rejection, or mount an effective response to intracellular pathogens like viruses. In mixed lymphocyte culture, their cells fail to respond to foreign histocompatibility antigens, either by proliferation or by the induction of cytotoxic T ($T_C$) cells.

One of the hallmarks of CMI is that it can be adoptively transferred to unprimed animals by injecting them with antigen-sensitized lymphocytes. However, prior treatment of the cell suspensions with anti-Thy-1 serum and complement destroys their capacity to transfer such cell-mediated responses as DTH and the accelerated rejection of allografts. The ability of a lymphocyte suspension to produce a graft versus host reaction is also destroyed by anti-Thy-1 treatment. In vitro manifestations of CMI, such as the mixed lymphocyte reaction (MLR) and cell-mediated cytotoxicity (CMC), are also completely abrogated if either the responding or the effector cell population is treated with anti-Thy-1. Thus every type of cell-mediated immune response involves T cells.

In some cell-mediated responses, *two* kinds of T lymphocytes participate: one type of T cell serving as the effector cell and the other, a helper T cell ($T_H$) serving to amplify the magnitude of the response. Helper T cells are certainly involved in the development of cytotoxic T cells ($T_C$). There is also evidence of the participation of $T_H$ cells in delayed-type hypersensitivity and in graft versus host reactions. In addition to T–T interactions, the response of most T cells to antigen (reviewed in Chapter 11) depends on their interaction with antigen-presenting cells (APCs). Antigen presentation can be performed by $Ia^+$ macrophages, dendritic cells, and even $Ia^+$ B cells. A third form of cell interaction occurs between $T_C$ cells and their targets. Let us now examine the details and rules by which (1) T cells interact with antigen-presenting cells, (2) $T_H$ cells interact with effector T cells, and (3) $T_C$ cells interact with their targets.

## 13.2 Interactions Between T Cells and Antigen-Presenting Cells

The so-called "mixed lymphocyte" reaction is something of a misnomer. The proliferative response that normally occurs when histo*in*compatible spleen cells are cultured together (Section 6.5) fails to take place if the adherent cells of the spleen (such as macrophages) are first removed. This is shown in Figure 13.1. The stimulus provided by 50,000 allogeneic spleen cells (consisting of 6% macrophages, a small number of dendritic cells, and the rest T and B lymphocytes) gives a stimulation index (SI) of 1.9. When the same number of purified adherent cells from the same allogeneic donor are used, the SI rises to 18. On the other hand, 50,000 allogeneic cells depleted of adherent cells give an SI of 1; i.e., the uptake of tritiated thymidine is no greater with allogeneic T and B lymphocytes than when syngeneic lymphocytes are used.

The dependency of T cells on the antigen-presenting properties of some other cell type is seen with conventional antigens as well. An excellent example of this is presented in the first figure of Chapter 11. Here the ability of OVA-specific T cells to proliferate when cultured with OVA requires the presence of dendritic cells as well as antigen. In fact, if the

**341**

*Section 13.2*
*Interactions Be-*
*tween T Cells and*
*Antigen-Presenting*
*Cells*

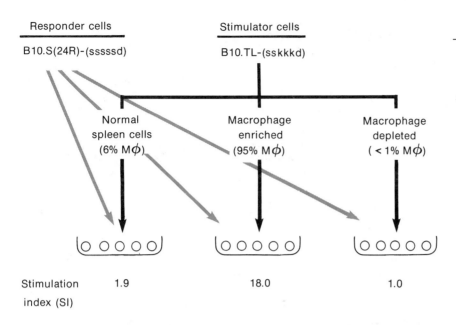

M $\phi$ = Macrophage

**Figure 13.1** Importance of adherent cells for a "mixed lymphocyte" response. Each culture contained $5 \times 10^4$ irradiated stimulator cells and $2.5 \times 10^5$ responder cells (normal lymph node cells from B10.S(24R) mice.) The B10.TL stimulator cells differ from the responding cells only at the loci between H-2K and H-2D. M$\phi$ = macrophages.

$$\text{Stimulation index (SI)} = \frac{\text{cpm in experimental (allogeneic) cultures}}{\text{cpm in control (syngeneic) cultures}}$$

[From M. Minami et al., *J. Immunol.* **124**:1314, 1980.]

dendritic cells are *precultured* (for 1 hour or so) with the antigen, washed, and then exposed to the T cells in the *absence* of soluble antigen, the T cell response is as strong as before. This suggests that the role of the dendritic cells is to "present" antigen to the T cells.

The presentation of antigen to T cells involves more than simply displaying antigen on the surface of the APC. Approximately 1 hour is needed after exposure to antigen for an APC to be able to perform its job. During this time, the antigen is taken into the cell and, in the case of protein antigens, some of it is degraded into peptides. Anything which interferes with these metabolic activities during this "processing" phase blocks APC function. Once done, however, the APCs can even be killed and still serve their function.

Antigen presentation involves the expression of the antigen (or its fragments) at the surface of the APC. These fragments are associated with MHC-encoded antigens providing the basis of the MHC restriction which is so characteristic of the response of T cells to antigen (Chapter 11). Only cells that express large amounts of class II antigens (dendritic cells, some macrophages and B cells) can serve as APCs.

## 13.3   Interactions Between $T_H$ Cells and Effector T Cells

T cells occur in several subsets that can be distinguished by a number of criteria. Among the most useful of these for mouse T cells are the Ly antigens on their surface (Section 7.7). Several correlations have been found between the profile of Ly antigens expressed by a T cell subset and the role played by that subset in immune responses. For example, the L3T4$^+$ helper cells in humoral immunity express high levels of the Ly-1 antigen (Section 12.3). Similar functional divisions occur in CMI. One striking example of this was discovered by Cantor and Boyse. They showed that a strong CMC reaction (Section 6.6) requires the synergistic cooperation of two distinct T cell subpopulations. One of these is strongly Ly-1$^+$, the other Ly-2$^+$.

Cantor and Boyse were able to prepare purified T cell subpopulations by treating lymphocyte suspensions with anti-Ly sera and complement. Thus, treating mouse spleen cells (they used BALB/c cells which have the H-2$^d$ haplotype) with anti-Ly-1 and complement produced a preparation containing mostly Ly-2$^+$ cells. Similarly, treatment with anti-Ly-2 serum produced a population composed mainly of Ly-1$^+$ cells. Each of these populations was placed in culture with irradiated allogeneic (H-2$^b$) cells and assayed five days later against $^{51}$Cr-labeled H-2$^b$ target cells. As Figure 13.2 shows, the Ly-2$^+$ population produced some cytotoxicity, while the Ly-1$^+$ population produced little or none. However, when the cultures were set up with a mixture containing the same numbers of Ly-1$^+$ and Ly-2$^+$ cells as had been used individually, a vigorous cytotoxic reaction followed (Figure 13.2). In demonstrating that the mixture of

**Figure 13.2**   A Ly-1 T cell provides help for the induction of Ly-2,3 cytotoxic T cells. The Ly-purified T cell subpopulations were prepared from BALB/c spleen cells (H-2$^d$) and were cultured in a one-way MLC with irradiated H-2$^b$ cells. Cytotoxicity was measured using H-2$^b$ target cells. [From H. Cantor and E. A. Boyse, *J. Exp. Med.* 141:1390, 1975.]

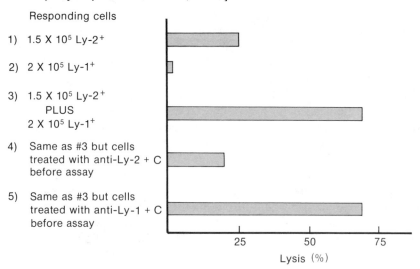

subpopulations responded far better than the sum of the individual responses, the need for T–T cooperation was established.

These experiments do not, however, show whether a division of labor occurs in the process; i.e., whether the different populations perform different functions in the CMC reaction. That this is true was demonstrated by using anti-Ly sera five days *after* the cells had been cultured with irradiated stimulator cells. In this case, anti-Ly-2 serum (plus complement) sharply reduces target cell lysis. Anti-Ly-1 serum does not interfere with cytotoxicity (Figure 13.2) This shows that the effector cells in CMC are Ly-2$^+$ cells. These are cytotoxic T lymphocytes (CTL) or $T_C$ cells.

The experiments of Cantor and Boyse clearly show that a population of Ly-1$^+$ T cells provides a powerful synergistic effect on the induction of $T_C$ cells although they do not themselves express cytotoxic activity. Therefore, we shall call these cells helper T cells or $T_H$ cells. You might argue that this nomenclature should be avoided because we have already used it for T cells that help in humoral immune responses. Some workers do prefer to use other terms for this cell. For example, these cells have been called T amplifier ($T_A$) cells. Nevertheless, we shall use the designation $T_H$ for two reasons. First, the designation $T_A$ for T amplifier cell is also used for cells that are clearly not the same as the population described here. Second, the $T_H$ cell in CMI resembles closely the $T_H$ cell in humoral immunity. As Cantor and Boyse themselves showed, the $T_H$ cells in both systems are Ly-1$^+$. But the analogy appears to be even closer than that, as we shall now see.

## $T_H$ Cells and $T_C$ Cells Respond to Different Antigenic Determinants

Evidence is presented in Section 12.3 that the $T_H$ cell in humoral immunity responds to a determinant ("carrier") on the antigen that is different from the determinant ("hapten") recognized by the B cell. A similar situation occurs in the CMC reaction.

The CMC assay begins as a mixed lymphocyte reaction (MLR). Cultured together, histoincompatible lymphocytes undergo a period of proliferation at the same time that $T_C$ cells are being generated (see Section 6.6). However, the antigenic stimuli for proliferation (as measured by the uptake of tritiated thymidine) and cell-mediated cytolysis (as measured by the release of $^{51}$Cr) are usually different. By coculturing spleen cells from recombinant strains of mice, it can be shown that the induction of $T_C$ cells depends upon genetic differences encoded by the K and/or D region of the H-2. Differences limited to other regions, such as I alone, yield very poor CMC responses. However, the best CMC responses occur when both K (and/or D) and I region differences exist (Figure 6.5).

On the other hand, the proliferative response in mixed lymphocyte culture is rather weakly stimulated by differences at K or D. Although such differences cause some proliferation, the most vigorous proliferative responses occur when the two cell types differ at I (Figure 6.5).

The same pattern is seen with conventional antigens. $T_H$ cells respond to conventional antigen in association with a class II MHC antigen, while $T_C$ cells respond to the antigen in association with a class I MHC antigen. An example of virus/class-I specificity in $T_C$ cells is given in Chapter 11. In that case, $T_C$ cells induced in a virus-infected H-2$^k$ mouse can lyse only virus-infected target cells that express the same H-2K$^k$ and/or H-2D$^k$ antigens (Figure 11.5). Killing by these class-I-restricted $T_C$ cells can be blocked by adding anti-H-2K/D antibodies to the CMC culture.

$T_H$ cells, on the other hand, respond to conventional antigen seen in association with class II MHC antigens. An example of this is shown in Figure 13.3. A population of $T_C$ cells specific for TNP-self can be generated in vitro over a period of five days. At the end of this time, the $T_C$ cells will kill TNP-modified syngeneic spleen cells. However, if antibodies against the I-A encoded antigens of these mice (I-A$^k$) are present throughout the culture period, there is no development of $T_C$ cells. Such anti-I-A antibodies have no effect on the killing ability of $T_C$ cells once they are formed. Rather the antibodies prevent the development of $T_C$ cells through their effect on the $T_H$ cell population.

How do $T_H$ cells help the $T_C$ cell precursors ($T_C$-P) to become mature $T_C$ cells? Evidently the antigen-stimulated $T_H$ cells provide the necessary help through the release of soluble mediators — certainly IL-2 and probably one or more others. Figure 13.3 shows that the presence of these factors (harvested from T cells stimulated with Con A) almost entirely overcomes the inhibitory effect of anti-I-A$^k$ antibodies during the culture period. The cellular interactions and different specificities leading to the formation of $T_C$ cells are summarized in Figure 13.4.

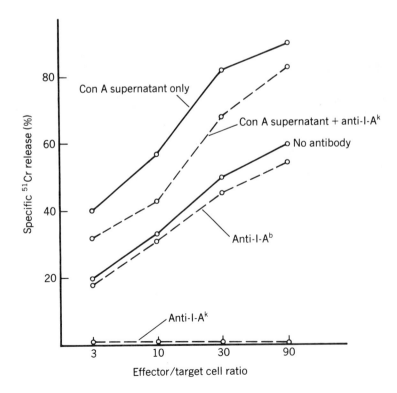

**Figure 13.3** Anti-I-A antibodies block the *induction* of $T_C$ cells. Although $T_C$ cells are restricted by class I MHC antigens (K/D), their *formation* requires $T_H$ cells that are restricted by class II antigens (Figure 13.4). In this case, all the cells were from B10.A(4R) mice *(kkkkbb)*. Anti-I-A$^k$ antibodies blocked the response; anti-I-A$^b$ antibodies did not. The inhibition by anti-I-A$^k$ could be overcome by helper factors (e.g., IL-2) present in the supernatant of cultures stimulated with Con A. [From Ada M. Kruisbeek et al., *J. Immunol.* 131:1650, 1983.]

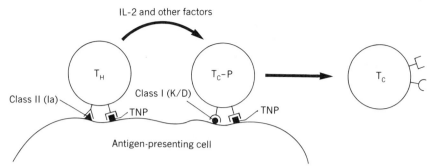

**Figure 13.4** Model of the induction of $T_C$ cells. Precursors of $T_C$ cells ($T_C$-P) specific for TNP associated with a class I antigen are helped by $T_H$ cells specific for TNP associated with a class II antigen. The help is mediated by IL-2 and probably one or more other lymphokines. Because most of the cells of the body express class I antigens, almost any TNP-conjugated cell can serve as an APC for the $T_C$-P. However, only Ia$^+$ cells, like dendritic cells, can serve as APCs for $T_H$ cells.

## Ly-1$^+$ and Ly-2$^+$ T Cells Respond to Different Antigenic Determinants

The immunization protocols that we have examined lead to the formation of $T_H$ cells directed against class II MHC antigens and $T_C$ cells directed against class I antigens. However, this turns out not to be an inviolable rule. With suitable manipulations, several workers have reported the generation of $T_H$ cells that respond to class I antigens (e.g., H-2D) and $T_C$ cells that kill class II-bearing (Ia$^+$) targets. In the first case, however, the cells ($T_H$) are now Ly-2$^+$ while in the second case, the cells ($T_C$) are Ly-1$^+$. Thus the common association between Ly phenotype and T cell function breaks down in these cases. Perhaps, then, the real association is not between Ly phenotype and function but between Ly phenotype and the nature of the MHC-restricting antigen: a class I molecule for Ly-2$^+$ cells; a class II molecule for Ly-1$^+$ cells.

We should also recall that *all* mature T cells express *some* Ly-1 on their surface. However, Ly-2$^+$ cells do not express enough Ly-1 to be killed by treatment with anti-Ly-1 and complement. Ly-2$^-$ cells, on the other hand, are richly coated with Ly-1 and are easily killed by anti-Ly-1 treatment. So as a practical matter, these treatments can be used to prepare nonoverlapping functional subsets of T cells, e.g., $T_H$ and $T_C$. But recent evidence (reviewed in Section 7.7) indicates that while Ly-2 uniquely defines a subset that includes $T_C$ cells, the $T_H$ cell subset in mice is defined not by Ly-1 but by the L3T4 antigen.

All the examples of T–T cooperation given in this section involve interactions between $T_H$ and $T_C$-P cells. However, other kinds of effector T cells also benefit from the help given by $T_H$ cells. The magnitude of both the **DTH** response and the **graft vs. host** response appears to be enhanced by $T_H$ cells. Once again, the nature of the help is probably the liberation of IL-2 (and perhaps other lymphokines) by $T_H$ cells responding to, in these examples, the same antigen as the effector cells. (Both the $T_D$ cell and the $T_{GVH}$ cell are Ly-1$^+$ cells and like the $T_H$ cell respond to class II antigens — either alone (e.g., $T_{GVH}$) or in association with conventional antigen (e.g., $T_{DTH}$).

There is still another subset of T cells, which are called T suppressor cells ($T_S$) because they exert suppressive effects on the immune system. $T_S$ cells are Ly-2$^+$. Their induction is also aided by the presence of Ly-1$^+$ T cells. The details of these T–T cell interactions are examined in Chapter 15.

## 13.4 Interactions Between $T_C$ Cells and Their Targets

The killing ability of most $T_C$ cells is dependent upon their recognition of a class I MHC antigen (in the mouse, H-2K or H-2D; sometimes H-2L) either alone (in allogeneic responses) or in association with a conventional antigen. As we have seen (Figure 11.5), the $T_C$ cells induced in a virus-infected mouse of a particular H-2 haplotype can lyse only virus-infected target cells that express *either* the same H-2K *or* the same H-2D antigens. That identity at either K or D is sufficient for effective cell-mediated cytotoxicity stems from the fact that virus infection leads to the induction of *two* separate populations of $T_C$ cells: one that recognizes

**Figure 13.5** Clonal restriction of $T_C$ cells to virus-infected cells carrying either the H-2K or the H-2D antigens of the immune donor. The haplotype of C3H.OH is H-2K$^d$ and H-2D$^k$. If every $T_C$ cell were capable of recognizing both V.K$^d$ and V.D$^k$, then unlabeled BALB/c cells (V.K$^d$) should have inhibited the attack against C3H targets (V.D$^k$) as well as C3H cells did. (V = viral portion of compound antigenic determinant.) [Based on R. M. Zinkernagel and P. C. Doherty, *J. Exp. Med.* 141:1427, 1975. Reprinted in V. L. Sato and M. L. Gefter, *Cellular Immunology*, Addison-Wesley Publishing Co., Inc., Reading, MA, 1982.]

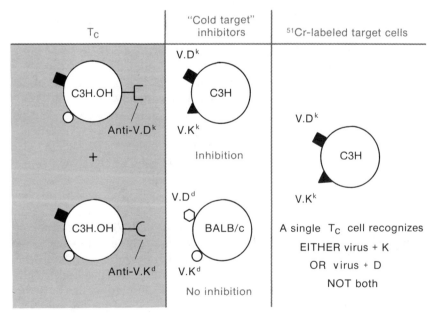

viral antigens in association with H-2K and a second that recognizes viral antigens in association with H-2D. This phenomenon has been demonstrated in several ways, one of which—"cold target inhibition"—is shown in Figure 13.5. The principle of this assay is that the mixing of unlabeled targets with $^{51}$Cr-labeled targets will inhibit chromium release as the unlabeled targets compete (as it were) for the lethal attentions of the T$_C$ cells. T$_C$ cells from virus-infected C3H.OH mice should, and do, lyse virus-infected C3H targets because they both express H-2D$^k$. The presence of virus infected but *unlabeled* C3H cells should, and does, reduce the amount of $^{51}$Cr released (Figure 13.5). However, if the same T$_C$ cell that recognizes virus in association with H-2D$^k$ also recognizes

**Figure 13.6** Clonal restriction of hybrid T$_C$ cells to hapten-modified cells of one or the other parental haplotype but not both. The suicide of the T$_C$ cells specific for TNP-H-2$^d$ leaves a population capable of responding to TNP-H-2$^k$. [Based on C. A. Janeway, Jr., et al., *J. Exp. Med.* **147**:1065, 1978.]

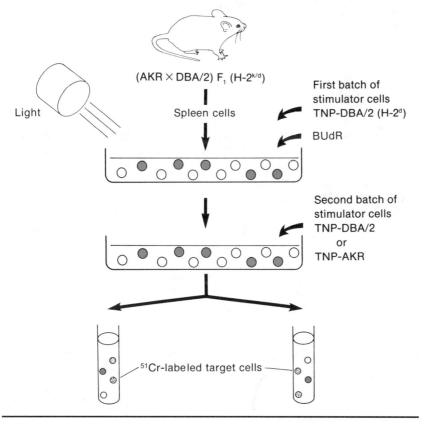

|  |  | Specific $^{51}$Cr release from target cells (%) | |
|---|---|---|---|
| First stimulators (suicide) | Second stimulators | TNP–BALB/c (H-2$^d$) | TNP–AKR (H-2$^k$) |
| TNP–DBA/2 | TNP–DBA/2 (H-2$^d$) | 3.7 | 2.6 |
| TNP–DBA/2 | TNP–AKR (H-2$^k$) | 0.8 | **16.0** |

virus in association with H-2K$^d$, then its activity should also be blocked by virus-infected cells carrying H-2K$^d$ (e.g., virus-infected BALB/c cells). But inhibition does not occur, leading us to conclude that the T$_C$ cell that recognizes the virus-H-2D combination is not the same cell that recognizes virus in association with H-2K.

The cold target inhibition technique (as well as others — see Figure 13.6) also reveals that hybrid animals — i.e., animals that inherit a different H-2 haplotype from each parent — recognize conventional antigens in association with one or the other set of parental H-2 antigens. As the antigen-suicide experiment in Figure 13.6 shows, an (AKR × DBA/2) hybrid (H-2$^{k/d}$) produces separate populations of T$_C$ cells which recognize and lyse TNP-conjugated H-2$^k$ and H-2$^d$ targets, respectively. Thus a hybrid animal develops a total of four separate populations of T$_C$ cells in response to a conventional antigen presented on the surface of its cells. As most mice (outside of laboratories) and most humans are heterozygous at the MHC, this means that the normal response to virus infections, for example, yields a diverse population of cytotoxic cells to deal with the infection.

## 13.5　How Does MHC Restriction Arise?

One of the most remarkable features of cell-mediated immune responses is that T cells respond to conventional antigens only when they are associated with the appropriate MHC-encoded antigens. This is the phenomenon of MHC restriction. Examples of the phenomenon are given in Sections 3.7, 11.3, 11.4, and 12.4, as well as in this chapter. The appropriate MHC antigen is either a class I antigen (for Ly-2$^+$ cells in mice; CD8$^+$ cells in humans) or a class II antigen (for L3T4$^+$ cells in mice; CD4$^+$ cells in humans). In the normal situation, the appropriate class I or class II antigen is, of course, self, i.e., the animal's own MHC-encoded antigens.

Two distinct theories have been proposed to explain how T cells become restricted to seeing conventional antigen in association with self-MHC molecules. One is that MHC restriction occurs during the normal development of the immune system prior to and independent of exposure to antigen. This is the *ontogeny* hypothesis. The second is that MHC restriction occurs at the time of the T cell's exposure to antigen. This is the *priming* hypothesis.

*The Ontogeny Hypothesis.*　This hypothesis supposes that the selection of T cell clones occurs in two distinct steps. First, a step during the early development of the animal when only those T cells with receptors capable of binding self-MHC antigens are selected for clonal expansion. Second, a step occurring at the time of antigen exposure when those T cells that are *also* specific for that antigen are selected for further clonal expansion. This two-step process fits well with the dual-receptor hypothesis: one receptor for self-MHC and a second for the conventional antigen.

What is considered self by the T cells of an animal could be an innate property of the T cells; in other words established by their own genotype. Alternatively, what is self could be *learned* by the T cells as they mature in an environment (e.g., the thymus) where they are surrounded by cells expressing a particular set of MHC antigens. In either case, however, T cells with high affinity receptors for self would have to be excluded from clonal expansion because of the threat they would pose of an autoimmune attack.

*The Priming Hypothesis.*  This hypothesis supposes that a particular T cell is selected for clonal expansion at the moment it encounters a combination of conventional antigen (Ag) and MHC-encoded antigen for which it bears the receptor or receptors needed to bind that particular Ag/MHC combination. It encounters the Ag/MHC combination on the surface of an antigen-presenting cell. The priming hypothesis can accomodate either a single receptor for Ag/MHC or separate receptors for Ag and MHC.

Whether clonal selection occurs in two steps (ontogeny) or in one (priming), the selected clones can generate a secondary response only if they encounter the same Ag + MHC combination at a later time. You may have noted that all our examples given of MHC restriction have involved secondary responses. What about the primary response? The ontogeny hypothesis leads to the prediction that an animal *cannot* be primed to a combination of conventional antigen and *foreign* MHC antigen. A response will be seen, to be sure, but it will be a response to the allogeneic MHC antigen alone. The priming hypothesis does not have this limitation. According to the priming model, it is theoretically possible to have the response to a conventional antigen restricted by a foreign MHC antigen. In contrast to the first model, the T cell repertoire should include cells capable of responding to a compound antigenic determinant containing the conventional antigen in association with a foreign MHC antigen. But to test this, we need to find a way to circumvent the normal vigorous response of T cells to foreign MHC antigens alone. Several approaches have been taken.

## 13.6  Testing Models of MHC Restriction

A number of circumstances—both natural and experimental—avoid the normal vigorous responses to tissue incompatibility. The long term, intimate coexistence of histo*in*compatible cells is called *tolerance*. Mechanisms that possibly maintain tolerance are explored in Chapter 16. Here we shall simply examine certain techniques by which it can be established—techniques that permit the testing of predictions generated by the different hypotheses to explain MHC restriction.

Lethal irradiation (about 900 rads for a mouse) has its most devastating effects on tissues containing rapidly dividing cells. Destruction of the bone marrow destroys the cells of the blood including the cells of the immune system. However, a lethally irradiated mouse can be saved by an injection of bone marrow. The stem cells in the injected marrow suspension take up residence in the marrow of the new host and gradually repopulate it. In due course, immune competence is restored. If care is taken that no mature T cells are present in the reconstituting marrow suspension (by treating it with anti-Thy-1 and complement), histoincompatible cells can successfully reconstitute the recipient without a graft vs. host reaction. Fully restored, the host is now a *chimera,* possessing lymphoid and other blood cells of one genotype in a body constructed of cells of a different genotype. It can be shown that in due course virtually all the lymphocytes in these *radiation chimeras* are derived from the donor of the bone marrow. Nevertheless, these cells live in apparent harmony in their allogeneic environment, a situation of true tolerance.

In the mid-1970s, Zinkernagel and his colleagues performed a number of experiments on radiation chimeras with the goal of deciphering the mechanism of MHC restriction. One of the first of these is shown in Figure 13.7. A suspension of bone marrow cells (from which T cells had

**Figure 13.7** Cytotoxic T lymphocytes of the A haplotype can lyse virus-infected cells of either their own haplotype (A) or of the second (B) haplotype they encountered in their hybrid host. These cells are not effective against virus-infected cells of third-party haplotypes. The low amount of lysis of uninfected B targets shows that the $T_C$ cells (A) are tolerant of B histocompatibility antigens. [Based on R. M. Zinkernagel, *Nature* **261**:139, 1976.]

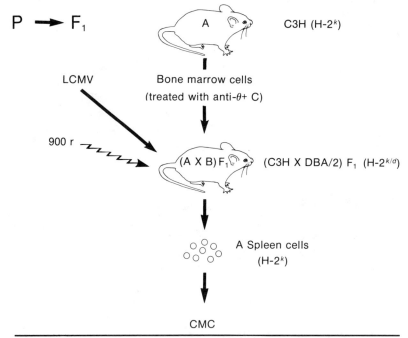

| $^{51}$Cr release from target cells (%) | | | |
|---|---|---|---|
| LCMV-infected A | Uninfected A | LCMV-infected B | Uninfected B |
| 67 | 24 | 98 | 41 |

been removed) taken from a C3H (H-2$^k$) mouse was used to restore an irradiated (C3H × DBA/2) hybrid (H-2$^{k/d}$). This type of reconstitution is described as parental to hybrid (P → F$_1$) or A → (A × B). When reconstitution was complete, the animal was injected with lymphocytic choriomeningitis virus (LCMV). Seven days later, the activity of its spleen cells was tested in CMC assays against several types of $^{51}$Cr-labeled targets. As expected, the spleen cells, which were exclusively of parental origin (A), lysed infected syngeneic (A) target cells ("self"). They also lysed infected DBA/2 (B) cells, but infected cells of third-party haplotypes (e.g., H-2$^b$) were not lysed efficiently. That the lysis of infected B targets was not simply the result of the histocompatibility difference was shown by the lower amount of lysis of *uninfected* B targets. Thus in a situation of tolerance to foreign MHC antigens *per se*, these cells showed MHC restriction—allo as well as self—in their response to viral antigens. This result indicates that recognition of "self" cannot be simply the expression of the genotype of the T$_C$ cell, for the H-2$^k$ T$_C$ cells lysed virus infected H-2$^d$ targets. However, the possibility remains that during their differentiation within the F$_1$ host, the T cell precursors in some way "learn" that all the histocompatibility antigens of the host represent "self." Such a possibility has been given the name "adaptive differentiation."

To test this hypothesis, Zinkernagel and his colleagues established

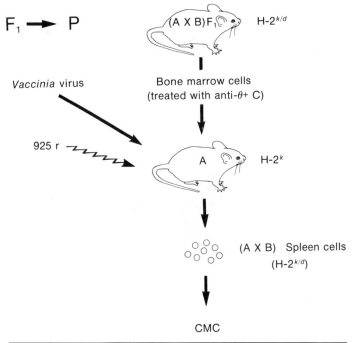

**Figure 13.8** Hybrid cytotoxic T cells (H-2$^{k/d}$) lyse infected targets carrying the MHC-encoded antigens of their host (H-2$^k$) only. [Based on R. M. Zinkernagel et al., *Nature* 271:251, 1978.]

| | $^{51}$Cr release from target cells (%) | | |
|---|---|---|---|
| Virus-infected A | Uninfected A | Virus-infected B | Uninfected B |
| 81 | 0 | 5 | 2 |

radiation chimeras consisting of parental-type hosts (A) reconstituted with hybrid bone marrow (A × B). This reconstitution is thus $F_1 \rightarrow P$ or (A × B) $\rightarrow$ A. Six days after immunizing these animals with vaccinia virus, their spleen cells were assayed against a variety of targets. No lysis occurred with either uninfected A or uninfected B targets because the spleen cells—being $F_1$—were intrinsically tolerant of both parental haplotypes. These spleen cells did lyse infected A targets (and infected hybrid targets) but were ineffective against infected B targets (Figure 13.8). Although the $T_C$ cells carried the H-2 antigens of B on their surface, they did not recognize these same antigens as self when they were expressed on infected targets. The result is certainly compatible with the notion that what T cells regard as self is determined by the genotype of the host in which they mature.

## Thymic Education

The same group of researchers went on to show that the genotype of the host thymus determines which histocompatibility antigens T cells will learn to regard as self. They thymectomized as well as lethally irradiated $F_1$ (A × B) mice and reconstituted these with $F_1$ bone marrow. They also implanted thymuses removed from parental-type (B) mice. The thymuses were irradiated before implantation to destroy the resident lymphocytes while leaving the nondividing epithelial cells intact. Later, the spleen cells from these reconstituted mice were able to lyse only virus-infected cells carrying the B haplotype (Figure 13.9).

Not only does this experiment reveal another crucial function of the thymus in the differentiation of T cells, but it also is difficult to reconcile with a theory of "altered self." If $T_C$ cells are selected at the time of antigen presentation, then $T_C$ cells active against virus-infected A should have been induced as well as cells active against virus-infected B. This is true whether the antigen-presenting cells are derived from the reconstituting bone marrow cells or whether they are derived from cells of the host because (in contrast to the earlier experiments) both of these carry the MHC antigens of the A type. Here, then, is evidence that seriously weakens the concept that T cells acquire their MHC restriction at the time of antigen presentation (priming). The evidence strengthens the concept that $T_C$ cells must interact with a separate MHC-encoded antigen that is determined by the MHC of the epithelial cells of the thymus in which they mature.

Before abandoning the idea that T cells are primed by a single compound antigenic determinant, let us examine some other experimental procedures designed to shed light on this question and which produced contrasting results.

## Removing Alloreactivity By Negative Selection

Populations of $T_C$ cells can be induced in vitro as well as in vivo. If T cells of one haplotype are cultured with irradiated, TNP-conjugated cells of

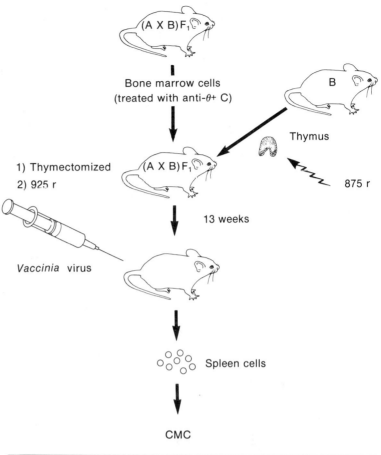

**Figure 13.9** The genotype of the thymus determines which MHC antigens T cells (which mature in the thymus) will recognize as "self." (Target cells incubated with medium alone gave 33% chromium release.) Irradiation of the thymus destroys its thymocytes and prevents it from eliciting a graft versus host reaction in the F₁ recipient. [Based on R. M. Zinkernagel et al., *J. Exp. Med.* **147**:882, 1978. Reprinted in V. L. Sato and M. L. Gefter, *Cellular Immunology*, Addison-Wesley Publishing Co., Inc., Reading MA, 1982.]

| | ⁵¹Cr release from target cells (%) | |
| Virus-infected A | Virus-infected B | Controls |
| --- | --- | --- |
| 36 | 100 | 33 |

the same haplotype (TNP–self), a population of TNP-specific $T_C$ cells arises. When the lytic activity of these cells is tested, it turns out to be restricted by the self-MHC. Just as Zinkernagel found with viral antigens, the $T_C$ cells lyse only TNP-coated targets bearing the same (self) haplotype. Thus cultures of parental-type (A) cells stimulated by TNP-conjugated self (TNP-A) develop $T_C$ cells effective against TNP-A targets but not normal A targets (self-tolerance) nor TNP-conjugated targets carrying foreign MHC antigens. However, when A cells are stimulated with TNP-B, they develop $T_C$ cells that lyse TNP-B targets and also unconjugated B targets as well (Figure 13.10). Here, then, is an illustration of the central dilemma we have been facing: the attack against TNP-B targets is simply the result of an allogeneic attack against B.

To circumvent this problem, Wilson and his colleagues used a "negative selection" technique to remove particular sets of alloreactive T cells from suspensions of lymph node cells. To do this, they exploited the property of that 0.5–10% of T cells which respond to a particular foreign

**353**

H-2 haplotype (see Section 11.9) to adhere to tissues expressing that haplotype. Thus when *mature* T cells from an animal of one parental haplotype (A) are injected into an irradiated $F_1$ (A × B) recipient, those T cells reactive against B are removed from the circulation. When the lymph is later collected from the thoracic duct of these animals, the lymphocytes it contains (almost exclusively T cells of the donor haplotype) are unreactive against B. Placed in mixed lymphocyte culture,

**Figure 13.10**  When strain A T cells from which all alloreactivity against strain B histocompatibility antigens has been removed (as tested in MLC) are stimulated with TNP-conjugated strain B cells (TNP-B), they recognize (by lysis) TNP-B but neither TNP-A nor B alone. These results are more easily explained by a single-receptor model of associate recognition than by a two-receptor model. [Based on D. B. Wilson et al., *J. Exp. Med.* **146**:361, 1977.

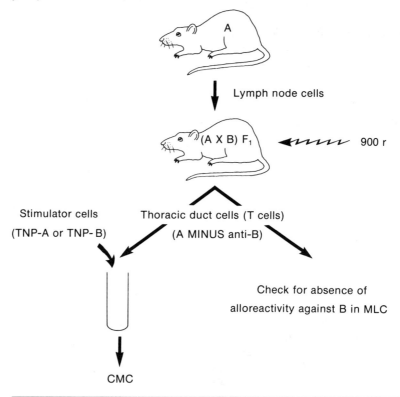

| Respond-ing cells | Stimu-lator cells | $^{51}Cr$ release from target cells (%) | | | | |
|---|---|---|---|---|---|---|
| | | A | TNP–A | TNP–B | B | |
| A | TNP–A | 0 | 33 | 3 | 3 | Restricted by A |
| A | TNP–B | 0 | 2 | 27 | 42 | Alloreactivity |
| A MINUS anti-B | TNP–A | 0 | 51 | 0 | 0 | Restricted by A |
| A MINUS anti-B | TNP–B | 0 | 2 | 21 | 0 | Antigen-specific response restricted by B |

these negatively selected A cells ("A minus anti-B") are not stimulated by cells of the B haplotype although they respond normally to stimulation by cells of other foreign haplotypes. When stimulated by TNP-conjugated parental (A) cells (TNP-A), they respond just as before; i.e., the response is restricted by A. However, when stimulated by TNP-B, they lyse TNP-conjugated B targets but still they cannot lyse unconjugated B targets (Figure 13.10). Thus, this response, too, is restricted by the MHC of the targets, but in this case it is a foreign MHC. This directly demonstrates that MHC restriction need not be confined to self. And note that no opportunity exists here for adaptive differentiation to occur. These $T_C$ cells are derived from a T cell population that differentiated totally within a normal A animal. Thus these results are difficult to reconcile with the ontogeny theory which stipulates that MHC restriction (in this

Figure 13.11 Although $F_1$ T cells preferentially lyse infected targets of the haplotype of the thymus in which they matured (thymic bias), they may show substantial activity as well against infected cells of the parental haplotype not present in the thymus. [Based on J. P. Lake *J. Exp. Med.* **152**:1805, 1980.]

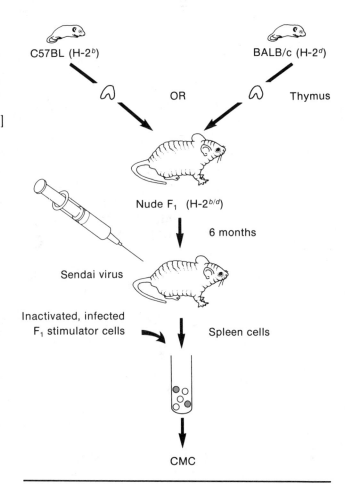

| Thymus donor | ⁵¹Cr release from target cells (%) | | | |
|---|---|---|---|---|
| | C57BL | Infected C57BL | BALB/c | Infected BALB/c |
| C57BL | 1 | 66 | 0 | 61 |
| BALB/c | 9 | 38 | 20 | 88 |

case, to B) is imposed during a T cell's transit through the thymus (which in this case is A).

Experiments performed by Zinkernagel and others with nude mice have cast further doubt on an absolute role for the thymus in establishing MHC restriction. These experiments took advantage of the fact that nude mice have no thymus. For example, Lake and his coworkers used nude mice that were hybrids of BALB/c and C57BL mice. These nude $F_1$ hybrids were implanted with a thymus taken from a neonatal, parental-type animal i.e., either BALB/c or C57BL. Six months later, the animals were infected with Sendai virus. Shortly thereafter, their spleen cells were harvested, restimulated with irradiated virus-infected $F_1$ cells, and assayed for CMC against virus-infected targets (Figure 13.11). Although the $T_C$ cells were $F_1$ and although the antigen-presenting cells were $F_1$ as well, the cells preferentially lysed infected targets of the haplotype of the implanted thymus. Nonetheless, substantial activity toward infected targets of the other (nonthymus) parental type was also seen. In this case, then, the role of the thymus in establishing MHC restriction appears to be partial, not absolute. This "bias" but not absolute restriction toward the haplotype of the host thymus has been observed in a number of other laboratories.

Even if the selection of MHC-restricted T cell clones takes place at the time of antigen priming, the pool of available precursors appears to be weighted in favor of T cells capable of recognizing self-MHC as the restricting element. If, as seems likely (Section 11.5), the recognition of Ag/MHC is mediated by a single receptor, we are left with the task of understanding how those T cells specific for Ag/thymic-MHC are favored over those specific for Ag/*non*thymic-MHC when the antigen-presenting cells have both types of MHC antigens on their surface (Figure 13.11). There is little likelihood that antigen presentation occurs within the thymus itself. Probably thymic bias is established before actual exposure to antigen occurs.

## 13.7 Biological Significance of MHC Restriction

Why do T cells not simply recognize antigen alone (as most antibodies do) rather than require that the antigen be associated with a histocompatibility antigen? For virus infections, a plausible case can be made for the utility of MHC restriction. It has been shown that $T_C$ cells can effectively limit the spread of virus infection by destroying infected cells before they can release progeny virus. For example, Lin and Askonas have demonstrated that an intravenous injection of $T_C$ cells specific for influenza A virus reduces virus replication in the lungs of mice and enables the mice to survive an otherwise lethal infection. As you would predict, the effect is restricted by the K and D regions of H-2; i.e., the adoptive transfer of virus-specific $T_C$ cells protects only mice that share K or D with the cell donor. If T cells bound free virus particles as antibodies do, their receptors could become occupied by these and no longer be available to "see" viral antigens on the surface of infected cells. The requirement for MHC restriction avoids this danger. Note, too, that the K/D

**357**

*Section 13.8*
*Summary*
restriction of $T_C$ cells makes good sense because almost all the cells of the body express class I antigens and so infected cells of any kind could be destroyed by $T_C$ cells.

What about class-II-restricted T cells? Class II antigens are only displayed by certain subsets of cells of the immune system such as dendritic cells, and some macrophages and B cells. In this case, then, the association of a conventional antigen with a class II MHC antigen assures that, for example, antigen-specific $T_H$ cells will interact with those cells — and only those cells — with which they can make a productive, functional association. Among these would be antigen-presenting cells to stimulate them (e.g., with antigen and IL-1) and antigen-specific B cells to which they can render help. It has also been suggested that the absence of class II antigens from most of the cells of the body keeps these cells from providing an immunogenic stimulus for $T_H$ cells and thus avoids triggering an autoimmune response to self cell-surface antigens.

## 13.8 Summary

Cell-mediated immune responses depend on the interaction of two or more kinds of cells. At least one of these is always a T lymphocyte. Murine $L3T4^+$ and human $CD4^+$ T lymphocytes can only be activated by antigen on the surface of an antigen-presenting cell (APC) such as a macrophage or dendritic cell. A secondary response by a clone of T cells to its priming antigen requires that the cells once again encounter the antigen associated with the same Ia (class II) antigen as before (MHC restriction).

The clonal development of at least some kinds of effector T cells ($T_C$, $T_D$, $T_{GVH}$, $T_S$) benefits from help provided by $T_H$ cells. In mice, most $T_H$ cells are $L3T4^+$; in humans they are $CD4^+$. These cells respond to conventional antigens in association with Ia (class II) histocompatibility antigens. As a result of this interaction, $T_H$ cells liberate lymphokines, such as IL-2, which stimulate the proliferation and differentiation of effector T cells (e.g., $T_C$). The requirement that $T_H$ cells respond to antigens in association with class II antigens ensures that they will respond only when they are associated with other cells of the immune system (e.g., APCs) with which they can establish a productive interaction.

Cytotoxic T cells ($T_C$) kill target cells expressing a conventional antigen on their surface associated with a class I histocompatibility antigen. Because class I antigens are found on most of the cells of the body, this form of MHC restriction ensures that $T_C$ cells will be able to kill targets of any cell type.

It is not yet known precisely how the MHC restriction of T cells arises. Perhaps it occurs in two steps: expansion of T cell clones capable of recognizing "self" MHC antigens followed later by selection of the subsets of these clones able to respond to a particular conventional antigen ("ontogeny hypothesis"). Alternatively, MHC restriction might arise at the moment of encountering conventional antigen, when a T cell bearing the appropriate receptor for a particular combination of conventional antigen and MHC antigen (Ag/MHC) is selected for clonal expansion.

## ADDITIONAL READING

1. Cantor, H., and R. Asofsky, "Synergy Among Lymphoid Cells Mediating the Graft-Versus-Host Response. III. Evidence for Interaction Between Two Types of Thymus-Derived Cells," *J. Exp. Med.* **135**:764, 1972.

2. Cantor, H., and E. A. Boyse, "Functional Subclasses of T Lymphocytes Bearing Different Ly Antigens. I. The Generation of Functionally Distinct T-Cell Subclasses Is a Differentiative Process Independent of Antigen," *J. Exp. Med.* **141**:1376, 1975. (Reprinted in V. L. Sato and M. L. Gefter, *Cellular Immunology*, Addison-Wesley Publishing Co., Inc., Reading, MA, 1982.)

3. Glasebrook, A. L., and F. W. Fitch, "Alloreactive Cloned T Cell Lines. I. Interactions Between Cloned Amplifier and Cytolytic T Cell Lines," *J. Exp. Med.* **151**:876, 1980. $T_H$ clones that help $T_C$ clones.

4. Lin, Y. -L, and Brigitte A. Askonas, "Biological Properties of an Influenza A Virus-Specific Killer T Cell Clone. Inhibition of Virus Replication in Vivo and Induction of Delayed-Type Hypersensitivity Reactions," *J. Exp. Med.* **154**:225, 1981.

5. Rosenthal, A. S., and E. M. Shevach, "Function of Macrophages in Antigen Recognition by Guinea Pig T Lymphocytes. I. Requirement for Histocompatible Macrophages and Lymphocytes," *J. Exp. Med.* **138**:1194, 1973. (Reprinted in V. L. Sato and M. L. Gefter, *Cellular Immunology*, Addison-Wesley Publishing Co., Inc., Reading, MA, 1982.) As assayed by the proliferative response to PPD.

6. Swain, Susan L., "Significance of Lyt Phenotypes: Lyt2 Antibodies Block Activities of T Cells That Recognize Class I Major Histocompatibility Complex Antigens Regardless of Their Function," *Proc. Natl. Acad. Sci. USA* **78**:7101, 1981.

7. Takai, Y., et al., "T-T Cell Interaction in the Induction of Delayed-Type Hypersensitivity (DTH) Responses: Vaccinia Virus-Reactive Helper T Cell Activity Involved in Enhanced in Vitro Induction of DTH Responses and Its Application to Augmentation of Tumor-Specific DTH Responses," *J. Immunol.* **134**:108, 1985.

8. Zinkernagel, R. M., et al., "The Lymphoreticular System in Triggering Virus plus Self-Specific Cytotoxic T Cells: Evidence for T Help," *J. Exp. Med.* **147**:897, 1978. Includes evidence that these $T_H$ cells are restricted by the H-2I region.

# The Effectors of Immunity

## 14.1  Introduction

Immune responses may be mediated by antibodies (humoral immunity) and/or by cells (cell-mediated immunity). In fact, many of the effector functions of antibodies are brought about by cells, such as macrophages

359

and neutrophils. What really distinguishes the effector functions of humoral and cell-mediated immunity is not whether cells are involved or not but what provides the specificity of the response. In humoral immune responses, the specificity is provided by antibody molecules; in cell-mediated responses, the specificity resides in cells — specifically T lymphocytes.

In a few situations, the simple binding of antibodies to antigen accomplishes the response. For example, viruses may be prevented from binding to susceptible target cells by antibodies binding to the virus. Similarly, toxins such as diphtheria toxin can be prevented from binding to cells by antibodies binding to the toxin molecule. In these cases, then, antibodies are able to produce a useful effect simply through their ability to recognize particular antigenic determinants.

In most cases, however, the interaction of antibodies and antigen by itself accomplishes nothing. Only if this interaction leads to the activation of some effector mechanism does a biologically significant outcome follow.

In the first part of this chapter, we shall examine the mechanism by which the interaction of antibodies and antigen activates a series of serum proteins collectively known as *complement*. Several of the complement proteins have specific effector functions. The role of antibodies in complement-mediated effects is to confer specificity on the response. We shall also explore the role played by antibodies in triggering effector functions mediated by the various white cells of the blood (neutrophils, basophils, eosinophils, monocytes, and lymphocytes of several types) and, in some cases, their tissue equivalents.

## 14.2 The Complement System

Late in the nineteenth century, it was discovered that the capacity of an antiserum to lyse cells is destroyed by heating the serum to 56°C for 30 minutes. However, the specific lytic ability of the antiserum can be restored by the addition of fresh *normal* (nonimmune) serum. For example, the heated serum of a rabbit immunized with sheep red blood cells (SRBC) will regain its ability to lyse SRBC when mixed with fresh nonimmune serum, even serum from some other species such as a guinea pig or human. Thus the specificity of the antiserum is heat stable but its capacity to trigger lysis is not. The nonspecific factor in fresh serum needed to bring about lysis is called complement (C).

As it turns out, complement is not a single factor but a complex system of serum proteins (Figure 14.1). We shall examine six proteins that are involved in the **classical pathway** of complement activation, the pathway that is activated by antigen–antibody complexes. Five more proteins participate in the **membrane attack complex** that leads to the lysis of antibody-coated cells. Complement activity can also be set off by the so-called **alternative pathway,** a pathway that need not involve antigen–antibody complexes. Three additional proteins participate in the alternative pathway, and these same proteins can also amplify the activity of

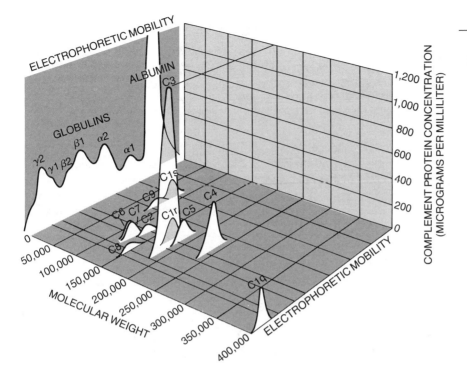

**Figure 14.1** Human complement proteins of the classical system. The molecular weight, electrophoretic mobility (at pH 8.6), and concentration in the serum of the 11 proteins are shown. The electrophoretic pattern of whole human serum is also shown for comparison. [From M. M. Mayer, "The Complement System." Copyright © 1973 by Scientific American, Inc. All rights reserved.]

the classical pathway. Finally we shall examine three proteins that regulate complement activity by inhibiting key steps in the pathways.

Prior to their activation, most of the components of the system are present in the serum as proenzymes; i.e., enzyme precursors. Activation of a complement molecule occurs as a *result* of proteolytic cleavage of the molecule and, in turn, confers proteolytic activity *on* the molecule. Thus many components of the system serve as the substrate of a prior component and, in turn, activate a subsequent component. This pattern of sequential activation has caused the system to be called the complement "cascade."

## The Classical Pathway

The classical pathway of complement activation is triggered by antigen–antibody complexes. Complexes of soluble antigens with antibodies, e.g., antigen–antibody precipitates, are fully effective. However, the model system we shall examine is one in which the antibodies have bound to antigenic determinants on the surface of a red blood cell. Such a system has played an important role in complement research because of the ease with which cell lysis can be quantitated (by the amount of hemoglobin released) and the requirement for *all* the components of the complement cascade to bring about cell lysis.

The classical pathway begins with the binding of C1q to an antibody molecule. C1q is present in the serum as part of a macromolecular complex which contains two molecules each of C1r and C1s. A binding site for C1q is present in the constant region of mu chains (IgM) and in the $C_H2$ domains of some gamma chains. A single molecule of IgM bound to the surface of a red cell is sufficient to bring about lysis of that cell. However, activation of the C1 complex requires that C1q bind to *two* adjacent IgG molecules (Figure 14.2). Hundreds of molecules of IgG must be available for each target cell in order to ensure that a suitably positioned IgG pair will occur on the cell surface. Thus IgG is several hundred times less efficient than IgM at activating the complement sys-

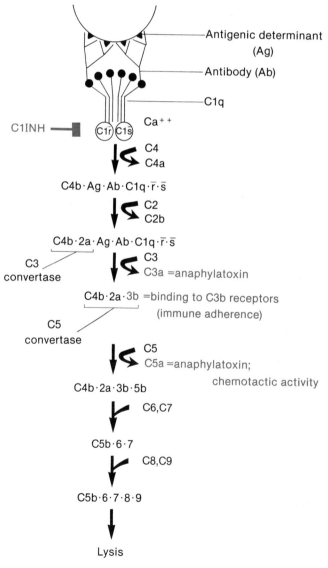

**Figure 14.2** The full complement sequence using the classical pathway. In this illustration, the complement sequence is initiated by the binding of antibodies to determinants on a cell surface and ends with lysis of the cell. C1 inhibitor (C1INH) blocks the proteolytic activity of C1r and C1s.

Antigenic determinant (Ag)

Antibody (Ab)

C1q

C1INH

$Ca^{++}$

C1r C1s

C4
C4a

$C4b \cdot Ag \cdot Ab \cdot C1q \cdot \bar{r} \cdot \bar{s}$

C2
C2b

$C4b \cdot 2a \cdot Ag \cdot Ab \cdot C1q \cdot \bar{r} \cdot \bar{s}$

C3
convertase

C3
C3a =anaphylatoxin

$C4b \cdot 2a \cdot 3b$ =binding to C3b receptors
(immune adherence)

C5
convertase

C5
C5a =anaphylatoxin;
chemotactic activity

$C4b \cdot 2a \cdot 3b \cdot 5b$

C6,C7

$C5b \cdot 6 \cdot 7$

C8,C9

$C5b \cdot 6 \cdot 7 \cdot 8 \cdot 9$

Lysis

tem. Furthermore, the efficiency of IgG varies among the several sub-classes. In humans, the efficiency of activation of the classical pathway is greatest for IgG3, somewhat less for IgG1, and very weak for IgG2. IgG4 does not normally bind C1q.

In no case does binding occur unless the antibody molecule has bound to its antigen or has been aggregated. These actions may cause some conformational change in the antibody molecule that exposes or other-wise alters the site so that it can bind C1q or they may simply bring several sites close enough together so that a C1q molecule can bind multivalently to them.

The binding of C1q activates the C1r and C1s molecules associated with it. Activated C1s is a protease that first cleaves C4 and then C2. Cleavage of C4 yields a small fragment (C4a) and a large fragment desig-nated C4b. As C4b is formed, a site is momentarily exposed on it which is capable of forming a covalent bond with, for example, a sugar residue on a cell-surface glycoprotein. The activity of a single C1s molecule will produce a number of C4b molecules which can bind to the cell surface near the C1 molecule (Figure 14.3).

C1s also cleaves C2 molecules into two fragments. Formation of the larger fragment, called C2a, momentarily exposes a hydrophobic region of the fragment which can bind to a site on C4b. The resulting complex —C4b2a—is called "C3 convertase" because it catalyzes the cleavage of C3.

C3 can well be considered the central component of the complement system. With a concentration in the serum of 1.3 mg/ml, it is the most abundant protein in the system (Figure 14.1). Because of its abundance and because of its ability to catalyze its own cleavage (by a mechanism discussed later), it magnifies an activity that begins at a pair of IgG molecules or a single IgM molecule into a response that spreads over the cell surface and even to nearby cells. Furthermore, C3 stands at the intersection of the second pathway of complement activation, the alter-native pathway.

The C4b2a complex cleaves C3 into two major fragments: C3b and C3a. Formation of the C3b fragment exposes a site on it that is able to form a covalent bond to, for example, OH groups on cell-surface glyco-proteins. Although the process is rather inefficient, the enzymatic activ-ity of C4b2a and the large concentration of substrate (C3) available ensures that many molecules of C3b will bind in the vicinity (Figure 14.3).

The binding of C3b to the surface of a particle (in this case a red cell) enables that particle to bind in turn to specific receptors for C3b found on such cells as macrophages and neutrophils. This phenomenon is called **immune adherence.** Binding of C3b-coated particles (which in vivo would include such things as bacterial cells and aggregates of antigen – antibody complexes) makes them more susceptible to phagocytosis. While antibodies alone bring about phagocytosis of antibody-coated particles (through Fc receptors on the phagocytes—Figure 14.8), the presence of C3b markedly enhances the effect.

The small C3a fragment produced during the cleavage of C3 is liber-ated into the surrounding fluids where it can exert a powerful inflamma-

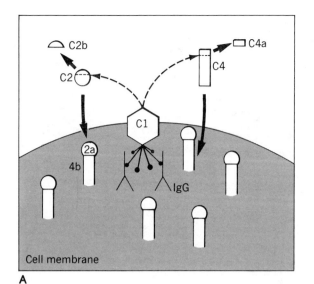

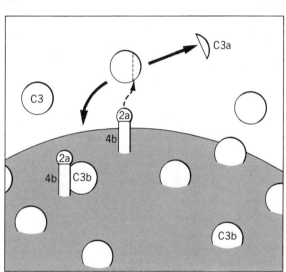

**Figure 14.3** A: Activation of the C1 complex causes it to cleave fluid phase C4. The resulting C4b fragments bind to the cell membrane in the vicinity. Activated C1 also cleaves C2, producing C2a fragments which bind to C4b. B: C4b·2a acts enzymatically on fluid phase C3, cleaving it into small anaphylatoxic fragments (C3a) and into C3b. C3b binds to the cell surface and also to the C4b·2a complex. The surface-bound C3b mediates binding to phagocytic cells (macrophages and neutrophils) through their receptors for C3b and stimulates phagocytosis. The trimolecular complex C4b·2a·3b is a C5 convertase and initiates the formation of the membrane attack complex.

tory effect. The C3a molecule triggers mast cells and basophils (Section 14.5) to release their content of vasoactive substances like histamine. Because of the role of these materials in anaphylaxis (see Section 18.2), C3a is called an **anaphylatoxin** (Figure 14.2).

Some of the C3b produced by C4b2a binds directly to C4b2a forming a trimolecular complex C4b·2a·3b. This complex is enzymatically active against C5 and for this reason is described as a C5 convertase. Cleavage of C5 by C5 convertase initiates the assembly of a set of complement proteins that constitute the **membrane attack complex.** The formation of the membrane attack complex can also be initiated by a C5 convertase produced by the alternative pathway. Thus the two pathways converge at this point.

# The Membrane Attack Complex

Cleavage of C5 by a C5 convertase produces two fragments. One, called C5a, is released into the fluid surroundings where, like C3a, it serves as a potent anaphylatoxin. C5a is also strongly chemotactic for neutrophils and stimulates them to express a high density of C3b receptors on their surface. Through these actions, C5a attracts phagocytes to the site and then primes them for immune adherence and phagocytosis.

The C5b molecule serves as the locus for the assembly of a single molecule each of C6, C7, and C8. The resulting C5b·6·7·8 complex appears to guide the polymerization of C9 molecules into a tubular hydrophobic structure that is inserted in the lipid bilayer of the cell membrane. Insertion of poly-C9 forms a transmembrane channel (Figure 14.4) through which ions and small molecules—but not macromolecules—are able to diffuse freely. The cell membrane now behaves like a simple semipermeable membrane. Water enters the cell by osmosis and the cell lyses.

It is tempting to view the drama of lysis as the apotheosis of this elaborate pathway of molecular interactions and all that precedes it as preliminary. Complement-mediated cell lysis does provide the immunologist with valuable assays (see Section 5.12 and 5.13) and a technique for preparing purified cell suspensions (see, e.g., Section 13.3). But lysis is only one function, and probably not the major one, of the complement system. What the complement pathway really provides is a well-integrated system for mobilizing the tissue defense mechanisms of the body. Immune adherence (acting through C3b) targets foreign particles for phagocytosis and/or destruction by lysosomal enzymes. Mobilization of

**Figure 14.4** Electron micrograph showing lesions in the cell wall of *Shigella dysenteriae* caused by the terminal components of the complement system (200,000×). Some of the holes have probably been enlarged by the later action of lysozyme. [Courtesy of Drs. J. H. Humphrey and R. Dourmashkin.]

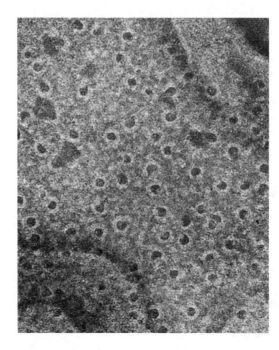

phagocytic cells to the site of damage is aided by increased vascular permeability (mediated by C3a and C5a) and the chemotactic action of C5a. The early complement components also have the important function of solubilizing antigen–antibody complexes and thus assisting in their catabolism and elimination from the body.

## The Alternative Pathway

The cleavage of C3 and the activation of the remainder of the complement cascade can also be triggered in the absence of complement-fixing antibodies. C3 in the serum and other body fluids is always subject to a low rate of spontaneous cleavage. Normally the C3b that is formed is quickly inactivated (by factors I and H — see Figure 14.7). However, if the spontaneously produced C3b comes in contact with certain foreign surfaces, it is protected from inactivation. Surfaces lacking sialic acid favor the binding of C3b. Because most eukaryotic cell surfaces express sialic acid and the surfaces of bacteria do not, C3b is able to engage in a primitive self–nonself discrimination.

*Surface-bound* C3b is able to bind a serum protein designated factor B

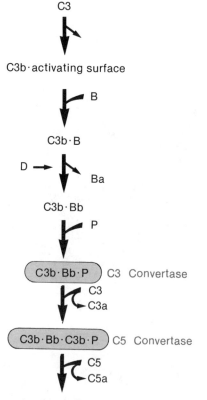

Figure 14.5 The alternative pathway of complement fixation. See text for details.

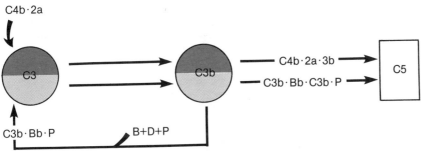

**Figure 14.6** The proteins of the alternative pathway also serve to amplify the conversion of C3 by the classical pathway.

(Figure 14.5). Once bound to C3, factor B is cleaved by factor D, another serum protease, leaving the cleavage fragment Bb still associated with C3b. The resulting complex — C3b·Bb — is stabilized by yet another protein called properdin (P). C3b·Bb·P — like C4b2a of the classical pathway — is a C3 convertase. It cleaves additional C3 to form a multi-molecular complex C3b·Bb·C3b·P. This complex is a C5 convertase and can activate the assembly of the membrane attack complex.

The proteins of the alternative pathway (B, D, and P) also play a major part in amplifying the effects of the classical pathway. Some of the C3b generated by the classical pathway interacts with factors B, D, and P to form additional C3 convertase activity that supplements that provided by C4b2a (Figure 14.6). This autocatalytic effect greatly amplifies the subsequent steps of the cascade starting with the enhanced cleavage of C5 by both the C4b·2a·3b complex (classical pathway) and the C3b·Bb·C3b·P complex (alternative pathway).

### Regulation of Complement Activity

The spontaneous generation of C3b and its autocatalytic effect through the proteins of the alternative pathway create the potential for an explosive triggering of the entire complement cascade. However, two regulatory proteins prevent this from occurring in the fluid phase. One of these proteins, designated factor I (formerly C3b inactivator), inactivates C3b *unless* it is bound to a surface. The action of factor I is enhanced by a second protein, factor H. Factor H also interrupts the positive feedback effect of the C3b·Bb·P complex by removing Bb from it (Figure 14.7).

The action of C1 in the classical pathway is also under regulatory control. Activated C1 is, you will recall, an enzyme and once formed on an antigen–antibody complex it could theoretically continue to cleave C4 and C2 molecules until they were entirely consumed. However, this does not occur because of the presence in the serum of C1 inhibitor (C1INH). C1INH binds to *activated* C1 (it binds to sites on activated C1r

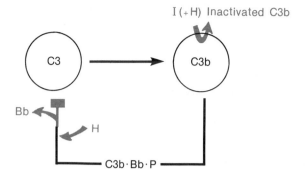

I (+H) Inactivated C3b

**Figure 14.7** Regulation of complement activity. Factors I and H inactivate any C3b that is not bound to a foreign surface. Factor H also blocks the amplification pathway. The site of the regulatory action of C1 inhibitor (C1INH) is shown in Figure 14.2.

and C1s—Figure 14.2). Thus when C1 is activated by an antigen–antibody complex, there is only a brief interval during which it can cleave C4 and C2 before it is deactivated by C1INH. Thus the classical pathway can be set in motion without the danger of its remaining turned on.

The complement system is certainly complex. But behind the myriad of factors and fragments there are some generalizations that can be made and that should not be obscured by the details of the system. The process of complement fixation involves the sequential activation of a series of water-soluble serum proteins. Activation of each member of the series is usually brought about by proteolytic cleavage of the molecule. Activation results in the transient exposure of a site or sites that (1) act enzymatically on the next member of the sequence, (2) bind covalently and/or through hydrophobic interactions to cell surfaces, and (3) bind through hydrophobic interactions to each other. Failure to achieve these effects leads to a rapid degradation of the molecule and the complement cascade is aborted. The enzymatic activity of a number of the components of the system provides a magnification of the response. What can start as a reaction triggered by single molecules of IgM and C1q can end with the lysis of a cell and even nearby cells.

The multiplicity of components in the complement cascade also provides a number of effector molecules that can mediate other defense mechanisms such as phagocytosis and walling off the site of infection through inflammation.

The need to discriminate between self and nonself is not limited to vertebrates. However, humoral immunity is found only in vertebrates. Perhaps the alternative pathway represents a primitive recognition system similar to that which invertebrates use to defend themselves against foreign invaders. Seen in this light, the classical pathway would represent a system for conferring a far higher degree of specificity on this defensive system.

In any case, it is certainly clear that many — if not most — of the physiological activities mediated by the humoral immune system are actually carried out by the complement system. The production of antibodies provides a means of identifying foreign molecules within the body. The complement system responds to the signals provided by this recognition system and mediates one or more effector activities, such as phagocytosis, inflammation, cell lysis, and the solubilization of immune complexes.

The phagocytic cells of the body are responsible for ingesting and destroying particulate matter. There are two major types of phagocytes: **neutrophils** and **macrophages.** Both are scavenging cells that are able to engulf foreign particulate matter, such as bacteria, that enters the body. In addition to microorganisms, these phagocytes also engulf aged or damaged tissue cells.

The process of phagocytosis begins when the cell surface makes contact with the particle. The cell membrane invaginates and the particle is engulfed in a **phagosome.** If all goes well, the phagosome fuses with one or more lysosomes forming a phagolysosome. Lysosomes contain a variety of hydrolytic enzymes capable of digesting all the types of macromolecules that might be present in the engulfed material.

Neither neutrophils nor macrophages are immune cells *per se.* They are able to engulf foreign particles without any assistance from the immune system. In fact, phagocytic cells represent one of the most primitive defense mechanisms in the animal kingdom, being found in invertebrates as well as vertebrates.

Although phagocytes can recognize and destroy foreign matter without the help of the immune system, the specificity of their action can be greatly enhanced by antibodies. Both neutrophils and macrophages have $Fc_\gamma$ receptors; i.e., receptors for the Fc portion of IgG molecules. The phagocytes bind to antibody-coated targets through these receptors enhancing phagocytosis (Figure 14.8). Aggregated IgG binds to the receptors far better than monomeric IgG ensuring that the receptors will be able to bind antigen–antibody complexes without having their sites blocked by circulating monomeric IgG.

Both macrophages and neutrophils also express surface receptors for

**Figure 14.8** Two mechanisms by which antibodies promote phagocytosis of particles such as bacteria. Once the complement sequence has been activated, C3b molecules bind directly to the surface of the particle and enhance its phagocytosis.

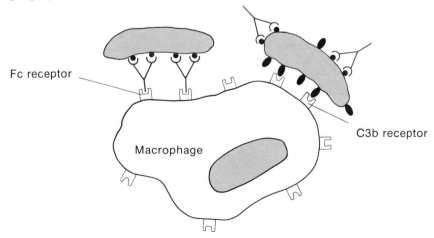

Fc receptor

C3b receptor

Macrophage

the C3b fragment of complement. These aid in the adherence of C3b-coated particles to the phagocyte (Figure 14.8) and this, too, enhances phagocytosis. Thus the humoral immune system confers not only specificity on this primitive defense mechanism but also magnifies its activity through the activation of the complement system.

While neutrophils and macrophages share many features, there are some differences between them. Neutrophils are the most abundant (~50%) of the circulating white blood cells. Thanks to their abundance and their chemotactic attraction to C5a (Section 14.2), they can be mobilized quickly to sites containing infectious agents and/or antigen–antibody complexes. Thus neutrophils are usually the dominant cell type early in an inflammatory response.

Macrophages are localized in such tissues as lymph nodes, spleen, skin, liver (Kupffer cells), lungs, and wherever foreign matter gains access to the body. While some macrophages are actively motile, others — such as the Kupffer cells of the liver — remain fixed in their position. Macrophages are recruited from the blood: their precursors are the monocytes. In addition to serving as part of the effector arm of humoral immunity, macrophages play an important part in cell-mediated immune responses (Section 14.8).

## 14.4   Killer (K) Cells

The lymphoid cells of both humans and mice contain a population of cells that mediate cytotoxicity but are quite distinct in their properties from $T_C$ cells. Because of their cytotoxic activity, these cells are called *killer* or *K cells*. K cells lyse targets that have been coated with antibodies directed against molecules on the cell surface (Figure 14.9). For example, cells infected by measles virus and exposed to antimeasles antiserum are lysed by K cells. Similarly, cells with TNP-conjugated proteins on their surface and exposed to anti-TNP antibodies become targets for K cells (Figure 14.10). Thus the specificity of killing resides in the antibodies,

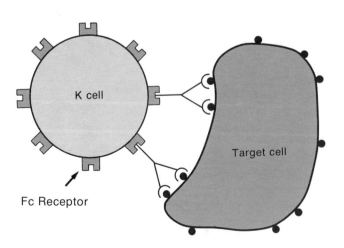

K cell

Fc Receptor

Target cell

**Figure 14.9**   Target cell killing by K cells. The specificity of killing is dictated by antibodies bound to determinants on the surface of the target cell. This phenomenon is called antibody-dependent cell-mediated cytotoxicity (ADCC). A number of other kinds of cells can also carry out ADCC.

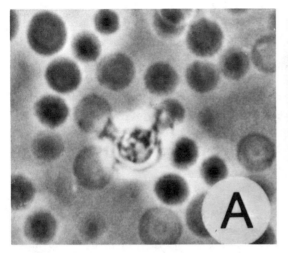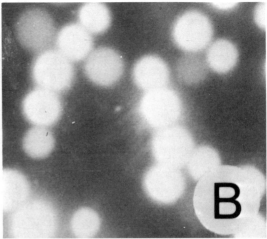

**Figure 14.10** Antibody-dependent attack by cytotoxic human lymphocytes. The targets are human red cells conjugated with TNP and treated to exchange their hemoglobin for a fluorescent dye. Anti-TNP antibodies were added to the culture. The lymphocyte in A is in contact with three targets. Fluorescence microscopy (B) reveals that two of these three (at 8 and 10:30 o'clock) have lost the fluorescent dye. [Courtesy of Charles B. Simone from C. B. Simone and P. Henkart, *J. Immunol.* **124**:954, 1980.]

not in the K cells. This mode of cell killing is called *antibody-dependent cell-mediated cytotoxicity* (ADCC). Complement plays no part in the killing process.

K cells are not as yet fully characterized. Although macrophages can also mediate ADCC, K cells are neither adherent nor phagocytic, so they are clearly distinct from macrophages. Although they appear to be a subpopulation of lymphocytes, they have little or no surface immunoglobulin (sIg) so are not B cells. Using special procedures, human K cells can be made to form rosettes with SRBCs, but this T cell property is weakly expressed at best. K-cell activity in mice is eliminated by anti-Thy-1 and complement, evidence of a T cell origin.

The surfaces of K cells carry receptors for IgG and for the third component of complement (C3b). The presence of the first type of receptor is demonstrated by the ability of K cells to form rosettes with IgG-coated erythrocytes (EA); the second by their ability to form rosettes with erythrocytes coated with IgM antibodies *and* complement (EAC — Figure 7.15). The receptors for IgG bind to the Fc portion of the molecule. Cells coated with F(ab')$_2$ fragments of IgG are not killed by K cells. However, the binding to the Fc region occurs only when the IgG molecule is bound to the antigenic determinant against which it is directed or if the IgG has been aggregated. Thus ADCC is not inhibited by the presence of free IgG but is blocked by the presence of aggregated IgG.

Cells other than K cells (as defined above) can mediate ADCC. Macrophages can kill virus-infected cells that have bound antibodies directed against viral antigens exposed on the cell surface. Neutrophils and **eosinophils** can also mediate ADCC. For example, schistosomula, the larvae of blood flukes, are rapidly killed in vitro by eosinophils when antischistosomula antibodies are present in the medium.

## 14.5  Basophils and Mast Cells

Basophils are the rarest of the circulating leukocytes ($<1\%$). Their cytoplasm is packed with granules containing vasoactive substances such as histamine and several leukotrienes (Section 17.2). When triggered by an appropriate stimulus, they discharge these granules causing vasodilation at the site and a rapid inflammatory response. Mast cells resemble basophils in both their morphology and their behavior, but are always localized in tissues (such as the lungs).

When white blood cells are incubated with $^{125}$I-conjugated IgE, autoradiography reveals that basophils are the only cells to become labeled. The binding of IgE to the basophil (or mast cell) occurs through receptors specific for the Fc portion of IgE. There are over 100,000 of these receptors per cell and their association constant for IgE is on the order of $10^8 - 10^{10}$ M$^{-1}$.

The binding to basophils (or mast cells) of IgE molecules of a particular antigen specificity sensitizes the cells to that antigen. When the antigen becomes bound to the antigen-binding sites of adjacent IgE molecules, a signal is transmitted into the cell that results in degranulation (Figure 14.11). In this way, basophils and mast cells serve as potent effectors for that portion of a humoral immune response mediated by IgE molecules. Unfortunately, these IgE-dominated responses are often associated with antigens such as pollen, insect venoms, many drugs, and a wide variety of foods. Many of these materials are innocuous in themselves but by producing IgE in response to them, the individual develops an **allergy** to them which may range in severity from annoying to life threatening. (The role of IgE, mast cells, and basophils in allergy is examined in Section 18.2.)

## 14.6  Effectors of Cell-Mediated Immunity

Several immune responses that are mediated primarily or exclusively by cells have been described in earlier chapters. Delayed-type hypersensitivities such as the classic tuberculin reaction, the rejection of allografts, and the graft versus host reaction are three examples of cell-mediated in vivo immune responses. The essential role played by cells in each case is established by the fact that injections of lymphoid cells, but not of serum, can transfer these responses to naive (nonimmune) recipients. Thus the tuberculin sensitivity of one guinea pig can be adoptively transferred to a naive guinea pig by the injection of lymphocytes but not by injection of serum. An allograft will be rejected in an accelerated fashion if the bearer of the graft is injected with lymphocytes from an animal previously sensitized to the histocompatibility antigens expressed on the graft. A graft versus host reaction is elicited by the introduction of immunocompetent lymphocytes lacking histocompatibility antigens that are present on the cells of the recipient. The injected lymphocytes rec-

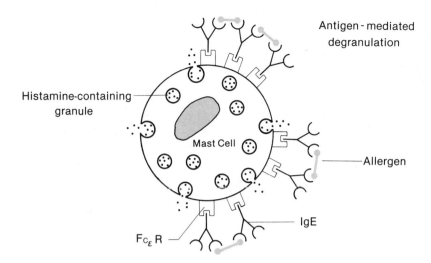

Antigen-mediated
degranulation

Histamine-containing granule

Mast Cell

Allergen

IgE

$Fc_\varepsilon R$

$Fc_\varepsilon R$ = [receptor for Fc region of IgE]

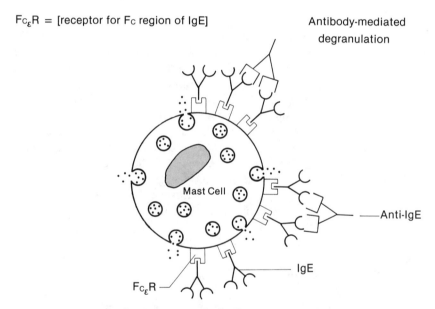

Antibody-mediated
degranulation

Mast Cell

Anti-IgE

IgE

$Fc_\varepsilon R$

**Figure 14.11** Anything that cross-links the $Fc_\varepsilon$ receptors on mast cells and basophils causes degranulation. This includes (1) exposure of IgE-sensitized cells to the allergen for which the IgE is specific (top), (2) exposure of IgE-sensitized cells to anti-IgE antibodies (bottom), and (3) exposure of unsensitized mast cells to antibodies directed against the $Fc_\varepsilon$ receptor (not shown). The importance of cross-linking is shown by the inability of Fab fragments to cause degranulation in cases 2 and 3.

ognize and respond to the "foreign" histocompatibility antigens of the host. In each of these in vivo manifestations of CMI, the responsible cells are T lymphocytes. With mice, treatment of the cell suspensions with anti-Thy-1 serum and complement destroys their capacity to transfer DTH, trigger accelerated graft rejection, or elicit graft versus host reactions, respectively.

Although T lymphocytes are responsible for triggering each of these cell-mediated responses, other cells may participate in the response. Macrophages are clearly implicated in the development of DTH lesions. Macrophages are probably also intimately involved in the rejection of allografts and perhaps in the host response (so often futile) to malignant tumors.

We have also examined several in vitro assays of cell-mediated immune reactivity (assays that one hopes reflect activities occurring within the living organism). These include the various assays of lymphokines released by antigen-stimulated T lymphocytes (Sections 3.2 and 6.2) and assays of cell-mediated cytotoxicity (CMC — Section 6.6). With one exception (NK cells — Section 14.10), the active cell in each case is a T lymphocyte. In mice, treatment of the effector cell population with anti-Thy-1 and complement eliminates the activity.

## 14.7 The $T_D$ Cell

$T_D$ cells are the T cells responsible for delayed-type hypersensitivity (DTH) reactions. Operationally, they can be defined as those cells that are able to transfer a state of DTH from an antigen-sensitized animal to a naive one (see Section 3.7). Murine $T_D$ cells are Thy-1$^+$ and Ly-1$^+$. They are killed by treatment with anti-Thy-1 and anti-Ly-1 antiserum plus complement but not by anti-Ly-2 or anti-Ly-3 serum.

The ability to transfer a state of DTH to a naive animal is restricted by the MHC. The evidence for mice is presented in Section 3.7. To recapitulate, the transfer of DTH in mice occurs only when the donor and the recipient of the cells are matched at the I region of the MHC (Figure 3.16). Presumably this reflects the fact that the $T_D$ cell can respond to an antigen only when it is presented (by a dendritic cell or macrophage) in association with the same I-region-encoded antigen(s) which were present when the cell was initially induced.

Once effectively stimulated by antigen, $T_D$ cells mediate the development of the typical skin lesion of DTH: a slow-developing, firm accumulation of lymphocytes and macrophages. However, 95% or more of the cells in a DTH lesion are not antigen-specific cells but nonspecific cells that have been recruited to the area. The effector function of $T_D$ cells thus appears to depend on their ability to recruit and activate nonspecific cells, like macrophages, to do the actual work. Let us see how this recruitment and activation process might work.

## 14.8 Lymphokines

When antigen sensitized Ly-1 T cells are exposed in vitro to the antigen, they proliferate and release into the culture medium a variety of physiologically active substances. These substances are collectively known as lymphokines. T cell mitogens like Con A also cause T cells to release lymphokines. In this case, the effect is nonspecific; i.e., the majority of T cells—regardless of their antigenic specificity—respond to the mitogen by releasing lymphokines. Section 3.2 examines some of the properties of one of the most thoroughly studied lymphokines: *migration inhibition factor* (MIF). It is one of over 50 different activities that have been ascribed to material in the supernatant of cultures containing antigen and T cells previously sensitized to that antigen. The nature of most of the molecules active in the various assays for lymphokines is poorly understood. In general, the active substances appear to be proteins or glycoproteins. In some cases, a particular lymphokine activity appears to be mediated by two or more distinct molecules. In other cases, the molecules active in one assay have later turned out to be the same as those active in another. We can do no more here than glance briefly at a small number of lymphokines.

## Macrophage Chemotactic Factor (MCF)

When lymphocytes taken from an antigen-sensitized animal are cultured with the antigen, they liberate a lymphokine that attracts macrophages and monocytes. The Boyden chamber—two compartments separated by a filter (Figure 14.12)—provides a convenient way to measure this activity. A cell suspension containing the lymphocytes to be tested is placed in one compartment along with the antigen. A suspension of normal macrophages is placed in the other compartment. If MCF is liberated, the macrophages move through the pores of the filter toward the source of MCF (Figure 14.13). Their presence can be quantitated by removing the filter, staining it, and counting the cells trapped within. Nonspecific mitogens like phytohemagglutinin (PHA) also trigger the release of MCF.

## Migration Inhibition Factor (MIF)

The assay system for MIF is shown in Figure 3.3. Like most of the lymphokines, MIF is liberated by (1) culturing antigen sensitized T cells with

**Figure 14.12** Assaying for macrophage chemotactic factor (MCF) in the Boyden chamber. The migration of macrophages toward the source of MCF can be determined by removing the filter, staining it, and counting the cells trapped within it. Macrophage chemotaxis through the filter will also occur if the supernatant from a culture of activated T lymphocytes is placed in the lower chamber.

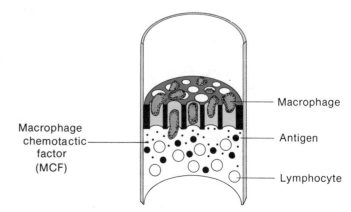

Macrophage

Antigen

Lymphocyte

Macrophage chemotactic factor (MCF)

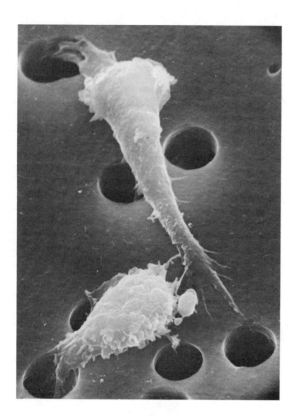

**Figure 14.13** Scanning electron micrograph (3400×) of two human monocytes migrating through the pores of a filter in response to MCF. The diameter of the filter pores is 5 μm. [Courtesy of Drs. Ralph Snyderman and C. A. Daniels from R. Snyderman and E. J. Goetzl, *Science* **213**:830, 1981.]

antigen or (2) culturing normal T cells with mitogens such as PHA and Con A. The ability of the lymphocytes from an immunized animal to liberate MIF correlates well with the ability of that animal to produce a DTH reaction when challenged intradermally with the antigen.

### Macrophage Activating Factor (MAF)

If a mixture of antigen-sensitized lymphocytes and normal macrophages is cultured with antigen for 2–3 days, the macrophages undergo many physiological changes. Their phagocytic (and pinocytotic) activity increases. The motility of their surface membrane and the rate of protein synthesis in the cell increases. Their ability to kill ingested intracellular parasites becomes markedly enhanced (Figure 14.14). All of these activities reflect a general state of vigorous activation. This nonspecific response by the macrophages occurs only if the lymphocytes in the culture are stimulated by the antigen to which they were primed or by a mitogen.

Macrophage activation does not require the physical presence of activated lymphocytes. The supernatant alone from a culture of antigen-activated (or mitogen-activated) lymphocytes will activate macrophages. The factor responsible is called *macrophage activating factor* (MAF). Attempts to characterize MAF in molecular terms suggest that in mice

376

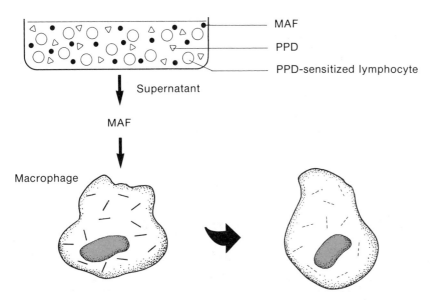

Supernatant

MAF

Macrophage

No killing of ingested mycobacteria       Bacteria killed

**Figure 14.14** Macrophages cannot kill ingested mycobacteria unless activated by macrophage-activating factor (**MAF**). MAF is a lymphokine liberated by antigen (as shown here) or mitogen-stimulated T lymphocytes. The physiological significance of this response is discussed in Section 3.8.

(and perhaps in humans) MAF is gamma interferon (**IFN-$\gamma$** — Section 17.2).

In addition to the lymphokine activities discussed here, many others have been described. These include B cell growth and differentiation factors (Section 12.7), IL-2 (Section 6.2), and factors that are chemotactic for granulocytes.

With few exceptions, lymphokine activities are measured by in vitro assays. This raises the question of whether these in vitro activities truly reflect what is occurring within the DTH lesions of a living animal. A plausible case can be made that they do. The activities enumerated above could (1) attract nonspecific cells like macrophages to the site (such as MCF), (2) keep them there (MIF), and (3) stimulate them to enhanced activity (MAF).

But plausibility is not proof. Direct evidence that $T_D$ cells achieve their effector functions through the release of these lymphokines remains scant. Some of the lymphokines that have been partially purified have physiological activity when injected into the skin. For example, the localized injection of **MIF** causes a drop in the number of circulating monocytes, perhaps as a result of their migration from the blood to the site of injection. Furthermore, factors active in several of the lymphokine assays can be recovered from the lymph draining the site of a DTH reaction or in extracts of the skin lesion.

Much remains to be done, but most of the data are consistent with the effector functions of $T_D$ cells being mediated by substances (the various lymphokines) that they release into their surroundings upon encountering the antigen to which they were sensitized. These lymphokines are responsible for the recruitment and activation of the nonspecific cells that make up the bulk of the DTH lesion. These nonspecific cells eventually produce the pathology of the lesion. In Chapter 18, we shall examine several examples of pathological conditions triggered by antigen-stimulated T cells but mediated by the nonspecific cells, like macrophages, brought to the site and put to work.

## 14.9  Cytotoxic T Lymphocytes (CTL or $T_C$)

The cytotoxic T lymphocyte or $T_C$ cell is a cell that destroys other cells in an antigen-specific fashion. In contrast to killer cells (K cells — Section 14.4), the specificity of the attack is mediated by a receptor for antigen on the T cell itself. The properties of this receptor are examined in Chapter 11 (Sections 11.5 – 11.8). While $T_C$ cells are induced in vivo, their activity is generally measured in the in vitro cell-mediated cytotoxicity (CMC) assay (Section 6.6).

$T_C$ cells respond only to antigens that are expressed on cell surfaces. The various kinds of cells that can induce, and subsequently be lysed by, $T_C$ cells are (1) virus-infected cells, (2) malignant cells, (3) allogeneic cells, and (4) cells carrying conventional protein antigens (e.g., KLH) or haptens (e.g., TNP) on their surface.

In most, perhaps all, of these examples, the specificity of the induced $T_C$ cell population is directed at both the conventional antigen (viral, tumor, TNP, etc.) and, simultaneously, at a class I MHC-encoded antigen. Thus, for example, the $T_C$ cells induced by cells infected with vaccinia virus can only lyse vaccinia-infected target cells that express at least one of the class I antigens (K, D, or L in the mouse) present on the inducing cell population. The MHC restriction of $T_C$ cells is examined in greater detail in Sections 11.4 and 13.4.

What about the $T_C$ cell response to allogeneic cells? The rule for *minor* histocompatibility antigens is the same as that for conventional antigens: the response is restricted by a class I MHC-encoded antigen. Thus $T_C$ cells elicited by a minor histocompatibility antigen can only recognize that antigen in association with a class I antigen. As for the response to allogeneic cells that differ at the MHC, the target antigen seen by the $T_C$ cell is usually a class I antigen itself. Thus there is no "restriction" in this case. But even here, the rule of associative recognition may be observed. Perhaps the $T_C$ cells induced by MHC-different stimulating cells actually see one or another *non*-MHC cell surface molecule present on both the inducing and the target cells *along with* the class I antigen. This might explain the observed failure of human $T_C$ cells directed against a human class I antigen to lyse *mouse* cells that express the same human antigen following DNA-mediated transfer of the human gene into the mouse cells. *Antibodies* directed against the class I antigen bind it just as well expressed on the surface of a mouse cell as on the surface of a human cell. The recognition of one or another of myriads of unknown cell surface molecules with a particular foreign class I molecule could also explain the extraordinary vigor of the $T_C$ cell response to foreign class I molecules (Section 11.9).

In all these examples, the cells responsible for the cytotoxic response are T cells. In mice, their cytotoxicity is destroyed by treatment with anti-Thy-1 serum and complement. Murine $T_C$ cells are also lysed by anti-Ly-2 serum and complement but not by anti-Ly-1. Therefore, $T_C$ cells belong to the Ly-2$^+$ subset of T cells in the mouse. The $T_C$ cells of humans express CD8 but not CD4.

We do not yet clearly understand the mechanism by which $T_C$ cells lyse their targets. The killing process does *not* resemble that caused by treatment with antiserum and complement. When lymphocytes, for example, are coated with antibodies (such as anti-Ly-1) and exposed to complement, the cell membrane is damaged and can no longer exert its normal control of the entry of molecules into the cell. Exposed to trypan blue, the mortally wounded cell takes up the stain. However, complement-mediated killing of white cells (unlike red cells) does not result in their lysis. Killing by $T_C$ cells, in contrast, quickly leads to the rupture of the target cell. Its cytoplasmic contents spill out, making possible the use of $^{51}$Cr release as a measure of $T_C$-mediated cytotoxicity in the CMC assay. The $T_C$ cell does not seem to be damaged by its activity; once having killed, it can kill again and again.

The biological significance of $T_C$ cells is uncertain. Although allografts elicit $T_C$ cells (detected in a CMC assay), some workers feel that graft rejection itself is actually mediated by $T_D$-like cells (Section 19.2) not $T_C$ cells. On the other hand, there is evidence that $T_C$ cells play an important role in protecting against virus infection. Experimental animals and humans with deficiencies in T cell function are notoriously prone to hard to control virus infections. It appears that $T_C$ cells kill virus-infected cells before they can release their load of mature, infective progeny virus. Such activity in vivo would limit the spread of virus through the host.

As for malignancies, one would like to think that the induction of a population of antitumor $T_C$ cells would represent a valuable defense mechanism against cancer. The presence of tumor-specific $T_C$ cells in the tumor-bearing host can be demonstrated in a CMC assay, but the evidence that these cells have a protective effect in vivo is weak. Here, too, it may be that $T_D$-like cells play a more important role than $T_C$ cells in attacking tumor cells within the host. There is also evidence that tumor cells can be destroyed by a class of non-T, non-B lymphocytes called natural killer (NK) cells.

## 14.10 Natural Killer (NK) Cells

The discovery of "natural killer" cells came about by chance. Cytotoxic T cells ($T_C$) specific for tumor-associated antigens (and "self") are induced in animals bearing tumors. Their presence can be detected by the usual CMC assay using chromium-labeled tumor cells as targets. In assaying the specificity and activity of such $T_C$ cells, one control that should logically be included is the measurement of the amount of target cell lysis caused by normal, unsensitized cells; i.e., lymphoid cells from non-tumor-bearing animals. But quite unexpectedly, lymphoid cells taken from normal animals turn out to be highly cytotoxic for tumor cells although not for normal cells. The cells responsible for this specialized form of killing have been named *natural killer* (NK) *cells*. The activity of these cells does not appear to represent a truly immune phenomenon. There is no evidence of specificity beyond the fact that only certain broad categories of cells, e.g., tumor cells, can serve as targets. And no evidence of a specific memory response exists, although NK activity against all tumor targets can be enhanced by prior sensitization to one type of tumor.

NK cells are neither phagocytic nor adherent, so they are not macrophages. They carry no immunoglobulin on their surface so they are not B cells. Human NK cells can form rosettes with SRBC but not nearly as easily as mature T cells do. Mouse NK cells carry small amounts of Thy-1 on their surface but treatment with anti-Thy-1 and complement does not usually kill them. Furthermore, NK cells in the mouse express none of the markers that distinguish the various subsets of mature T cells (e.g., Ly-1, Ly-2, L3T4). We would not expect NK cells to be mature T cells because nude mice have very high levels of NK activity although they have no thymus and no T-cell-mediated immune responses.

Some NK cells also have receptors for the Fc portion of IgG, and these cells can also mediate antibody-dependent cell-mediated cytotoxicity (ADCC). In other words, some NK cells can also act as K cells.

The mechanism of natural killing is as yet unknown. However, it clearly differs from the killing mediated by $T_C$ cells. Ordinarily, each NK cell is able to lyse only a single target and no MHC restriction is imposed; NK cells lyse allogeneic tumor cells as well as syngeneic tumor cells. Natural killing is greatly enhanced by interferon or by anything (virus infection, certain chemicals) that induces interferon production. When exposed to interferon, NK cells are able to lyse several target cells.

Could a cell that destroys tumor cells in vitro do the same in the intact organism? Nude mice, which have none of the normal T-cell-mediated immune responses, are no more susceptible to spontaneous or induced tumors than are normal mice. For some years, this observation was puzzling to immunologists who had proposed that one of the major functions of T cells was to destroy neoplastic cells arising in the host. Perhaps they were looking at the wrong cell. The high levels of NK activity in nude mice may, in fact, provide them with protection against tumors. Cantor and his collaborators (see reference 6 at the end of the chapter) have been able to protect mice against tumor cells by injecting a purified suspension of NK cells along with the tumor cells. Perhaps, then, it is the NK cell that performs surveillance of the cells of the body, finding and destroying (usually) neoplastic cells as they arise. Human victims of the Chediak–Higashi syndrome have unusually low levels of NK activity and, at the same time, suffer a high incidence of lymphomas. Possibly some of the beneficial effects attributed to interferon in tumor therapy are the result of its role as a stimulator of NK activity. Now that large amounts of pure, well-characterized interferon are becoming available, it should be possible to test this hypothesis more thoroughly.

1. Brown, E. J., et al., "Complement," in W. E. Paul (ed.), *Fundamental Immunology*, Raven Press, New York, 1984.

2. Gery, I., and B. Waksman, "Potentiation of the T-Lymphocyte Response to Mitogens. II. The Cellular Source of Potentiating Mediator(s)," *J. Exp. Med.* 136:143, 1972. (Reprinted in V. L. Sato and M. L. Gefter, *Cellular Immunology*, Addison-Wesley Publishing Co., Inc., Reading, MA, 1982.) On IL-1.

3. Gillis S., et al., "The *in vitro* Generation and Sustained Culture of Nude Mouse Cytolytic T-Lymphocytes," *J. Exp. Med.* 149:1460, 1979. (Reprinted in V. L. Sato and M. L. Gefter, *Cellular Immunology*, Addison-Wesley Publishing Co., Inc., Reading, MA, 1982.) On IL-2.

4. Ishizaka, K., and T. Ishizaka, "Identification of $\gamma$ E-Antibodies as a Carrier of Reaginic Activity," *J. Immunol.* 99:1187, 1967.

5. Joiner, K. A., et al., "Complement and Bacteria: Chemistry and Biology in Host Defense," *Ann. Rev. Immunol.* 2:461, 1984.

6. Kasai, M., et al., "Direct Evidence That Natural Killer Cells in Nonimmune Spleen Cell Populations Prevent Tumor Growth *in vivo*," *J. Exp. Med.* 149:1260, 1979.

7. Kiessling, R., Eva Klein, and H. Wigzell, " 'Natural' Killer Cells in the Mouse. I. Cytotoxic Cells with Specificity for Mouse Moloney Leukemia Cells. Specificity and Distribution According to Genotype," *Eur. J. Immunol.* 5:112, 1975. (Reprinted in V. L. Sato and M. L. Gefter, *Cellular Immunology*, Addison-Wesley Publishing Co., Inc., Reading, MA, 1982.)

8. Matzinger, P., and G. Mirkwood, "In a Fully H-2 Incompatible Chimera, T Cells of Donor Origin Can Respond to Minor Histocompatibility Antigens in Association with Either Donor or Host H-2 Type," *J. Exp. Med.* 148:84, 1978. (Reprinted in V. L. Sato and M. L. Gefter, *Cellular Immunology*, Addison-Wesley Publishing Co., Inc., Reading, MA, 1982.)

9. Rocklin, R. E., et al., "Mediators of Immunity: Lymphokines and Monokines," *Adv. Immunol.* 29:55, 1980.

10. van de Rijn, M., et al., "Recognition of HLA-A2 by Cytotoxic T Lymphocytes After DNA Transfer into Human and Murine Cells," *Science* 226:1083, 1984. Mouse cells expressing a human class I antigen (complete with human $\beta_2$-microglobulin) were not lysed by human $T_C$ cells specific for that antigen when it is expressed on human cells.

# PART V

# Regulation of Immune Responses

# CHAPTER 15

# Homeostatic Control of Immunity

## 15.1 Introduction

A primary immune response often seems a pretty straightforward affair. Antibodies appear in the blood some days after the administration of antigen. Their appearance usually hastens the disappearance of residual

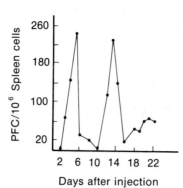

**Figure 15.1**  Cyclical production of IgG (indirect) plaque-forming cells in the spleens of rabbits immunized on day 0 with a single injection of aggregated human IgG. [From C. G. Romball and W. O. Weigle, *J. Exp. Med.* 138:1426, 1973.]

antigen as antigen – antibody complexes are formed and catabolized. With the disappearance of the last of the antigen, the concentration of antibodies wanes.

But a closer examination of the dynamics of an immune response reveals that the situation may be more complex than it first appears. Figure 15.1 shows the humoral response in rabbits that follows a *single* injection of aggregated human IgG. The number of specific plaque-forming cells rises rapidly two days after the administration of antigen, reaches a peak at four days, and then declines sharply. However, 12 days after the initial injection of antigen, a second burst of antibody production occurs and this, in turn, is followed by a third. Data such as these suggest that something other than simply the presence of antigen is turning antibody production on and off. The curves suggest some form of homeostatic regulatory mechanism that turns antibody production down when it reaches a high level and turns it back up when it declines to a low level.

A similar phenomenon is shown in Figure 15.2. In this case, a fixed dose of antigen (killed type 3 pneumococci) was given once each week over the course of a year. Despite the constancy of antigenic stimulation, the concentration of antipneumococcal antibodies is seen to rise and fall repeatedly during this period.

Cell-mediated immune responses are probably subject to some form of homeostatic control as well. For example, the characteristic skin lesion of DTH reaches a peak 24 hours or so after its first appearance and then

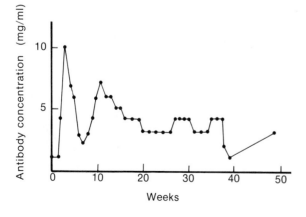

**Figure 15.2**  Concentration of antipneumococcal antibodies in the serum of a single rabbit receiving 1 dose of vaccine ($5 \times 10^9$ killed type 3 pneumococci) each week for a year. [From J. W. Kimball, *Immunochemistry* 9:1169, 1972.]

fades. Nevertheless, it can often be shown that the eliciting antigen is still present at the site.

In this chapter we shall examine several mechanisms that operate in a homeostatic fashion to suppress or "down regulate" the magnitude of immune responses.

**387**

*Section 15.2
Suppression of
Humoral Immunity
by Antibodies
Directed Against
Antigen*

## 15.2 Suppression of Humoral Immunity by Antibodies Directed Against Antigen

In 1961 Uhr and Baumann demonstrated that passively administered diphtheria antitoxin suppresses the active humoral response to diphtheria toxoid. When guinea pig antitoxin was administered simultaneously with, or a few days after, the administration of diphtheria toxoid, the response of the injected animals was reduced almost 1000-fold. This suppression lasted for several weeks.

This type of antibody-mediated feedback suppression operates at the level of the individual antibody-producing cells. Figure 15.3 shows the decline over time of the anti-SRBC PFC response of mice receiving a single injection of SRBC. The rate of decline becomes much steeper any time that anti-SRBC antibodies are administered to the animal.

A simple explanation for antibody-mediated feedback is that the passively administered antibodies bind to the antigen and hasten its catabolism and elimination from the animal. But this simple mechanism cannot be the whole story. Consider the response of an animal to two different haptens coupled to the same carrier. If such a simple mechanism were at work, then administration of antibodies directed against *either* hapten should hasten the elimination of the antigen and the response to both haptens should be suppressed. But as Brody and his colleagues demonstrated in 1967, this is not the case (Figure 15.4). The administration of antiarsonate antibodies suppresses the antiarsonate response but not the anti-DNP response to a conjugate of the two haptens coupled to the *same*

**Figure 15.3** Accelerated decline of anti-SRBC plaque-forming cells in the spleens of SRBC-immune mice receiving passively administered anti-SRBC antibodies. All the mice were immunized on the days shown and their indirect (IgG) PFC response compared one week later with that of untreated immune mice. [From H. Wigzell, *J. Exp. Med.* 124:953, 1966.]

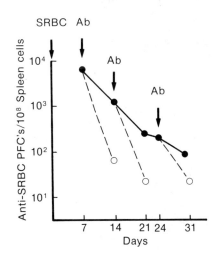

| Antigen[1] | Antibodies (mg/ml) | |
| | Anti-DNP | Anti-ABA |
|---|---|---|
| DNP–RGG | 0.97 | 0 |
| ABA–RGG | 0 | 0.90 |
| Mixture of above | 0.33 | 0.08 |
| DNP–RGG–ABA conjugate | 0.46 | 0.10 |
| Anti-ABA + mixture | 0.71 | **0.01** |
| Anti-ABA + conjugate | 0.56 | **0.02** |

[1] ABA = azobenzenearsonate; RGG = rabbit gamma globulin.

**Figure 15.4**   The administration of anti-ABA antibodies to rabbits suppresses the response to ABA but not to DNP even when both haptens are presented on the same carrier molecule ("anti-ABA plus conjugate"). Thus the suppressive effect of these passively administered antibodies cannot be caused by accelerated elimination of the antigen. A similar effect is seen with passively administered anti-DNP antibodies. [Data from N. I. Brody et al., *J. Exp. Med.* **126**:81, 1967.]

carrier just as it does when each hapten is presented on a separate carrier (Figure 15.4).

What alternative mechanism might be at work? One possibility is that passively administered antibodies suppress active immunity by competing with the antigen-binding B cells (ABCs) for limiting amounts of antigen. If antibodies and ABCs are competing for the same determinant, then we would predict that the higher the $K_0$ of an antibody preparation, the more suppressive its effect. This turns out to be the case as Walker and Siskind have demonstrated. They found that it took 67 mg of passively administered, low affinity ($K_0 = 2 \times 10^6$ M$^{-1}$), anti-DNP antibodies to exert the same suppressive effect provided by 6 mg of high affinity ($K_0 = 10^{11}$ M$^{-1}$) anti-DNP antibodies.

A mechanism based on competition leads to a further prediction. To the extent that a suppressed animal can synthesize any antibodies at all, these should be of higher affinity than those produced by nonsuppressed animals. In a competition between antigen-binding cells and passively administered antibody molecules, those cells bearing receptors of highest affinity should be most successful at winning the competition. Able to bind antigen, they are stimulated to grow up into clones of plasma cells secreting antibodies of high affinity. Siskind et al. showed that animals injected with both antigen and anti-DNP antibodies *synthesized* anti-DNP antibodies with a $K_0$ ten times greater than those synthesized by animals receiving antigen alone.

The phenomenon of antibody-mediated suppression of active immunity has practical as well as theoretical consequences. For six months or so following birth, an infant retains substantial levels of IgG antibodies received from its mother during gestation. The mechanism described here suggests that so long as these antibodies — reflecting as they do the lifetime antigenic experiences of the mother — remain, the child will respond poorly to active immunization. For some antigens, at least, this is true. Therefore, live measles, mumps, and rubella vaccines are usually not given until the child is 15 months of age.

389

*Section 15.3*
*Suppression of*
*Humoral Immunity*
*by Anti-Immuno-*
*globulin Antibodies*

## 15.3 Suppression of Humoral Immunity by Anti-immunoglobulin Antibodies

The antigen-binding receptors on B cells, like antibody molecules, represent a mosaic of isotypic, allotypic, and idiotypic determinants. Recall that isotypic determinants are chiefly found on the constant regions of heavy and light chains. The allotypic determinants are formed by structural variants — chiefly confined to constant regions (see, e.g., Sections 9.5 and 9.6) — whose expression in a given animal is inherited as a single gene trait. Idiotypic determinants are those determinants characteristic of a particular $V_H$ region or, commonly, a combination of unique $V_H$ and $V_L$ regions.

The passive administration of anti-isotypic, anti-allotypic, or anti-idiotypic antibodies produces, in each case, a profound effect on the immune system. Injecting newborn mice with anti-IgM antibodies suppresses the ability of the animals to mount any sort of humoral response. Presumably this suppression reflects the fact that the isotypic determinants of mu chains are present on the antigen-binding receptors of ABCs. The administration of anti-allotypic antibodies to an animal heterozygous for a

**Figure 15.5** Allotype suppression. Heterozygous (b4/b5) rabbits injected at birth with anti-b4 antibodies fail to synthesize normal levels of antibodies with b4 light chains. The preponderance of b5 antibodies in the untreated littermates in the first few weeks after birth represents the antibodies transferred across the placenta during gestation in their b5/b5 mother. [Based on R. G. Mage, *Cold Spring Harbor Symposia on Quantitative Biology*, Vol. XXXII: 203, 1967.]

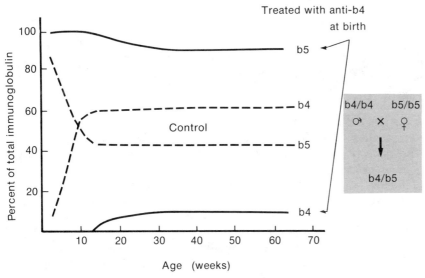

particular allotype suppresses the animal's ability to synthesize antibodies of that allotype (Figure 15.5). Again, the mechanism presumably operates at the level of the receptors on the ABCs.

## Idiotype Suppression

While isotype and allotype suppression have been useful investigative tools, they probably do not reflect normal control mechanisms. However, suppression of particular *idiotypes* may indeed be an important homeostatic control mechanism in the normal animal. And because idiotypes are so often correlated with particular antigenic specificities, the suppressive effects of antibodies directed against idiotypic determinants could be antigen specific. For these reasons, we shall examine the effects of anti-idiotypic serum in some detail.

TEPC-15 is an IgA myeloma protein that arose in BALB/c mice. It binds phosphorylcholine (PC), the major antigenic determinant of the C-polysaccharide found in the cell *walls* (not the capsule) of pneumococci. Injection of BALB/c mice with rough pneumococci elicits a vigorous anti-PC response. Most of the anti-PC antibodies express the same idiotype as TEPC-15. (But note that these are almost exclusively IgM and IgG antibodies while TEPC-15 is IgA.) Antibodies raised against the TEPC-15 protein inhibit the anti-PC PFC response of immunized mice when added to the assay dish. Administered to BALB/c mice, the same anti-idiotypic antibodies suppress the ability of the mice to produce anti-PC antibodies expressing the idiotype (see Section 8.5). The anti-TEPC-15 antibodies appear to act as antireceptor antibodies that block the induction of cells carrying the PC receptors of the TEPC-15 idiotype.

## 15.4 The Network Theory

Anti-idiotypic (anti-id) antibodies thus have the potential to suppress a particular antibody response in a highly specific fashion. Could they play a role in the down regulation of antibody responses? In 1974 Niels Jerne based his "network" hypothesis on this assumption. In its simplest form, the hypothesis proposes that the introduction of antigen into an animal stimulates the synthesis of antibody molecules bearing particular idiotypes associated with the antigen-binding sites. As these idiotypes become more prevalent in the animal, they induce, in turn, the synthesis of molecules directed against the idiotype, that is, anti-idiotypic molecules. As the level of anti-idiotypic antibodies (or cells) increases, they exert a specific suppressive effect on the further production of those idiotypes. Here, then, would be a specific homeostatic control mechanism.

The examples cited in the previous section of suppression by anti-idiotypic (anti-id) antibodies employed heterologous antibodies. That is, the anti-idiotypic antibodies were produced by immunizing another animal (in this case a rabbit) with the idiotype and passively transferring these anti-id molecules to BALB/c mice. The network hypothesis, on the other hand, rests on the assumption that an animal can make its own anti-id molecules. Is there evidence for this?

Indeed there is. As described in Section 2.3, Rodkey demonstrated that antibodies harvested from immunized rabbits and stored for 16 months in the freezer, could — upon reintroduction into the rabbit that had made them — stimulate it to synthesize antibodies that precipitated the injected antibodies. He demonstrated that the new population of antibodies were, indeed, anti-idiotypic. We would have expected them to be so inasmuch as molecules bearing all the "self" isotypic and allotypic determinants were still present in the animal. So clearly there is no innate or genetic limitation on the animal's ability to recognize self-idiotypic determinants as new to the immune system and to mount a response against them.

The immunization protocol used by Rodkey involved injection of a protein — along with complete Freund's adjuvant — into an animal no longer synthesizing that protein. The network theory requires that an animal produce anti-id antibodies *spontaneously.*

In 1974 Kluskens and Köhler reported on a series of experiments that provided strong evidence that anti-idiotypic antibodies arise spontaneously during the course of an immune response to antigen. Once again, the PC-TEPC-15 system was used. Normal spleen cells were cultured with antigen and the number of anti-PC PFCs induced was measured by the hemolytic plaque assay. When serum from animals immunized four days earlier with rough pneumococci was added to the cultures, their PFC response was sharply suppressed (just as it is in vivo). The suppression was specific because the response of these cultures to horse red blood cells (HRBC) was unaffected by the treatment (Figure 15.6). Serum taken from mice repeatedly immunized over a period of 200 days also exerted a specific suppressive effect on the response of these cultures to PC.

Closer analysis revealed that the suppressive effects of day 4 antiserum and day 200 antiserum were mediated by different mechanisms. When day 4 antiserum was first absorbed with rough pneumococci (to remove all anti-PC antibodies), its suppressive effect was eliminated. This treatment had no effect on the day 200 antiserum.

However, when the antisera were absorbed with the TEPC-15 myeloma protein, the effects were reversed. Absorption with the myeloma protein had no effect on the suppressive effect of day 4 antiserum but almost eliminated the suppression produced by the day 200 antiserum.

These results indicate that the early suppression is caused by anti-PC antibodies and thus resembles the suppression described in Section 15.2. However, the late suppression was caused by anti-idiotypic antibodies. This shows that the mice which received multiple injections of antigen spontaneously produced anti-id antibodies. Not only did the serum from these mice have the suppressive effect shown in Figure 15.6, but it was also able to specifically agglutinate red cells coated with the idiotype. The agglutination could be blocked by the presence of soluble TEPC-15 molecules but not by the presence of other BALB/c myeloma proteins. Furthermore, the spontaneous production of anti-id antibodies coincides with a decline in the animal's production of anti-PC antibodies

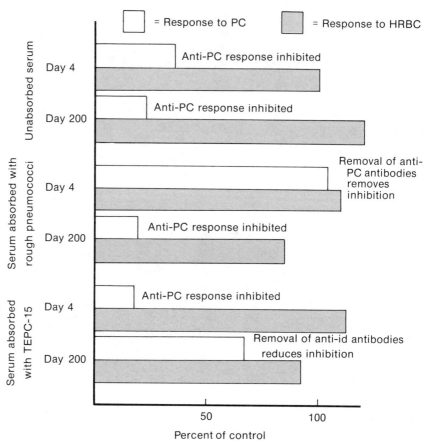

Figure 15.6  Response of cultures of normal **BALB**/c spleen cells to immunization with rough pneumococci (or HRBC) in the presence of serum from mice immunized once (day 4) or 5 times (day 200) with rough pneumococci. The suppressive effect of day 4 serum could be removed by absorption with antigen; that of day 200 serum by absorption with the **TEPC**-15 myeloma protein. HRBC = horse red blood cells. [From L. Kluskens and H. Köhler, *Proc. Natl. Acad. Sci. USA* **71**:5083, 1974.]

(Figure 15.7). The decline does not seem to reflect a loss of B cells responsive to PC, for when the spleen cells from these multiply immunized animals are washed and placed in culture, they respond vigorously to PC.

## 15.5  Some Anti-idiotypic Antibodies Mimic Antigens

Idiotypic determinants are expressed on the V domains of antibody molecules (Section 2.3). At least three distinguishable categories of idiotypic determinants ("idiotopes") might be expected to occur (Figure 15.8).

1. Some idiotypic determinants should occur close to the antigen-binding site of the molecule, a region where many of the amino acid residues

**Figure 15.7** Response of BALB/c mice to a single injection of rough pneumococci. As the number of anti-PC plaque-forming cells in the spleen began to decline, spleen cells secreting anti-TEPC-15 antibodies appeared. Anti-PC plaques were assayed with sheep red cells coated with C-polysaccharide (from rough pneumococci); anti-TEPC-15 plaques with sheep red cells coated with the TEPC-15 myeloma protein. [From H. Cosenza, *Eur. J. Immunol.* 6:114, 1976. Reprinted in V. L. Sato and M. L. Gefter, *Cellular Immunology,* Addison-Wesley Publishing Co., Inc., 1982.]

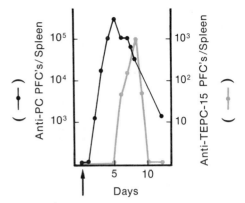

found in complementarity-determining regions (CDRs) are exposed at the surface of the molecule (Figure 9.31). We might well expect that binding of antigen to its site would interfere with the ability of an anti-idiotypic antibody to bind this type of determinant. Binding of the anti-idiotype in such cases is hapten inhibitable (Figure 2.16). If conformational changes should occur upon antigen binding, then even idiotopes remote from the binding site might be inhibited by hapten.

2. Some idiotopes are located in portions of the V domains that do not participate in antigen binding. Binding of anti-idiotypic antibodies to these determinants is not hapten inhibitable. Presumably these determinants are created by framework (FR) residues present on those antibody V regions associated with a particular antigen specificity.

3. The antigen-binding site itself could serve as an idiotypic determinant. If so, anti-idiotypic antibodies (Ab2) elicited by such determinants should have special properties. Because their binding site is the topological complement of the antigen-binding site, it should have properties like those of the antigenic determinant or epitope to which the idiotype (Ab1) binds. Thus such anti-idiotypic antibodies present an "internal image" of the antigen. If anti-id antiserum contains this third subset of antibodies, this subset should mimic the properties of the antigen. If so, we might predict that (a) if the antigen has biological effects (e.g., a hormone), then the anti-idiotypic antibody might mediate the same effects, and (b) if the internal image subset of Ab2 is used as an antigen to elicit *anti-anti*-idiotypic antibodies (Ab3), some of these should—like Ab1—bind antigen. Both of these predictions have been tested successfully.

**Figure 15.8** Schematic representation of various types of idiotypic determinants and the anti-idiotypic antibodies directed against them. A: A hapten-inhibitable interaction; B: a nonhapten-inhibitable interaction; C: this anti-idiotypic antibody (Ab2) is specific for the antigen-binding site (sometimes called the paratope) of Ab1. The binding site of this Ab2 represents the "internal image" of the antigen to which Ab1 binds.

## Internal Images Can Mimic Hormones

Many types of vertebrate cells carry surface receptors for the hormones adrenaline (epinephrine) and noradrenaline (norepinephrine). These $\beta$-adrenergic receptors also bind such clinically important hormone antagonists as the "beta blocker" drugs propanolol and alprenolol.

Strosberg and his colleagues produced monoclonal antibodies (Ab1) against alprenolol by immunizing BALB/c mice with an alprenolol–BSA conjugate (Figure 15.9). The hybridoma cells producing these antibod-

**Figure 15.9** Production of (1) monoclonal antibodies (Ab1) against alprenolol, a drug that binds to $\beta$-adrenergic receptors, and (2) monoclonal anti-idiotypic antibodies (Ab2) against Ab1. The anti-idiotypic antibodies bind to the $\beta$-adrenergic receptor, stimulating the adenyl cyclase system (Figure 15.11). Although shown here with only two binding sites, the Ab2 in these experiments is IgM. [Based on S. Chamat et al., *J. Immunol.* **133**:1547, 1984, and J. G. Guillet et al., *Proc. Natl. Acad. Sci. USA* **82**:1781, 1985.]

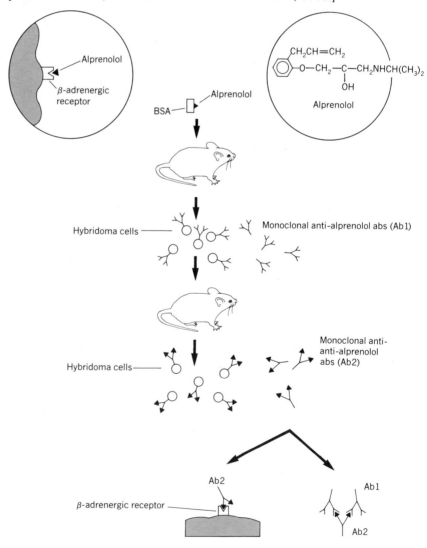

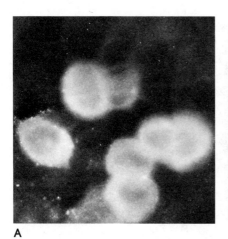

**A**                                **B**

**Figure 15.10**   A: Binding of anti-idiotypic antibodies to $\beta$-adrenergic receptors on cultured human cells. Antibody binding is revealed by indirect immunofluorescence (Section 5.14) using rabbit antimouse IgM and fluorescein-labeled goat antirabbit antibodies. B: Isoproterenol, an adrenaline-like drug that binds to $\beta$-adrenergic receptors, inhibits the binding of anti-idiotype antibodies. [From J. G. Guillet et al., *Proc. Natl. Acad. Sci. USA* **82:**1781, 1985.]

ies were then used to immunize other BALB/c mice and hybridomas secreting monoclonal anti-idiotypic antibodies (Ab2) were derived from them. Not only did the Ab2 molecules bind Ab1, the antigen that elicited them, but they also bound to the $\beta$-adrenergic receptor (Figure 15.10). Furthermore, binding of these anti-id antibodies mimicked the physiological effects of hormone binding, activating — as hormone binding does — the adenyl cyclase system. However, the anti-idiotypic antibodies failed to stimulate adenyl cyclase in the presence of the beta blocker propanolol (Figure 15.11).

At first glance, the existence of antibodies with combining sites that resemble the epitopes of antigens may seem odd. Much of the work on the nature of the antigen-binding site that we have examined suggests that these sites consist of a cleft into which the appropriate ligand fits. X-ray analysis of the antigen-binding fragments of McPC-603 and the human myeloma New reveal such a conformation. Thus most diagrammatic representations of ag–ab interactions show epitopes projecting

**Figure 15.11**   Response of cultured human cells to stimulation with (1) isoproterenol, an adrenaline-like drug that binds to $\beta$-adrenergic receptors, (2) a mixture of isoproterenol and the "beta-blocker" propanolol, and (3) a monoclonal anti-idiotypic antibody raised against anti-alprenolol antibodies. The response to the anti-idiotypic antibodies, like the response to isoproterenol, is inhibited by propanolol (4). Thus the anti-idiotypic antibody mimics the effects of hormone binding (even though it was raised as the "internal image" of alprenolol, a beta-blocker). [Based on J. G. Guillet et al., *Proc. Natl. Acad. Sci. USA* **82:**1781, 1985.]

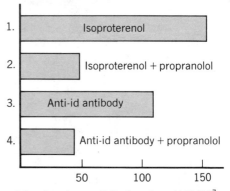

1. Isoproterenol

2. Isoproterenol + propranolol

3. Anti-id antibody

4. Anti-id antibody + propranolol

50     100     150

Adenyl cyclase activity (pmoles cAMP/$10^7$ cells)

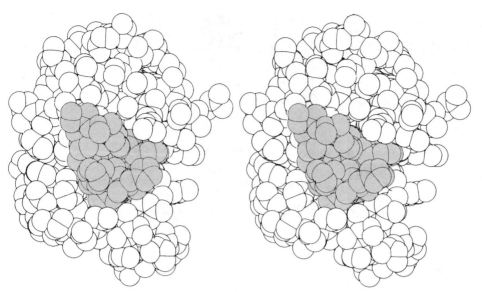

**Figure 15.12** Stereoscopic view of Fab Kol. Kol has 9 more residues (shaded) than McPC-603 (Figure 9.31) in CDR3 of the H chain, and these entirely fill what would otherwise be a cleft between $V_L$ (top) and the rest of $V_H$ (bottom). The specificity of Kol is unknown, but antibodies with this type of binding site would be able to bind in the clefts of antibodies with a cleft-type site and thus could serve as "internal images" of antigen. [Courtesy of Robert Huber.]

out, antigen-binding sites projecting in. But that subset of anti-idiotypic antibodies that represent the internal image of an antigenic determinant like TNP or PC cannot be built this way. And there is no structural reason that they have to be. A glance at Figure 9.31 will remind us that many of the amino acid residues in such cleft-forming antibodies as McPC-603 are present around the margins of the cleft. Six CDRs clustered at the tip of an Fab fragment could provide abundant opportunities for noncovalent interactions with concave or even interdigitating complementary surfaces on other molecules.

The Fab fragment of a monoclonal human IgG1 designated Kol has been analyzed by x-ray crystallography. In contrast to Fab' New and Fab McPC-603, the CDRs of Kol do not form a cleft. In fact, the residues of CDR3 of the H chain project above the surrounding surface formed by the other CDRs (Figure 15.12). Although the antigen specificity of Kol is not known, molecules of this type are good candidates for "internal images."

### Internal Images as Vaccines

Just as immunization with Ab1 yields anti-id antibodies (Ab2), so immunization with Ab2 should elicit antibodies directed against the unique determinants on Ab2. Such a population would be anti-anti-idiotypic antibodies or Ab3. If Ab2 represents an internal image of antigen, then might not some Ab3 molecules bind not only the eliciting Ab2 but the original antigen as well? In other words, immunization with the *image* of antigen might produce antibodies specific for the actual antigen.

Once again, the TEPC-15 system provides an instructive example. Kohler and his colleagues (reference 6) immunized mice with TEPC-15, the phosphorylcholine-binding myeloma. They derived a hybridoma from these mice that secreted a monoclonal antibody (Ab2) that was specific for the binding site of TEPC-15. When mice were immunized with this Ab2, they produced almost as high a titer of anti-PC antibodies as mice immunized with PC–KLH itself. Furthermore, these Ab2-immune mice were able to survive a challenge with doses of living type 3 pneumococci 100 times greater than needed to kill unimmunized mice. In other laboratories, immunization with anti-id antibodies has been used to protect mice against trypanosome infection and to induce neu-

**Figure 15.13** Procedure for making monoclonal anti-idiotypic antibodies (Ab2) that represent the "internal image" of an antigenic determinant on reovirus. Thus Ab2 binds to the same cell receptor that reovirus does. Furthermore, immunization of a mouse with the Ab2 hybridoma elicits $T_D$ cells able to generate DTH against reovirus infected cells. [Based on A. H. Sharpe et al., *J. Exp. Med.* **160**:1195, 1984.]

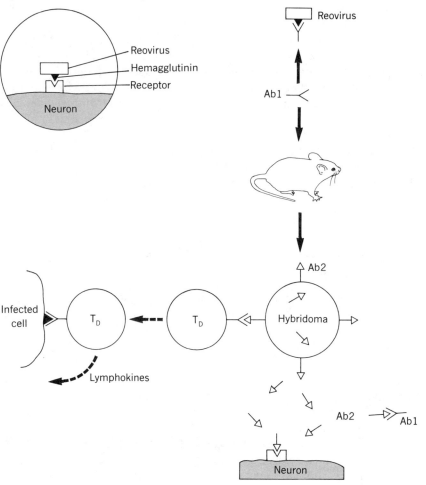

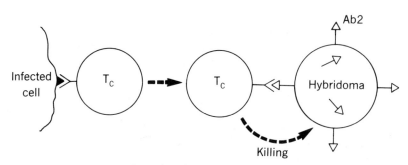

**Figure 15.14** Mice infected with reovirus generate cytotoxic T cells ($T_C$) which not only lyse reovirus-infected cells (not shown) but also the hybridoma cells producing the "internal image" (Ab2) of the reovirus hemagglutinin (see Figure 15.13). [Based on H. C. J. Ertl et al., *Proc. Natl. Acad. Sci. USA* 79:7479, 1982.]

tralizing antibodies against several types of viruses. Will immunization with anti-idiotypic antibodies provide a new generation of vaccines?

Greene and his colleagues have shown that immunization with internal-image Ab2 can also induce cell-mediated immunity. Their system employs a reovirus that infects mice by binding to specific receptors on the animal's neurons. First these investigators developed a monoclonal antibody (Ab1) against a capsid protein of the reovirus (Figure 15.13). Ab1 was then used to produce a monoclonal Ab2 that (1) binds to Ab1 and (2) binds to the same receptors on neurons to which the reovirus itself binds. Furthermore, immunization of mice with this Ab2 elicited a population of $T_D$ cells that generated a DTH response when challenged with reovirus. Conversely, $T_C$ cells induced in mice by reovirus infection were able to lyse the Ab2-secreting hybridoma itself (Figure 15.14). These latter findings are of particular interest because they suggest that T cells can also participate in idiotype–antiidiotype networks even though the T cell receptor for antigen is not an antibody molecule.

## 15.6  T Cells Participate in the Network

One of the earliest demonstrations that T cells can be specific for idiotype was provided by Eichmann and his colleagues. When mice of the A/J strain (a subline of strain A mice) are injected with killed group-A streptococci, they produce antibodies directed against the carbohydrate (A-CHO) present in the cell walls of the bacteria. A substantial fraction of these antibodies express an idiotype called A5A that can be detected with an anti-idiotypic antiserum raised in guinea pigs.

These investigators found that the guinea pig anti-A5A serum — when administered in vivo — exerts a powerful idiotype-specific suppression. Mice immunized with the carbohydrate after being pretreated with the antiserum go on to synthesize almost normal concentrations of antiA-CHO antibodies but *not* of the A5A idiotype (Figure 15.15). When mice are given a high dose (60 $\mu$g) of purified anti-A5A antibodies, the sup-

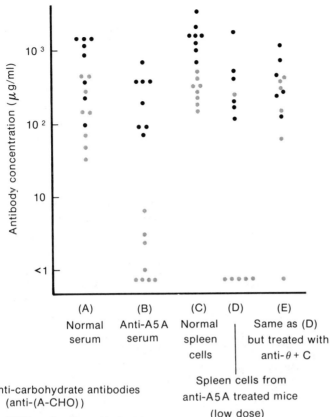

• Total anti-carbohydrate antibodies
  (anti-(A-CHO))

• Anti-(A-CHO) antibodies with A5A idiotype

**Figure 15.15**  Idiotype (A5A)-specific and total anticarbohydrate antibody production in A/J mice treated as shown. Anti-idiotypic antibodies suppressed the production of antibodies with the A5A idiotype (column 2). Furthermore, the transfer of spleen cells from mice treated months earlier with a low dose of anti-A5A antibodies also caused idiotype-specific suppression (column 4). Treatment of the spleen cells with anti-$\theta$ serum and complement abolishes the effect showing that the suppressor cells are T cells. The response of each mouse is shown by one open circle and one closed circle. [From K. Eichmann, *Eur. J. Immunol.* **4**:296, 1974, and **5**:511, 1975.]

pression reaches a peak in one week and wanes by the end of three weeks. During this interval, it can be shown that *both* B cells and $T_H$ cells are suppressed. B cells from suppressed mice cannot be helped by $T_H$ cells from unsuppressed mice when the two populations are cultured together. On the other hand, T cells from suppressed mice cannot help B cells mount an anti-TNP response when the carbohydrate is used as the "carrier" for the TNP.

When the mice are treated with small (0.1 $\mu$g) doses of purified anti-A5A antibodies, the response is quite different. Such a dose produces maximum suppression after seven weeks, and this level of suppression continues for a year or more. In the second case, only $T_H$ cells appear to be targets of suppression. B cells from suppressed animals mixed with T cells from nonsuppressed mice synthesize the A5A idiotype without difficulty.

The mechanism of *high dose* suppression is not clear. Perhaps this suppression follows a direct interaction between the anti-A5A antibodies and those B and $T_H$ cells expressing receptors with the A5A idiotype. One could visualize such an interaction preventing access of the antigen to these receptors and thus inhibiting stimulation of the clones. But the simple masking of receptors cannot be the whole story because $F(ab')_2$ fragments of anti-id antibodies have none of the suppressive activity of the intact molecules although their ability to bind is unimpaired. Suppression must also depend in some way on the Fc region of the anti-id molecules.

In the case of *low dose* suppression, the suppression is mediated by *cells*. A/J mice that are lightly irradiated and reconstituted with normal spleen cells respond normally to immunization with group A streptococci. However, if the mice also receive as few as $10^5$ spleen cells from a suppressed (low dose) mouse, the A5A-specific response is eliminated (Figure 15.15). Thus low dose suppression of the idiotype specific humoral response can be adoptively transferred by cells. The inability of the cell suspension to suppress after it is treated with anti-Thy-1 and complement reveals these are T cells.

Thus we meet another member in our panoply of T cells: the suppressor T cell or $T_S$ cell. Eichmann's finding that anti-id serum induces $T_S$ cells intersected with an increasing number of reports from other laboratories that $T_S$ cells play an important role in the response to antigens as well. Let us examine some of this evidence.

## 15.7 Suppression of Humoral Immunity by $T_S$ Cells

The earliest evidence that humoral responses can be suppressed by T cells was indirect. You may recall the statement (in Section 8.9) that nude mice *(nu/nu)* respond better to pneumococcal polysaccharide than do their phenotypically normal, heterozygous *(nu/+)* littermates. The polysaccharide is a T-independent (TI) antigen so we would expect nude mice to respond as well as normal mice, but why should they respond *better* than animals with a functioning system of T cells? Furthermore, when normal mice are treated with antilymphocyte serum (ALS), which is powerfully cytotoxic for T cells, their response to pneumococcal polysaccharide is increased some 100-fold. These observations led to the notion that among the many subsets of T cells in the animal there exists a population that exerts suppressive effects on immune responses.

A direct demonstration of the existence of suppressor T cells would be achieved if T cell suspensions could exert specific suppressive effects when adoptively transferred into a nonsuppressed host. In the early 1970s, a number of laboratories devised methods for inducing $T_S$ cells and demonstrating these by adoptive transfer. For example, Tada and Takemori showed that the intraperitoneal injection of KLH without adjuvant induces a population of suppressor cells in the spleen and thymus. A normal mouse immunized with DNP–KLH *and adjuvant* produces, after six days, some 11,000 anti-DNP plaque-forming cells (PFC) per

**Figure 15.16** Suppression of a primary humoral response to DNP–KLH by the transfer of KLH-primed spleen cells. The suppressor cells in the spleen are T cells (suppression is eliminated by anti-$\theta$ plus complement) and their effect is carrier specific. [From T. Tada and T. Takemori, *J. Exp. Med.* **140**:239, 1974.]

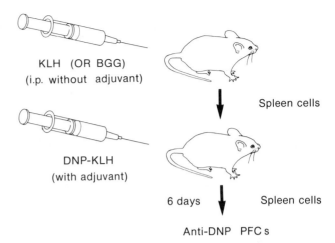

KLH (OR BGG)
(i.p. without adjuvant)

DNP-KLH
(with adjuvant)

Spleen cells

6 days    Spleen cells

Anti-DNP PFC s

RESULTS

| Cells transferred | IgG PFC/spleen (day 6) |
|---|---|
| None | 11,000 |
| KLH-primed spleen | 89 |
| KLH-primed spleen treated with anti-$\theta$ + C | 20,600 |
| BGG-primed spleen | 11,600 |

spleen. However, if the animal is immunized, and simultaneously given an intravenous injection of spleen cells from a KLH-suppressed animal, its ability to mount a DNP response is virtually abolished (Figure 15.16). The ability of anti-Thy-1 and complement to abolish the suppressive effect shows that the spleen cells are T cells. The suppression is specific for the carrier; spleen cells from BGG-suppressed mice do not suppress the response to DNP–KLH (Figure 15.16).

## $T_S$ Cells Are Ly-2$^+$

The so-called "B" mouse is an experimental system which provides a convenient method for studying the effects of T cell populations. B mice are created by lethal irradiation, *thymectomy,* and reconstitution with bone marrow cells that have been treated with anti-Thy-1 and complement to remove T cells. Such animals survive but having no thymus and thus no mature T cells, they cannot respond to T-dependent antigens like SRBC. However, they do respond well to SRBC if at the same time they are given antigen, they are also given T cells from an animal primed earlier with SRBC (Figure 15.17). By the use of the appropriate anti-Ly sera and complement, purified subsets of these T cells can be prepared and tested for their activity. Ly-2$^+$ cells generate no response at all, while two million Ly-1$^+$ cells give a response that is almost three times as great as that given by the same number of unfractionated T cells. The en-

**401**

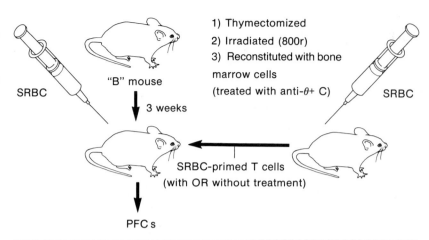

SRBC

"B" mouse

1) Thymectomized
2) Irradiated (800r)
3) Reconstituted with bone
   marrow cells
   (treated with anti-$\theta$+ C)

SRBC

3 weeks

SRBC-primed T cells
(with OR without treatment)

PFC s

| SRBC-primed T cells | | Anti-SRBC PFC/spleen |
|---|---|---|
| Dose | Subclass | |
| $2 \times 10^6$ | All | 32,000 |
| $2 \times 10^6$ | Ly-2$^+$ | 0 |
| $2 \times 10^6$ | Ly-1$^+$ | 90,000 |
| $\left\{ \begin{array}{l} 2 \times 10^6 \\ 2 \times 10^6 \end{array} \right.$ | $\left. \begin{array}{l} \text{Ly-1}^+ \\ \text{Ly-2}^+ \end{array} \right\}$ | 28,000 |
| $\left\{ \begin{array}{l} 2 \times 10^6 \\ 4 \times 10^6 \end{array} \right.$ | $\left. \begin{array}{l} \text{Ly-1}^+ \\ \text{Ly-2}^+ \end{array} \right\}$ | 18,000 |

**Figure 15.17** Demonstration that suppressor T cells belong to the Ly-2$^+$ subset. "B" mice cannot respond to T-dependent antigens unless they are reconstituted with the appropriate T cells. [Based on H. Cantor et al., *J. Exp. Med.* 143:1391, 1976.]

hanced response provided by purified Ly-1 T cells can be partly explained by the enrichment of the suspension with $T_H$ cells which belong to this subset. But there is more to the story than that because injection of a *mixture* of $2 \times 10^6$ Ly-1$^+$ cells—which by themselves can help produce 90,000 PFCs per spleen—with an equal number of Ly-2$^+$ cells, suppresses the helper effect by almost 70% (Figure 15.17). The suppressive effect of the Ly-2$^+$ cells is dose dependent: a doubling of the number of Ly-2$^+$ cells suppresses the response still further (Figure 15.17). Thus the administration of antigen seems to elicit two populations of T cells: the familiar $T_H$ cells and a population of Ly-2$^+$ $T_S$ cells.

Cytotoxic T cells ($T_C$) are Ly-2$^+$ cells (see Section 14.9). Are, then, suppression and cytotoxicity simply different activities mediated by the same population of T cells? Probably not. $T_S$ cells react with antibodies against an antigenic specificity called I-J. $T_C$ cells do not.

The I-J specificity received its name when it was thought to be expressed on molecules encoded in a subregion of H-2 distinct from (and between) the I-A and I-E subregions. Although the story turns out not to be that straightforward (see Section 15.13, "The I-J Enigma"), these antibodies clearly distinguish between $T_S$ cells (Ly-2$^+$, I-J$^+$) and $T_C$ cells (Ly-2$^+$, I-J$^-$). In humans, $T_S$ cells belong (as do $T_C$ cells) to the CD8$^+$ subset.

## 15.8   Suppressor Cells in Cell-Mediated Immunity

Suppressor T cells affect the magnitude of delayed-type hypersensitivity (DTH) responses. Figure 15.18 shows a convenient assay system with which to study this phenomenon. Mice are primed with an antigen, in this case the hapten (4-hydroxy-3-nitrophenyl)acetyl or "NP" coupled to bovine gamma globulin (BGG). At the time of antigen priming, the

**Figure 15.18**   Suppression of a cell-mediated response (DTH) by the transfer of $T_S$ cells. The NP-specific suppressor cells are induced in the donor by injection of NP-conjugated syngeneic spleen cells. Pretreatment of the recipient with cyclophosphamide reduces its ability to generate its own suppressor cells and thus maximizes the response of the positive controls to antigen challenge. [Based on J. Z. Weinberger et al., *J. Exp. Med.* **150:**761, 1979.]

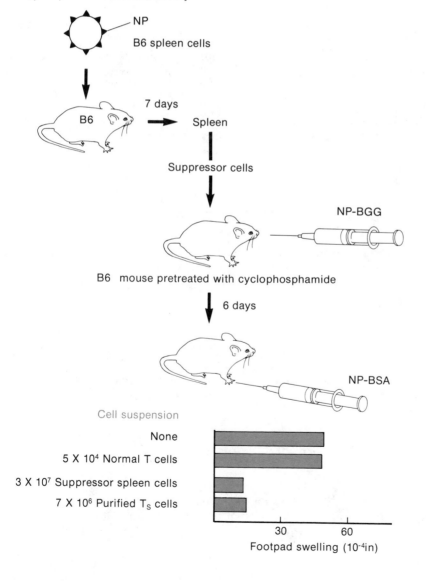

animals are also given an intravenous injection of the cell suspension to be tested. Six days later the animal's left foot is injected with a challenge dose of antigen consisting of the same hapten coupled to a different carrier (NP – BSA). Twenty-four hours after that, the thickness of the left foot is measured with an engineer's micrometer and compared with the thickness of the untreated (right) foot. The degree of swelling in the left foot is a measure of the strength of the reaction.

Two further points about the assay should be noted. (1) If the mice are pretreated with cyclophosphamide, their DTH reaction is enhanced. Cyclophosphamide is a cytotoxic compound and one might expect it to suppress an immune response rather than enhance it. However, at low doses, this agent seems to exert its cytotoxic effect primarily on the induction of $T_S$ cells. Therefore, treatment with cyclophosphamide removes host suppressor cells and maximizes the DTH response in the positive controls. (2) The antigen used for priming is NP – BGG while the antigen used for challenge is NP – BSA so any reaction is specific for the hapten.

NP-specific $T_S$ cells can be induced by intravenously injecting normal mice with *syngeneic* spleen cells to which the hapten has been coupled. When the spleen cells from such suppressed animals are then injected along with the priming antigen (NP – BGG) into normal recipients, the response of the recipients to antigen challenge (given six days later) is substantially reduced. Purified T cell suspensions from the suppressed animals produce the same effect at a lower cell dose (Figure 15.18). The suppression is specific: NP-specific suppressor cells have no effect on the DTH response in an animal primed and challenged with some other antigen.

### Suppressor T Cells Bind Antigen Alone

One of the most remarkable properties of $T_S$ cells is their ability to bind to antigen alone. This behavior contrasts sharply with that of the other subsets of T cells ($T_D$, $T_H$, and $T_C$) which can bind antigen only when it is presented on a cell surface which also carries the "correct" MHC-encoded antigen (Section 11.3). In this respect, then, $T_S$ cells behave like B cells (Section 8.3).

Figure 15.19 gives an example. TNP-specific $T_S$ cells can be enriched by adsorbing them to the surface of a dish coated with TNP – BSA. Cells that adhere to the dish can adoptively transfer suppression of a DTH response to the TNP group; nonadherent cells cannot.

### 15.9 The Induction of Suppression

The cells used in the experiment shown in Figure 15.19 must be given six days prior to antigen challenge in order for suppression of the DTH response to occur. During this interval, the first set of cells induces a

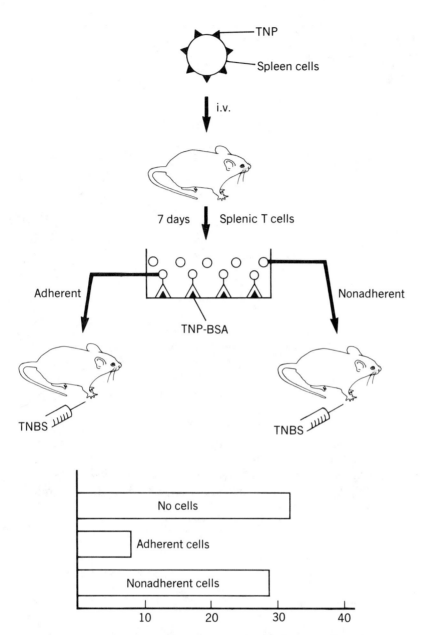

**Figure 15.19**   The DTH response to TNP is suppressed by TNP-binding T cells. These $T_S$ cells are Ly-1$^+$ and belong to the $T_{SI}$ ($T_S1$) subset. $T_S$ cells differ from the other kinds of T cells (e.g., $T_C$, $T_D$) in being able to bind antigen alone. The recipients are challenged with TNP injected as the water-soluble molecule trinitrobenzene sulfonic acid (TNBS). [Based on M. Tsurufuji et al., *J. Exp. Med.* **158**:932, 1983.]

| SRBC-immune Ly-1 T cells ($0.3 \times 10^6$) | Nonimmune T cells ($8 \times 10^6$) | PFC/$10^6$ spleen cells | Interpretation |
|---|---|---|---|
| None | None | 8 | $T_H$ cells needed |
| Yes | None | 145 | $T_H$ cells present in SRBC-primed Ly-1 population |
| Yes | Yes | 22 | Nonimmune population contains precursors of $T_S$ cells |
| None | Yes | 361 | Ly-1 cells ($T_{SI}$) needed to induce $T_S$ cells |
| Yes | Ly-1 + Ly-2,3[1] | 155 | Responding cells in nonimmune population are Ly-1,2,3 |

[1] Mixture of separate populations treated with anti-Ly-2 and anti-Ly-1, respectively (plus complement).

**Figure 15.20** Evidence that (1) the precursors of $T_S$ cells are Ly-1,$2^+$ cells and (2) antigen-specific Ly-$1^+$ T cells ($T_{SI}$) are needed to induce these to become mature suppressor cells. "B" mice (thymectomized, irradiated, and reconstituted with B cells) were given the cell mixtures indicated—all prepared from spleens—and immunized with sheep red blood cells. [From H. Cantor et al., *J. Exp. Med.* 147:1116, 1978.]

second population of *effector* $T_S$ cells (sometimes designated Tse or $T_S2$ cells) that can act immediately to suppress the DTH response. The first set of cells are called T suppressor-inducer cells ($T_{SI}$) or, by some workers, $T_S1$ cells.

$T_{SI}$ cells are Ly-$1^+$ cells. Figure 15.20 demonstrates this. The experimental animal is, once again, the "B" mouse, which, like the nude mouse, has no T system and thus cannot respond to such T-dependent antigens as SRBC. The mouse is reconstituted with the T cell suspension to be tested, given a dose of SRBC, and its spleen cells assayed for PFCs five days later.

When the animal is given no T cells at all, it produces very few plaques (Figure 15.20). However, a purified suspension of Ly-$1^+$ T cells from an animal primed with SRBC gives a good response. We should expect that $T_H$ cells would be present in this population. However, when the animal is given the same number of $T_H$ cells along with $8 \times 10^6$ *nonimmune* T cells, the response is severely depressed. Evidently the nonimmune T cell suspension contains a population of $T_S$ cell precursors. However, these precursors of $T_S$ cells cannot be turned on in the absence of the Ly-$1^+$ cell population because nonimmune T cells alone give an excellent response. This experiment thus reveals the existence of a Ly-$1^+$ T cell, the $T_{SI}$ cell, that is required to induce effector $T_S$ cells.

The target of the Ly-$1^+$ $T_{SI}$ cell is a Ly-1,$2^+$ T cell. A *mixture* of nonimmune Ly-$1^+$ cells (nonimmune cells treated with anti-Ly-2 and complement) and nonimmune Ly-$2^+$ cells (those left after treating a suspension with anti-Ly-1 and complement) does not yield suppression. The only cells missing from such a mixture are those carrying both of these Ly antigens. They are part of the large (50% of all peripheral T cells) pool of Ly-1,$2^+$ cells. These Ly-1,$2^+$ cells are also extremely sensitive to cyclophosphamide and are presumably the precursors of the effector $T_S$ cells.

The $T_{SI}$ cell is a Ly-$1^+$ cell and the question naturally arises whether its suppressor-inducer activity is simply another manifestation of help. However, $T_{SI}$ cells differ from $T_H$ cells in several ways. (1) They bind soluble antigen as we have seen. (2) They react with anti-I-J antibodies.

(3) They also express an MHC-encoded antigen called Qa-1 (see Figure 3.12). In humans, $T_{SI}$ cells belong to the $CD4^+$ subset.

## 15.10   Idiotype-Specific $T_S$ Cells

When mice of the A/J strain are immunized with azobenzenearsonate (ABA), most of the antibodies they produce express an idiotype designated $CRI_A$ (Section 8.8). If A/J mice are pretreated with rabbit anti-$CRI_A$ serum, they still respond well to immunization with ABA but the antibodies they synthesize do not carry the $CRI_A$ idiotype. This suppression of idiotype by heterologous anti-id serum thus resembles the A5A system described in Section 15.6. And as was the case in the A5A system, the effect is mediated by $T_S$ cells. T cells harvested from mice treated with anti-$CRI_A$ serum before being immunized with ABA–KLH can adoptively transfer idiotype suppression to naive recipients. The cells responsible for this suppression can be isolated by allowing them to bind to an immunoadsorbent, in this case red blood cells coated with the Fab fragments of anti-ABA antibodies of the $CRI_A$ idiotype. Removal of the rosettes leaves a T cell population unable to suppress the idiotype response (Figure 15.21). Injection of the rosettes, however, profoundly inhibits the appearance of the $CRI_A$ idiotype even though the recipients produce normal amounts of anti-ABA antibodies.

Idiotype-specific $T_S$ cells have been found in a number of other experimental systems where the response of the strain to a particular antigen is normally dominated by one idiotype. The response of C57BL/6 mice to NP, for example, is dominated by the $NP^b$ idiotype (Section 10.3). Appropriate immunization of C57BL/6 mice induces a population of $T_S$ cells specific for the $NP^b$ idiotype. These cells express receptors for the idiotype; i.e., they are anti-idiotypic. Like the $CRI_A$ $T_S$ cells, they can bind to antibodies expressing the idiotype and, in the presence of complement, be lysed by them.

**Figure 15.21**   Results of the adoptive transfer of T cells on the production of $CRI_A$-positive antibodies in A/J mice immunized with ABA–KLH. The T cell suspensions were prepared from A/J mice treated with anti-$CRI_A$ antibodies before they were immunized with ABA–KLH. T suppressor cells were isolated by having them form rosettes with RBCs coated with Fab fragments of $CRI_A$-positive anti-ABA antibodies. The $CRI_A$ component of the anti-ABA response was measured in a radioimmunoassay using the serum from the recipients to displace $^{125}$I-anti-ABA from rabbit anti-$CRI_A$ antibodies. [Based on F. L. Owen et al., *J. Exp. Med.* 145:1559, 1977.]

| Cell suspension | Total anti-ABA (mg/ml) | $CRI_A$-positive anti-ABA |
|---|---|---|
| Unfractionated T cells | 1.3 | +/− |
| T minus $T_S$ | 1.4 | + + + + |
| $T_S$ | 1.8 | +/− |

Antigen-specific $T_S$ cells could exert their effect on either B cells or $T_H$ cells, and evidence for both types of interaction has been found. With either target, the $T_S$ cell probably binds to one determinant on the antigen while the $T_H$ or B cell binds to a second determinant. Using cloned $T_S$ and $T_H$ cells, Asano and Hodes have found that suppression of the anti-TNP response of B cells requires that the $T_S$ cells interact with *both* the $T_H$ and B cells. They cultured TNP-primed B cells with a clone of KLH-specific $T_S$ cells and a clone of $T_H$ cells specific for fowl gamma globulin (FGG). Suppression of the anti-TNP response of the B cells occurred only when the cell mixture was cultured with a conjugate containing all three antigens covalently linked (TNP – FGG – KLH). Mixtures such as TNP – KLH with FGG – KLH did not work.

We would expect **idiotype-specific $T_S$** cells to be able to react with targets expressing the idiotype. Thus id⁺ B cells should be targets of id-specific (i.e., anti-idiotypic) $T_S$ cells, and this has been demonstrated

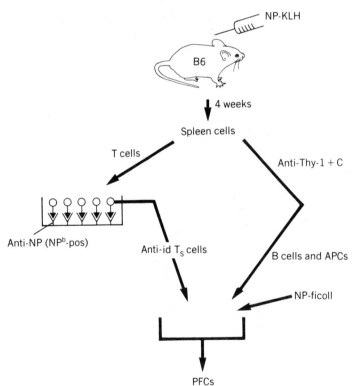

**Figure 15.22**   Idiotype-specific $T_S$ cells. The NPᵇ-positive anti-NP B cells are suppressed by $T_S$ cells that bind to NPᵇ-positive antibodies. These $T_S$ cells are Ly-2⁺ and seem to act directly on id⁺ B cells. B cells were removed from the T-cell preparation by allowing them to adhere to rabbit anti-mouse immunoglobulin antibodies. The NPᵇ-positive plaques are shown as the % of total anti-NP PFCs. [Based on D. H. Sherr et al., *J. Immunol.* **133**:1142, 1984.]

| T cells | NPᵇ-positive PFCs (%) |
|---|---|
| None | 40 |
| Unfractionated | 8 |
| NPᵇ-adherent | 6 |
| NPᵇ-nonadherent | 43 |

(Figure 15.22). In this case, NP-primed B cells respond to a T-independent form of NP (NP-ficoll) with plaque-forming cells many of which secrete antibodies that are $NP^b$ positive. When purified $NP^b$-adhering T cells are added to the culture, the production of $NP^b$ positive plaques is suppressed. There are no $T_H$ cells to serve as potential targets because (1) the NP-primed responding spleen cells are treated with anti-Thy-1 and C to remove all T cells, and (2) $T_H$ cells would not adhere to the immunoadsorbent used to purify the $T_S$ cells.

Idiotype-specific $T_S$ cells may also act on a third type of $T_S$ cell designated $T_S3$. Such a cell has been identified in mice whose response to a particular antigen is dominated by one idiotype (e.g., C57BL/6 to NP; A/J mice to ABA). The $T_S3$ cell is antigen specific ($id^+$) and seems to require the anti-idiotypic $T_S$ cell (or its factor) in order to be activated. $T_S3$ cells have been detected in both humoral and cell-mediated immune responses. In the latter case, the target is the $T_D$ cell.

## 15.12 Suppressor Factors

There is a great deal of experimental evidence that $T_S$ cells synthesize soluble factors ($T_SF$) that can mimic many or all of the effects of intact $T_S$ cells. The existence of a $T_SF$ can be (and was) shown by using the same experimental system shown in Figure 15.16. The only difference is that the mice immunized with DNP–KLH receive cell *extracts* — with or without further treatment — instead of cell suspensions (Figure 15.23). The extract is prepared by disrupting thymus or spleen cells taken from KLH-primed mice. Such an extract is almost as suppressive of the anti-DNP response as a suspension of intact cells (compare the results in Figure 15.16). The effect is specific. The extract has no suppressive effect on an animal's response to DNP–BGG, and extracts of BGG-primed spleen cells have no suppressive effect on the response to DNP–KLH. The cells producing the $T_SF$ belong to the $Ly-2^+$ subset of T cells. Presumably they are the $T_S$ cells themselves.

With an extract in hand, the next step is to characterize the properties of the active material. This $T_SF$ binds specifically to the antigen, KLH, for which it is specific. When the cell extract is passed through an immunoadsorbent column containing KLH, its activity is removed (Figure 15.23). This would, of course, occur if the active factor were anti-KLH antibodies. But that hardly seems possible. For one thing, the factor is too small: its molecular weight is approximately 70,000 — much smaller than an antibody molecule. Furthermore, antisera raised against mouse immunoglobulins fail to remove the activity. However, anti-I-J serum completely removes the suppressive activity of $T_SF$. Thus this $T_SF$ appears not to be an immunoglobulin even though it binds specifically to antigen.

T cell hybridomas have been made that secrete this KLH-specific $T_SF$. Taniguchi et al. have found that the factor consists of two polypeptide chains linked by disulfide bridges. One chain reacts with anti-I-J antibodies; the other chain binds the antigen (KLH).

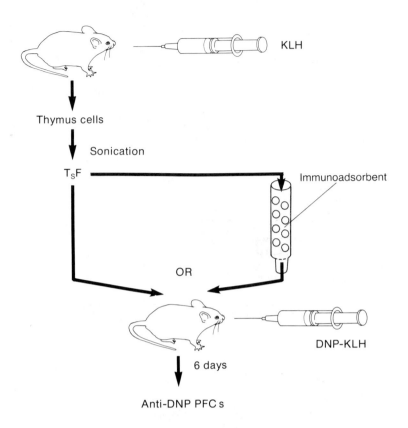

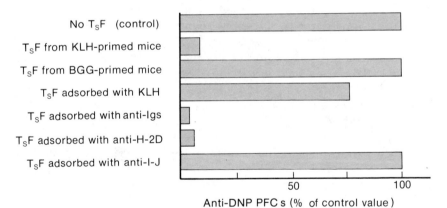

**Figure 15.23** Preparation and activity of a KLH-specific suppressor factor. The suppressive activity of the factor (which could also be prepared from spleen cells) is removed by absorption with antigen (KLH) or with anti-I-J antibodies. However, the factor was not absorbed by a rabbit antimouse immunoglobulin serum nor by an antiserum specific for the H-2D determinants of BALB/c mice. The anti-I-J serum was prepared by immunizing B10.A(3R) mice with B10.A(5R) cells (Figure 15.24). [From T. Takemori and T. Tada, *J. Exp. Med.* **142**:1241, 1975, and T. Tada et al., *J. Exp. Med.* **144**:713, 1976.]

Several other groups of investigators have isolated T suppressor factors. In some cases, these, too, consist of molecules of approximately 70 kd made up of two S—S linked chains: one that binds the antigen and one that reacts with anti-I-J antibodies. Both chains are necessary for the molecule to be active. In other cases, the active factor is a single polypeptide chain.

T suppressor factors mimic the activities of the cells that produce them. Thus, a factor from $T_{SI}$ cells induces a population of effector $T_S$ cells. Similarly, factors harvested from effector $T_S$ cells exert their suppressive effect immediately. In fact, the properties of suppressor factors suggest that they represent a solubilized form of the receptor for antigen on the $T_S$ cell. But the factors do not resemble immunoglobulins (the B cell receptor for antigen). On the other hand, neither their structure nor their behavior suggests that these molecules are like the antigen/MHC-binding receptors of other subsets of T cells. Are we, then, looking at yet a third category of specific antigen-binding receptors found on the cells of the immune system?

When tested both in vivo and in vitro, T suppressor factors seem capable of carrying out all the functions of the cells that produce them. It is possible, in fact, that $T_S$ cells naturally accomplish their activities through the release of these factors. Although some factors, such as the KLH-specific factor in Figure 15.23, are prepared by disrupting the cells that synthesize it, many workers have used factors that are released spontaneously into the cell culture medium.

## 15.13 The I-J Enigma

Both $T_S$ cells and the factors they produce react with anti-I-J antibodies. These antibodies bind to most of the suppressor factors that have been studied. They also bind to $T_S$ cells and, when complement is present, lyse them efficiently.

Anti-I-J antibodies are generated by immunizing one mouse strain with cells from a second strain thought to differ from the first in a limited region of H-2 designated I-J. For example, immunization of B10.A(3R) mice with cells from B10.A(5R) mice produces an antiserum designated anti-I-J$^k$. The reciprocal immunization yields an anti-I-J$^b$ serum. Each of these strains is the result of an intra-H-2 recombination that occurred while strain A mice *(kkkkkd)* were being backcrossed to C57BL/10 mice *(bbbbbb)* to produce congenic strains (Section 3.5). In both cases, the recombination occurred between the I-A and I-E subregions (Figure 3.12). Thus both strains appeared to be *bbbbkd* for the K, $A_\beta$, $A_\alpha$, $E_\beta$, $E_\alpha$, and D loci, respectively (Figure 15.24). Since both strains have the same genetic background (C57BL/10), it was only logical to assume that the antibodies were directed against one or more molecules encoded in a portion of chromosome 6 between the I-A and I-E subregions. On this basis, a new subregion, I-J, was established.

The B10.A(3R) strain was assumed to have retained the I-J$^b$ subregion of the C57BL/10 parent while a crossover further to the left had left the

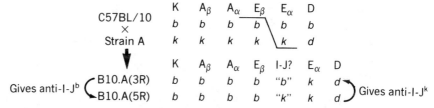

Figure 15.24   Derivation of the congenic recombinant inbred B10.A(3R) and B10.A(5R) mouse strains. Reciprocal immunization with each other's cells is used to elicit anti-I-J antisera. The only apparent genetic difference in these congenic strains was thought to occur between the $E_\beta$ and $E_\alpha$ loci, and this region was designated I-J. However, no structural genes have been detected in the DNA of this region.

B10.A(5R) mice with an I-$J^k$ subregion derived from the strain A parent. A number of other recombinant strains have also been found to yield anti-I-J serum. (The region between I-A and I-E appears to be unusually prone to recombination.)

The genetic evidence for I-J has not been supported by molecular analysis. Examination of the DNA in the I region of various mouse strains has failed to provide any evidence of a structural gene that could encode an I-J molecule. In fact, there does not seem to be any difference whatsoever between the I region DNA of the B10.A(3R) and B10.A(5R) strains. So what can account for the generation of such potent antisera by these two strains which appear to be identical in H-2 as well as in their background genes? A great many possibilities have been suggested (see, for example, reference 4 at the end of the chapter), but as yet the enigma of I-J remains unsolved.

## 15.14   Summary

In this chapter we have examined mechanisms by which the magnitude of immune responses—both humoral and cell mediated—are subjected to homeostatic control. The introduction of antigen appears to induce two distinct pathways: one leading to immunity, the other to its suppression. Immunity can be expressed as the product of B cells (antibodies) or as a T-cell mediated activity like DTH. Both can be suppressed by antibodies and also by a pathway of suppressor T cells and their factors.

In the case of humoral immunity, the very production of antibody molecules can act in a homeostatic fashion to suppress further production of those molecules. Two mechanisms appear to be at work. (1) By interfering with the binding of antigen to antigen-specific clones of ABCs, their participation in further synthesis of antibody is blocked. (2) The accumulation of antibodies bearing a particular idiotype induces the synthesis of anti-idiotypic antibodies and subsequent suppression of the idiotype.

Among the idiotopes expressed by an antibody molecule is the antigen-binding site itself. The V regions of the subset of anti-idiotypic antibodies able to bind this idiotope must express a structure complementary to it. Thus this subset of anti-idiotypic antibodies represents an "internal image" of the antigen. For example, anti-idiotypic antibodies that represent the internal image of a hormone may be able to mimic the effects of the hormone. The internal image set of anti-idiotypic antibodies can be used to elicit a set of anti-anti-idiotypic antibodies (Ab3) some of which have the antigen-binding properties of Ab1. Thus, immunization with Ab2 can, at least in some cases, substitute for antigen in eliciting protective antibodies.

Suppression of both humoral immunity and CMI can be mediated by T-suppressor ($T_S$) cells. $T_S$ cells differ from the other subsets of T cells in being able to bind to soluble antigen (as B cells do). In the mouse, effector $T_S$ cells are Ly-2$^+$; in the human they are CD8$^+$. Effector $T_S$ cells can suppress humoral immunity by acting directly on either or both $T_H$ and B cells. The induction of effector $T_S$ cells depends on helper T cells ($T_{SI}$ or $T_S1$). Murine $T_{SI}$ cells are Ly-1$^+$ but are distinct from the $T_H$ cells that enhance immunity. Unlike $T_H$ cells, they can bind soluble antigen, and they react with anti-I-J antibodies.

Idiotype-specific $T_S$ cells can be detected in certain inbred animals whose normal humoral response is dominated by antibodies of a particular idiotype (e.g., the $CRI_A$ idiotype on the anti-ABA antibodies of A/J mice). Idiotype-specific $T_S$ cells can act directly on id$^+$ B cells or on a population of id$^+$, antigen-specific $T_S$ cells ($T_S3$).

Many, if not all, the effects of the cells in the T suppressor pathway can be mediated by soluble factors (TsF) liberated by the cells.

## ADDITIONAL READING

1. Eichmann, K., et al., "Absolute Frequencies of Lipopolysaccharide-Reactive B Cells Producing A5A Idiotype in Unprimed, Streptococcal A Carbohydrate-Primed, Anti-A5A Idiotype-Sensitised and Anti-A5A Idiotype Suppressed A/J Mice," *J. Exp. Med.* **146**:1436, 1977. (Reprinted in V. L. Sato and M. L. Gefter, *Cellular Immunology*, Addison-Wesley Publishing Co., Inc., Reading, MA, 1982.)

2. Gershon, R. K., and K. Kondo, "Infectious Immunological Tolerance," *Immunology* **21**:903, 1971. (Reprinted in V. L. Sato and M. L. Gefter, *Cellular Immunology*, Addison-Wesley Publishing Co., Inc., Reading, MA, 1982.) The discovery of T suppressor cells.

3. Hart, D. A., et al., "Suppression of Idiotypic Specificities in Adult Mice by Administration of Antiidiotypic Antibody," *J. Exp. Med.* **135**:1293, 1972. (Reprinted in V. L. Sato and M. L. Gefter, *Cellular Immunology*, Addison-Wesley Publishing Co., Inc., Reading, MA, 1982.)

4. Hayes, Colleen E., et al., "Chromosome 4 *Jt* Gene Controls Murine T Cell Surface I-J Expression," *Science* **223**:559, 1984.

5. Jerne, N. K., "Towards a Network Theory of the Immune System," *Ann. Immunol. (Inst. Pasteur)* **125** C:373, 1974. (Reprinted in V. L. Sato and M. L. Gefter, *Cellular Immunology*, Addison-Wesley Publishing Co., Inc., Reading, MA, 1982.)

6. McNamara, Mary K., et al., "Monoclonal Idiotype Vaccine Against *Streptococcus pneumoniae* Infection," *Science* **226**:1325, 1984.

7. Owen, F. L., et al., "Presence on Idiotype-Specific Suppressor T Cells of Receptors That Interact with Molecules Bearing the Idiotype," *J. Exp. Med.* **145**:1559, 1977. (Reprinted in V. L. Sato and M. L. Gefter, *Cellular Immunology*, Addison-Wesley Publishing Co., Inc., Reading, MA, 1982.)

8. Rodkey, L. S., "Studies of Idiotypic Antibodies. Production and Characterization of Autoantiidiotypic Antisera," *J. Exp. Med.* **139**:712, 1974.

9. Siskind, G. W., et al., "Studies on the Control of Antibody Synthesis. II. Effect of Antigen Dose and of Suppression by Passive Antibody on the Affinity of the Antibody Response," *J. Exp. Med.* **127**:55, 1968.

10. Takemori, T., and T. Tada, "Properties of Antigen-Specific Suppressive T-Cell Factor in the Regulation of Antibody Response of the Mouse. I. *In vivo* Activity and Immunochemical Characterizations," *J. Exp. Med.* **142**:1241, 1975. (Reprinted in V. L. Sato and M. L. Gefter, *Cellular Immunology*, Addison-Wesley Publishing Co., Inc., Reading, MA, 1982.)

11. Taniguchi, M., et al., "Functional and Molecular Organisation of an Antigen-Specific Suppressor Factor from a T-Cell Hybridoma," *Nature* **283**:227, 1980. (Reprinted in V. L. Sato and M. L. Gefter, *Cellular Immunology*, Addison-Wesley Publishing Co., Inc., Reading, MA, 1982.)

12. Uhr, J. W., and Joyce B. Baumann, "Antibody Formation. I. The Suppression of Antibody Formation by Passively Administered Antibody," *J. Exp. Med.* **113**:935, 1961.

13. Walker, J. G., and G. W. Siskind, "Studies on the Control of Antibody Synthesis. Effect of Antibody Affinity upon Its Ability to Suppress Antibody Formation," *Immunology* **14**:21, 1968.

14. Yamauchi, K., et al., "Analysis of Antigen-Specific, Ig-Restricted Cell-Free Material Made by I-J$^+$ Ly-1 Cells (Ly-1 TsiF) That Induces Ly-2$^+$ Cells to Express Suppressive Activity," *Eur. J. Immunol.* **11**:905, 1981.

# Immunological Tolerance

## 16.1  Introduction

Immunological tolerance is a specific lack of immune responsiveness to an antigen induced by prior contact with the antigen. In considering this definition, perhaps it will help to give examples of what tolerance is *not*.

Tolerance is not the failure of an animal to be immunized following exposure to a general immunosuppressive agent like x-irradiation or a cytotoxic drug. Such treatments suppress all immune reactivity, and thus our criterion of specificity is not met. (However, general immunosuppressants may be useful adjuncts in the induction of immune tolerance.) Tolerance is not the failure to respond to a particular antigen because of an inherited genetic defect (e.g. an Ir gene). Thus the inability of strain 13 guinea pigs to respond to DNP coupled to poly-L-lysine is not an example of tolerance. This inability exists prior to contact with the antigen. Thus, immunological tolerance is really the converse of immunity; it shares with immunity the characteristics of specificity and memory.

Tolerance occurs in both antibody-mediated and cell-mediated immune responses. In the following sections of this chapter, we shall first examine how humoral tolerance is induced and how it can be broken. We shall then turn our attention to possible mechanisms by which tolerance is created and maintained. Subsequent sections will examine the special features of tolerance in the cell-mediated branch of the immune system and possible mechanisms that may operate there. Finally, we shall examine those special aspects of tolerance that (1) permit a mother to tolerate her histoincompatible fetus (for nine months or so) and (2) normally keep us from mounting an immune response against our own molecules (self-tolerance).

## 16.2 Humoral Tolerance

The first systematic study of humoral tolerance was made by Lloyd Felton and his colleagues in the 1940s. They used pneumococcal polysaccharides as antigens. One week after receiving 0.5 $\mu$g of purified pneumococcal polysaccharide of a given type, a mouse can normally withstand challenge with $10^5 - 10^6$ minimum lethal doses (MLD) of virulent pneumococci of the *same type*. However, if the mouse is first treated with a 1000-fold larger dose (0.5 mg) of the polysaccharide, a subsequent dose of 0.5 $\mu$g is no longer able to immunize the animal. The mouse now succumbs to as little as one MLD of virulent pneumococci. The larger dose has tolerized the mouse. The tolerance is type specific as is immunity. Thus a mouse tolerized by 0.5 mg. of the type 3 pneumococcal polysaccharide can later be successfully immunized with small doses (0.5 $\mu$g) of type 1 or type 2 pneumococcal polysaccharide. Notice the operational definition of tolerance used in this work: the inability of an animal to be immunized by a normally immunizing dose of an antigen following a tolerogenic dose of the same antigen.

### Factors Predisposing to Tolerance

*Antigen dose.* The tolerance induced by large doses of antigen is called **high zone tolerance.** High zone tolerance has been demonstrated with many antigens, including T-dependent antigens like soluble proteins as well as T-independent (TI) antigens like the pneumococcal polysaccharides.

Tolerance to TD antigens can also be induced by repeated injections of subimmunogenic doses of the antigen. The resulting tolerance is called, appropriately enough, **low zone tolerance.** A number of factors beside dose play a role in the ease with which tolerance—rather than immunity—results.

*Nature of the Antigen.* The response to protein antigens is critically dependent upon the physical state of the antigen. Preparations containing aggregates of protein molecules (the usual situation in solutions of proteins) are highly immunogenic. However, if all aggregates are carefully removed, the preparation becomes tolerogenic. A routine method for removing aggregates is to subject the protein solution to ultracentrifugation and to use the resulting supernatant. Deaggregated proteins are less likely to be ingested by macrophages and thus may interact directly with B and/or $T_H$ cells without the immunogenic signals provided by macrophage processing (see Section 12.1). In fact, the serum from an animal that was previously injected with an immunizing dose of antigen has a powerful tolerogenic effect when injected into a second animal. This is because macrophages remove the aggregated (immunogenic) antigen from the circulation and leave only the monomeric (tolerogenic) form of the antigen in the serum.

Antigens that are difficult for the host to degrade are apt to be excellent tolerogens. The type 3 pneumococcal polysaccharide and such synthetic antigens as the copolymer of D-glutamic acid and D-lysine are not degraded in mammalian tissue. Thus they remain in the tissues long after administration, and this persistence seems to play an important part in the maintenance of tolerance toward them.

Haptens, by themselves, are not immunogenic (Section 1.4). In fact, when injected intravenously, haptens may induce a state of tolerance. Tolerance to haptens such as TNP and NIP is also routinely achieved by injection of the hapten coupled to nonimmunogenic carriers. These include (1) strong tolerogens like the pneumococcal polysaccharides, (2) "self" molecules such as the recipient's own gamma globulins, and (3) syngeneic cells. (Figures 15.18 and 15.19 show the use of hapten-conjugated syngeneic spleen cells for inducing $T_s$ cells.)

The administration of antigen along with an **adjuvant** induces immunity instead of tolerance. One of the most widely used and potent adjuvants is Freund's "complete adjuvant." This is an emulsion of the antigen solution in mineral oil to which killed mycobacteria are added. The emulsion prolongs the release of the antigen to the lymphoid tissues and the mycobacteria induce an intense inflammatory response. Freund's complete adjuvant is particularly effective at stimulating cell mediated immune responses as well as humoral responses to weakly immunogenic molecules.

*Site of Administration.* Antigens that are immunogenic when given to the animal by one route (e.g., subcutaneously or intramuscularly) may be tolerogenic when given by another (such as intravenously or intraperitoneally). The feeding of antigen is especially apt to lead to tolerance rather than immunity (and may provide some basis for such items of folklore as eating poison ivy leaves to prevent allergy to the plant). Probably any method of antigen administration that tends to bypass macrophages predisposes the animal to a tolerogenic response.

*Immunological Immaturity.* Animals are far easier to tolerize before or shortly after birth than they are later. Adult animals that are immunosuppressed or otherwise immunodeficient are more easily tolerized than their normal counterparts. Exposure to antigen when an animal is beginning to recover from irradiation often leads to tolerance of that antigen. In this case as well as in the case of neonatal animals, it is probably a matter of the immaturity of the emerging antigen-sensitive cells. It has often been observed that immature B cells are much more easily tolerized than are mature B cells. The mechanism underlying this difference is uncertain.

### Tolerance Is Directed Toward Specific Determinants

Tolerance, like immunity, is not directed against the entire antigen but only at specific determinants on the antigen. Let's look at one example. A common way to produce anti-idiotypic antibodies is to immunize another species with the idiotype. Section 15.6 describes how Eichmann used guinea pigs to raise anti-id serum against the A5A idiotype in A/J mice. The drawback of such a procedure is that the guinea pig responds not only to idiotypic determinants on the mouse immunoglobulin but to a mosaic of isotypic and any allotypic determinants as well. This is because all of these are foreign to the guinea pig. To make the resulting antiserum specific for the idiotype, it must then be absorbed with pooled A/J serum to remove antibodies directed against isotypic and allotypic determinants. An alternative procedure is to tolerize the guinea pig to the pooled immunoglobulins of the donor species. When the idiotypic antibodies are then given in immunogenic form, the animal is able to respond only to the idiotypic determinant(s) on the molecules. Although tolerized to most of the molecule, it is able to respond to determinants that were not involved in the tolerization process.

### Both B Cells and T Cells Can Be Tolerized

The collaboration of B and T cells in the response to such antigens as HGG raises the question of whether one or both cell types become tolerized. Weigle and his colleagues solved this problem using the protocol shown in Figure 16.1. As you can see, the answer turns out to be "both." Neither the B cells nor the T cells taken from a tolerized donor

**Figure 16.1** Demonstration by adoptive transfer that both B cells and T cells can be tolerized. HGG = human gamma globulin. Deaggregated HGG is tolerogenic; aggregated HGG is immunogenic. Normal animals receiving the dose of aggregated HGG used in these experiments produce some 74,000 PFCs per spleen. [From J. M. Chiller et al., *Proc. Natl. Acad. Sci. USA* **65**:551, 1970.]

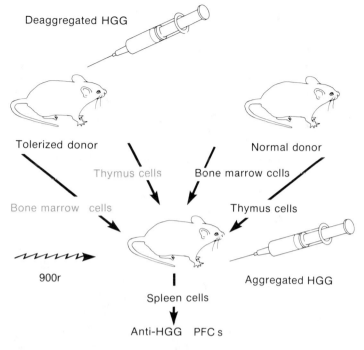

RESULTS

| Bone marrow | Thymus | PFC/spleen |
|---|---|---|
| Normal | Normal | 2250 |
| Normal | Tolerized | 0 |
| Tolerized | Normal | 0 |
| Tolerized | Tolerized | 0 |

can collaborate with normal cells when adoptively transferred into an irradiated recipient.

Although both B cells and $T_H$ cells can be tolerized, the kinetics and sensitivity to tolerization are different for the two cell types. By testing T and B cells at various times after tolerization, Weigle's group was able to show that two weeks are required for B cells to become fully tolerant and by the end of seven weeks, this tolerance is completely broken (Figure 16.2). $T_H$ cells, on the other hand, become rapidly unresponsive upon exposure to the tolerogen (deaggregated HGG) and this tolerance remains unbroken after many weeks.

As for sensitivity, they found that even at their highest doses (2.5 mg) of tolerogen, B cells were not fully tolerized whereas $T_H$ cells were completely tolerized at all doses used, even ones as low as 0.1 mg (Figure 16.3). These results (and others like them) suggest that high zone tolerance eliminates both B and $T_H$ cells while low zone tolerance acts on $T_H$ cells only.

Another useful way of detecting the end of B cell tolerance while $T_H$ cells remain tolerized is to give the immunogen either in T-independent form or along with a B cell mitogen like LPS. Thus mice that are still

**419**

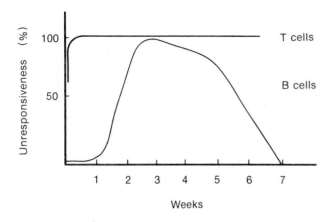

**Figure 16.2** Differences between thymus (T) cells and bone marrow (B) cells in the speed of tolerance induction and in the duration of the tolerant state. Tolerance was induced and each cell population was tested using the procedures shown in Figure 16.1. [From J. M. Chiller et al., *Science* **171**:813, 1971.]

unresponsive to aggregated HGG 13 weeks after being tolerized by deaggregated HGG are able to give a perfectly normal anti-HGG PFC response when LPS is given along with the immunogen. Or, to cite another example, injections of DNP–POL (a TI antigen) can reveal the presence of anti-DNP B cells in mice tolerized earlier with DNP–HGG. The interpretation in each case is that B cells are the first to recover from tolerance. However, their potential for antibody synthesis can be revealed only by providing them with a substitute for the $T_H$ cells that remain tolerized.

### Breaking Tolerance

The discussion above shows that time is one factor needed for breaking tolerance. How much time seems to be dictated by the dose of tolerogen used and the ease with which it can be catabolized and eliminated from

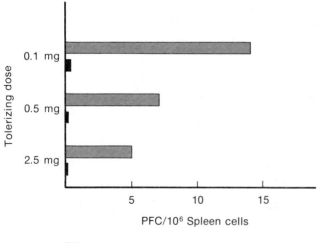

**Figure 16.3** Differential sensitivity of bone marrow and thymus cells to a tolerogen (deaggregated HGG). Mice receiving normal bone marrow and normal thymus cells produced approximately 16 PFCs per $10^6$ spleen cells. The experimental protocol is shown in Figure 16.1. [Based on J. M. Chiller et al., *Science* **171**:813, 1971.]

▨ = Tolerizing dose given to bone marrow donors only.

■ = Tolerizing dose given to thymocyte donors only.

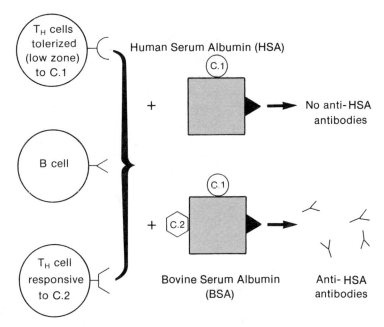

**Figure 16.4** Mechanism by which tolerance to a thymus-dependent antigen could be broken by giving a cross-reacting antigen. This mechanism assumes that at the time the cross-reacting antigen is given, the animal's B cells are no longer tolerized.

the body. So long as substantial amounts of undegraded tolerogen remain, tolerance persists.

Tolerance to TD antigens can also be broken by giving the animal a cross-reacting form of the antigen. Thus a rabbit tolerized to human serum albumin (HSA) will begin to synthesize anti-HSA antibodies when immunized with bovine serum albumin (BSA). This interesting result makes sense when we recall that proteins display a mosaic of determinants, each of which can serve as a haptenic determinant (for B cells) and as a carrier determinant (for $T_H$ cells) — see Figure 12.8. After B cell tolerance to HSA has waned, the animal is still unresponsive because the $T_H$ cells specific for each determinant on HSA are still tolerized. BSA shares some determinants with HSA as well as having some of its own. The *latter* can trigger nontolerized $T_H$ cells. These turn on all those no longer tolerized B cells that are specific for determinants shared by BSA and HSA (Figure 16.4).

## 16.3  Mechanisms of B Cell Tolerance

Many theories have been proposed to account for B cell tolerance. These fall roughly into two categories.

1. Antigen reactive B cells are present in the tolerant animal but an extrinsic agent blocks their activity. This suggests that continuing tolerance depends upon the continuing presence of some inhibitory agent.
2. All the B cells specific for the tolerogen have been eliminated or permanently inactivated. This intrinsic B cell defect has been called

**421**

clonal deletion. It suggests that B cell tolerance merely reflects the absence of the appropriate B cells.

Adoptive transfer provides a technique with which to try to discriminate between these two possibilities. If an injection of cells from a normal animal restores immunocompetence to a tolerized animal, we conclude that the normal cells have replaced the deleted B cells in the recipient; if not, we conclude that the normal cells have in their turn fallen under the action of inhibiting influences in the tolerant recipient. As we shall see, the results of many such experiments suggest that both mechanisms can play a part.

## Tolerance Caused by Residual Antigen

One simple explanation for the failure to detect serum antibodies in a tolerized animal is that they become complexed with residual antigen as fast as they are formed. This phenomenon (sometimes called the "treadmill effect") has been demonstrated many times. One example can be seen in Figure 16.6. But if that were all there was to tolerance, then antibody-secreting cells would be present in tolerized animals. Therefore tolerized animals should produce normal numbers of PFCs when their spleen or lymph node cells are tested in hemolytic plaque assays. But they don't. In the tolerized animal, there is a marked reduction in PFCs, not simply a reduction in the titer of circulating antibodies.

## Receptor Blockade

One of the earliest events in the induction of a humoral response is the binding of antigen to those B cells bearing receptors for the antigen. Following binding, the antigen is "capped" and engulfed by endocytosis (see Section 8.7). Tolerogenic forms of antigen also bind to B cells. However, a number of laboratories have reported that the binding of a tolerogen is not followed by capping and endocytosis of the antigen – receptor complexes. As long as the cells remain with tolerogen stuck on their surface, their receptors are unavailable for binding to an immunogenic form of the antigen. This is called, appropriately enough, *receptor blockade*.

## Clonal Anergy

Physical occupation of the antigen receptors by tolerogen is probably not the whole story of tolerant B cells because subsequent removal of the tolerogen may not restore immunocompetence. Exhaustive washing, cultivating the cells in antigen-free medium, stripping the blockaded receptors away with proteolytic enzymes like pronase, and using anti-immunoglobulins to bind to the receptor and trigger capping and endocytosis have all been used successfully to remove tolerizing antigen. And still the cells often remain tolerized. Perhaps the binding of tolerogen to the ABCs transmits some form of permanent inactivating signal to the cell which cannot be reversed by later removal of the tolerogen.

Nossal and Pike have demonstrated that tolerant mice continue to harbor B cells capable of *binding* an immunogenic form of the antigen but the cells cannot be activated by it. These workers have coined the term *clonal anergy* (unresponsiveness) for this effect. As far as the tolerant animal is concerned, it is equivalent to clonal deletion.

## Tolerance Mediated by $T_S$ Cells

If it were possible to tolerize a normal animal by injecting it with cells from a tolerized donor, this would be strong evidence for the existence of an active suppressor mechanism in tolerized animals. Although it is very difficult to tolerize normal mice in this way, it is sometimes possible to do so if huge doses (e.g., $250 \times 10^6$) of "tolerant" cells are used. The adoptive transfer of tolerance can be demonstrated more easily by protocols similar to the one shown in Figure 16.5. In this case, 15 million tolerized spleen cells greatly suppress the response of the same number of normal spleen cells when the mixture is given to an irradiated, immunized recipient. The suppression is specific: the response to an unrelated antigen is

**Figure 16.5** Suppression of normal spleen cells by spleen cells from tolerized donors. Treatment with anti-Thy-1 plus complement shows that the suppressor cells are T cells ($T_S$). FGG = fowl gamma globulin. Spleen cells from donors tolerized to FGG had no suppressive effect on the recipient's ability to respond to unrelated antigens. [Based on A. Basten et al., *J. Exp. Med.* **140**:199, 1974.]

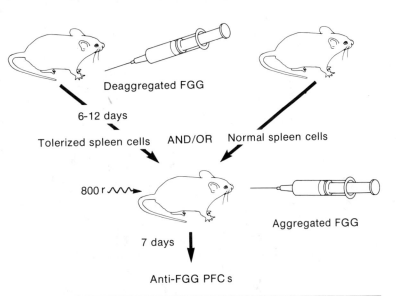

Deaggregated FGG

6-12 days

Tolerized spleen cells    AND/OR    Normal spleen cells

800 r

Aggregated FGG

7 days

Anti-FGG PFCs

| Donor spleen cells | PFC/spleen |
|---|---|
| $1.5 \times 10^7$ normal | 1195 |
| $1.5 \times 10^7$ tolerized | 105 |
| $1.5 \times 10^7$ normal + $1.5 \times 10^7$ tolerized | 30 |
| $1.5 \times 10^7$ normal + $1.5 \times 10^7$ tolerized cells treated with anti-$\theta$ + C | 4645 |

unimpaired. No suppression occurs if the tolerized suspension is first treated with anti-Thy-1 and complement. What we are looking at, of course, is another demonstration of the existence of T suppressor ($T_s$) cells.

Basten and his coworkers, who performed these experiments, also looked for the presence of antigen-binding cells (ABCs) in the tolerized and normal animals. They found no significant difference in the frequency of antigen-binding cells in the two groups. This reinforced their conviction that tolerance in this system could not be explained by the absence of antigen (FGG)-sensitive B cells, but was explained instead by the induction of a population of $T_s$ cells that blocked the production of anti-FGG PFCs.

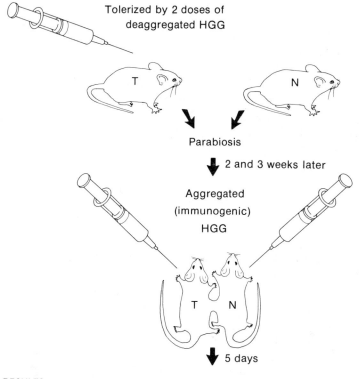

Tolerized by 2 doses of
deaggregated HGG

Parabiosis

2 and 3 weeks later

Aggregated
(immunogenic)
HGG

5 days

**Figure 16.6** A normal mouse can restore immunocompetence to its tolerized parabiotic partner. But note that restoration of immunocompetence is revealed only by examining individual spleen cells (PFCs). The titers of anti-HGG antibodies remain low because of the binding of antibodies to the large amount of residual antigen in the circulation. [Based on Susan Zolla and D. Naor, *J. Exp. Med.* **140**:1421, 1974.]

RESULTS

|  | Anti-HGG PFC in spleen of each partner | Anti-HGG titer in serum of each partner |
|---|---|---|
| Normal | +++ | ± |
| Tolerant | +++ | ± |
| Normal | ++ | ++ |
| Normal | ++ | ++ |
| Tolerant | ± | ± |
| Tolerant | ± | ± |

Most workers have failed to restore immune competence to tolerized animals by injections of normal cells. However, Zolla and Naor reported in 1974 that they were able to achieve the same effect through parabiosis of a normal animal with a tolerant one. In parabiosis, two animals are surgically united so that they share a common circulation. If suppression is mediated by some active agent, like $T_s$ cells, then both animals should become tolerant. If, on the other hand, tolerance results from the absence of certain cells, then both animals should show normal immunity. Zolla and Naor found the latter. When mice tolerized to HGG were linked by parabiosis to normal partners, each partner responded well to an immunogenic dose of aggregated HGG (Figure 16.6). Note, however, that the normal response of the previously tolerant partner was seen only when its spleen cells were examined in a hemolytic plaque assay. When the titers of the circulating antibodies were measured, normal–tolerant pairs appeared just as tolerant as tolerant–tolerant pairs (Figure 16.6). Here is an example of apparent tolerance occurring because large amounts of residual antigen in the tolerant animals (which these workers demonstrated) was soaking up anti-HGG antibodies as fast as they were released. Only by looking at the numbers of individual PFCs were Zolla and Naor able to show that the normal mouse was able to restore immunocompetence to its tolerant partner.

## Analysis of the Frequency of B Cell Precursors

The results of Zolla and Naor lend support to the view that tolerance results from the absence of antigen-specific B cells; i.e., clonal deletion. One way to test this notion is to examine the frequency of antigen-specific cells in normal (unprimed) and in tolerized animals. This can be done by enumerating the frequency of antigen-binding cells using radio-labeled antigen and autoradiography (see Section 8.3). Many laboratories have performed such studies but with contradictory results. Some groups (like Basten's) find that there are just as many specific antigen-binding B cells (ABCs) in tolerized as in normal animals. Others find a sharp reduction in the number of ABCs in tolerized animals.

There may be many reasons for such contrasting results. Until the issue can be resolved, perhaps we should turn instead to a *functional* analysis of the frequency of B cell precursors in tolerant animals. To support the concept of clonal deletion, we need evidence that tolerant animals have a lower frequency of precursor B cells capable of *responding* to the antigen than do normal animals. The technique of limiting dilution analysis provides such evidence. The technique (more fully described in Section 8.8) involves (1) setting up a series of dilutions of a cell suspension, (2) culturing aliquots of these dilutions with the antigen, and (3) scoring each culture as positive or negative. Negative cultures had no cells capable of responding to the antigen; positive cultures had at least one, perhaps more, responding cells. For statistical reasons, that cell dilution that yields 37% negative cultures establishes the frequency of responding cells in the original cell suspension (see Section 8.8).

When limiting dilution analysis is applied to a preparation of B cells

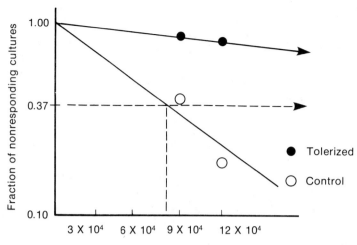

Figure 16.7 Reduction in the frequency of TNP-sensitive B cells in cultures treated with a tolerogenic dose of TNP–BSA. Untreated cultures had a precursor frequency of $1.25 \times 10^{-5}$. The principles of limiting dilution analysis are described in Section 8.8. [From C. Desaymard and H. Waldmann, *Nature* **264**:780, 1976.]

from CBA mice, approximately 1 in 80,000 B cells responds to TNP–LPS (a TI antigen) and develops into a clone of anti-TNP PFCs. However, when the B cells are precultured with a tolerogenic dose (0.5 mg/ml) of TNP–BSA, the precursor cell frequency declines to less than 1 in 400,000 cells (Figure 16.7). These results indicate that B cells exposed to tolerogenic (high zone) doses of antigen become intrinsically incapable of responding later to immunogenic doses of the antigen. Just how this inactivation occurs remains to be established.

So how are we to reconcile such conflicting data? Is tolerance the result of clonal deletion or an externally imposed active suppression? The answer appears to be that specific suppression of humoral immunity can be mediated by either or, more often, both mechanisms. Evidence of $T_S$ cells usually appears early in the induction of tolerance; clonal deletion without the presence of $T_S$ cells appears to be the rule later in the response. It may be that the role of $T_S$ cells is to provide an auxiliary suppression mechanism during the period when the balance between the induction of immunity and the induction of tolerance is being decided in favor of tolerance. If this turns out to be the case, perhaps the role of $T_S$ cells in tolerance is simply another — albeit extreme — expression of the regulatory role that they play in all immune responses (examined in Chapter 15). In that case, the concept of tolerance might better be restricted to the lack of antibody response that occurs when B (perhaps $T_H$) cells become irreversibly inactivated by exposure to tolerogen.

## 16.4 Tolerance in Cell-Mediated Responses

Immunological tolerance can be induced in all types of cell-mediated immune responses. Animals can be tolerized to conventional antigens to which they would otherwise mount a DTH response. Animals can be tolerized to alloantigens which would otherwise elicit graft rejection or a graft versus host reaction. Tolerance in the cell-mediated branch of the immune system can also be detected by such in vitro assays as the mixed lymphocyte reaction (MLR) and cell-mediated cytotoxicity (CMC).

One of the major rules in immunobiology is that immunocompetent animals reject foreign tissue. An exception to this rule emerged in the mid 40s as a result of a study by Owen of red cell antigens in cows. Owen found that fraternal (dizygotic) cattle twins often share exactly the same antigens on their red blood cells although the pattern of inheritance would make this an extremely unlikely event. It turned out that each twin was chimeric; i.e., each twin carried two populations of red cells — those of its own genotype and those of its twin's genotype. The chimerism was lifelong, indicating that the bone marrow was permanently inhabited by stem cells of each genotype. When the chimeric twins are of separate sexes, the female often remains sexually undeveloped and is called a *freemartin.* Freemartins, and blood cell chimerism, arise during fetal development if the blood vessels of the two placentas become joined. The shared circulation allows the bone marrow of each twin to be colonized by the stem cells of the other. Here, then, is a case of lifelong immunological tolerance of foreign tissue. It appears to be made possible by exposing the animal to allogeneic cells *before* the animal develops immunocompetence.

If these cattle twins are tolerant of each other's blood cells, what about other tissues? It turned out that skin grafts between such chimeras were retained. But for several reasons (only one of which is size) cattle are not ideal animals with which to explore transplantation tolerance. So attention quickly turned to mice.

**Figure 16.8** Two adult strain A mice with CBA skin grafts. Both recipients had been neonatally tolerized by intravenous injection of (CBA $\times$ A)F$_1$ lymphoid cells. The CBA skin is still healthy 60 days after grafting. [Courtesy of Rupert B. Billingham.]

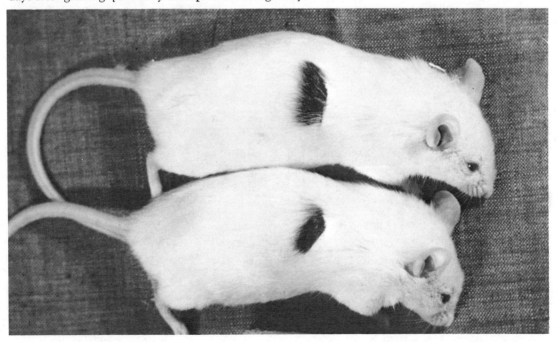

In 1953 Billingham, Brent, and Medawar reported that they had been able to induce lifelong tissue tolerance in mice (Figure 16.8). They accomplished this by mimicking the situation in the cattle twins: infusing allogeneic cells into newborn mice, a period before they have gained immunocompetence. Attempts to establish tolerance by injecting adult allogeneic cells into neonatal mice usually fail. The reason for this is that the donor cells *are* immunocompetent and they mount a graft vs. host reaction (GVHR) in the recipients that usually kills them. A GVHR can be avoided by using *embryonic* allogeneic cells, but the standard procedure is to use semiallogeneic cells (Figure 16.9). Thus, adult $(CBA \times A)F_1$

**Figure 16.9** *Left:* Induction of tolerance to CBA histocompatibility antigens. The use of semiallogeneic cells avoids the danger of a graft versus host reaction. *Right:* Demonstration of cellular chimerism in animals given semiallogeneic cells at the time of birth. The persistence of $(CBA \times A)F_1$ cells in the strain A adults is shown by the ability of their lymphoid cells to trigger accelerated rejection of CBA as well as A skin when transferred to mice of a third strain.

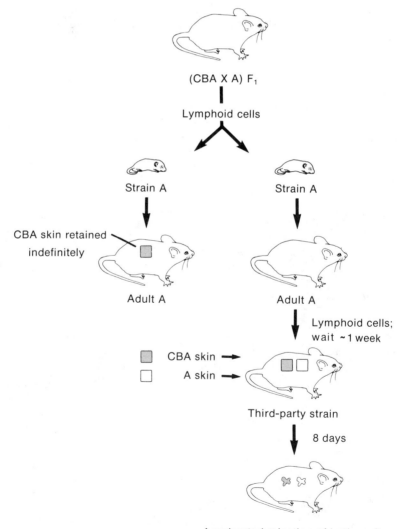

Accelerated rejection of both grafts

lymphoid cells (lymph node, spleen) can be safely injected into a new-born strain A mouse because the injected cells—though fully immunocompetent—see no foreign antigens. When the recipient matures, it is completely tolerant of the CBA histocompatibility antigens and accepts CBA skin grafts indefinitely (Figure 16.8).

Several features of allograft tolerance should be emphasized.

1. Allograft or transplantation tolerance, like tolerance to conventional antigens, is specific and is induced by the specific antigenic stimulus. An animal that maintains an allograft following generalized immunosuppression is not tolerant in the sense used here. Nor is the nude mouse that retains allografts and xenografts because of the absence of T-dependent immunity.
2. The maintenance of allograft tolerance depends upon the continuing presence of the alloantigens. This implies that tolerant mice—like Owen's cattle twins—are chimeras. This can be tested and turns out to be the case. Lymphoid cells from a strain A mouse neonatally tolerized to CBA cells will sensitize a mouse of a third strain to *both* A and CBA histocompatibility antigens (Figure 16.9) since both cell types now exist in the tolerized animal.

**Figure 16.10** Once tolerance has been broken by an injection of sensitized lymphoid cells (which ends the chimeric state), a normal animal regains immunocompetence *(left)*, a thymectomized animal does not *(right)*. This suggests that alloreactive T cells have been eliminated (clonal deletion) in chimeras and cannot be regenerated in the absence of a thymus. [Based on W. K. Silvers et al., *J. Exp. Med.* 142:1312, 1975.]

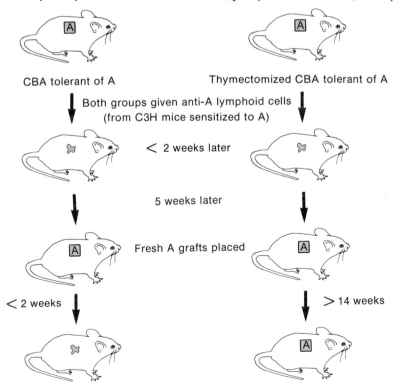

CBA tolerant of A    Thymectomized CBA tolerant of A

Both groups given anti-A lymphoid cells
(from C3H mice sensitized to A)

< 2 weeks later

5 weeks later

Fresh A grafts placed

< 2 weeks    > 14 weeks

Allograft tolerance is easily broken by the injection of lymphoid cells from an animal previously *sensitized* to the alloantigens. The lymph node cells from a C3H mouse that has already rejected a strain A graft will trigger the rejection of an A graft previously accepted by a CBA recipient (Figure 16.10). The rejection is mediated by the sensitized donor cells, not the cells of the CBA host. With the loss of the A graft and thus the loss of antigen stimulation, tolerance wanes, and the host gradually becomes capable of rejecting a strain A graft with its own cells. However, this restoration of immunocompetence requires the presence of the thymus. Thymectomized mice tolerant to strain A skin remain tolerant even after one A graft has been rejected by the adoptive transfer of sensitized cells (Figure 16.10).

## 16.5 Mechanisms of Tolerance in Cell-Mediated Responses

The proposals to explain humoral tolerance that are examined in Section 16.3 have also been proposed to explain cellular tolerance. These are (1) cells capable of reacting with the tolerated antigen have been deleted from the animal; (2) the cells are still there but they are prevented from attacking their target by serum-borne factors; (3) the cells are still there but they are inhibited by T suppressor cells. The third mechanism could work at the effector phase (like the $T_s2$ cells discussed in Section 15.9). Serum-borne factors (e.g., antibodies) or suppressor cells might also — or alternatively — induce tolerance by blocking the *induction* of immunocompetent T cells. This would be tantamount to a mechanism of clonal deletion.

When lymphoid cells from an animal tolerized to strain B are cultured with irradiated strain B cells, they fail to respond with proliferation

**Figure 16.11** T cells from tolerized rats fail to respond in mixed lymphocyte culture to the tolerated alloantigens. This failure could be caused by the absence of potentially reactive cells (clonal deletion) and/or the presence of T suppressor cells. [From R. N. Smith and J. C. Howard, *J. Immunol.* **125:**2289, 1980.]

| Responding cells[1] | Stimulator cells[2] | Incorporation of $^3$H-TdR (cpm) |
|---|---|---|
| Normal A | A | 1,000 |
| Normal A | B | 31,000 |
| Normal A | C | 23,000 |
| A tolerized to B[3] | A | 1,200 |
| A tolerized to B | B | 1,300 |
| A tolerized to B | C | 37,000 |

[1] Thoracic duct lymphocytes (T cells).
[2] Irradiated spleen cells.
[3] Thoracic duct lymphocytes harvested from animals neonatally tolerized to B (and able to retain a graft of B skin indefinitely).

(Figure 16.11). If tolerance were mediated by serum-borne factors, we would expect such cells — washed free of any serum of the donor — to respond vigorously. The lack of response is specific: cells from an animal tolerized to B respond vigorously to third-party (C) alloantigens (Figure 16.11).

Assays of cell-mediated cytotoxicity (CMC) tell the same story. Cytotoxic $T_C$ cells are not generated by strain B alloantigens in cell suspensions taken from animals made neonatally tolerant to these antigens. However, these animals have the precursor cells to mount vigorous CMC responses against third-party (C) cells (Figure 16.12). Again, if serum factors were interfering with the induction or expression of $T_C$ cells, then we would expect these cultured cells to respond well to the previously tolerated alloantigens once the cells were removed from the body of the donor and washed thoroughly.

Lymphoid cells from animals tolerant of B cannot — even after thorough washing — elicit a GVHR when injected into strain B recipients. All of these findings suggest either that there is an absence of reactive clones of T cells in neonatally tolerant animals or that suppressor cells are also present.

If tolerance *is* mediated by $T_S$ cells, then we would expect that when cells from tolerant animals are mixed with normal cells, the normal cells would be suppressed. In fact, this is very difficult to demonstrate: cells from fully tolerant animals do not reduce the activity of normal cells when the two are mixed together (group 4 in Figure 16.13).

It is possible, however, to demonstrate the existence of $T_S$ cells in tolerant animals. When cell suspensions from tolerized rats are injected into *irradiated* recipients, they greatly prolong the time that it takes the recipient to reject a graft carrying the tolerated antigens (group 3 in Figure 16.13).

**Figure 16.12**  Inability of thoracic duct lymphocytes from neonatally tolerized rats to generate substantial cell-mediated cytotoxicity against the tolerated alloantigen. [Based on R. N. Smith and J. C. Howard, *J. Immunol.* **125**:2289, 1980.]

| $T_C$ cells | Sensitized by | Target cells |
| --- | --- | --- |
| Normal A | A | A |
| Normal A | B | B |
| Normal A | C | C |
| A tolerant of B | A | A |
| A tolerant of B | B | B |
| A tolerant of B | C | C |
| Spontaneous release | | |

$^{51}$Cr release (%)

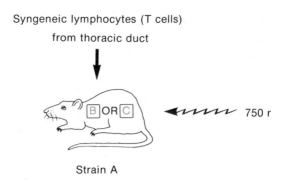

Strain A

| Thoracic duct lymphocytes | Graft | Average survival time (days) | Interpretation |
|---|---|---|---|
| None | B | 19 | Delayed rejection by irradiated hosts |
| | C | 19.5 | |
| T cells from normal donor | B | 10.5 | Normal rejection by reconstituted host |
| T cells from donor neonatally tolerized to B | B | 100+ | Neonatally tolerized donor contains B-specific $T_S$ cells |
| | C | 10.5 | |
| Mixture of normal AND tolerized cells | B | 13 | $T_S$ cells do not suppress normal cells |

**Figure 16.13** Adoptive transfer of allograft tolerance by antigen-specific T suppressor cells. [Based on R. N. Smith and J. C. Howard, *J. Immunol.* **125**:2289, 1980.]

So $T_S$ cells can be demonstrated in animals tolerant of an allograft. Chapter 15 describes examples of DTH responses that are suppressed by $T_S$ cells. Whether either or both of the examples here of $T_S$ cells should be considered as mechanisms for inducing and/or maintaining tolerance or simply homeostatic mechanisms for reducing the strength of the immune response is debatable.

A number of workers through the years have also found evidence for the presence of protective serum factors in animals that are tolerant of allografts. When lymphoid cells are removed from these animals, washed, and placed in mixed lymphocyte culture, they show strong alloreactivity. However, this reactivity is blocked by adding *serum* from the cell donor to the culture. The inhibitory factors in the serum may be free antibody or antigen – antibody complexes. In either case, the factors might exert their inhibitory effect by binding to the alloantigens on the surface of the stimulator/target cells and masking them from alloreactive cells.

Can these conflicting observations be reconciled? I think so. Serum-borne factors and/or $T_S$ cells that act to hold alloreactive cells in check are more likely to be found in situations of partial tolerance. They are found, for example, in animals given a tolerizing regimen as adults. In that case, these may simply be another example of the homeostatic regulatory mechanisms discussed in Chapter 15. There is also evidence that $T_S$ cells, perhaps even antibodies, can act to suppress the *appearance* of alloreactive cells. But how does this differ from clonal deletion?

It appears that animals neonatally tolerized to alloantigens specifically lack the T cells capable of reacting with those antigens. As long as the antigens persist, alloreactive clones fail to appear. This is clonal deletion. The mechanism by which the clones are deleted is not understood. Possibly $T_S$ cells play a role in blocking the formation of alloreactive cells from their precursors. Perhaps antibodies can play this role as well. However, if any alloreactive cells can be detected in an animal — albeit held in check by serum or $T_S$ cells — it is probably better to consider these cases as examples of a regulatory suppression of immunity rather than examples of true tolerance.

## 16.6 Tolerance of the Fetus

The fetus is an allograft. Except for inbred animals, the probability that a fetus will have the same set of histocompatibility antigens as its mother is virtually nil. Even in inbred animals, male fetuses differ from their mother at one minor histocompatibility locus responsible for the expression of the H-Y antigen on male tissue.

In many mammals, including humans and mice, the trophoblast cells of the placenta are in direct contact with the circulation of the mother. Why, then, does the mother not mount an attack against the fetus as she would against any other allograft?

There seems little doubt that the mother is potentially capable of such an attack. During pregnancy, the mother becomes sensitized to the paternal histocompatibility antigens expressed by the fetus. This sensitization is revealed by the formation of antibodies against HLA antigens. In fact, women that have borne several children of the same father are often excellent sources of anti-HLA serum for use in tissue typing. Pregnant women also develop cytotoxic T cells directed against paternal histocompatibility antigens. The effectiveness of these mechanisms is shown by how easily the female rejects skin grafts expressing the same paternal histocompatibility antigens as the fetus.

Not only does the mother not damage the fetus, but there is evidence that strong histocompatibility differences between them are actually beneficial to the fetus. In mice, a hybrid fetus (A × B) in a homozygous mother (A) develops a larger placenta than does a homozygous (A) fetus. If the mother has been presensitized to the foreign antigens (B), the placenta becomes larger still. Some complications in human pregnancies have been attributed to insufficient histocompatibility differences between mother and fetus.

What mechanism(s) protect fetal tissues from immunological attack? A number of explanations have been suggested to explain this puzzling but essential phenomenon.

1. The placenta is shielded from immunological attack. The major histocompatibility antigens appear very early in embryonic development. After implantation, however, the cells of the trophoblast lose

much of their immunogenicity. This seems to occur because the cells express class I but not class II antigens. The importance of class II antigens in the development of cell-mediated immunity is examined in Section 13.3

2. One of the major gene products expressed during embryonic development is alpha fetoprotein (AFP). A number of studies have indicated that this substance exerts a generalized immunosuppressive effect, and thus might help protect the fetus.

3. Although most maternal IgG molecules can cross the placenta and enter the fetal circulation, anti-MHC antibodies produced by the mother may not be able to reach the fetus to harm it. Wegmann and others have shown that cytotoxic antibodies directed against paternal class I H-2 antigens expressed by the fetus are specifically absorbed by the placenta and thus denied entrance into the fetal circulation.

So long as they are not cytotoxic, anti-MHC antibodies might protect the placenta itself from a cell-mediated immune attack. Bound harmlessly to antigens on the cell surface, these antibodies might shield the cells from attack by the mother's T cells. The existence of such protective antibodies has long been observed in tumor immunology. Their ability to enhance tumor growth has given them the name *enhancing antibodies.* The humoral anti-MHC response in pregnant mice seems to be dominated by the IgG1 subclass, which does not fix complement, and thus cannot trigger complement-mediated cytotoxicity.

When lymphocytes from a mother presensitized (by repeated pregnancies) to the father's alloantigens are cultured for two days with his lymphocytes (thus an MLC), they release migration inhibition factor (MIF — see Section 3.2). However, when serum taken from the mother late in pregnancy is added to the cultures, it blocks the release of MIF. Rocklin and his coworkers have shown that the effect is specific: pregnancy serum from other mothers does not block the effect. The blocking effect of the serum can be absorbed with the father's lymphocytes and appears to be mediated by IgG directed at his class II antigens.

4. Suppressor cells in pregnancy. Mixed lymphocyte cultures are usually established by mixing a population of inactivated (for example, by mitomycin C or irradiation) stimulator cells with an equal number of normal responder cells. This is the classic "one-way" MLR (see Section 6.5). However, if neither population is inactivated, then each responds to the other by proliferation ("two-way"). Normally, the two cell populations respond about equally. Thus when male lymphocytes are cultured with female lymphocytes, approximately one-half of the cells that enter mitosis will carry the Y chromosome, the remainder will not. Curiously enough, this situation does not occur when lymphocytes from a newborn male baby are cultured with his mother's lymphocytes. Some 95% of the cells entering mitosis will carry the Y chromosome (Figure 16.14). (Presumably the same phenomenon occurs with the lymphocytes of baby girls but there is no convenient way to distinguish their cells from their mother's.) There is nothing intrinsically wrong with the mother's lymphocytes. They are perfectly responsive to other allogeneic cells and to mitogens.

The suppressive effect of the baby's lymphocytes is not specific. His cells will inhibit mitosis when cultured with the cells of other adults as

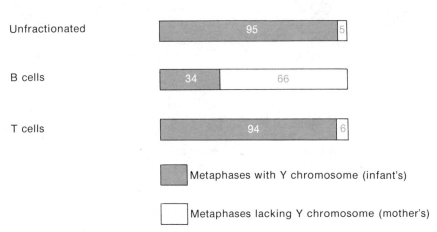

Figure 16.14 Inhibition of mitosis of the lymphocytes of the mother by the T cells of her newborn son. Mixed lymphocyte cultures were set up with equal numbers of the mother's cells and her male baby's cells ($2.5 \times 10^6$ of each). Mitogens were added to the cultures (phytohemagglutinin for T cells; pokeweed mitogen for the B cell cultures.) After several days, the cultures were treated with colchicine and metaphase cells examined for the presence of the Y chromosome. When cultured alone, the baby's and the mother's lymphocytes had similar rates of mitosis. [Based on L. B. Olding and M. B. A. Oldstone, *J. Immunol.* **116**:682, 1976.]

well. The cells responsible for suppression are T cells; the baby's B cells are not suppressive.

So it appears that the human fetus may play an active role in defending itself from its mother's immune system. Upon encountering her T cells —perhaps at the placenta, perhaps within the mother's tissues—the $T_s$ cells of the fetus could prevent the mother's T cells from becoming activated and mounting an allogeneic attack.

## 16.7  Self-tolerance

From the earliest days of immunology as an experimental science, it was apparent that animals could not be immunized with their own body constituents. The serum albumin of a cow (BSA) that acts as so powerful an immunogen in the rabbit or mouse is not immunogenic in the cow. Paul Ehrlich expressed this inability of the immune system to respond to self as "horror autotoxicus." The concept of lack of self-reactivity occupied a central position in the further development of the theory of clonal selection. Burnet proposed that during the ontogeny of the organism, all self-reactive clones of cells are destroyed. In the early 70s, Jerne suggested that the original pool of immunocompetent cells consists of cells directed against all the histocompatibility antigens of the species. Those cells directed against the histocompatibility antigens of the *individual* are stimulated to proliferate and then destroyed *unless* they mutate to a slightly different receptor specificity. In this way, the repertoire of anti-gen-sensitive cells for the conventional antigens in the world outside develops.

While self-tolerance describes a phenomenon that needs explaining, it is certainly not an absolute truth. Humans may have antibodies against all sorts of self components. These include soluble molecules like thyro-globulin, intrinsic factor (which is responsible for the transport of vita-min $B_{12}$), and IgG. They also include cell-surface molecules found on red cells, platelets, and many other cell types. Often these antiself antibodies are associated with disease states, the so-called autoimmune diseases. But they can also be found, usually in lower concentration, in the serum of persons with no obvious signs of disease. This is particularly true of the elderly.

Clearly we must harbor B cells specific for self. What, then, normally keeps them in check? At least three mechanisms seem responsible.

## B Cell Tolerance

The high concentration of soluble proteins like serum albumin might be expected to mediate high zone tolerance of B cells. Attempts to identify antigen-binding cells (ABCs) for such self antigens have failed. It appears, then, that through some mechanism (for possibilities see Section 16.3), these self-reactive clones have been deleted. At least this appears to be the case for those cells with receptors of high affinity for the antigen. When human lymphocytes are exposed to B-cell mitogens like LPS, a variety of anti-self antibodies are produced. But these are generally of low affinity. We would not expect to have been able to see their precursors through the standard technique of binding to radiolabeled antigen.

## T Cell Tolerance

Radiolabeled antigen and autoradiography does reveal ABCs for some self components. Characteristically these are molecules like thyroglobu-lin present in the circulation in very low concentrations. The failure of antigen-specific B cells to respond in these cases could result from (1) the absence of $T_H$ cells or (2) the presence of suppressor cells which actively prevent $T_H$ and/or B cells from responding to the self antigen. There is evidence that both mechanisms are at work in T cell self-tolerance.

One of the most interesting systems with which to explore this question is a mutant mouse strain designated B10.D2 OSN. This strain lacks the gene needed to manufacture the fifth component of complement (C5). The congenic B10.D2 NSN strain is genetically identical to the mutant strain except that it has normal amounts of C5 in its serum (50 – 85 $\mu$g/ml).

As you would expect, the normal strain is tolerant of its own C5. Immunization with C5 and adjuvant fails to elicit any anti-C5 antibodies.

The mutant, on the other hand, responds to injections of C5 with a vigorous production of anti-C5 antibodies.

Figure 16.15 shows the results of experiments in which various combinations of T and B cells from tolerant and nontolerant donors were mixed in an attempt to identify the cells responsible for the tolerant state. The cell mixtures were injected into a tolerant recipient that had been irradiated to prevent its own lymphocytes from participating in the response. The recipient's own supply of circulating C5 serves as the source of antigen. A drop in the amount of circulating C5 was used in these experiments as a measure of the production of anti-C5 antibodies.

As Figure 16.15 shows, it is the T cells, not the B cells, that are tolerized in the tolerant animals. B cells from tolerant animals are able to produce antibodies when exposed to nontolerant T cells. Clearly, then, there has been no clonal deletion of B cells in the tolerant mice.

As for the tolerant T cells, they could arise from (1) a missing or unresponsive set of C5-specific $T_H$ cells and/or (2) the presence of a population of suppressor T cells capable of actively suppressing $T_H$ or B

**Figure 16.15** T cells are responsible for natural self-tolerance to C5, the fifth component of the complement system. When B cells and T cells from mice lacking C5 find themselves in an environment with C5 present, they make anti-C5 antibodies (expt. 1). B cells from a tolerant (normal) mouse are also able to make anti-C5 antibodies when helped by T cells from a nontolerant donor (expt. 4). Thus the B cells in a tolerant animal are not tolerant. Transfer of B cells or T cells alone from a nontolerant mouse gives little or no response, showing that the response is a T-dependent humoral one. Anti-C5 production was measured by the drop in circulating C5 in the recipients. In other experiments, using injected C5 and nontolerant recipients, tolerance lasted only so long as antigen was present. [Based on D. E. Harris et al., *J. Exp. Med.*, **156**:567, 1982.]

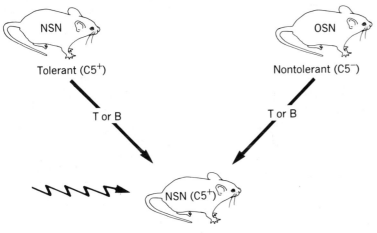

| T-cell donor | B-cell donor | Anti-C5 |
|---|---|---|
| 1. Nontolerant (OSN) | Nontolerant (OSN) | + |
| 2. Tolerant (NSN) | Tolerant (NSN) | − |
| 3. Tolerant (NSN) | Nontolerant (OSN) | − |
| 4. Nontolerant (OSN) | Tolerant (NSN) | + |

cells (or both). The use of purified T cell subsets in other experiments suggests that both mechanisms are at work. Ly-1$^+$ cells from tolerant mice, which in nontolerant animals would be expected to contain T$_H$ cells, are unable to provide help to B cells. On the other hand, no antibodies are produced in animals receiving B cells and a *mixture* of T cells from nontolerant mice (containing T$_H$ cells) with T cells from tolerant mice. This shows that tolerant animals also contain a population of suppressor T cells that actively suppresses the immune response to self antigen.

## Autoreactive T Cells

The various assays for cell-mediated responses normally do not reveal any sign of autoreactivity. Thus placing syngeneic cells in culture does not cause them to proliferate nor do syngeneic cells mount GVH reactions. But as is the case with B cells, there is accumulating evidence that the normal lack of T cell activity against self is not because of any intrinsic lack of potential autoreactive clones. In the early 1970s, Cohen and Wekerle found that rat T cells could be sensitized to self antigens. They cultured thymus or lymph node cells with autologous (i.e., taken from the same animal) thymus reticulum cells. Removed from culture, these T cells were able to (1) mount a GVHR when injected into syngeneic recipients, and (2) lyse $^{51}$Cr-labeled syngeneic fibroblasts. The cytotoxicity was quite specific: the lysis of allogeneic targets was less than half that of syngeneic targets. These results suggest that the normal self-tolerance of T cells can be circumvented and a population of T cells capable of attacking self can be uncovered. A similar phenomenon has been found in humans. When human T cells are cultured in vitro with autologous non-T cells that express class II MHC antigens, the T cells become activated and proliferate. This response is called the autologous mixed lymphocyte reaction (AMLR).

Clearly autoreactive T cell clones exist. What keeps them from normally mounting an attack against self? In the system explored by Cohen and Wekerle, a serum factor in the rats appears to be responsible for preventing the activation of T cells in vivo. In mice evidence exists that T cells prevent autosensitization. Muraoka and Miller have shown that mice have a population of T cells that prevents attack against self H-2 antigens. Figure 16.16 shows a few of the cell-mixing experiments that revealed the presence of such cells. These workers found that the bone marrow of *normal* mice contains a cell population that blocks cytotoxicity directed against target cells that display the H-2 antigens of the bone marrow cells. Suppression by these cells occurs only when they are added early in the five-day period during which the responding and stimulating cells are cultured together. This (and other) evidence indicates that the suppression acts on the precursors of the T$_C$ cells generated in the culture. So the normal intact animal appears to have a population of cells, which have been named "veto" cells, that specifically block attacks against its own histocompatibility antigens — i.e., attacks against self.

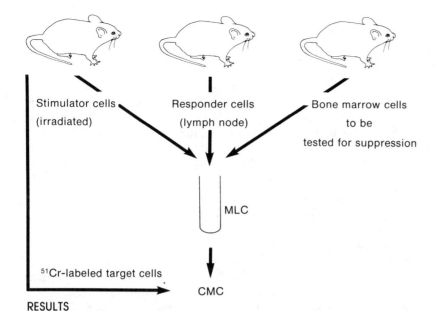

RESULTS

| Stimulator and target | Responder | Bone marrow | Cytotoxicity (% specific $^{51}$Cr release) |
|---|---|---|---|
| B6 | RNC | None | 28 |
| B6 | RNC | RNC | 28 |
| B6 | RNC | B6 | 11[1] |
| (B6 × C3H) F$_1$ | C3H | None | 22 |
| (B6 × C3H) F$_1$ | C3H | C3H | 15 |
| (B6 × C3H) F$_1$ | C3H | B6 | 4[1] |

[1] Bone marrow cells block development of cytotoxicity against their own haplotype.

**Figure 16.16**  Antiself suppressor cells. Normal bone marrow contains cells ("veto" cells) that suppress the development of cytotoxicity against cells of their own haplotype. [Based on S. Muraoka and R. G. Miller, *J. Exp. Med.* **152**:54, 1980.]

In one sense, many (if not most) T cells are autoreactive. The response of most subsets of T cells ($T_H$, $T_D$, $T_C$) to conventional antigens requires that the conventional antigen be displayed along with self histocompatibility antigens. (Refer, e.g., to Sections 3.7, 11.3, and 11.4.) Furthermore, even alloreactivity may be the fortuitous outcome of associative T cell specificity directed against a particular combination of conventional and self antigens (see Section 11.9).

## 16.8  Summary

Both tolerance and immunity meet the same criteria of specificity and memory. Tolerance is the converse of immunity. The tolerant state can exist in a population of B cells and also in T cells. While more details must be discovered, the present evidence points to there being more than one mechanism that can lead to tolerance. Both humoral factors (i.e., antibodies, antigens, complexes of each) and $T_s$ cells have been implicated in the establishment and maintenance of tolerance.

Tolerance is a relative term. By glancing back over the data given in this chapter, you can see that what is often called tolerance is a *reduction* in normal immune responsiveness. Where easily measurable responses remain, tolerance may be no more than an extreme example of the sort of homeostatic down regulation of immunity that is examined in Chapter 15. Thus many of the same mechanisms discussed in Chapter 15 reappear in this chapter. Perhaps, then, the term tolerance should be reserved for those cases where present assays fail to detect any immune response at all. But even in these cases, tolerance is clearly the result of an active mechanism, not some sort of intrinsic defect.

Tolerance can often be broken and replaced by immunity. When self-tolerance is broken, the result is autoimmunity. An autoimmune response may cause — and is certainly often associated with — pathological changes in the body. But autoimmune responses are not the only mechanisms by which the immune system produces damage. The general topic of damage mediated by the immune system is examined in Chapter 18.

## ADDITIONAL READING

1. Aldo-Benson, M, and Y. Borel, "The Tolerant Cell: Direct Evidence for Receptor Blockade by Tolerogen," *J. Immunol.* **112**:1793, 1974.

2. Billingham, R. E., L. Brent, and P. B. Medawar, "'Actively Acquired Tolerance' of Foreign Cells," *Nature* **172**:603, 1953. (Reprinted in V. L. Sato and M. L. Gefter, *Cellular Immunology,* Addison-Wesley Publishing Co., Inc., Reading, MA, 1982.)

3. Cohen, I. R., and H. Wekerle, "Regulation of Autosensitization. The Immune Activation and Specific Inhibition of Self-recognizing Thymus-Derived Lymphocytes," *J. Exp. Med.* **137**:224, 1973.

4. Felton, L. D., et al., "Studies on the Mechanism of Immunological Paralysis Induced in Mice by Pneumococcal Polysaccharides," *J. Exp. Med.* **74**:17, 1955.

5. Jerne, N. K., "The Somatic Generation of Immune Recognition," *Eur. J. Immunol.* **1**:1, 1971.

6. Mitchison, N. A., "Induction of Immunological Paralysis in Two Zones of Dosage," *Proc. Roy. Soc. Med.* **161**:275, 1964.

7. Nossal, G. J. V., and Beverley L. Pike, "Clonal Anergy: Persistence in Tolerant Mice of Antigen-Binding B Lymphocytes Incapable of Responding to Antigen or Mitogen," *Proc. Natl. Acad. Sci. USA* **77**:1602, 1980.

8. Owen, R. D., "Immunogenetic Consequences of Vascular Anastomoses Between Bovine Twins," *Science* **102**:400, 1945.

9. Pence, H., W. M. Petty, and R. E. Rocklin, "Suppression of Maternal Responsiveness to Paternal Antigens by Maternal Plasma," *J. Immunol.* **114:**525, 1975.

10. Wegmann, T. G., et al., "Allogeneic Placenta is a Paternal Strain Antigen Immunoabsorbent," *J. Immunol.* **122:**270, 1979.

11. Wegmann, T. G., and T. J. Gill III (eds.), *Immunology of Reproduction,* Oxford University Press, New York, 1983.

12. Weigle, W. O., "The Production of Thyroiditis and Antibody Following Injection of Unaltered Thyroglobulin Without Adjuvant into Rabbits Previously Stimulated with Altered Thyroglobulin," *J. Exp. Med.* **122:**1049, 1965.

13. Weksler, M. E., and R. Kozak, "Lymphocyte Transformation Induced by Autologous Cells: V. Generation of Immunologic Memory and Specificity During the Autologous Mixed Lymphocyte Reaction," *J. Exp. Med.* **146:**1833, 1977. The AMLR in humans.

# PART VI

# Immunity and Disease

# CHAPTER 17

# Immunity and Infectious Disease

## 17.1  Introduction

The immune system is the ultimate defense of vertebrates against infectious disease. Without a functioning immune system, the vertebrate host eventually and inevitably succumbs to infection. No combination of antibiotics and chemotherapy can keep a totally immuno-incompetent host alive. The only way to circumvent this rule is to raise the subject from birth in a sterile environment. The immune system not only protects us from such well-recognized pathogens as pneumococci or polioviruses but also enables us to live amicably with the many species of microbes that inhabit various niches in our bodies. In the immunodeficient patient, these normally harmless saprophytes can establish invasive and lethal infections.

The human body can serve as the host for viruses, bacteria, fungi, protozoans, and helminths (flukes, tapeworms, and roundworms). The clinician often limits the term "parasite" to protozoans and metazoans, but we will apply the term to all infectious agents that cause disease.

The encounter of parasite with its host has two possible outcomes. The parasite may cause an acute but transitory illness that ends with either the death of the host or the death and elimination of the parasites. This is the pattern seen with such diseases as measles and influenza. If the host survives, it is immune to a subsequent invasion by that parasite for some period of time. On the other hand, many parasites establish persistent infections in the host. Once within the body, *Plasmodium malariae*, the protozoan that causes quartan malaria, may survive for decades. Most metazoan parasites also live within the body for long periods. From our perspective, the most curious aspect of the persistent infections is the inability of the immune system to eradicate the parasite. In Sections 17.7 and 17.8, we shall examine two mechanisms by which persistent parasites evade the immune response. These mechanisms are simply two of many examples of the interplay between the defenses of the host and the countermeasures by which parasites evade them.

## 17.2 Nonimmune Host Defenses

The vertebrate host does not depend solely on its immune system to protect it from the agents of disease. Many nonimmune defense mechanisms play important roles as well. Some of them, phagocytosis for example, represent a more ancient and primitive method of defense than immunity. It is mechanisms such as these that enable invertebrates to survive without an immune system.

### Mechanical and Chemical Barriers

Unbroken skin and, to a lesser extent, mucous membranes provide a physical barrier to the entrance of most bacteria and many other parasites. The effectiveness of these barriers is often enhanced by the presence of chemical barriers as well. Tears, saliva, and the secretions of the nasopharynx contain lysozyme, an enzyme that digests the peptidoglycan of bacterial cell walls. The low pH of the gastric juice and of the vaginal secretions inhibits invasion by many pathogens. The bile salts delivered into the intestine in the flow of bile inhibit the growth of several intestinal pathogens. The protective chemistry of the skin and vagina are, in large measure, created by harmless saprophytes that colonize these locations and create unfavorable conditions for harmful parasites.

## Phagocytosis

The major scavengers of the body are the neutrophils and the macrophages. There is a steady traffic of both of these phagocytic cells throughout the tissues of the body. In addition, many macrophages, such as the Kupffer cells of the liver, carry out their function while relatively immobilized as part of the architecture of the tissue.

Phagocytes respond to and, if possible, engulf an enormous variety of materials: particulate matter that is foreign to the body as well as the debris of the host's tissues. Often phagocytosis occurs without the intervention of any immune mechanism. However, immunity as expressed by both antibodies (Figure 14.8) and activated T cells (Figure 14.14) greatly enhances the efficiency of phagocytosis.

## Interferons

Interferons (IFNs) are a family of proteins that share the property of interfering with the replication of viruses. There are three main types.

1. IFN-$\alpha$, secreted by leukocytes,
2. IFN-$\beta$, secreted by fibroblasts, and
3. IFN-$\gamma$ ("immune interferon"), secreted by antigen- or mitogen-stimulated lymphocytes.

Secretion of both IFN-$\alpha$ and IFN-$\beta$ is induced by virus infection of the cells and can also be induced by certain chemical stimuli (e.g., double-stranded RNA). Because it is a product of activated lymphocytes, IFN-$\gamma$ qualifies as a lymphokine.

Interferons play an important part in limiting the spread of viruses within the host. When experimental animals are injected with anti-interferon antibodies, their susceptibility to viral diseases increases greatly. Interferons also increase the phagocytic activity of macrophages and the cytotoxicity of $T_C$ cells. Interferons increase the activity of NK cells (see Section 14.10) and this may be an important defense mechanism against virus-infected cells.

## Inflammation

The tissue damage caused by invading parasites initiates a constellation of events that collectively cause the tissue to become inflamed. The blood supply to the site is increased. The permeability of the capillary walls increases, causing edema as fluids and proteins leak into the tissue spaces. Phagocytic cells, especially neutrophils and monocytes, leave the circulation and begin work at the site.

The complex events of inflammation are orchestrated by a large number of chemical mediators. These are generated by mast cells, macrophages, neutrophils, the clotting system, the kinin system, and the complement system. Although the interaction and regulation of these factors are only poorly understood, a few features stand out clearly. Tissue damage causes the degranulation of mast cells, and the subsequent liberation of histamine and leukotrienes is responsible for the rapid increase in the blood supply to and accumulation of fluid in the area. The activation of the clotting system causes fibrin to be deposited at the site and helps wall it off from undamaged tissue.

Prostaglandins and leukotrienes are derivatives of arachidonic acid (AA), an unsaturated fatty acid produced from membrane phospholipids (Figure 17.1). The principal pathways of arachidonic acid metabolism are the 5-lipoxygenase pathway, which produces a collection of leukotrienes (LT), and the cyclo-oxygenase pathway which yields a number of prostaglandins (PG) and thromboxanes (Tx). The products of both pathways act in concert to bring about inflammation. (Aspirin, ibuprofen, and certain other anti-inflammatory drugs achieve their effect by blocking the enzymatic activity of cyclo-oxygenase.) Macrophages and neutrophils are major sources of these inflammatory metabolites.

The complement system can be activated by nonimmune mechanisms (as well as by antigen–antibody complexes — see Section 14.2 and Figure 18.10). Molecules on the surface of such diverse pathogens as protozoans *(Entamoeba)*, helminths *(Schistosoma)*, and many bacteria activate the complement system by the alternative pathway. In addition, tissue damage causes the liver to release C-reactive protein (CRP). Although CRP is not an immunoglobulin, it binds to the C-polysaccharide of bacterial cell walls and triggers the complement cascade by the classical pathway. Whether initiated by the classical or the alternative pathway, the

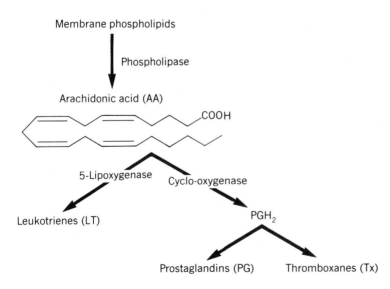

Membrane phospholipids

Phospholipase

Arachidonic acid (AA)

COOH

5-Lipoxygenase     Cyclo-oxygenase

Leukotrienes (LT)

PGH$_2$

Prostaglandins (PG)     Thromboxanes (Tx)

**Figure 17.1** Pathways of arachidonic acid metabolism. All three pathways occur in macrophages and monocytes. Mast cells and basophils generate a mixture of leukotrienes collectively responsible for the "slow-reacting substance of anaphylaxis" (SRS-A). Prostaglandins mediate fever and the pain and swelling associated with inflammation. The activity of cyclo-oxygenase is blocked by aspirin and such other anti-inflammatory drugs as ibuprofen.

production of C3a and C5a increases vascular permeability and attracts phagocytes to the site.

We emphasize here nonimmune tissue responses. However, immune responses can also produce tissue inflammation. Examples are given in Sections 18.3 and 18.6.

## Fever

Most microbial infections produce fever. This response is triggered by the release of IL-1 from activated macrophages. IL-1, in turn, causes the release of prostaglandins (Figure 17.1) which act directly on the temperature control center of the hypothalamus. Fever occurs not only in endotherms (mammals and birds) but also in ectotherms like fishes and reptiles. Kluger, Bernheim, and their associates have clearly shown that the ability of lizards to develop fever greatly enhances their ability to cope successfully with infection. It has been more difficult to show conclusively that fever is beneficial to mammals.

## 17.3 Parasite Countermeasures to Nonimmune Defenses

Pneumococci and some other pathogenic bacteria synthesize a polysaccharide capsule that makes them less easily ingested by phagocytes. It is the presence or absence of this capsule that determines whether pneumococci are virulent (the S forms) or not (the R forms — see Figure 2.2).

Many pathogenic bacteria secrete enzymes that digest host components that might otherwise serve to limit the spread of infection. Pathogenic clostridia secrete collagenase which, by softening connective tissue, probably contributes to their ability to spread rapidly through muscles. Streptococci and staphylococci secrete kinases that digest fibrin. Many pathogenic bacteria secrete hyaluronidase, which degrades the hyaluronic acid in connective tissue. To what degree these latter activities contribute to the invasiveness of these pathogens is not certain.

A number of bacterial pathogens (e.g., *Staphylococcus aureus*) secrete substances that decrease inflammation. These materials also inhibit the activity of phagocytes.

## 17.4 Immune Defenses

Infection of an immunocompetent host usually sets an elaborate complex of immune defense mechanisms into action. These defenses are mediated by antibodies, by cells and most often by both.

## Humoral Defenses

The synthesis of antibodies directed against determinants on the invader can protect the host in several ways. The secretion of antibodies (chiefly IgA) on the surface of mucous membranes interferes with the adherence of microorganisms and thus makes it more difficult for them to invade the underlying tissue. IgA antibodies serve such a protective function on the surfaces of the conjunctiva, nasopharynx, lungs, gut, and genitourinary tracts. The binding of antibodies to gram-negative bacteria triggers the full complement sequence and, at least in vitro, lyses them.

The binding of antibodies to the surface of microorganisms opsonizes them for more efficient phagocytosis. Two mechanisms contribute to this phenomenon (Figure 14.8). First, antibodies can link the microorganism to the phagocyte by binding, by means of their Fab regions, to an antigenic determinant on the microbe and binding to the phagocyte surface through its receptors for the Fc region. Both macrophages and neutrophils have receptors for the Fc region of IgG. Second, the binding of IgG to determinants on the microorganism initiates the complement sequence through the classical pathway. The accumulation of C3b on the surface of the microbe causes it to be bound by the receptors for C3b on macrophages and neutrophils (Figure 14.8). Antibodies, especially those of the IgM class, also agglutinate bacteria, and this may aid in clearing them from the site of infection. Antibodies also inactivate toxins (e.g., tetanus and diphtheria toxins) and viruses.

In general, humoral immunity plays a more important part in combating bacterial infections than viral infections. We see this in patients with agammaglobulinemia, who are dangerously susceptible to bacterial infections but usually manage to cope successfully with viruses. However, antibodies are an important defense against those viruses, like the polio viruses, that spread through the blood. Initially, polio virus invades the gastrointestinal tract. However, it does not cause serious disease unless it is carried to the central nervous system by way of the blood. Antipolio antibodies in the blood block this transmission and prevent damage to the central nervous system.

## Cellular Defenses

The fixed and mobile phagocytic cells of the body represent a major defense against foreign invaders. Phagocytosis by both neutrophils and macrophages is enhanced by the presence of antimicrobial antibodies and also complement components. Invading organisms that are too large to be ingested by phagocytes may nevertheless be killed by them. Antibody-coated protozoans and worms may be destroyed by neutrophils, macrophages, certain lymphocytes (K cells), and eosinophils. The mechanism of killing, called antibody-dependent cellular cytotoxicity (ADCC — see Section 14.4) does not involve the complement system. In the case of neutrophils and eosinophils, antibodies link these cells with their targets. Both IgG and IgE can serve this purpose, and these leukocytes have receptors for the Fc region of each of these isotypes. Following contact between the cytotoxic cell and its target, the cytoplasmic granules of the cell are discharged onto the surface of the target and kill it. The mechanism of killing used by K cells (lymphocytes) is not clearly understood nor is its in vivo significance fully established.

A similar uncertainty exists for cytotoxic T cells ($T_C$) cells and for NK cells. We find abundant evidence for the existence of these cells, and their activity in vitro has been amply demonstrated. However, it has not been easy to demonstrate that these cells play an important role in protecting the intact organism from virus infection. Indirect evidence of an important role for these cells is provided by the fact that humans deficient in T cells are notoriously prone to unchecked virus infections. The high levels of NK cells in nude mice may give them some protection from a similar fate. Lin and Askonas have provided direct evidence that $T_C$ cells serve a protective function in vivo. They have shown that an intravenous injection of $T_C$ cells specific for influenza A virus reduces virus replication in the lungs of mice and enables the mice to survive an otherwise lethal infection. As you would predict, the effect is restricted by the K and D regions of H-2; i.e., the adoptive transfer of virus specific $T_C$ cells only protects mice that share K and D with the cell donor.

## 17.5 Enhancing Immune Defenses

### Active Immunization

Since Jenner's introduction of vaccination almost 200 years ago, the greatest practical benefit to come from immunology has been the development of safe and effective vaccines against a variety of infectious agents (Figure 17.2). Vaccination appears to have eliminated smallpox from the world. In developed countries, vaccines against tetanus, diphtheria, and poliomyelitis have made these diseases extremely rare. In the United States, an intensive vaccination program promises to do the same for measles (rubeola) and rubella. A number of other vaccines are available for persons exposed to particular risks (e.g., travel to a country where yellow fever is endemic, or exposure to a rabid animal).

The procedure for making a vaccine varies from case to case. Protection against pertussis (whooping cough) and typhoid *(Salmonella typhi)* is generated by the use of the killed organism. Vaccines against virus diseases consist of either inactivated virus particles (e.g., the Salk polio vaccine, and influenza vaccines) or specially attenuated strains of the virus (measles and the Sabin polio vaccine). Protection from the deleterious effects of the tetanus and diphtheria bacilli is given by vaccination with their toxoids (inactivated toxins). A common principle underlies all of these vaccines. In every case, the object is to render the infectious or harmful material safe while still retaining at least some of its antigenic determinants intact. The most direct, if unsophisticated, approach is simply to kill the organisms by high temperatures, formaldehyde treat-

| Disease | Preparation | Notes |
|---|---|---|
| 1. Diphtheria | Toxoid ⎫ | Often given to children in a single preparation |
| 2. Tetanus | Toxoid ⎬ | (DTP; the "triple vaccine") |
| 3. Pertussis | Killed bacteria ⎭ | |
| 4. Polio | Inactivated virus | Inactivated polio vaccine; IPV (Salk) |
| | Attenuated virus | Oral polio vaccine; OPV (Sabin) Both vaccines trivalent (types 1, 2, and 3) |
| 5. Measles | Attenuated virus ⎫ | Often given as a mixture (MMR) |
| 6. Mumps | Attenuated virus ⎬ | |
| 7. Rubella | Attenuated virus ⎭ | |
| 8. Influenza | Hemagglutinins | Contains hemagglutinins from the type B and type A viruses recently in circulation |
| 9. Pneumococcal pneumonia | Capsular polysaccharides | A mixture of the capsular polysaccharides of 23 common types |
| 10. Meningococcal disease | Polysaccharides | Used chiefly to prevent outbreaks among the military |
| 11. Hepatitis B | HBsAg | Particles isolated from blood of human carriers of the disease |
| 12. Rabies | Inactivated virus | Vaccine prepared from human diploid cell cultures (HDCV) has replaced the duck vaccine (DEV) |
| 13. Smallpox | Attenuated virus | Now recommended only for laboratory workers exposed to smallpox or related viruses |
| 14. Typhoid | Killed bacteria | |
| 15. Yellow fever | Attenuated virus | |
| 16. Tuberculosis | Attenuated bacteria (BCG) | Rarely used in the United States |

**Figure 17.2**  Some of the vaccines currently used in humans.

ment, etc. and use the killed organisms as the active ingredient in the vaccine. A more difficult procedure is to purify a surface antigen from the organism. The present pneumococcal vaccine contains purified capsular polysaccharides from 23 types of pneumococci. A vaccine against hepatitis B, using purified hepatitis B surface antigen (HBsAg) was approved by the United States Food and Drug Administration in 1981. In both of these cases, protective immunity is elicited without the danger of introducing extraneous or potentially infectious material into the patient. The rapid advances in genetic engineering provide another promising approach to vaccine manufacture. One procedure is to clone the gene for an antigenically important molecule on the pathogen and insert this gene into an organism like *E. coli* so that it can express it efficiently. In this way, large quantities of a single, fully characterized antigen can be produced.

Successful vaccines often require the incorporation of adjuvants. These are agents, like alum or aluminum hydroxide, that—for reasons not entirely understood—enhance the immunogenicity of the material. (Freund's adjuvant is not used in humans because it provokes an intense inflammatory response.) In the case of DTP, the "triple" vaccine (diphtheria, tetanus, pertussis), the killed pertussis cells have an adjuvant effect as well as serving as an immunogen in their own right.

The practical and safe use of vaccines also requires close attention to such details as

1. The duration of protection and the scheduling of booster doses.
2. The avoidance of allergic responses to extraneous components (such as egg proteins) in the vaccine.
3. The avoidance of the complications that occur when live virus vaccines are given to immunodeficient patients or to pregnant women (because of possible damage to the fetus).

### Passive Immunization

Passive immunization involves the administration of an antiserum to the patient. This is usually done when a nonimmune patient has been, or is likely to be, exposed to a disease and there is not time to achieve active immunization. Passive immunization is still frequently used for those exposed to tetanus, hepatitis A ("infectious" hepatitis), measles, rabies, diphtheria, and some other diseases. (It is also used to provide immediate protection against snake venoms, black widow spider bites, and to prevent Rh-negative mothers from becoming sensitized to the Rho (D) antigen of their newborn child—see Section 18.4.)

Some protective antisera are raised by actively immunizing large animals like horses but these antisera have two serious drawbacks.

1. The large quantity of extraneous foreign protein in the preparation tends to elicit an active immune response which may, on further use of the material, produce anaphylaxis and/or serum sickness (see Section 18.6).
2. They are catabolized much more rapidly than human immunoglobulins.

Therefore, pooled *human* globulin ("immune globulin" or IG) is used for such common diseases as measles, rubella, and hepatitis A. For diseases in which the level of antibodies in the general population is low, the gamma globulin is prepared from *individuals* who have either recently recovered from the disease, such as varicella (chicken pox), or who have been deliberately and intensively immunized against it (the $Rh_0$ or D antigen).

The advantages of monoclonal antibodies have raised the hope that they might be used for human therapy. However, the immunogenicity of mouse monoclonal antibodies when given to humans has been a serious drawback to such use. And, unfortunately, the techniques for producing monoclonal antibodies, which work so well for mouse cells (Section 4.8) have been difficult to apply to human cells. However, using recombinant DNA technology, it has been possible to construct both heavy and light chain genes that combine a mouse V region with a human C region (reference 7). Such hybrid genes can be expressed in mouse myeloma cells, and their product should prove to be much less immunogenic in humans than are "all-mouse" monoclonal antibodies.

## 17.6 Parasite Countermeasures to Immune Defenses

For many human diseases, the interactions of parasite and host have gone on for millennia. Over a long span of time we might well expect natural selection to have produced parasites with adaptations that blunt the immune defenses of the host. Looking over the spectrum of human parasites, we do find a variety of techniques by which such protection is accomplished. For persistent parasites, like the protozoans that cause malaria, an optimal condition seems to exist when the defenses of the host are blunted but not destroyed. If the parasite is too efficient at avoiding immunological attack, it may well kill its host before the parasite has had a chance to pass on to a fresh one.

Thus persistent parasites seem to have worked out a *modus vivendi* with their hosts. For example, blood flukes *(Schistosoma)* elicit an immune reaction that the adult worms evade successfully (by a mechanism that we shall examine in the following section) but which is effective against a fresh crop of infectious larvae (called schistosomula). In this way, the early arrivals close the door on the late arrivals that might threaten their meal ticket with an overwhelming infection. (A little like the present residents of a town passing more stringent zoning regulations.) *Plasmodium falciparum* also induces an immunity that reduces the chances of additional infection but is ineffective against the first invaders. This phenomenon is called **concomitant immunity**. A similar effect is sometimes seen with malignant tumors and is described in Section 20.7.

One approach by which parasites evade attack by antibodies is to take up residence where antibodies cannot reach them. Many accomplish this by living within cells. The malaria organisms spend much of their lives within red cells and are only exposed to antibodies during the brief period when merozoites are in transit from one red cell to another. Some other protozoans and the mycobacteria that cause tuberculosis and leprosy live inside macrophages, protected from antibodies and undamaged by the normal lysosome-mediated killing machinery of their host cells.

A number of parasites liberate materials that cause a generalized immunosuppresssion in their host. Persons heavily infected with *Plasmodium* (malaria) or *Trypanosoma* (trypanosomiasis) usually give poor responses to vaccines and other antigens.

Several different species of pathogenic bacteria secrete proteases that cleave human IgA1 (and, as far as is known, no other protein). Each protease cleaves a particular peptide bond in the hinge region (Figure 17.3), breaking the molecules into Fab and Fc fragments. All of these organisms infect mucous membranes, and the suspicion is that the remarkable specificity of their enzymes represents a defense against the IgA antibodies that normally coat these surfaces. However, IgA2 molecules, which have a deletion in the hinge region (a counter-countermeasure?), are not degraded by these enzymes.

Some parasites evade immune attack by covering themselves with antigens that look to the immune system like "self." Adult schistosomes

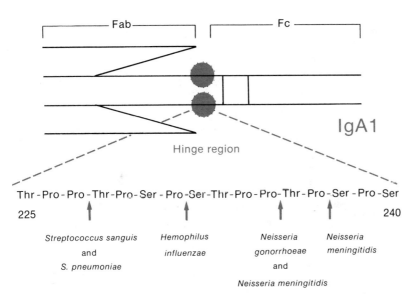

**Figure 17.3**  Cleavage sites in the hinge region of human IgA1 of proteases secreted by several pathogenic bacteria. Each of these organisms infects mucous membranes. IgA2 molecules, which have a deletion in the hinge region, are not degraded by these enzymes. [From Martha H. Mulks et al., *J. Exp. Med.* **152**:1442, 1980.]

do this as we shall see in the following section. Some parasites elude immune attack by periodically changing the antigens on their surface. The trypanosomes do this by a mechanism we will examine in Section 17.8. The virus of influenza A does so by mechanisms described in Section 17.9.

## 17.7  Schistosomiasis

Schistosomes are parasitic flat worms that live within blood vessels and hence are commonly called blood flukes. Perhaps as many as 300 million humans presently harbor blood flukes. With the increasing use of irrigation in arid lands, this number will probably rise because the parasite is acquired by contact with water containing cercariae: the free-swimming stage in the life cycle of the parasite (Figure 17.4). When cercariae come in contact with human skin, they are able to invade it after first softening a spot on the skin with enzymes. As they enter the skin, they shed their tails. At this stage, they are called *schistosomula*. The schistosomula enter the blood vessels of the skin, are carried to the heart, and from there travel to the lungs. After residing within the lungs for a few days, they return to the heart and are carried in the arterial blood throughout the body. However, they can only lodge successfully in the liver. Here the schistosomula mature into adult flukes. Finally the adults move into the hepatic portal veins and, depending on the species, take up permanent residence in the veins draining the bladder *(S. hematobium)*, the large intestine *(S. mansoni)*, or the small intestine *(S. japonicum)*. Once estab-

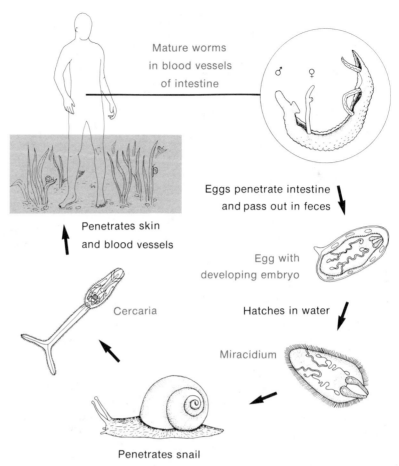

**Figure 17.4** Life cycle of the blood fluke *Schistosoma mansoni*. Once within the alternate host, a snail, a single miracidium may produce as many as 200,000 infectious cercariae. Both sexes must infect the human if the cycle is to continue.

lished, the worms mate and the females begin to lay large numbers of spiny eggs. The accumulation of these irritant eggs in the liver and the tissue damage caused as the eggs break through the walls of the bladder or intestine cause the debilitating effects of the disease.

Adult schistosomes may live for decades bathed in the blood of their host. How, then, do they escape immune attack? Infection by schistosomes elicits the formation of antischistosome antibodies. Butterworth and his colleagues have shown that these antibodies are capable of damaging schistosomula in vitro even though they appear to have no effect on adult worms. The mechanism of in vitro killing is antibody-dependent cell-mediated cytotoxicity (ADCC). Neither antibodies alone nor cells alone are effective (Figure 17.5). Complement is not needed. ADCC is mediated by both macrophages and eosinophils. If ADCC also operates in the host, it would provide the basis for concomitant immunity; that is, protection from superinfection caused by later batches of schistosomula.

If infection elicits an immune response, how are adult worms spared?

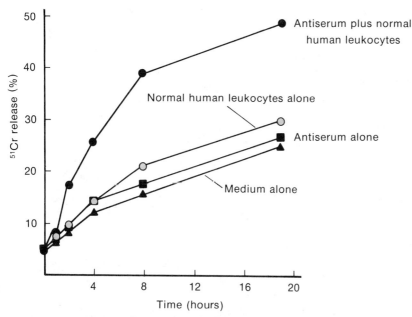

**Figure 17.5** Killing of schistosomula by antibody-dependent cell-mediated cytotoxicity (ADCC). Schistosomula were labeled with $^{51}$Cr and incubated under the conditions shown. The antiserum was from infected patients; the leukocytes from healthy donors. Neither antiserum alone nor leukocytes alone caused any more damage than occurred with control cultures containing medium alone or serum from uninfected donors (not shown). [From A. E. Butterworth et al., *Nature* **252**:503, 1974.]

They appear to protect themselves by coating their exposed surface with antigens acquired from their host. Smithers and his colleagues developed a technique by which they could introduce worms into several laboratory animals and later recover those that had survived. They found that worms that had been living in a mouse were destroyed when transferred to monkeys that had previously been immunized against tissue antigens of the mouse. These monkeys could not destroy worms that they received from other monkeys (Figure 17.6). This suggested that during their residence within the mouse, the worms had acquired tissue antigens of their host.

The accumulation of host antigens is reversible. When "mouse" worms were transferred to normal monkeys for seven days and *then* transferred to mouse-immune monkeys, their final host was no longer able to destroy them. Evidently during their seven-day residence in the normal monkey, they had lost their mouse-derived antigens.

The ability to kill adult worms in vivo, like the ability to kill schistosomula in vitro, is antibody dependent. The passive transfer of antimouse serum to a normal monkey enables it to destroy adult worms that have previously resided within mice.

A number of host antigens may be acquired by schistosomes. These include blood-group antigens (e.g., ABO) and, at least in the case of mice, histocompatibility antigens. The presence of host antigens on the surface

All donors harboring adult *Schistosoma mansoni*

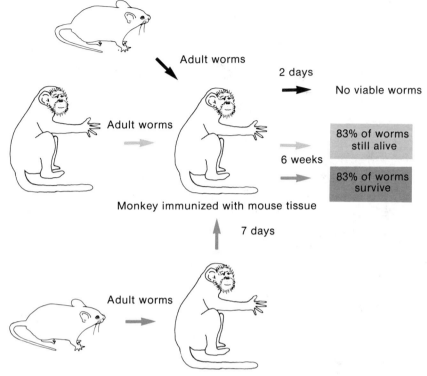

Adult worms

Adult worms

2 days

No viable worms

6 weeks

83% of worms
still alive

83% of worms
survive

Monkey immunized with mouse tissue

7 days

Adult worms

**Figure 17.6** Evidence that adult schistosomes acquire surface antigens of the host in which they reside. Worms removed from mice are killed when transferred directly *(top)* to monkeys immunized against mouse tissue antigens. However, after 7 days residence in a normal monkey, "mouse" worms are no longer killed when transferred to a mouse-immune monkey *(bottom)*. Presumably the "mouse" worms lose their mouse antigens during this period (and probably replace them with monkey antigens). In separate experiments, these workers showed that killing was mediated by antibodies: normal monkeys given antimouse serum also killed worms that had previously resided in mice. [Based on S. R. Smithers et al., *Proc. Roy. Soc. B.* **171**:483, 1969.]

**Figure 17.7** Demonstration of mouse H-2 antigens on the surface of a schistosomulum harvested from a CBA mouse (H-$2^k$) (900×). The schistosomulum was treated with mouse anti-H-$2^k$ serum and then with fluorescein-labeled rabbit antimouse Ig antibodies. [Courtesy of Alan Sher from A. Sher et al., *J. Exp. Med.* **148**:46, 1978.]

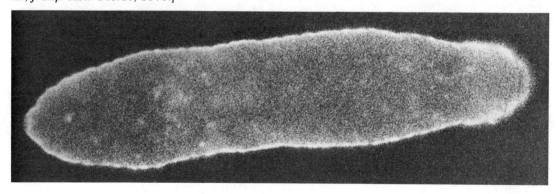

of the schistosomula can be demonstrated with fluorescence-labeled antibodies (Figure 17.7). At the same time that the organisms acquire the host antigens, they lose their ability to be bound by antischistosomula antibodies.

The story that emerges from all this is that adult blood flukes are able to survive indefinitely in their host by hiding from the host's immune response. They do this by acquiring a surface coat of host antigens which masks the presence of their own antigens. However, the infection does provoke an immune response effective against later arrivals. This concomitant immunity reduces the risk of accumulating such an overwhelming level of infection that the host's life is in grave danger.

## 17.8 Trypanosomiasis

Trypanosomes are flagellated protozoans that swim freely in the bloodstream (Figure 17.8). In a belt that extends across sub-Saharan Africa, they cause nagana, a debilitating disease of domestic ungulates and, in humans, sleeping sickness. They are transmitted to their hosts by the bite of the tsetse fly. The human parasites are subspecies of *Trypanosoma brucei, T. b. rhodesiense* in East Africa and *T. b. gambiense* in Central and West Africa.

Once introduced by the bite of the tsetse fly, the organisms multiply rapidly in the blood and may quickly reach a density in excess of $10^6$ organisms per milliliter. Soon, however, the number of parasites drops

**Figure 17.8** Scanning electron micrograph of *Trypanosoma brucei*. This is the metacyclic stage found in the salivary glands of the tsetse fly and injected into the mammalian host when the fly bites. The specimen is 12 $\mu$m long. [Micrograph by L. Tetley; courtesy of Keith Vickerman, *Nature* 273:613, 1978.]

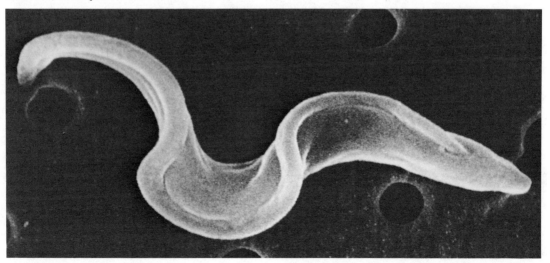

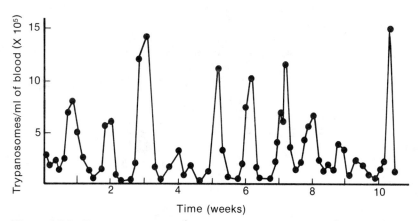

**Figure 17.9** Recurring waves of parasitemia in a patient with trypanosomiasis. Each peak represents the development of a clone of trypanosomes expressing a new variant surface glycoprotein (VSG). [From K. Vickerman, *Ciba Foundation Symp.* **25**:53, 1974.]

precipitously only to be followed a week or so later by another wave of parasitemia (Figure 17.9). This pattern continues indefinitely.

Living in the blood, we should expect that trypanosomes would be susceptible to immune attack. And so they are. The appearance of antibodies is responsible for the periods of remission. The antibodies that appear in the serum are specific for and destructive to the trypanosomes responsible for the present wave of parasitemia, but they are not effective against the organisms that appear at the next wave. The reason for this is that the organisms in each fresh wave are covered with a glycoprotein coat that is antigenically quite distinct from the one worn by the parasites of the previous wave. The coat consists of a 12nm thick layer of "variant surface glycoprotein" (VSG) molecules. The molecular weight of the VSGs is about 60,000.

Although the initial inoculum of trypanosomes is heterogeneous with respect to their VSGs, the successive dominance of new variants does not depend on such initial heterogeneity. A mouse infected with a *single* trypanosome of, say, "VSG-1" will — after its first wave of parasitemia by VSG-1 — have relapses dominated by trypanosomes expressing one or another new VSGs ("VSG-2", "VSG-3", etc.). Trypanosomes expressing new VSGs arise spontaneously in the host. They do so at a frequency of approximately $10^{-4}$. The presence of antibodies against a temporarily dominant VSG does not influence the *emergence* of new VSGs but does provide a selective advantage for the new variants enabling them to create a new wave of parasitemia.

Contrary to what a bacteriologist or virologist might expect, new VSGs are not produced simply by gene mutation. Partial amino acid sequences have been determined for several VSGs, and these sequences are quite different, with little or no evidence of homology. Furthermore, the order in which particular VSGs appear in a freshly infected host is predictable to some degree. This sort of behavior would be unlikely with a process of random mutation.

The evidence suggests instead that trypanosomes contain a large (at least several hundred) family of genes, each member of which encodes one VSG. Only one of these genes is *expressed* in a single cell. This is reminiscent of the story for immunoglobulin V genes. Several laboratories have succeeded in cloning cDNA to use as probes for genes encoding particular VSGs. These probes always recognize at least one — sometimes several — restriction fragments in the DNA of *all* clones of trypanosomes irrespective of the particular VSG they are expressing at the time. This tells us that each trypanosome carries all the genes for the VSG repertoire of the species. When the cDNA probe derived from one clone is annealed to the DNA of that clone — and only that clone — one additional copy of the gene, on a restriction fragment of a different size, is sometimes seen (Figure 17.10). This finding suggests that on some occasions the VSG gene *expressed* in a given clone has been copied from one of a master set of genes and translocated to a new location in the genome to be transcribed.

This new location is always at the end of a chromosome. At least three, perhaps more, specific chromosome ends can serve as sites for VSG gene

**Figure 17.10** Autoradiogram of Southern blots of nuclear DNA from clones of *Trypanosoma brucei* expressing different variant surface glycoproteins (VSGs). The DNA was digested with PstI in every case. The probe was a fragment of cDNA from a clone designated 118. The probe binds to a 2.1 kb fragment in every clone examined. It also binds to a second fragment in clones expressing the 118 gene (lanes 3 and 8 (which are duplicates) and lane 9). The clone represented in lane 9 was derived from a clone (lane 6) that had not been expressing the 118 gene. The clones in lanes 6 and 7 were derived from a 118 clone (lane 3) but no longer expressed the 118 VSG nor possessed the second gene fragment. [Courtesy of P. Borst; from P. A. M. Michels et al., *Nucleic Acids Research* **10**:2353, 1982.]

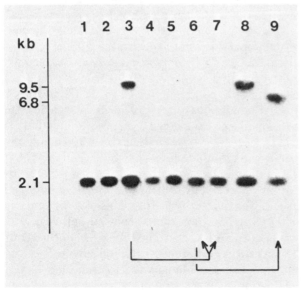

expression. Some VSG genes are normally located at these chromosome ends, and these genes do not need to be copied and translocated to be expressed.

In addition to a large repertoire of germline VSG genes, additional diversity is generated by point mutations occurring in the expressed copy of a particular gene. This, too, is reminiscent of the story for immunoglobulin V genes.

Thus *Trypanosoma brucei* maintains itself indefinitely in the face of repeated attempts by its host to eliminate it by periodically switching to the expression of a new VSG gene. If at the time a trypanosome appears with a new VSG, there are no antibodies present directed against that VSG, the organism is selectively favored to establish a new clone of organisms. The result is a fresh wave of parasitemia that lasts until the immune system responds anew.

## 17.9 Influenza

Probably the most devastating plague in human history was the "Spanish flu" of 1918 and 1919. The disease (which may have arisen in the United States, certainly not in Spain) swept around the world three times causing skyrocketing death rates. The most conservative estimates put the final death toll at 21 million. Over one-half million persons died in the United States alone. A disease that attacks a large proportion of the population in every region is called a **pandemic.**

Two pandemics of influenza have occurred since 1919. These were the "Asian" flu of 1957 and the "Hong Kong" flu of 1968. Although the number of victims in 1957 was higher than in 1918–19, the fatality rate was much lower. The main reason for this was the availability of antibiotic therapy in 1957. The influenza virus seldom kills directly. Instead it weakens the victim so that secondary invaders, like pneumococci, become established and cause a pneumonia that may end fatally. In fact, until the viral cause of influenza was established in the 1930s, some of these secondary invaders, especially *Hemophilus influenzae*, were mistakenly thought to be the causative agent.

In retrospect, it is clear that the pandemics of 1918, 1957, and 1968 had been preceded by other pandemics for at least several centuries. On the average, influenza pandemics occur every 13 years, although there is considerable variation in the interval between them (the 1918 pandemic was the first to occur since the great pandemic of 1889).

In 1918, virology was in its infancy. An influenza-like disease of birds (fowl plague) was known to be caused by a virus. In 1930 Shope showed that a flu-like illness in pigs was caused by a virus. This was particularly interesting because in 1918 it had been noted that an outbreak of a flu-like illness in pigs often occurred close to the time of an outbreak of influenza in humans. (It was a virus very similar to Shope's swine flu virus that caused several outbreaks among humans in 1976 and led to the massive program of vaccination against swine flu.)

In 1933, after failing with such standard lab animals as rabbits and guinea pigs, Smith and his collaborators found that they could transmit human influenza to ferrets, and that the agent was a virus. Thus it became possible for the first time to propagate the virus in the laboratory. The use of ferrets was (and continues to be) also useful in that the antisera from infected animals can be used to analyze the antigenicity of the various isolates of influenza virus. In time it was possible to distinguish three distinct types of virus that cause influenza in humans: A, B, and C. Only influenza A causes pandemics.

In 1940 Burnet discovered that flu viruses grow vigorously in chick embryos. This made virtually unlimited amounts of virus available for research work and, in due course, for the preparation of vaccines.

The influenza virion is a spherical particle with a diameter of about 100 nm (Figure 17.11). It is enveloped within a lipid bilayer membrane derived from the cell membrane of its host. Two proteins are inserted in the membrane (Figure 17.12): a hemagglutinin (H) and a neuraminidase (N). Beneath the lipid bilayer is a shell of protein (the matrix protein). The interior of the virion contains eight separate RNA molecules (single stranded), a protein closely associated with these, three different RNA

**Figure 17.11** Influenza virions (284,000×). Note the surface projections of hemagglutinin and neuraminidase molecules. [Courtesy of Dr. K. G. Murti.]

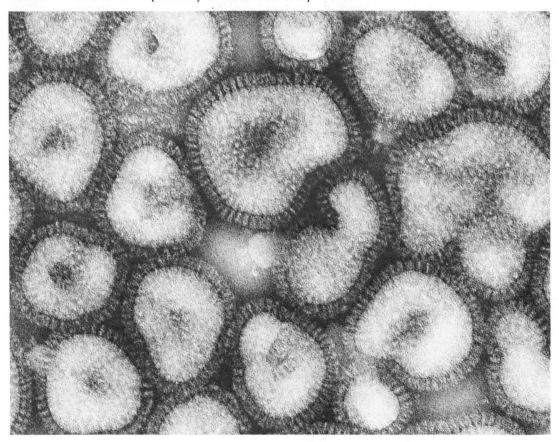

polymerases, and a protein of unknown function. Each of the eight pieces of RNA encodes one of the eight proteins found in or on the virion.

The hemagglutinin is present as trimers which project like spikes from the surface of the virion (Figure 17.12). The hemagglutinin is responsible for binding to receptors on host cells, a function essential for infection. The neuraminidase digests the complex polysaccharides found at the surface of the host cells and this aids in the release of progeny virus from infected cells. Thus the neuraminidase facilitates the spread of the virus through the infected host. Exposed as they are at the surface of the virion, the H and N molecules are the major immunogens.

Influenza virions also stick to chicken red blood cells and agglutinate them. This makes possible a convenient hemagglutination assay (see Section 5.7) for determining virus titers. The hemagglutination reaction is inhibited by the presence of antibodies against H, thus providing the basis for a hemagglutination inhibition (HAI) assay for measuring *antibody* titers.

Analysis by HAI reveals that influenza viruses differ antigenically. In influenza A, these differences occur at two levels. The hemagglutinin (H) on some viruses is entirely different from that on others. For example, antibodies against the flu virus that circulated in the years immediately

**Figure 17.12** Schematic representation of an influenza virus. The lipid bilayer is derived from the cell membrane of the host cell. Each of the 8 single-stranded RNA molecules encodes one of the 8 proteins from which the virus is constructed.

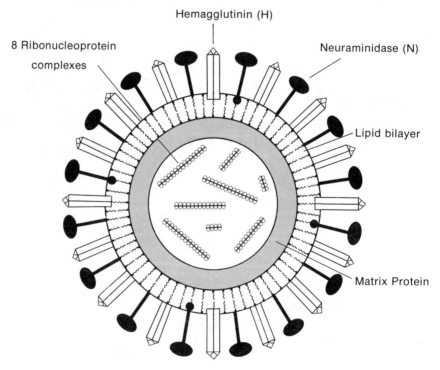

prior to 1957 did not react at all with the hemagglutinin that was present on the Asian flu virus that appeared in 1957. The hemagglutinin on the "Hong Kong" virus that appeared in 1968 shared no determinants with either of the other two. These major changes are called *antigenic shifts*. Antigenic shift has also occurred in the neuraminidase. Antigenic shift in H or in both H and N establishes a distinct "subtype" (Figure 17.13). The influenza virus that immediately preceded the Asian flu is designated H1N1. Both the H and N of the Asian flu were completely different and are designated H2N2. The Hong Kong flu of 1968 had a new hemagglutinin but retained the same neuraminidase (H3N2). The occurrence of pandemic influenza coincides with the emergence of a new subtype. Because of the totally new antigenic structure, the population (or at least the more youthful members of it) will have no residual immunity from prior influenza infections.

Influenza *epidemics*, which are more localized outbreaks of the disease, occur at two to three year intervals in the periods between pandemics. Each new epidemic is usually caused by a variant of the subtype that has been circulating since the last pandemic. The variants express some new antigenic determinants on their hemagglutinin (and, to a lesser extent, on their neuraminidase). However, some of the determinants are shared with the preceding variants. This more gradual change in antigenic structure is called *antigenic drift*.

The mechanism of antigenic drift is quite clear. The amino acid sequences of the hemagglutinins of a number of variants of A/Aichi/68 (the first "Hong Kong" subtype, H3N2) have been determined. In addition, the *nucleotide* sequences of two H genes (A/Aichi/68 and A/Victoria/75

**Figure 17.13**  Representative subtypes of influenza A.

| Date | Strain | Subtype | Notes |
|------|--------|---------|-------|
| 1889 | — | H3N? | Pandemic |
| 1918 | — | H1N1 | Pandemic of "Spanish flu" |
| 1930 | A/swine/30 | H1N1 | Isolated from pigs |
| 1933 | A/England/33 | H1N1 | First isolate from humans |
| 1957 | A/Singapore/57 | H2N2 | "Asian" flu pandemic; antigenic shift |
| 1962 | A/Japan/62 | H2N2 | Antigenic drift |
| 1964 | A/Taiwan/64 | H2N2 | Further antigenic drift |
| 1968 | A/Aichi/68 | H3N2 | "Hong Kong" flu pandemic; antigenic shift |
| 1972 | A/Memphis/72 | H3N2 | Antigenic drift: 18 amino acid residues different from A/Aichi/68 |
| 1975 | A/Victoria/75 | H3N2 | Further antigenic drift: 29 amino acid residues different from A/Aichi/68 |
| 1976 | A/New Jersey/76 | H1N1 | Swine flu in recruits |
| 1977 | A/Texas/77 | H3N2 | |
| 1977 | A/USSR/77 | H1N1 | "Russian" flu |
| 1982 | A/Philippines/82 | H3N2 ⎫ | Two subtypes have continued to |
| 1983 | A/Chile/83 | H1N1 ⎭ | cocirculate since 1977 |

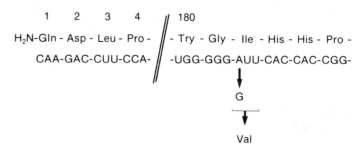

A/Aichi/68

A/Victoria/75

**Figure 17.14** *(above and opposite)* Antigenic drift of the hemagglutinin of the "Hong Kong" influenza virus. Although the nucleotide sequence shown here (which represents only a small part of the entire gene) is for the RNA, the actual sequencing was done on the cDNA of the two H genes. The amino acid sequence has been deduced from the gene sequence. From 1968 to 1975, 64 nucleotide substitutions occurred within the entire gene. Many of these were "silent"—i.e., specified the same amino acid as before (e.g., see residue 194). Others, however, produced 28 changes in the amino acid sequence. [Based on M. Verhoeyen et al., *Nature* **286**:771, 1980.]

—see Figure 17.14) have been established. The picture these data present is that

1. Antigenic drift occurs as a result of the gradual accumulation of point mutations in the H gene (and presumably in the N gene as well).
2. Within a subtype, mutations giving rise to amino acid substitutions occur at an average rate of two to four per year.
3. Although some amino acid substitutions are antigenically neutral (i.e., they affect a portion of the molecule that does not form or influence any antigenic determinant), others create altered antigenic determinants.
4. The presence of new determinants gives the virus a selective advantage as it circulates in a host population that has been increasingly exposed to earlier variants of the subtype.
5. By the time that drift has produced several (perhaps four) new antigenic determinants, the stage is set for a major epidemic.
6. Eventually the potentiality for further significant drift within a subtype may become reduced. At this time, the world stage is set for another antigenic shift—the emergence of an entirely different subtype.

In contrast to antigenic drift, the mechanism of antigenic shift is still puzzling. It is as if the virus has suddenly acquired an entirely new gene for H or for both H and N. Where could such genes come from? There are two possibilities. One is that with the emergence of a new subtype, the previous subtype goes into hiding for a few decades, perhaps residing in some animal host. It is reasonably certain that animals can contract influenza from humans (and vice versa). The appearance of A/USSR/77 (H1N1), twenty years after H1N1 had last been seen suggests that a reservoir exists awaiting the opportunity to reappear and reestablish dominance. Studies of antisera from persons who were first infected in the pandemic of 1889 suggest that the hemagglutinin at that time may have been H3, which reappeared in 1968.

A second possibility (and one that does not exclude the first), is that

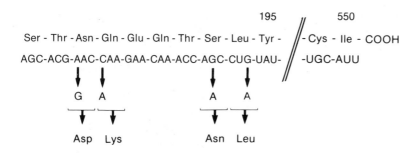

new subtypes appear by the reassortment of H genes and N genes between human flu viruses and similar A type viruses found in domestic mammals (e.g., horses and pigs) and birds, both domestic and wild (mallard ducks, arctic terns). Reassortment of flu genes certainly occurs in the laboratory. When tissue culture cells are simultaneously infected with two types of flu virus, they produce progeny viruses that contain various combinations of the genes of the parental strains. For example, in order to make a vaccine against the latest strain in circulation, the practice is to coinfect cells with that strain (such as a variant of H3N2) and with A/PR8/34, an H1N1 strain that grows especially well in chick embryos. Antiserum against H1N1 is added to the medium. This system selects for virions that have acquired the genes for H3N2 and the gene or genes responsible for vigorous growth in chick embryos (from which the vaccine is prepared). The fact that the eight influenza genes are located on separate molecules of RNA probably facilitates this reassortment.

Genetic reassortment can also occur in vivo. By simultaneously infecting a pig with the swine flu virus (H1N1) and a Hong Kong virus (H3N2), Webster and Campbell were able to isolate viruses that were H3N1. Genetic assortment of H and N genes has not been observed in humans, although some of the H1N1 strains that were circulating in 1978 and 1979 show evidence of reassortment having occurred among the other six genes.

Ten subtypes of hemagglutinin (H3→H12) have been detected in birds; two of these (H3 and H7) are also found in horses. Five subtypes of N (N3→N6, and N9) are found in birds, and two others (N7 and N8) have been found in horses. The H3 subtype was first detected, in both birds and horses, in 1963, five years before it emerged in the human population in the first of the Hong Kong viruses. Like the swine flu hemagglutinin (H1), these bird and horse antigens are not identical with their human counterparts. But they do share antigenic determinants with them and so belong to the same subtype. They also raise the possibility that these animal viruses might serve as the reservoir on which antigenic shift draws. The close association between humans and their domestic animals and the migratory abilities of wild birds suggest the means by which animal flu viruses might periodically infect humans and how they might be spread so rapidly across the globe.

Infection by influenza virus provides a solid, probably lifelong immunity. The protection is most likely dependent on IgA antibodies which block infection through the mucous membranes of the respiratory system. Subsequent infections by related viruses elicit a memory (secondary) response against cross-reacting determinants on the first virus and also a primary response against new epitopes on the new virus. This lifelong imprint of one's first encounter, which has been called "original antigenic sin," may not keep you from getting sick, but it has provided fascinating clues as to the nature of the virus that caused pandemics before the discovery of the influenza virus in 1933. By analyzing the memory response of survivors of the pandemics of 1889 and 1918–19, those viruses can be tentatively identified as H3 and H1N1, respectively (see Figure 17.13). Original antigenic sin also explains why the swine flu vaccine of 1976 (H1N1) was less effective in persons under 20 years of age than in older persons, most of whom had encountered variants of H1N1 in the years prior to their replacement by Asian flu (H2N2) in 1957.

The immune response to an infection by a strain of influenza virus is probably just as effective as the response to the measles and variola (smallpox) viruses. The reason that we suffer periodic attacks of influenza is not, then, the inadequacy of our immune response but rather the ability of the influenza virus to evade the growing level of immunity in a population through antigenic drift and, from time to time, antigenic shift.

## ADDITIONAL READING

1. Bernheim, H. A., and M. J. Kluger, "Fever: Effect of Drug-Induced Antipyresis on Survival," *Science* **193**:237, 1976.

2. Capron, A., and J. P. Dessaint, "Effector and Regulatory Mechanisms in Immunity to Schistosomes: A Heuristic View," *Ann. Rev. Immunol.* **3**:455, 1985.

3. Davies, P., et al., "The Role of Arachidonic Acid Oxygenation Products in Pain and Inflammation," *Ann. Rev.Immunol.* **2**:335, 1984.

4. Dinarello, C. A., et al., "Role of Arachidonate Metabolism in the Immunoregulatory Function of Human Leukocyte Pyrogen/Lymphocyte-Activating Factor/ Interleukin 1," *J. Immunol.* **130**:890, 1983.

5. Gerhard, W., et al., "Antigenic structure of influenza virus hemagglutinin defined by hybridoma antibodies," *Nature* **290**:713, 1981.

6. Lin, Y.-L., and Brigitte A. Askonas, "Biological Properties of an Influenza A Virus-Specific Killer T Cell Clone. Inhibition of Virus Replication in Vivo and Induction of Delayed-Type Hypersensitivity Reactions," *J. Exp. Med.* **154**:225, 1981.

7. Morrison, S. L., et al., "Chimeric Human Antibody Molecules: Mouse Antigen-Binding Domains with Human Constant Region Domains," *Proc. Natl. Acad. Sci. USA* **81**:6851, 1984.

8. Myler, P. J., et al., "Antigenic Variation of African Trypanosomes by Gene Replacement or Activation of Alternate Telomeres," *Cell* **39**:203, 1984.

9. Palese, P., and J. F. Young, "Variation of Influenza A, B, and C Viruses," *Science* **215**:1468, 1982.

10. Stuart-Harris, C., "The Epidemiology and Prevention of Influenza," *American Scientist* **69**:166, 1981.

11. Webster, R. G., et al., "Molecular Mechanisms of Variation in Influenza Viruses," *Nature* **296:**115, 1982.

12. Wiley, D. C., et al., "Structural Identification of the Antibody-Binding Sites of Hong Kong Influenza Hemagglutinin and Their Involvement in Antigenic Variation," *Nature* **289:**373, 1981.

# Immunopathology

The immune system is essential to life. No regimen of antibiotic and antiviral therapy can keep a person alive who is totally incapable of mounting an immune response. But the immune system can be the cause of disease as well as its cure. In this chapter we shall examine three general categories of pathological disorders produced by the immune system.

1. Hypersensitivities.
2. Autoimmune disorders.
3. Immunodeficiency diseases.

The hypersensitivities are immune responses that produce tissue injury upon subsequent exposure to an agent that is *not intrinsically harmful*. Like all immune responses, hypersensitivities display specificity and memory. One milligram of ovalbumin can be administered to an unprimed guinea pig with no harmful effects. But a second dose given 14 days later triggers a rapid and dramatic onset of shock. Intravenous injection of this innocuous material usually kills the guinea pig within a few minutes. A similar injection of some other antigen has no harmful effect. Two important points emerge from this demonstration. First, the responsiveness of the animal to OVA—and only to OVA— has obviously been altered by prior exposure to it. Second, the response leads to such gross pathological changes that the animal dies. But in a real sense, the animal's own immune system killed it, not a harmful property intrinsic to the antigen.

The term hypersensitivity is not entirely satisfactory to describe these disorders. In some cases, the damage *is* caused by an excessive response, but this is not always the case. Often, the damage simply results from an "inappropriate" response. The term *allergy* is often used as a synonym for hypersensitivity. Unfortunately, allergy has been used in a number of different ways in the past. Here we shall use it in the lay sense of a damaging immune response to an environmental antigen. Antigens that trigger allergic responses are often called **allergens.**

One or more of several different immune mechanisms may be at work in hypersensitivities. Some are mediated by antibodies; some by cells; some by both. Gell and Coombs have proposed a classification scheme to aid in delineating the different mechanisms (Figure 18.1). Their scheme encompasses four types of hypersensitivities.

*I. Immediate Hypersensitivities.*    These are sudden allergic responses mediated by antibodies, usually of the IgE class. These will be discussed in Sections 18.2 and 18.3.

*II. Antibody-Mediated Cytotoxicity.*    In the strict sense, Type II reactions produce cell damage which is mediated by complement-fixing antibodies directed against cell-surface antigens. These will be discussed in

| | Gell & Coombs classification | Mechanism | Examples |
|---|---|---|---|
| Immediate hypersensitivity | Type I | Release of vasoactive substances from antigen-sensitized mast cells; mediated by reaginic abs (IgE in humans) | Drug allergies; hay fever |
| Antibody-mediated cytotoxicity | Type II | Cell damage caused by antibodies directed against cell-surface antigens | Hemolytic disease of the newborn; Goodpasture's syndrome |
| Immune complex disorders | Type III | Deposits of antigen–antibody complexes activate complement pathway causing inflammation and other tissue damage | Serum sickness; extrinsic allergic alveolitis |
| Cell-mediated hypersensitivity | Type IV | T lymphocytes interact with antigen and liberate lymphokines, which recruit macrophages to the site | Contact dermatitis; tubercular lesions |

Figure 18.1  Hypersensitivities.

Section 18.4. However, antibodies directed against some cell-surface antigens do not kill the cell but instead alter its physiological activity. The antigens in these cases are receptor structures that ordinarily respond to chemical signals within the body. Examples of these disorders will be discussed in Section 18.5.

*III. Immune Complex Disorders.* The tissue damage in Type III hypersensitivities is caused by activation of the complement system following the formation of antigen–antibody complexes. Mechanisms and examples are treated in Section 18.6.

*IV. Cell-Mediated Hypersensitivities.* These are reactions mediated by T cells. The classic examples are the delayed-type hypersensitivities (DTH) that occur when antigen triggered $T_D$ cells release lymphokines. But in Section 18.7 we shall also examine cell-mediated disorders in which other subsets of T cells play a role.

## 18.2  Systemic Anaphylaxis

The response of the OVA-primed guinea pig to a second injection of OVA is a classic example of systemic anaphylaxis. Shortly after receiving the second ("shocking") dose of antigen, the animal's breathing becomes

472

labored, it defecates and urinates, and there is a sharp drop in blood pressure. These reactions are brought about by generalized vasodilation, increased capillary permeability, and contraction of smooth muscle. The immediate cause of death is usually asphyxiation brought on by the marked constriction of the bronchioles. If the animal does not die in a few minutes, recovery is usually speedy and complete.

Systemic anaphylaxis can be passively transferred to unprimed animals by the injection of serum from a sensitized animal. Thus the response is a humoral one. However, only a minor fraction of the circulating immunoglobulins is capable of sensitizing an animal for anaphylaxis. For years these elusive antibodies were called **reagins.** Their low concentration in the serum made their study difficult. An early breakthrough came with the Ishizakas' discovery that reaginic antibodies represent a previously unknown class of immunoglobulin. They immunized a rabbit with "reagin-rich" serum from hay fever sufferers. They then subsequently absorbed the antiserum with myeloma proteins or purified immunoglobulins of each of the then known classes: IgG, IgA, IgM, and IgD. Even after these absorptions, the rabbit antiserum still retained the ability to absorb reaginic antibody activity. This suggested that reaginic antibody represented a unique class of antibody. The discovery of a human IgE myeloma opened the way for structural studies of this fifth antibody isotype (see Section 9.10).

**Figure 18.2** Systemic anaphylaxis triggered by the sting of a single honeybee. This highly allergic patient required cardiac massage and intravenous epinephrine at the times shown. [From Dr. J. Vick in L. M. Lichtenstein, "Allergic Responses to Airborn Allergens and Insect Venoms," *Fed. Proc.* **36**:1727, 1977.]

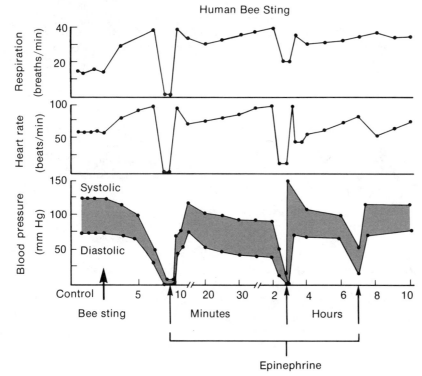

The binding to mast cells of IgE molecules of a particular specificity sensitizes the cell to the corresponding allergen. When the allergen becomes bound to the antigen-binding site of the IgE molecules, a signal is transmitted into the cell that results in degranulation (Figure 14.11). The basophilic granules are filled with histamine and other vasoactive materials. The release of these substances elicits the various signs of anaphylaxis.

Systemic anaphylaxis is a frequent occurrence in humans. Insect stings, many drugs (e.g., penicillin), and a wide variety of foods (e.g., sea food) may trigger systemic anaphylaxis that, if not treated promptly, can be fatal. Allergic reactions to food seem to be triggered by sensitized mast cells in the intestinal mucosa and/or the transfer into the circulation of undigested allergenic proteins.

Treatment of systemic anaphylaxis centers on the prompt administration of adrenaline (Figure 18.2), antihistamines, and—in the case of shock—intravenous fluid replacement.

## 18.3 Local Anaphylaxis

Local anaphylaxis is different from systemic anaphylaxis in only one important respect: the anaphylactic response is limited to certain tissues or organs. The most common manifestations of local anaphylaxis are (1) allergic rhinitis (hay fever), (2) urticaria (hives), and (3) bronchial asthma. In the case of hay fever, airborne allergens—often plant pollens—react with IgE-sensitized mast cells in the conjunctiva and nasal mucosa. Hives are usually elicited by food. Bronchial asthma may be triggered by airborne allergens reaching sensitized mast cells in the bronchi or by allergens reaching the lungs by way of the circulation. The list of allergens that can trigger asthmatic attacks is enormous. House dust (rich in the feces of house dust mites), animal dander, and fungal spores are notorious offenders. Leukotrienes (Section 17.2) are probably the most important pharmacological agents involved in the development of hives as well as in the constriction of the bronchi during attacks of asthma. Leukotrienes are far more potent than histamine in mediating both of these reactions. As little as 0.1 nmol of certain leukotrienes will elicit a wheal and flare reaction (Figure 5.17) when injected into the skin.

Why are some of us so prone to allergies when others are not? Part of the answer is genetic. A predisposition to allergies often runs in families. In some cases, the allergy is restricted to one or a few closely related allergens but, more often, the victim becomes sensitized to a wide variety of allergens. An inherited predisposition to allergic responses is called **atopy**. Atopic persons usually have higher levels of circulating IgE (up to 12 $\mu$g/ml) than are found in normal individuals ($\sim$0.3 $\mu$g/ml). Whereas only 20–50% of the receptors are occupied by IgE on mast cells from normal persons, all the receptors may be occupied in atopic individuals.

Sometimes the offending allergen(s) can be identified by a marked association between contact (e.g., to lobster) and anaphylaxis. Where the cause is not immediately apparent, the usual recourse is to attempt to identify the allergen by skin testing the sufferer with a variety of different allergens. Each is introduced into a separate site in the skin and each site is observed for the development of a wheal and erythema (Figure 5.17) over the next few minutes.

As we have seen, anaphylactic responses can be transferred by serum. The Prausnitz–Küstner (P-K) test in humans and passive cutaneous anaphylaxis (PCA — see Section 5.8) are examples. The P-K test was once widely used in diagnosis. Serum from the allergic individual is introduced into the skin of a normal recipient. After allowing a latent period of several hours to elapse, the suspected allergen is introduced into the same site. The development of a wheal and erythema indicates a positive response. The advantage of the P-K test is that there is no danger of inadvertently precipitating systemic anaphylaxis by introducing antigen into the allergic patient. The disadvantage is the possibility of transmission of serum hepatitis (hepatitis B) to the recipient.

The need for a latent period before the P-K test can be completed can be accounted for by (1) the time required for IgE molecules to become bound to the mast cells and (2) the time required for other classes (such as IgG) of antibodies of the same specificity to diffuse away from the site so that they will not interfere with ("block") the interaction of allergen with the mast cells.

What, besides efforts at providing immediate relief of symptoms, can be done for atopic patients? The time-honored approach is to attempt desensitization. At present this consists of administering repeated, graded doses of the allergen. The procedure is time consuming, hence expensive, and often only marginally effective. The procedure was developed empirically, but we are now in a position to explore the immunological basis for such success as it achieves. One possibility for which there is considerable evidence is that the desensitization schedule deflects the immune response away from IgE production in favor of IgG production. The IgG antibodies presumably act as "blocking" antibodies, intercepting the allergen before it can reach the sensitized mast cells. Another possibility is that repeated, minute doses of the allergen bring on a state of tolerance in $T_H$ cells (see Section 16.2). A third possibility is that the desensitization process stimulates the development of T suppressor ($T_S$) cells. There is some evidence, in humans as well as in experimental animals, of the existence of $T_S$ cells that suppress IgE responses irrespective of the antigen specificity involved.

## 18.4 Humoral Cytotoxicity

These Type II hypersensitivities are mediated by antibodies directed against cell-surface antigens. The binding of antibody to the cell usually activates the complement system (see Section 14.2). Four modes of damage to the cell can follow (Figure 18.3).

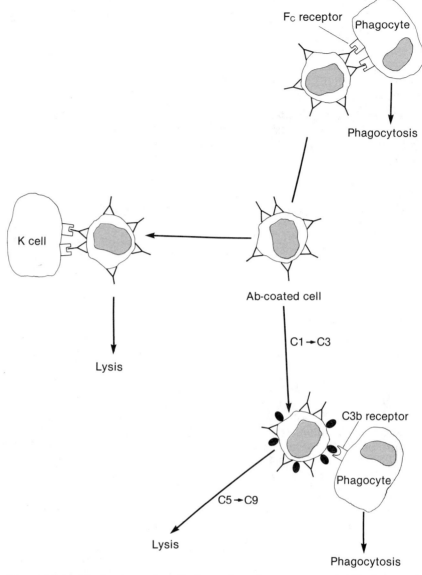

**Figure 18.3** Mechanisms of antibody-mediated cytotoxicity. Antibody-coated cells may be lysed by K cells *(left)* or through activation of the full complement sequence. Phagocytosis of antibody-coated cells may be mediated by receptors for the Fc region of the antibodies or by receptors for C3b *(right)*.

1. The binding of antibody to the cell surface leads to a cytotoxic attack by K cells. This is antibody-dependent, cell-mediated cytotoxicity (ADCC — see Section 14.4).
2. The antibody-coated cell binds to macrophages through their receptors for the Fc portion of IgG and initiates phagocytosis.
3. Activation of the complement system leads to the deposition of C3b on the cell surface. The C3b-coated cells are bound by phagocytic cells through their receptors for C3b, and phagocytosis follows.

**4.** If complement fixation continues to the terminal stages of binding C8 and C9, the cell is lysed.

Let us examine four examples of these Type II hypersensitivities that occur in humans.

### Hemolytic Disease of the Newborn (Rh Disease)

In this disease, the antibodies are IgG antibodies synthesized by the mother and directed against red cell antigens — usually Rh — of her fetus. The Rh system of red cell antigens is quite complex. However, most of the problems arise when an Rh-negative mother becomes sensitized to a major Rh antigen designated $Rh_0$ or D. This can occur at the time she gives birth to an Rh-positive child (who has inherited the antigen from its father). At the time of parturition, there is often a flush of fetal blood cells into the maternal circulation. If these cells are $Rh^+$, the mother will develop antibodies (chiefly IgG) against them. With a subsequent $Rh^+$ fetus, these antibodies, which readily cross the placenta, bind to the fetal red cells and cause their destruction. The outcome is anemia and jaundice from the accumulation of bilirubin, a product of the catabolism of hemoglobin. The disease may be sufficiently severe to kill the fetus.

Although red cell antigens other than $Rh_0$ are sometimes implicated in this disorder, an ABO incompatibility between mother and fetus generally does not present any problem. One reason for this is that the anti-A and anti-B antibodies are mostly IgM, and these do not cross the placenta to enter the fetal circulation. In fact, sensitization of Rh-negative mothers to $Rh_0$ is less likely to occur when the mother lacks the A or B antigen found on the fetal cells. Presumably this is because she quickly destroys any fetal red cells that get into her circulation before she can become sensitized to them. This phenomenon has led to an extremely effective preventive measure to avoid Rh sensitization (Figure 18.4). Soon after each birth of an $Rh^+$ child, the mother is given an injection of anti-$Rh_0$ (D) antibodies (Rh immune globulin, RhIG). These passively acquired antibodies prevent an active immune response to the red cells,

**Figure 18.4** Incidence of Rh hemolytic disease of the newborn in the United States, 1970–1979. Rh immune globulin (RhIG) came into common use in 1968. [U.S. Public Health Service.]

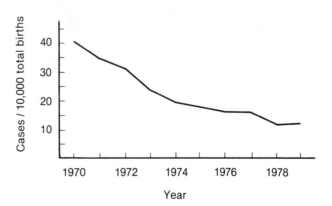

perhaps operating through a homeostatic mechanism like that described in Section 15.2.

## Immune Hemolytic Anemia

In this disorder, the individual synthesizes antibodies, usually of the IgG class, against his own red cells. Binding of these antibodies to the cells activates the complement system, which can opsonize the cells (by C3b) for phagocytosis or, in some cases, proceed to their lysis (by C8 and C9). The presence of IgG-coated red cells is revealed by the Coombs antiglobulin test (see Section 5.7).

In many cases, this disorder is idiopathic; i.e., no underlying cause can be found. However, this autoimmune disorder is often found associated with other diseases, including infections, malignancies, and other autoimmune disorders like systemic lupus erythematosus (SLE). A wide variety of drugs — penicillin, methyldopa, quinidine, and many others — may trigger attacks of immune hemolytic anemia. Where there is no immediate cause to be treated (like stopping use of the eliciting drug), corticosteroids and splenectomy are often effective.

## Immune Thrombocytopenic Purpura

The antigens in this disorder are on the platelet surface. Antibodies coat the platelets and opsonize them for phagocytic destruction in the spleen. Platelet life time may be reduced from the normal of eight days to as little as one hour, and platelet counts may drop from a normal of 250,000/$\mu$l to 20,000/$\mu$l. This greatly reduces clotting efficiency and results in both external bleeding (e.g., from the nose) and internal bleeding into the skin, causing purple patches (purpura).

Although infections and certain other autoimmune disorders are

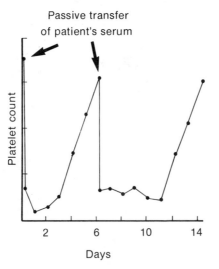

Figure 18.5 Decline and recovery in the platelet count of a normal human subject receiving two transfusions of serum from a patient with thrombocytopenic purpura. [From W. J. Harrington et al., *J. Lab. Clin. Med.* 38:1, 1951.]

sometimes associated with this disease, in many cases its cause is unknown. The victim's blood contains antibodies that bind to naturally occurring antigens on the platelet surface. The patient's serum can be used to passively transfer the disorder to a normal recipient, with a rapid but temporary decline in the platelet count of the recipient (Figure 18.5).

Some cases of thrombocytopenic purpura are drug induced. Quinidine, sulfonamides, aspirin, digitoxin, methyldopa, and others have been implicated. Often in these cases, platelet destruction occurs because of antibodies directed against drug molecules bound to the platelet. Such cases cannot be passively transferred because the antibodies are ineffective in the absence of the drug. Drug-induced thrombocytopenic purpura is alleviated by withdrawing the drug. The idiopathic form of the disease can often be helped by corticosteroids and/or splenectomy.

## Goodpasture's Syndrome

This rare disorder is characterized by antibodies directed against determinants on the basement membrane of the glomeruli of the kidney.

**Figure 18.6** A: Smooth, linear deposits along the basement membrane of a glomerulus from the kidney biopsy of a patient with Goodpasture's syndrome. The deposits, which contain antibodies directed against determinants on the glomerular basement membrane, have been visualized with a fluorescent antihuman IgG. B: Irregular, lumpy deposits along the glomerular basement membrane of a patient with nephrotic syndrome and membranous glomerulonephritis. The deposits have been visualized with fluoresceinated rabbit antihuman IgG. These deposits are presumably immune complexes containing antigen and complement components as well. Such deposits have been shown to contain C1q, C3, C4, C5, and C6. [Courtesy of Dr. Frank J. Dixon, "The importance of immunologic mechanisms," in *Controversy in Internal Medicine, II,* Saunders, Philadelphia, 1974.]

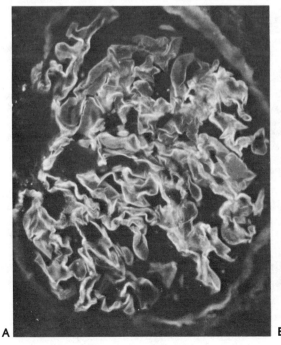 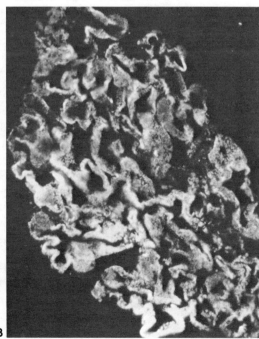

A          B

Binding of antibodies activates the complement sequence, which leads, to a severe glomerulitis. The integrity of the basement membrane is destroyed, allowing blood and protein to leak into the urine. Total kidney failure often follows.

The presence of antibodies and complement on the inner surface of the basement membrane can be revealed by immunofluorescence. The pattern of immunofluorescence faithfully follows the contour of the membrane as we would expect if the antibodies have bound to its surface (Figure 18.6). Antibodies, mostly IgG, can be eluted from these specimens and these will subsequently bind to slices of normal human kidney tissue.

The precipitating cause of Goodpasture's syndrome is unknown. But like the immune hemolytic anemias and thrombocytopenic purpura, it clearly represents a disorder mediated by the patient's own antibodies and thus is another example of an autoimmune disorder (see Section 18.9).

## 18.5  Antireceptor Antibodies

Antibodies directed against cell-surface antigens do not necessarily lead to destruction of the cell. In some cases, binding of antibodies to the cell surface may alter the physiology of the cell without destroying it. Two particularly illuminating examples are myasthenia gravis and Graves' disease. In each case, the antigen is a receptor which normally mediates chemical communication between cells.

### Myasthenia Gravis (MG)

This autoimmune disorder is characterized by weakness and fatigue of skeletal muscles. The defect occurs at the neuromuscular junction. In order to understand the immunopathology of myasthenia gravis, let us review the physiology of skeletal muscle excitation. Contraction of skeletal muscle is triggered by the release of acetylcholine (ACh) by motor neurons terminating at the surface of the muscle fiber (Figure 18.7). When a nerve impulse reaches the axon terminal, ACh is released. The ACh molecules bind to receptors (AChR) on the adjacent portion of the membrane covering the muscle fiber (the *end plate*). This opens channels that permit the rapid influx of sodium ions into the fiber. A potential of about 90 mV exists across the membrane of a resting fiber. The influx of sodium ions causes this potential to drop, a drop called the **end-plate potential (EPP)**. If, as it normally does, the EPP drops sufficiently to reach the threshold of the fiber, an action potential is generated and contraction of the fiber follows. With a volley of nerve impulses, the later impulses release less ACh than the first impulses. Nonetheless, the normal neuromuscular junction has sufficient capacity to respond, and adequate EPPs continue to be generated. Diffusion of ACh away from the

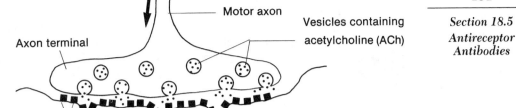

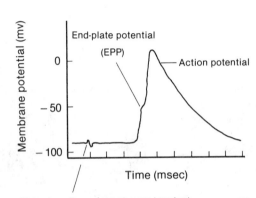

**Figure 18.7** Structure of the neuromuscular junction. The binding of ACh to receptors on the muscle fiber triggers an end plate potential (EPP). If the EPP reaches the threshold of the fiber, an action potential is generated *(bottom)* and contraction follows. In myasthenia gravis, the number of ACh receptors is reduced and this reduces the ability of the muscle to respond to repeated stimulation. The destruction of the AChR appears to be caused by autoantibodies.

site and its hydrolysis by acetylcholinesterase removes the ACh, closes the ion channels, and permits the fiber to return to its resting state ready for the arrival of a fresh volley of nerve impulses.

Victims of myasthenia gravis have smaller EPPs than normal. With repeated stimulation, the EPPs become too small to trigger further action potentials and the fiber ceases to contract. Administration of an inhibitor of acetylcholinesterase usually restores contractility by allowing more ACh to remain at the site.

In victims of myasthenia gravis, the number of ACh receptors is only 20% or so of the number found in normal neuromuscular junctions. Thus the capacity to continue to respond in the face of declining amounts of ACh is reduced.

The loss of AChR appears to be caused by antibodies directed against them. Binding of the antibodies causes (probably with the aid of complement) the AChR to be degraded faster than they can be resynthesized.

Several lines of evidence indicate that myasthenia gravis is an autoimmune disorder, which is mediated primarily (if not exclusively) by anti-AChR antibodies. (1) An experimental disease much like MG can be induced in rabbits, rats, etc. by injection of purified AChR along with adjuvant. (2) Anti-AChR antibodies can usually be detected in the serum of MG patients. (3) A series of injections of MG serum into a mouse leads in a few days to signs of muscle weakness. (4) The passive transfer of MG by antibodies also accounts for the occasional occurrence of transient MG in children born to myasthenic mothers.

The essential role of autoantibodies in this disorder also provides a therapeutic approach that has been used with some success. Plasmapheresis, a procedure in which the patient's plasma is exchanged while all the formed elements of the blood are returned to the circulation, lowers the concentration of AChR autoantibodies and provides temporary relief from the symptoms.

### Graves' Disease (Thyrotoxicosis)

This is a hyperthyroid condition in which an overactive thyroid produces a rise in metabolic rate, goiter, and a number of other unpleasant symptoms. To help us understand the mechanism at work in Graves' disease, let us review the normal operation of the thyroid. The thyroid gland takes up iodine from the blood and uses it to synthesize its two hormones, triiodothyronine ($T_3$) and thyroxin ($T_4$). The activity of the thyroid is driven by the thyroid-stimulating hormone, TSH, released from the anterior lobe of the pituitary (Figure 18.8). TSH binds to receptors on the secretory cells of the thyroid, activates the adenyl cyclase system, and turns on synthesis and release of $T_3$ and $T_4$. In addition to their manifold effects throughout the body, these hormones act on the hypothalamus to suppress the release of thyrotropin-releasing hormone (TRH) which, in

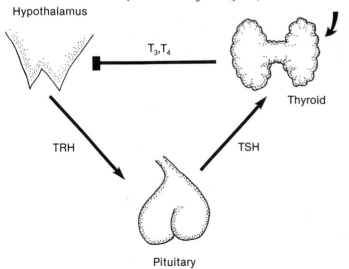

Binding of autoantibodies to TSH receptors stimulates synthesis of $T_3$ and $T_4$ despite low levels of TSH.

Hypothalamus

$T_3, T_4$

Thyroid

TRH

TSH

Pituitary

**Figure 18.8**  Negative feedback loop that regulates the level of circulating thyroid hormones. A rising level of $T_3$ and $T_4$ suppresses the releasing factor activity of the hypothalamus (bar). This leads to a drop in the level of $T_3$ and $T_4$. Antibodies directed against the receptors for TSH stimulate the production of $T_3$ and $T_4$ despite low levels of TSH.

turn, leads to a reduction in the release of TSH. Thus a negative feedback loop exists to maintain homeostatic control of the levels of $T_3$ and $T_4$ (Figure 18.8). In victims of Graves' disease, this feedback loop is broken. Despite high levels of $T_3$ and $T_4$, their thyroid continues to synthesize and release the hormones.

The problem appears to stem from autoantibodies that bind to the TSH receptors on the thyroid cell membrane. The binding of these antibodies causes the receptors to transmit the same stimulatory signal to the cell that TSH would elicit. The antibodies are not cytotoxic. In fact, their Fab fragments, which cannot bind complement, stimulate the gland as well as intact antibodies. The fact that these antibodies compete for the TSH binding site can be shown by their ability to block the binding of radiolabeled TSH to the cells.

The humoral basis for Graves' disease is also revealed by the transient hyperthyroidism found in infants born to mothers with Graves' disease. As the maternal IgG is degraded in the infant, the symptoms disappear.

## 18.6  Immune Complex Disorders

We ordinarily think of the binding of antibody to antigen as a final step in the immune response and the "cure" of the host. And it often is. But in some circumstances, the formation of antigen – antibody complexes triggers pathological changes in the host, the Type-III hypersensitivities.

### Serum Sickness

Passive immunization through the administration of antiserum was once widely used for patients at risk of diphtheria or tetanus infections. The source of the antiserum was usually an actively immunized horse. While the antitoxin in the horse serum could save the patient's life, the injections often produced their own special pathology. A week or two after receiving the horse serum, the patient developed a syndrome that usually included fever, hives, arthritis, and protein in the urine. This syndrome was called *serum sickness.* After another week or two, the symptoms subsided and the patient's health was restored.

The serum sickness syndrome can be produced in animals. A rabbit is given a large dose of a foreign protein (e.g., 250 mg BSA). If the antigen is radiolabeled, its fate within the body can be monitored. Over a period of days, it is slowly degraded and excreted from the body. After a week or two, the rate of catabolism becomes sharply accelerated (Figure 18.9). During this period of accelerated removal, the animal develops the signs associated with serum sickness, including fever and inflammatory kidney damage. During this entire period, no anti-BSA antibodies can be detected in the serum. Not until the last of the antigen is gone does circulating anti-BSA appear (Figure 18.9). Antibody *synthesis* actually precedes its appearance in the serum, but in the early stages of synthesis, the

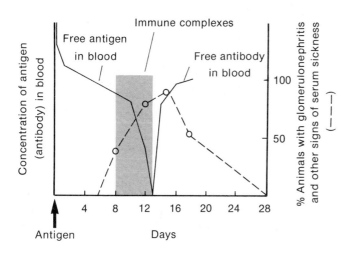

Serum Sickness

**Figure 18.9** Serum sickness in the rabbit. A large (0.5 g) dose of antigen (BSA) was given at day 0. The production of antibodies leads to the formation of immune complexes (day 8) and accelerates the clearance of antigen from the blood. The complexes are deposited in the kidneys, causing glomerulonephritis, and elsewhere. Antibodies are not seen in the blood until all the antigen in it has been complexed. [Based on F. G. Germuth, Jr., *J. Exp. Med.* 97:257, 1953.]

anti-BSA antibodies combine with residual antigen as fast as they are formed. Antigen is in great excess during this initial phase, so the complexes that form (e.g., $Ag_3Ab_2$) are soluble (you may wish to refer to the discussion on ag–ab complexes in Section 4.1).

These complexes are carried by the circulation and deposited in blood vessel walls, including the glomeruli of the kidneys. The complexes fix complement with the resulting production of the **anaphylatoxins** C3a and C5a. These molecules act on mast cells and basophils eliciting the release of histamine and leukotrienes. These mediators produce vasodilation, increased capillary permeability, and thus inflammation. The inflammatory effect of mast cells is magnified by their release of platelet-activating factor (**PAF**) which triggers the release of histamine and serotonin from platelets (Figure 18.10). C5a is also chemotactic for neutrophils which gather at the site and mediate further damage to the vessel walls.

As more antibody is synthesized, the system shifts into *antibody* excess. The complexes that form become larger and are now easily ingested by phagocytic cells. With the appearance of free antibody, the animal is well on the road to recovery.

The huge blood supply of the kidney and the function of the glomerular membrane as a filter makes the kidney particularly vulnerable to damage by immune complexes. Their presence can be revealed by immunofluorescence with antiserum directed against either antibody or complement components (such as C3). The fluorescence appears as a lumpy pattern along the walls of the glomeruli. This pattern is quite different from the smooth, linear pattern seen with antibodies directed against the glomerular basement membrane (Figure 18.6).

Thanks to widespread *active* immunization against tetanus and diphtheria, serum sickness is no longer commonly seen. However, glomerulonephritis produced by deposits of immune complexes is found in a number of other human ailments. Infectious organisms that can persist for long periods within the body often bring on glomerulonephritis. These include protozoans (e.g., *Plasmodium*, the agents of malaria), helminths

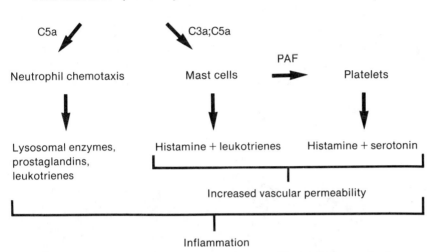

**Figure 18.10** Pathways to inflammation triggered by antigen–antibody complexes. PAF = platelet activating factor.

(as in schistosomiasis and filariasis), and some persistent viruses like hepatitis B. In each case, the continuing presence of the pathogen provides a continuing supply of antigen to combine with the antibodies synthesized by the host. Kidney biopsies reveal the presence of both antigen and antibody. Their presence can be revealed not only by immunofluorescence but by eluting both antigen and antibodies from the tissue.

Endogenous antigens that stimulate the formation of autoantibodies can also produce glomerulonephritis and other manifestations of immune-complex disease. In **rheumatoid arthritis,** complexes of IgG and anti-IgG antibodies are deposited in the joints. Their presence elicits the inflammatory reactions leading to swelling and pain in the joint. Victims of systemic lupus erythematosus (SLE) develop antibodies against a broad array of self antigens. These include antibodies against DNA, RNA, IgG, red cells, platelets, and ribosomes. Antigen–antibody complexes form, and these are deposited in the skin, joints, and kidneys. At each site, the complexes trigger inflammatory reactions.

## The Arthus Reaction

The formation of antigen–antibody complexes in the skin produces a characteristic lesion named after the investigator who first studied it.

The complexes can be formed by injecting antigen into the skin of a hyperimmune animal. Alternatively, both antigen and antibody can be injected into the skin. In either case, the complexes that form initiate the reaction. Complement is fixed by the complexes, and C3a and C5a increase vascular permeability. C5a also attracts neutrophils to the site. The neutrophils ingest the complexes and release a variety of lysosomal enzymes. The result is inflammation and tissue damage that reaches a peak some four to eight hours after the reaction is initiated. Thus the Arthus reaction develops more slowly than does immediate (IgE-mediated) hypersensitivity and more rapidly than delayed-type hypersensitivity (DTH). The histology of the skin lesion differs as well from that seen in the other two conditions. In the Arthus reaction, the site becomes infiltrated with neutrophils, and there is extensive injury to the walls of the local blood vessels.

### Extrinsic Allergic Alveolitis

Persons repeatedly exposed to airborne organic particulates may develop serum antibodies (chiefly IgG) to antigens contained in the dusts. Upon subsequent inhalation of the particles, a characteristic inflammatory response develops in the lungs. Over a period of four to six hours, the sufferer develops a cough, fever, and his breathing becomes labored. The cause is an Arthus reaction occurring within the lungs. The formation of antigen–antibody complexes initiates the inflammatory reaction in the alveoli. Once removed from the source of antigen, the attack usually subsides in a few days.

One of the most thoroughly studied examples of allergic alveolitis occurs in farmers exposed to moldy hay. The spores of actinomycetes growing in the hay are the eliciting antigen for this so-called "farmer's lung." Sugarcane workers, mushroom growers, cheesemakers, pigeon fanciers, and a number of other occupational and hobby groups are apt to develop allergic alveolitis from exposure to the spores and dusts associated with their activities. In cases where the eliciting antigen is not immediately apparent from the patient's history, it can be pinpointed by skin testing. Intradermal injection of the offending material produces the characteristic Arthus reaction.

### 18.7 Cell-Mediated Hypersensitivities

As the name indicates, the tissue damage in these hypersensitivities ("Type IV") is produced by the action of cells, not antibodies. Perhaps the best studied examples are the delayed-type hypersensitivities (DTH) such as the tuberculin reaction. The properties of DTH are examined in some detail in Sections 3.1 and 6.1. The antigen-specific cells in DTH are T cells which, in the mouse, belong to the Ly -1$^+$ subset. Other types of T cells (such as $T_C$) can, in some hypersensitivities, also participate in causing tissue damage.

Cell-mediated hypersensitivities differ from antibody-mediated hypersensitivities in several ways. The development of the response is usually slower (hence "delayed"). The lesions produced are heavily infiltrated with lymphocytes and macrophages, in contrast to, for example, the accumulation of neutrophils seen in the Arthus reaction.

The major criterion for establishing a hypersensitivity as cell mediated is the ability to transfer the response to an unprimed animal by an injection of cells (T lymphocytes) but not by injections of serum. We have seen that in order for a transfer of DTH to be successful, the recipient must share at least one class II antigen with the donor (see Section 3.7).

The pathological changes seen in DTH are mediated by lymphokines. The interaction of antigen with sensitized $T_D$ cells causes the cells to release a number of these substances. The properties of several lymphokines and the way in which these properties can produce tissue damage are reviewed in Section 14.8. In short, some of the lymphokines recruit nonspecific effector cells, like macrophages, to the site while other lymphokines produce direct inflammatory and cytotoxic effects at the site.

There is an exception to the rule that DTH can only be transferred by cells. In 1954, Lawrence and his coworkers reported that tuberculin sensitivity in humans could be passively transferred to unprimed recipients using an extract of the leukocytes of a sensitized donor. They called the active material **transfer factor.** Transfer factor appears to have antigen specificity; i.e., cell extracts from tuberculin-sensitized donors transfer tuberculin sensitivity only. The factor is dialyzable and thus is a relatively small molecule (or molecules). Transfer factor may contain nucleotides. The lack of suitable animals in which to study transfer factor has greatly limited the type of studies which can be performed. Nonetheless, the material has been tested empirically in a number of human diseases. Injections of transfer factor have been reported to enhance T cell function in immunodeficient patients and to induce an effective antitumor immunity in some victims of osteosarcoma.

## Contact Sensitivity

There are a number of chemicals that produced dermatitis when applied to the skin. These include certain dyes, metals (e.g., nickel), the catechols found in poison ivy and poison oak *(Rhus)*, and many others. The tissue damage that results can range from mild to extremely severe and, in every case, is the result of the action of the immune system. The response is totally unrelated to any intrinsic toxicity of the eliciting chemicals themselves. Contact sensitivities are thus exceptionally clear-cut examples of immunopathology.

Probably all substances capable of causing contact sensitivity can form covalent bonds with proteins. Thus the actual immunogen may be a complex of self-protein (in the skin) acting as the "carrier" and the contact sensitizer acting as a hapten. There is some evidence that the immunogen must be processed or presented to the immune system by the phagocytic, macrophage-like Langerhans cells of the skin.

Contact sensitivity meets most, if not all, of the criteria of a DTH response. The skin lesion takes about 48 hours to develop and is characterized by an accumulation of mononuclear cells. Contact sensitivity can be passively transferred by the injection of cells, but not by serum. (As early as 1942, Landsteiner and Chase showed that lymphocytes taken from a guinea pig sensitized to picryl chloride could transfer this sensitivity to unprimed guinea pigs.) The cells responsible for contact sensitivity appear to be the same as those responsible for the typical DTH response to soluble antigens, that is, $T_D$ cells. The rules of MHC restriction are also the same.

The eliciting allergen can often be determined from the history given by the patient, for example, recent exposure to poison ivy, wearing of nickel-containing jewelry, or job-related exposure to organic compounds. A more systematic analysis involves the use of a patch test. Pieces of gauze impregnated with suspected allergens are placed on the skin. After 48 hours, they are removed and each site is examined for a positive response (a reddened, itching, eczematous area).

### Experimental Allergic Encephalomyelitis (EAE)

Experimental allergic encephalomyelitis (EAE) is a disease that can be induced in guinea pigs, rats, rabbits, and a number of other animals (but not very reliably in mice). The disease process can be initiated by a single injection of spinal cord tissue emulsified in Freund's complete adjuvant. In two or three weeks, the animal's hind legs become weak. The disease often progresses to complete paralysis of the hind legs, incontinence, and death. But if not, the animal usually recovers completely.

Histological examination reveals extensive injury to the central nervous system. Patches of the myelin surrounding axons in the spinal cord are destroyed. The sites of damage are heavily infiltrated with lymphocytes and macrophages.

The eliciting antigen in spinal cord tissue is a protein. This protein is called the **basic protein** (**BP**) because of its high content of arginine, histidine and lysine (its isoelectric point is approximately pH 10.5). BP constitutes some 30% of the protein in myelin. The structures of the BPs from different mammals are quite similar. Most contain 170 amino acid residues (and have a MW of 18,200). Their interspecies similarity accounts for the ease with which any source of BP — syngeneic, allogeneic, or xenogeneic — can be used to elicit EAE. The ability of BP to elicit EAE appears to be localized in a single short stretch of nine amino acids (#114–122) in the molecule. Mixed with Freund's complete adjuvant, a peptide of this sequence can elicit the disease.

Although anti-BP antibodies are found in EAE, the disease process itself seems to be mediated almost entirely by cells. EAE can be passively transferred to unprimed animals by injecting them with T cells harvested from donors immunized with BP. Serum from the same donors does not work. Thus EAE is another example of an autoaggressive attack by the cell-mediated branch of the immune system.

Although T cells are clearly implicated as the damaging agents in EAE, it is still uncertain as to whether the damage is caused by $T_D$ cells, $T_C$ cells, or both. The presence of $T_D$ cells sensitized to BP can be shown by skin testing animals that have EAE. In addition, the abundance of macrophages in the lesions suggests their recruitment by lymphokines liberated by $T_D$ cells. But there is also evidence for the presence of $T_C$ cells (cells capable of lysing syngeneic BP-coated target cells in vitro).

EAE has been intensively studied in a number of different laboratories. Why? The major reason is that as an autoimmune, demyelinating disease, it may be able to teach us something about **multiple sclerosis (MS)** a demyelinating disease in humans with many features suggesting autoimmunity. While some clear differences exist between EAE and MS (e.g., MS is a chronic disease, while EAE generally is not), the similarities are sufficient to keep interest kindled. Studies with EAE have shown that treatment with certain nondisease producing peptides isolated from BP can prevent or even reverse the symptoms of EAE. This, of course, raises the hope that a similar approach might be useful in MS. The pathogenesis of EAE is also of interest because it appears to account for the frequent occurrence of encephalomyelitis in persons who have received rabies vaccine prepared from central nervous system tissue (e.g., the Pasteur treatment). As rabies vaccine produced from human diploid cell cultures becomes more widely available, the problem of postvaccination encephalomyelitis should become a thing of the past.

## Lymphocytic Choriomeningitis (LCM)

Lymphocytic choriomeningitis (LCM) is another disorder in which most of the damage is confined to the central nervous system. The eliciting agent of LCM is an RNA virus, LCMV (see Section 11.4). The host range of the virus includes not only laboratory rodents (mice, hamsters) but humans who come in contact with these infected animals or their tissues.

Depending upon the circumstances (some of which we shall examine), the disease can vary greatly in its severity. In humans, the effects of viral infection can range from a brief, flu-like illness to severe, even fatal, meningitis and encephalitis. Injection of LCMV into a newborn mouse produces no obvious signs of disease (Figure 18.11). The mouse grows up and has almost a normal life span. However, living virus can be recovered from its tissues at any time during its life, and late in life there are usually signs of immune complex disease.

An intracerebral inoculation of virus into an adult mouse produces quite a different story. The animal becomes increasingly ill and in a little over a week goes into convulsions and dies. Autopsy reveals edema in the brain and extensive inflammation of the meninges. These tissues are filled with lymphocytes and macrophages.

One might first assume that the virus is cytopathic in the adult mouse; i.e., it causes extensive cell damage and this is what produces death. But

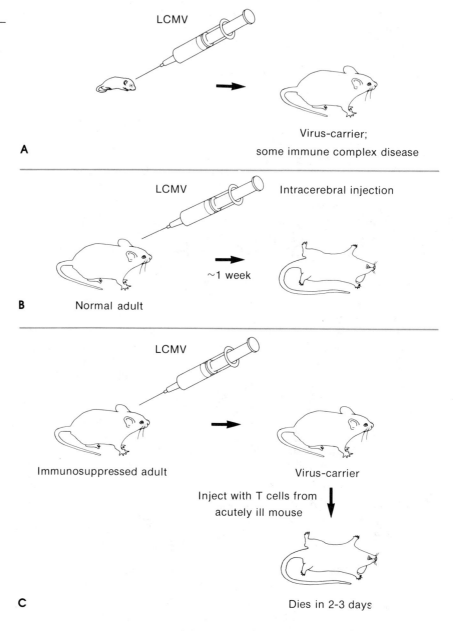

**Figure 18.11** A: Injection of lymphocytic choriomeningitis virus (LCMV) into a newborn mouse produces a persistent infection with only minor pathological changes. B: Intracerebral injection of a normal adult mouse produces a fulminating disease that quickly kills the animal. C: However, a T-deficient mouse (e.g., neonatally thymectomized or treated with antithymocyte serum) tolerates an intracerebral injection of LCMV. This carrier state can be broken by an injection of T cells (but not serum) from a mouse acutely ill with LCM.

careful investigation since the pioneering work of Rowe in the 1950s shows that this is not the case. Rowe demonstrated that *immunosuppressed* adult mice do *not* succumb as do normal adult mice. If the animal is first irradiated, or treated with cyclophosphamide or antithymocyte serum, it survives injection of the virus and becomes a carrier just like the newborn mouse (Figure 18.11). Furthermore, neither nude mice nor neonatally thymectomized mice are made ill by LCMV. All of this suggests that the fatal disease is not "caused" by the virus but by the immune system and specifically by T cells.

Figure 18.12   The adoptive transfer of active disease to an immunosuppressed LCMV carrier requires that the donor immune spleen cells share the same K and/or D region with the recipient. Identity in the I region only is not sufficient (not shown). The cells active in this adoptive transfer are T cells (the effect is abrogated by anti-Thy-1 plus complement) and are probably $T_C$ cells. They are harvested just before the donor would otherwise die of its infection. [Based on P. C. Doherty and R. M. Zinkernagel, *J. Immunol.* **114**:30, 1975.]

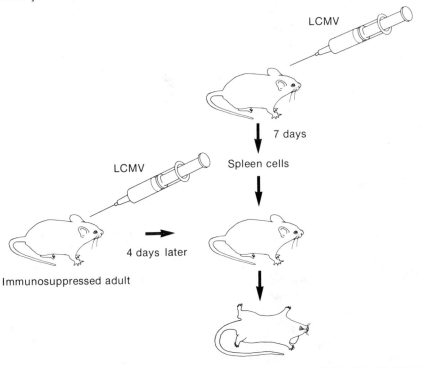

| Donor | Recipient | Days to death | | |
|---|---|---|---|---|
| | | Immune spleen cells | Normal spleen cells | |
| C57BL | C57BL | 2 | 10 | Syngeneic |
| (C57BL × CBA)F₁ | C57BL | 2 | 9 | Semiallogeneic |
| CBA | C57BL | 11 | 11 | Allogeneic |
| (B10.A × C57BL)F₁ (KᵏDᵈ/KᵇDᵇ) | CBA (KᵏDᵏ) | 4 | 8 | Single identity at K |

The argument can be made even stronger. If an immunosuppressed, LCMV-carrying adult mouse is given an injection of T cells from an acutely ill mouse, the recipient also becomes acutely ill and usually dies in two or three days (Figure 18.11). The passive transfer of serum or of B cells from an infected donor has no such effect.

The ability of T cells to trigger acute disease in a recipient is restricted by their respective H-2 haplotypes. The disease is induced most rapidly and reliably if donor and recipient are syngeneic or semisyngeneic. Allogeneic cells are not effective (Figure 18.12)). The use of H-2 recombinants shows that the critical alleles are at H-2K and H-2D. The donor and recipient must share at least one of these. Lack of identity at the I region does not seem to be important.

The fatal autoaggressive attack in LCM is probably mediated by $T_C$ cells; i.e., T cells able to lyse infected, $^{51}$Cr-labeled targets in vitro. The cerebrospinal fluid of acutely ill animals is filled with these cells. The greater the concentration of $T_C$ cells in a cell suspension, the lower the dose needed to induce disease in the recipient. The restriction to H-2K and/or D for the successful adoptive transfer of the disease also suggests that $T_C$ cells are at work. This is just what is found for the in vitro activity of $T_C$ cells (see Section 11.4). (The phenomenon of the MHC restriction of $T_C$ cells was first discovered in the LCM system.) The minor role played by the H-2I region also suggests that $T_D$ cells are not the important effectors of the disease process. In order to transfer DTH, the cells ($T_D$) must be matched with the recipient at H-2I but not at H-2K or H-2D (see Section 3.7)

## Summary

Many other examples of cell-mediated hypersensitivities could be cited. Some represent natural disorders. Others have been deliberately induced, both in experimental animals and in humans. In the latter group, we might well include allograft rejection and graft versus host (GVH) disease. Although cytotoxic T cells ($T_C$) have been implicated in allograft rejection, a Ly-1 T cell (perhaps the $T_D$ cell) appears to be the dominant effector in mice of both allograft rejection (see Section 19.2) and GVHR.

Cell-mediated hypersensitivities can be produced in response to both exogenous antigens (e.g., the catechol of poison ivy or an allograft) and endogenous (self) antigens (such as the basic protein of myelin). Hypersensitivities directed against self antigens are examples of **autoimmune disorders** (see Section 18.9). Some, perhaps many, hypersensitivities may involve a response to both exogenous and self antigens such as occurs in the attack by $T_C$ cells against LCMV-infected self.

The cells that have been implicated in cell-mediated hypersensitivities include (1) $T_D$ cells (i.e., in delayed-type hypersensitivity), (2) the macrophages they recruit, and (3) cytotoxic T cells ($T_C$).

Despite the diversity of examples, one common thread binds them all. In every case, the cell-mediated response damages the host totally out of proportion to any intrinsically harmful properties of the eliciting agent. The pathology is created *by* — not in spite of — the immune system.

We usually think of the immune system in terms of the protection it affords us, and rightly so. How, then, can we account for those occasions when the system turns against us? Are occasional hypersensitivities the inevitable price we must pay for the protection afforded by immunity?

There is no clear answer yet. Many of the features of DTH suggest a process that might well protect against infection by microorganisms. In tissues like the skin, the recruitment of macrophages and other cells leads to (1) the walling off of the site of infection and (2) the scavenging of the infectious organisms by phagocytosis. These mechanisms, presumably orchestrated by $T_D$ cells, thus act together to confine and eventually eliminate the invading organisms. In a different context, the same mechanisms can produce extensive tissue injury. When Mantoux-negative persons contract tuberculosis, the progress of the disease is often sharply limited. The organisms grow slowly; they produce no toxins and little direct tissue damage. Often the disease becomes fully arrested, leaving simply two telltale traces: a nodule or two (within which living tubercle bacteria may still reside) in the lungs and a positive Mantoux test, i.e., DTH to tuberculin. If this sensitized person should become exposed to the organism again, either through a fresh infection or by a recrudescence of the disease from the nodules, the outcome is quite different. The response in the lung tissue is violent: tissue damage may be so extensive that cavities form in the lungs. The bacteria are no longer walled off and are released from the site of infection. They are now free to spread elsewhere in the lung and may even spread into the pulmonary circulation from whence they disseminate throughout the body. What was once a mild, limited disease becomes transformed into a life-threatening one. The organism is the same. But the immune response that led to the healing of the first infection has been transformed into a cell-mediated hypersensitivity that is largely responsible for the disastrous (if untreated) outcome of the second attack of the disease.

A similar situation may exist in lymphocytic choriomeningitis (LCM). There is some evidence that the $T_C$ cells that develop in response to the virus perform the very useful function of limiting the propagation of the virus in such organs as liver and spleen. But the mechanism that appears to work well in the liver and spleen becomes lethal when it attacks virus-infected tissue at the blood–brain barrier.

There is even a good word to be said for IgE. David and his colleagues have demonstrated that suppression of IgE synthesis makes rats more susceptible to infection by the nematode *Trichinella spiralis*. One of the products released from mast cells is a chemotactic factor for eosinophils. IgE-deficient rats fail to mobilize the usual concentration of eosinophils around the invading worms. Eosinophils are probably important in coping with many helminth infections. Perhaps, then, the unpleasant symptoms of hay fever and other IgE-mediated allergies are the legacy of a system that evolved in response to the challenges of parasitic worms.

The view that emerges is that the hypersensitivities respresent a compromise. Each of the mechanisms we have examined in this chapter probably serves some useful, protective function in the appropriate context. The price we pay for this function is the occasional threat of tissue damage when the same machinery encounters antigen under inappropriate circumstances.

## 18.9   Autoimmune Disorders

The preceding sections of this chapter should have made it quite clear that Ehrlich's "horror autotoxicus" is by no means absolute. Antibodies directed against self-determinants and autoreactive T cells are frequently observed. The presence of either or both establishes autoimmunity. Evidence of autoimmunity is often found in humans and animals that are unquestionably ill, but apparently healthy individuals may also reveal signs of autoimmunity. Where illness exists along with autoimmune phenomena, the question is whether the autoimmunity caused the disease or whether the autoimmunity is simply one of the consequences of an illness caused by unrelated factors.

The pathological effects of some autoimmune disorders are quite localized. Thus the antibodies in Grave's disease are directed exclusively against receptors on the surface of thyroid cells. Other autoimmune disorders, particularly those that generate immune complexes, produce damage at many locations. For reasons that are not yet clear, a single patient often suffers from multiple autoimmune disorders. Victims of SLE, for example, often suffer simultaneously from autoimmune hemolytic anemia, thrombocytopenic purpura (Section 18.4), and rheumatoid arthritis (Section 18.6). The tendency to develop autoimmunity also runs in families. Even when close kin show no signs of disease symptoms, they often have autoantibodies similar to those of the patient. This suggests a genetic predisposition, especially when the kin have not been exposed to the same environmental influences. Certain autoimmune disorders are associated with the MHC, especially HLA-D, the human counterpart of the I region in the mouse. For example, persons who carry the DR3 antigen are three to four times more likely to develop Grave's disease than those who do not. The risk of developing multiple sclerosis and Goodpasture's syndrome is higher in persons that inherit the DR2 antigen. (The DR antigens are discussed in Section 19.3.) But obviously not everyone with a particular set of MHC antigens develops an autoimmune disorder. So we must look for precipitating mechanisms.

A once popular theory to explain the onset of autoimmunity held that certain self antigens are normally sequestered (hidden) from the immune system. Thus they are not available to elicit tolerance — i.e., to become recognized as "self" — at the time immunocompetence is being established. As long as they remain sequestered, everything is fine. But if something like trauma or infection exposes them to the immune system later in life, then autoimmunity develops. Some tissues, in the eye and the central nervous system for example, do seem to be isolated from the immune system. Such tissues lack lymphatic drainage and/or reside behind a barrier (e.g., the blood-brain barrier) which isolates them from the immune system. Such a mechanism was also postulated for the development of autoimmunity to thyroglobulin. But radioimmunoassay reveals that low concentrations of thyroglobulin are present in the blood and thus exposed to the immune system. Perhaps some antigens (proteins within the eye for example) *are* normally sequestered in this way, but we cannot use such a mechanism to account for the majority of autoimmune disorders.

The absence of autoimmunity is far more likely the result of self-tolerance. And self-tolerance is a response of the immune system (see Section 16.7). So the question of autoimmunity comes down to looking for the mechanism or mechanisms that break self-tolerance.

The possible mechanisms by which tolerance is created are examined in Chapter 16. For self antigens, T cell tolerance is probably the rule. This is true for humoral as well as cell-mediated autoimmunity. Normal persons have lymphocytes, presumably B cells, that are able to bind self components like thyroglobulin and the basic protein of myelin. The presence of these cells is revealed by autoradiography following exposure to radiolabeled antigen. Furthermore, when suspensions of B cells are treated with polyclonal stimulators like LPS, antibodies against a large number of self antigens are produced. The absence or suppression of $T_H$ cells probably keeps these B cells from secreting antiself antibodies.

In experimental situations, it is clear that where $T_H$ cells are tolerized and B cells are not, tolerance can be broken by the introduction of a cross-reacting antigen. The mechanism is reviewed in Section 16.2. Briefly, determinants to which $T_H$ cells are not tolerant elicit T help for B cells specific for determinants shared by the two antigens (see Figure 16.4). Considerable clinical evidence suggests that a similar mechanism accounts for some autoimmunity. Certain exogenous antigens are cross-reactive with self antigens. For example, some antigens found in group A streptococci (including the carbohydrate, A-CHO, see Section 15.6) cross-react with antigens in cardiac tissue. This may account for the heart damage that is a frequent complication of rheumatic fever, which is caused by group A streptococci.

Extrinsic agents that are not in themselves cross-reactive with self antigens may nonetheless alter self antigens in such a way as to break self-tolerance. Both viruses and chemicals have been implicated. Earlier in the chapter we noted how acute autoimmunity can be produced in mice by LCMV (see Section 18.7). Mononucleosis (which is associated with the Epstein–Barr virus) occasionally produces signs of autoimmunity, for example, antibodies against the patient's own red cells. These antibodies gradually disappear when the virus is eliminated from the body. Autoimmune disorders can also be elicited by drugs; thrombocytopenic purpura (Section 18.4) and SLE are common examples. Here the signs of autoimmunity disappear when use of the drug ceases.

Can chemicals or viruses trigger self-sustaining autoimmunity? The answer is uncertain. Lifelong autoimmunity is found in NZB mice and in mice infected at birth with LCMV (see Section 18.7). But probably in the first case and certainly in the second, the animals harbor virus throughout their lives. Persistent viral infection has also been implicated in human autoimmunity. *Subacute sclerosing panencephalitis* (SSPE) is associated with persistent measles (rubeola) infection and several viruses, most often measles, have also been implicated in multiple sclerosis. In each case, the association is usually based on the high antibody titers in the patients. Only rarely has live virus been actually demonstrated in the victim.

### $T_S$ Cells and Autoimmunity

A number of lines of evidence lead to the conclusion that autoimmune disorders are the outcome of a defect in the activity of T suppressor ($T_S$) cells. Experimental procedures that selectively depress the levels of $T_S$ cells. (e.g., treatment with cyclophosphamide or steroids, adult thymectomy, low doses of radiation) lead to the appearance of autoantibodies and/or autoreactive T cells in mice. The NZB mouse, that classic victim of autoimmunity, has reduced numbers of the Ly-1,2$^+$ suppressor cell precursors (see Section 15.9). As for humans, evidence exists of a defect in SLE patients in their ability to generate $T_S$ cells, and some patients with juvenile rheumatoid arthritis appear to lack $T_S$ cells.

No evidence suggests that any of these postulated causes of autoimmune disorders are mutually exclusive. In all likelihood, the occasional onset of a full-blown autoimmune disorder requires the unhappy interaction between a hereditary predisposition—perhaps manifested through improper regulation by T cells—and some extrinsic agent such as a virus infection.

### 18.10 Immunodeficiency Diseases

In most cases, immunodeficiency diseases reveal themselves by the inability of the victims to cope with infectious organisms. However, other pathological effects (e.g., malignancies and immune complex disease) are seen in some kinds of immunodeficiencies.

The immunodeficiency diseases are not only important in their own right. When it has been possible to pinpoint the source of the problem, they have provided important insights into the normal operation of the immune system. In this section, we shall briefly review a few examples of immunodeficiency diseases that reveal defects in (1) B cells, (2) T cells, (3) both B and T cells, (4) $T_S$ cells, and (5) components of the complement system.

### Infantile X-Linked Agammaglobulinemia

In 1952, Bruton described the first immunodeficiency disorder recognized in humans. This was a case of agammaglobulinemia, a lack of circu-

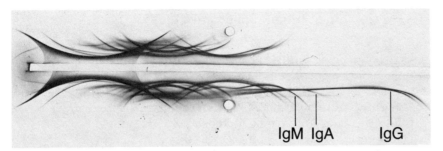

**Figure 18.13**  Immunoelectrophoresis of normal human serum *(bottom)* and serum from an agammaglobulinemic patient. [Courtesy of Dr. Fred S. Rosen.]

lating gamma globulins. This and most subsequent cases were found in young boys, and these cases show X-linked inheritance. The disorder is characterized by the development in male infants of a series of bacterial infections commencing at five to six months of age. At this time most of the antibodies acquired from the mother have disappeared. The concentration of IgG in these patients is extremely low and the other isotypes are usually not detectable at all (Figure 18.13). These patients do not make antibodies in response to vaccines or test antigens. Tests for the presence of B cells are negative. The B-dependent areas of the spleen and lymph nodes are poorly developed and no plasma cells can be found. T cell functions and the ability to cope with viral infections are normal. Many victims of this disorder have been kept alive through the use of antibiotics and periodic injections of human immune globulin (IG). Although mature B cells are missing from these patients, they have normal numbers of pre-B cells in their bone marrow. In some cases, at least, the $\mu$ chains that these pre-B cells synthesize lack V regions suggesting that the primary defect in these cases is the inability to translocate the $V_H$ gene segment successfully (see Section 10.8).

## Thymic Hypoplasia (DiGeorge Syndrome)

This disease is characterized by failure of the thymus and of the parathyroid glands to develop normally. The various tests for T cells (DTH, MLR, response to PHA, the formation of rosettes with SRBC — see Section 7.7) are seriously depressed or negative. Curiously, the primary response to antigens, even supposedly thymus-dependent ones, is often normal. However, the secondary, IgG-dominated humoral response is usually absent, showing the importance of $T_H$ cells for this response.

Victims of this defect are bothered more by viruses, protozoans, and fungi than they are by bacterial infections. Live-virus vaccines are usually fatal for them. However, a number of victims of this disorder have survived for long periods following treatment with thymic hormones or the successful implantation of a fetal thymus.

## Severe Combined Immunodeficiency (SCID)

This is not a single entity but a set of disorders all characterized by a serious reduction in or complete absence of both B cell and T cell function. The victims are prey to all sorts of infections, often by organisms that normally reside harmlessly within the body. Untreated, victims of this disorder rarely survive beyond one year of age.

One approach taken to cope with this disease is to raise the youngster in a sterile environment. As long as the child can be kept isolated from all microorganisms, all goes well. But clearly this presents enormous and confining technological barriers to a normal existence. A more practical approach has been the use of bone marrow transplants. In successful cases (one recipient is alive and well after 16 years), the transplanted marrow produces functioning T cells and, usually, B cells as well. Presumably, the transplanted marrow restores a supply of stem cells that contains precursors of both the B and T lineages. Ideally, the donor of the bone marrow should be identical to the recipient at the MHC; otherwise a fatal graft vs. host reaction (GVHR) may follow. In practice, though, a perfect match is often unavailable. Even so, the procedure may work if the GVHR can be controlled. This has been achieved by treating the donor bone marrow with complement and antibodies directed against mature T cells. Such treatment destroys the immunocompetent T cells without damaging their precursors.

A substantial fraction of the victims of SCID suffer from a lack of the enzyme adenosine deaminase. These patients have elevated levels of ATP and dATP in their body and, for reasons that are not thoroughly understood, this has a peculiarly toxic effect on lymphoblasts. Because these cases involve a single gene defect that needs to be corrected in lymphoblasts only, this disease is a prime candidate for gene therapy: an attempt to introduce a functioning adenosine deaminase gene into the bone marrow cells of the patient.

### Common Variable Hypogammaglobulinemia

This is a set of disorders that are all characterized by a marked suppression of immunoglobulin production that begins in late adolescence or adulthood. The victims become prone to bacterial infections. Their level of circulating IgG drops to 10% or less of normal. Curiously, though, some victims have normal numbers of B cells. The problem *in these particular cases* appears to be an excessive activity of T suppressor ($T_S$) cells. When the patient's B cells and T cells are separated, the B cells respond normally to pokeweed mitogen (PWM) (Figure 18.14). Remixing of the isolated cell populations once again turns off the capacity of the culture to respond to PWM. Purified T cells from these patients also suppress immunoglobulin secretion when cultured with the lymphocytes from a normal person.

**Figure 18.14** Response to pokeweed mitogen of lymphocyte populations from a patient with common variable hypogammaglobulinemia. When freed of T cells, the patient's own B cells synthesize normal amounts of immunoglobulins when cultured with pokeweed mitogen. The synthesis of immunoglobulins by B cells from healthy donors is inhibited by culturing them with T cells from the hypogammaglobulinemic patient. Thus the defect in this patient appears to be caused by $T_S$ cells. [From T. A. Waldmann et al., *Fed. Proc.* **35**:2067, 1976.]

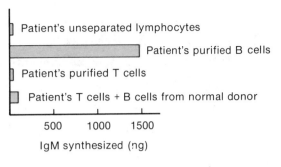

## Acquired Immune Deficiency Syndrome (AIDS)

From 1981 through April 30, 1985, 10,000 cases of an apparently new disease were diagnosed in the United States. This disease, named acquired immune deficiency syndrome (AIDS), is characterized by (1) life-threatening "opportunistic" infections, i.e., infections by organisms (e.g., *Pneumocystis carinii, Candida*) that are rarely serious pathogens in immunocompetent hosts; (2) a high incidence of cancer, the most common being Kaposi's sarcoma, which develops in almost one-third of the patients; (3) high levels of antibodies to cytomegalovirus (CMV) and/or Epstein–Barr virus (EBV); and (4) evidence of profound immunodeficiency in the cell-mediated—but not the humoral—branch of the immune system. The level of circulating T lymphocytes in these patients is depressed. This is especially evident for the T helper cell subset. Whereas the ratio of $T_H$ to $T_S$ cells in normal humans averages 2.3, the $T_H/T_S$ ratio in AIDS patients is less than 0.9.

The disease is thought to be caused by one of three newly characterized retroviruses which bind specifically to receptors on $T_H$ cells (CD4+). Because of this property, these viruses have been designated *human T cell lymphotropic viruses* or HTLV. Two of these viruses (HTLV-I and -II) transform the infected cells and have been implicated as agents of leukemia. Infection by the third (HTLV-III) kills the $T_H$ cells, and it appears to be the causative agent of AIDS.

Approximately 75% of the victims of AIDS are male homosexuals and most of the remainder have a history of intravenous drug use. In addition, some recipients of blood transfusions have contracted AIDS. The preparations of factor VIII that are so essential for hemophiliacs are manufactured from human blood, and a number of hemophiliacs have contracted the disease. Most have antibodies against the virus. All this evidence points to a virus present in body fluids like blood and semen. The prognosis for those with full-blown cases of the disease is poor. Three-quarters of the patients diagnosed prior to January 1983 had died by the end of 1984.

## Complement Deficiencies

The many components of the complement system (see Section 14.2) provide several possible sites for deficiencies to occur. And, in fact, specific, inherited deficiencies of one or another of most of the components in the classical pathway have been identified. As you might expect, some of these deficiencies (e.g., of C3 and C5) are associated with increased susceptibility to infection. However, deficiencies of the early components (C1, C2, and C4) are most often associated with immune complex disease. This suggests that one of the functions of the complement system is to dissolve immune complexes. Inherited deficiencies of molecules that control the complement system (such as C1INH and factor I — see Figure 14.7) are also found and each is associated with pathological symptoms.

## ADDITIONAL READING

1. Buchmeier, M. J., et al., "The Virology and Immunobiology of Lymphocytic Choriomeningitis Virus Infection," *Adv. Immunol.* **30:**275, 1980.

2. Dessein, A. J., W. L. Parker, S. L. James, and J. R. David, "IgE Antibody and Resistance to Infection. I. Selective Suppression of the IgE Antibody Response in Rats Diminishes the Resistance and the Eosinophil Response to *Trichinella spiralis* Infection," *J. Exp. Med.* **153:**423, 1981.

3. Ishizaka, K., and T. Ishizaka, "Identification of $\gamma$ E-Antibodies as a Carrier of Reaginic Activity," *J. Immunol.* **99:**1187, 1967.

4. Landsteiner, K., and M. W. Chase, "Experiments on Transfer of Cutaneous Sensitivity to Simple Compounds," *Proc. Soc. Exp. Biol. Med.* **49:**688, 1942.

5. Lane, H. C., and A. S. Fauci, "Immunologic Abnormalities in the Acquired Immune Deficiency Syndrome," *Ann. Rev. Immunol.* **3:**477, 1985.

6. Lawrence, H. S., "Transfer Factor," *Adv. Immunol.* **11:**195, 1969.

7. Lewis, R. A., and K. F. Austen, "Mediation of Local Homeostasis and Inflammation by Leukotrienes and Other Mast Cell-Dependent Compounds," *Nature* **293:**103, 1981.

8. Lindstrom, J., "Immunobiology of Myasthenia Gravis, Experimental Autoimmune Mysathenia Gravis, and Lambert-Eaton Syndrome," *Ann. Rev. Immunol.* **3:**109, 1985.

9. Nardella, F. A., D. C. Teller, and M. Mannik, "Studies on the Antigenic Determinants in the Self-association of IgG Rheumatoid Factor," *J. Exp. Med.* **154:**112, 1981.

10. Reinherz, E. L., et al., "Reconstitution after Transplantation with T-Lymphocyte-Depleted HLA Haplotype-Mismatched Bone Marrow for Severe Combined Immunodeficiency," *Proc. Natl. Acad. Sci. USA* **79:**6047, 1982.

11. Rosen, F. S., et al., "The Primary Immunodeficiencies," _New Engl. J. Med._ **311:**235–242, 300–310, 1984.

12. Samuelsson, B., "Leukotrienes: Mediators of Immediate Hypersensitivity Reactions and Inflammation," _Science_ **220:**568, 1983.

13. Weigle, W. O., "Analysis of Autoimmunity Through Experimental Models of Thyroiditis and Allergic Encephalomyelitis," _Adv. Immunol._ **30:**159, 1980.

# CHAPTER **19**

# Transplantation Immunity

## 19.1 Introduction

Surgeons have long wished for the ability to replace damaged or worn-out organs. As early as the seventeenth century, attempts were made to transfuse blood. But only in this century, thanks to the pioneering work of Landsteiner, has blood transfusion become a safe and reliable procedure. Organ transplants, especially kidney transplants, have become routine in the last two decades. However, transplants of heart, liver, and lungs are still only rarely performed. If progress has been slow, it has not been because of surgical barriers. The surgical techniques for organ transplants were developed early in this century and are quite straight-forward. The great stumbling block has been the immune system, which reacts with great vigor against the introduction of foreign tissue.

Not all transplants fail. Transplanted tissue genetically identical with the host survives indefinitely. This is the case for autografts and isografts (see Section 3.3). An **autograft** is host tissue (e.g., a layer of skin) transplanted from one area of the body to another. **Isografts** are grafts between genetically identical individuals. For humans this means identical (monozygotic) twins. For inbred strains of mice and rats, it means members of the same inbred strain. (However, identity of strain *designation*, such as BALB/c, may not be enough. Separate breeding colonies of the same strain often develop genetic disparities and cease to tolerate each other's tissues.)

As a general rule, **allografts** fail because of rejection by the immune system. There are, however, some exceptions to this rule. Allografts placed in immunologically privileged sites are sometimes retained for unusually long periods. These are sites, like the brain, that have no lymphatic drainage and sites, like the cornea, where blood vessels may not reach the graft. In the first case, no immunogenic stimulus is given; in the second, no immunological response can be carried out. Grafts of allogeneic (even xenogeneic) cartilage, bone, and segments of blood vessels are often successful. In these cases, only the connective tissue matrix of the graft is needed. The matrix provides a mechanical support for eventual recolonization by host cells.

Allografts of such organs as kidney, liver, pancreas, and lungs pose much greater difficulties. In all of these cases, continued functioning of the graft depends upon continued functioning of the allogeneic cells that make up the graft. But these allogeneic cells elicit an immune reaction on the part of the host which, if unchecked, leads to the destruction of the organ.

The transplant of allogeneic bone marrow represents a special twist to the basic immunological problem. Bone marrow transplants are given to recipients who are either naturally immunodeficient (e.g., victims of SCID—see Section 18.10) or who have been made immunodeficient (by x-irradiation). In either case, the problem is not rejection of the graft by the host but the reverse: immunological damage to the host triggered by the immunocompetent cells of the donor's bone marrow. This is the graft vs. host reaction (GVHR—see Section 6.4).

## 19.2  The Immunological Basis of Allograft Rejection

Graft rejection meets the criteria of immunity: specificity and memory. The rejection of a first graft takes a characteristic period of time; e.g., it takes a mouse (**A**) about 14 days to reject a first graft of allogeneic skin

(B). However, a second graft of skin from the same donor (B) is rejected in an accelerated fashion. This is the "second set" reaction (see Section 3.3). The specificity of this "learned" response is revealed by grafting third-party (C) skin on the primed recipient. *This* graft (C) is rejected in 14 days, even when it is put on at the same time as the second graft of B skin.

Graft rejection is a cell-mediated immune response. It can be adoptively transferred by injections of cells (T lymphocytes) but not (except in special circumstances) by injections of serum. Thus neonatally induced tolerance to a graft of allogeneic skin is quickly broken by an injection of T cells from a mouse that has been previously sensitized to the same kind of skin (Figure 19.1).

Organ grafts elicit humoral responses as well as cell-mediated responses. However, the antibodies produced usually do not play a major role in graft rejection. But if prior to receiving the graft, the recipient already has a high titer of antibodies against the antigens of the donor, destruction of the organ begins almost immediately. Although the mechanism of rejection is different, the threat is sufficiently great that each patient awaiting a graft should be tested for preexisting antibodies against the histocompatibility antigens of a potential donor.

Graft rejection is mediated by T cells. Both $T_D$ and $T_C$ cells have been implicated. The spleen of an animal in the process of rejecting a graft contains a sizeable population of $T_C$ cells; i.e., cells that will specifically lyse donor-type cells in the CMC assay (see Section 6.6). However, the same population of cells also contains $T_D$ cells. Their presence is revealed by injecting them into the skin of the graft donor where they elicit a typical DTH response. Histological examination of a graft in the process of being rejected shows the same accumulation of lymphocytes and macrophages seen in DTH reactions.

The ability to transfer graft rejection adoptively makes it possible to identify the effector T cells involved. One approach is shown in Figure

**Figure 19.1** Adoptive transfer of accelerated graft rejection.

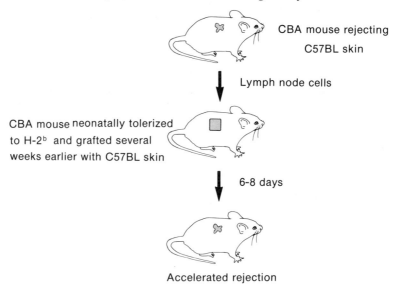

CBA mouse rejecting
C57BL skin

Lymph node cells

CBA mouse neonatally tolerized
to H-2$^b$ and grafted several
weeks earlier with C57BL skin

6-8 days

Accelerated rejection

19.2. The graft recipient is a "B" mouse; i.e., an irradiated, thymecto-mized mouse reconstituted with B cells. Left alone, this mouse is able to retain an allograft for months. However, when the animal is given lymph node and spleen cells from an animal previously sensitized to the histo-compatibility antigens of the graft, the mouse rejects the graft swiftly. If the cell suspension is depleted of all T cells, rejection does not occur. Furthermore these workers found that removal of only the Ly-1$^+$ T cells from the suspension also removes its capacity to elicit rejection. Removal of only the Ly-2$^+$ cells does not delay rejection. These results indicate that the active cell in this example of allograft rejection is a Ly-1$^+$,2$^-$ cell like the $T_D$ cell. Other investigators have found, in contrast, that Ly-2$^+$ cells (presumably $T_C$ cells) play the more important role in graft rejec-tion. It may well be that a first-set rejection is dominated by $T_D$-like cells; a second-set rejection by $T_C$ cells.

The antigens responsible for provoking rejection are *histocompatibil-ity antigens.* In addition to eliciting graft rejection, histocompatibility antigens can be studied by all the other assays for cell-mediated immu-

**Figure 19.2** Evidence that graft rejection is mediated by Ly-1$^+$ T cells. [Based on B. E. Loveland et al., *J. Exp. Med.* **153**:1044, 1981.] Evidence that Ly-2$^+$ ($T_C$) cells play the more important role is presented in J. D. Tyler et al., *J. Exp. Med.* **159**:234, 1984.

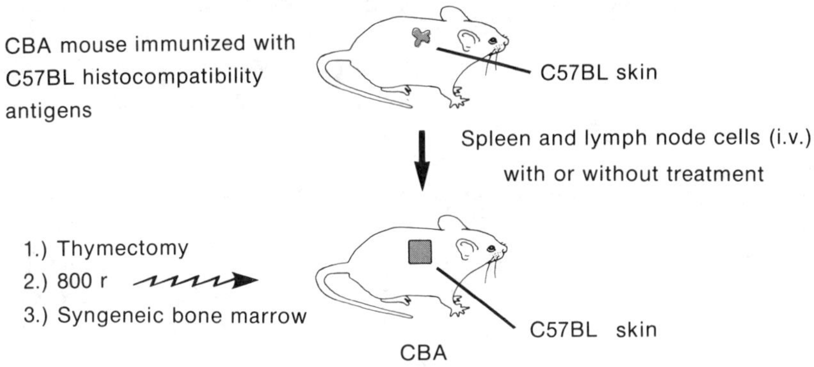

CBA mouse immunized with C57BL histocompatibility antigens — C57BL skin

Spleen and lymph node cells (i.v.) with or without treatment

1.) Thymectomy
2.) 800 r
3.) Syngeneic bone marrow
CBA
C57BL skin

| Cell dose | Treatment | Graft survival (days) | Interpretation |
|-----------|-----------|-----------------------|----------------|
| None | — | >80 | T-deficient recipient is immunoincompetent |
| 1 × 10⁶ | None | 13 | Rejection adoptively transferred by primed lymphoid cells |
| 1 × 10⁶ | Anti-Thy-1.2 + C | >60 | Removal of T cells abrogates response |
| 1 × 10⁶ | Anti-Ly-2 + C | 12 | Removal of Ly-2$^+$ cells (e.g., $T_C$) does not abrogate response |
| 2 × 10⁶ | Anti-Ly-1 + C | >40 | Removal of Ly-1$^+$ cells (e.g., $T_D$) abrogates response |

nity, which are described in Chapter 6: mixed lymphocyte culture (MLC), CMC, DTH, graft vs. host reaction, and the production of lymphokines. Antisera can also be produced against many histocompatibility antigens, and these provide important reagents for their study.

The histocompatibility antigens of an animal are inherited. They are, then, the products of genes. The structures of some of these antigens — glycoproteins in every case — have been determined and are described in Section 3.6.

## 19.3 HLA: The Major Histocompatibility Complex of Humans

The MHC of humans is located on chromosome 6. Like the MHC of mice, it consists of a number of genes which encode class I and class II histocompatibility antigens as well as some of the proteins (class III) used in the complement system (Figure 19.3).

### The Class I Genes

Three class I genes of the human MHC are expressed on each chromosome: HLA-A, HLA-B, and HLA-C. Each encodes a glycosylated polypeptide of approximately 45,000 daltons. All of these polypeptides are integral membrane proteins. Each is noncovalently associated with a molecule of $\beta_2$-microglobulin (Figure 3.14).

The sequence of these molecules reveals a high degree ($\sim$75%) of homology to the class I polypeptides of mice. HLA-A, HLA-B, and HLA-C appear to be the homologues of the mouse H-2K, D, and L genes, respectively (Figure 19.3). The class I antigens are expressed at the surface of most of the cells of the body.

The HLA-A and -B loci are extremely polymorphic; HLA-C is less so. Some 20 alleles have been identified at HLA-A; approximately 50 at HLA-B. Undoubtedly more remain to be discovered. Often a person expresses only a single allelic specificity at HLA-A or -B. This could mean that the person is homozygous at the locus. But it could mean instead that the person carries a second allele which awaits development of the appropriate antiserum to detect it.

Each allele at HLA-A, -B, and -C is identified by using an appropriate antiserum (often harvested from women who have become immunized, after repeated pregnancies, to paternal HLA antigens expressed on their fetuses). As in mice, each allele is recognized as a distinct antigenic specificity expressed on the surface of lymphocytes. Each specificity is given an alphanumeric designation, such as HLA-B7. The capital letter after the hyphen designates the locus (A, B, C, or D) and the number identifies the antiserum used to define the specificity. The practical consequences of HLA typing for organ transplants are such that workers throughout the world are engaged in this pursuit. This means that anti-

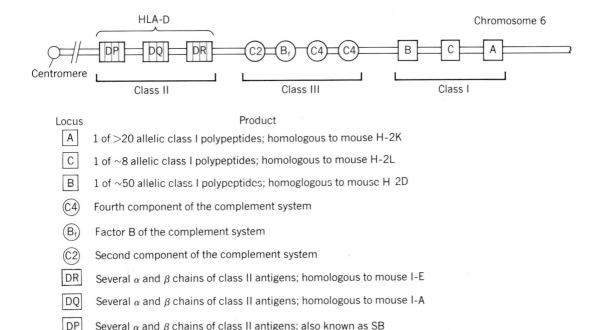

**Figure 19.3** The HLA region of humans and the gene products associated with each locus. DP, DQ, and DR are not single loci but clusters of several loci encoding α and β chains of class II antigens. Several allelic versions of β chain genes have been discovered; the α chain genes are less polymorphic. One or more additional class II loci are probably located between DR and C2. Not shown are additional class I genes which have been identified telomeric to the A locus and which may represent the human counterparts of the Qa/Tla genes of mice.

sera used for typing must be exchanged regularly between laboratories to determine when different antisera are detecting the same specificities. Until a given specificity is fully established as representing a unique allele, its designation includes a lower case w to indicate its provisional ("workshop") status.

## The Class II Genes

The HLA-D region, like the I region in mice, contains genes that were initially defined by their control over the strength of the mixed lymphocyte reaction. Later, antisera and monoclonal antibodies became available that detected antigens that mapped to this same region and thus were called "D related" or DR antigens. The strong possibility exists, as it does in mice, that the DR antigens are actually the same molecules encoded by the D loci and are simply being detected by a different assay method.

A substantial number of expressed structural genes have been found in the D region. Each of these encodes either an α chain (~32 kd) or a β chain (~28 kd) for a class II antigen (Figure 3.15). The loci are clustered in three subregions: DP, DQ, as well as the original DR (Figure 19.3). The sequence of the chains encoded in DR suggests that this region is homologous to the I-E subregion of mice. DQ appears to be the human

**507**

equivalent of the mouse I-A subregion. As is the case in mice, the $\alpha$ chains are less polymorphic than the $\beta$ chains.

The expression of class II genes is far more limited than is the case for class I genes. Dendritic cells, activated macrophages, and mature B cells all express substantial amounts of class II antigens (as they do in the mouse). We have reviewed the roles that class II antigens play in the induction of humoral and cell-mediated immunity. In all likelihood, these antigens play equivalent roles in the human. Whereas class I antigens serve to identify almost all the cells of the body as "self," the role of class II antigens is to mediate the productive interaction of the cells involved in immune responses. However, some cells other than those of the immune system, e.g., the endothelial cells of blood vessels, express class II antigens. Such cells may play a significant role in the rejection of allografts.

### The Class III Genes

The class III genes encode (1) the second component (C2) of the classical pathway of complement activation, (2) factor B, which particpates in the alternative pathway (Section 14.2), and (3) two forms of C4, the fourth component of the complement system.

It is interesting to note that both the mouse and human MHC contain these three classes of genes. However, the class II and class III genes of the mouse are located between class I genes (H-2K and H-2D) while in the human they are all centromeric to them.

---

### 19.4  The Biological Significance of the MHC

Our topic is transplantation. But surely the MHC regions of mice and men did not evolve in response to the evolutionary pressure exerted by transplant surgeons. What evolutionary benefits does this extraordinarily polymorphic collection of genes confer? Let us examine this question in two parts. First, what useful role do these genes play in the organism? Second, why are their products so diverse?

The first question is the easier one to answer. Virtually every immunological activity that involves the interaction of cells is influenced by genes in the MHC. These include the activity of $T_C$ cells, the activity of $T_D$ cells, the interaction of macrophages with $T_H$ cells and of $T_H$ cells with B cells. The ability of an animal to respond to certain antigens is also controlled by the MHC (the Ir genes). Class I and/or class II molecules are involved in each of these activities. For example, antisera or monoclonal antibodies raised against class II molecules interfere with such MHC-dependent activities as the mixed lymphocyte reaction and the expression of Ir gene control. Thus the ability of most T cells to perform their normal functions depends upon their interacting with a self histocompatibility antigen. Seen in this light, the function of these antigens could be to provide recognition signals that enable T cells to discriminate between normal cell surfaces within the body and those that have become altered by such things as virus infection, the ingestion of foreign molecules (macrophages), or possibly even neoplastic transformation. The ubiquitous distribution of class I molecules ensures that any altered cell in the body can be eliminated by $T_C$ cells. The limited distribution of class II molecules, on the other hand, ensures that $T_H$ cells will respond to only those antigens expressed on specialized antigen-presenting cells. (This may help maintain tolerance to one's own cell surface molecules.)

The second question is more difficult. Possibly the extraordinary genetic diversity between individuals that is embodied in the MHC provides a sufficient variety of immune reactivity so that no outside agent (a virus, for example) could be equally pathogenic for every member of the species. One could envisage the appearance of a virus that could elude the immune defenses by expressing antigens that fail to make an immunogenic complex with certain MHC-encoded molecules. While some individuals would be at the mercy of such an organism, the great diversity of MHC molecules would ensure that not all members of the species would be equally susceptible to the pathogen.

Curiously, while susceptibility to particular pathogens has been difficult to correlate with the possession of particular HLA antigens, close correlations have been found with certain "organic" diseases. HLA-B27, for example, is strongly associated with certain arthritic conditions. Some autoimmune disorders also occur more frequently with certain HLA genes than would be expected by the frequency of these genes in the population (Section 18.9). Why these correlations exist is not yet understood.

In any case, the number and variety of class I and class II molecules provide the basis for the biochemical uniqueness that is the hallmark of all outbred animals (except identical twins). Unfortunately, they also stand ready to ultimately frustrate the good intentions and dexterity of the transplant surgeon.

## 19.5  Matching Organ Donor and Recipient

The number of alleles currently identified at HLA-A, -B, -C, and -D totals over 80. The list is certainly incomplete, especially for HLA-D. Such diversity provides for thousands of possible combinations of these alleles. In a study of over 1000 blood and organ donors in the San Francisco area, over half had an HLA phenotype that was unique, yet this study only examined the antigens encoded by HLA-A and HLA-B. Another 111 donors had a set of HLA-A and -B antigens shared with only one other person in the group. The most frequently observed phenotype (HLA-A1, A3, B7, and B8) was found in only 11 donors. What hope do such data hold for the dialysis patient awaiting a kidney transplant?

If the patient has a large family of willing donors, the odds for the availability of a good match are not too bad thanks to the tight linkage between these loci. Assuming that no crossing over occurs within the

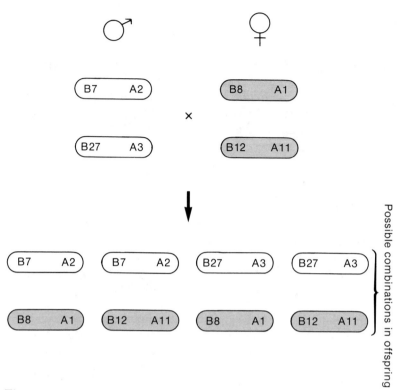

**Figure 19.4** Patterns of inheritance of the HLA-A and HLA-B antigens in humans. Assuming that no recombination occurs, there is a 1 in 4 chance that any child will be HLA-identical with one of its siblings. Although disparity at HLA-A and -B may be less significant than disparity at HLA-D for a successful transplant, the tight linkage of all of these loci makes it worthwhile to match *family members* for HLA-A and HLA-B alone.

HLA region of either of the mother's or the father's two number 6 chromosomes, there are four possible combinations in which they may transmit their haplotypes to their children (Figure 19.4). Even if the parents carry different alleles at each locus (which is often the case), there is a one-in-four chance that any one of their children will be an exact HLA match with any other. Even if no sibling qualifies, one of the parents or even an uncle or aunt could provide identical haplotype. What is needed, then, is a method for screening potential donors. Let us examine several techniques that have been used for this purpose. Although some are no longer in use, they each illustrate valuable immunological principles.

## Skin Grafting the Recipient

A tiny piece of skin from each of the potential donors is engrafted on the recipient. The graft that lasts the longest reveals the most compatible donor. This is certainly a direct approach to the problem, but it suffers the grave defect that it sensitizes the recipient to the antigens of the

selected donor. Subsequent grafting of an organ threatens the organ with
accelerated (second set) rejection.

**511**

*Section 19.5*
*Matching*
*Organ Donor*
*and Recipient*

## Skin Grafting the Donor

Here a tiny piece of the recipient's skin is engrafted on each of the
potential donors. The one who retains the graft the longest *may* be the
most suitable donor, but as we shall see in the next paragraph, is not
inevitably so.

## The Third-Man Test

A piece of the recipient's skin is first engrafted on the arm of any third
party. After the graft is rejected, this person is then engrafted with pieces
of skin from all the potential donors. In this case, the graft that is rejected
*first* ought to identify the best donor. The initial graft sensitizes the third
person to the histocompatibility antigens of the recipient; the skin most
closely matching these antigens is then rejected in an accelerated manner. Unfortunately, while tests two and three demonstrate antigens
shared between donor and recipient, they may fail to reveal an antigen
present in the donor but absent in the recipient. They are also cumbersome to perform and have been replaced by serological methods.

## Tissue Typing

At the present time, most tissue typing is done using a cytotoxicity assay.
The principles of this assay are described in Section 5.13. Briefly, leukocytes are harvested from the person to be tested and distributed in a
series of wells in a microtiter plate. A specific (monospecific if possible)
anti-HLA serum is added to each well. After a preliminary incubation,
complement is added along with a reagent to distinguish living cells from
dead. For example, the ability of a cell to exclude such dyes as eosine or
trypan blue from its cytoplasm shows that it is still alive.

Tissue typing makes it possible to establish the distribution of haplotypes among family members. It has been of great value for establishing
the best possible organ donor within a family because the sharing of two
haplotypes produces better results than the sharing of one (Figure 19.5).
(Tissue typing is also now used frequently in cases of disputed paternity.)

Unfortunately, HLA typing has not been as useful a predictor of graft
success when used to test organs from unrelated donors. One reason for
this is that most of the serological specificities for which antisera are
available are controlled by HLA-A and -B. However, there is evidence
that disparity between donor and recipient at HLA-D is more likely to
lead to failure of the graft. Because of the tight linkage of these loci,
failure to type for HLA-D usually does not present a problem within a

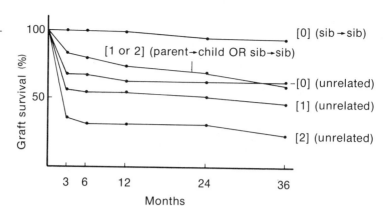

[ ] = # incompatibilities   (HLA-A & -B only)

**Figure 19.5**  Representative survival curves for kidney transplants in humans. The total number of incompatibilities for HLA-A and HLA-B is given in brackets. The greater success of transplants between relatives than between unrelated persons with the *same number of incompatibilities* reflect (1) the influence of other nontested loci (e.g., HLA-D) that are closely linked to HLA-A and -B and therefore will most likely be matched along with them in family members and (2) the fact that unrelated kidneys are almost always cadaver kidneys and conditions for their transplantation may not be ideal.

Within the unrelated group, the differences associated with number of incompatibilities are not so pronounced in genetically heterogeneous populations (e.g., in the United States) as they are in more homogeneous populations (Denmark in this case). This, too, suggests that HLA-A and HLA-B are not themselves so significant for transplant survival, but are closely linked to a locus (HLA-D?) that is. [Curves for family members from J. Dausset and J. Hors, *Transplantation Proceedings* V:223, 1973; those for cadaver kidneys from F. Kissmeyer-Nielsen et al., "The HLA System, Serology and Transplantation" in *HLA System—New Aspects*, G. B. Ferrara (ed.), Elsevier, 1977.]

family. If a suitable haplotype has been identified by anti-HLA-A and anti-HLA-B sera, the D locus is probably matched as well.

With unrelated donors, there is no reason to expect such an outcome. What is needed for unrelated donors is a means of typing for the antigens of HLA-D. But until recently HLA-D antigens (like H-2I) were identified by the proliferation they cause in mixed lymphocyte culture, and this test takes 6 days to perform. Virtually all organs from unrelated donors come from cadavers. If the death of the donor was unexpected, there is simply not time to await the results of an MLC if the condition of the organ is not to deteriorate. Thus in the situation where matching for HLA-D might really improve graft survival, the test is too slow to be of value. Efforts are being made to develop more rapid assays of proliferation. In addition, a number of defined antisera and monoclonal antibodies are now becoming generally available for D-related (DR) antigens; that is, antigens that map to the D region and elicit antibodies. These antisera can be used in the more rapid cytotoxicity assay. If the DR antigens turn out to be a major factor in rejection, the availability of a quick test for the HLA-DR specificities should improve the rate of success with cadaver organs.

Aside from HLA matching, there are two other tests that should be run before transplantation. The donor and recipient must be compatible for the ABO antigens. Also, the serum of the recipient should be checked to be sure that it does not contain high levels of antibodies cytotoxic for the cells of the donor. This cross-matching is necessary because the recipient might have become sensitized to certain foreign HLA antigens as a result of prior transfusions of whole blood. [Curiously, though, patients who have received blood transfusions often retain their transplants better than those who have not (Section 19.7).]

Unfortunately, even with the most careful tissue typing, some histoincompatibility always remains (except for grafts between identical twins). This is probably due to minor histocompatibility antigens about which we know virtually nothing. In any case, the practical consequence is that allograft transplantation *must* be accompanied by some degree of immunosuppression if the transplant is to succeed.

## 19.6  Immunosuppression

A variety of agents have been used to suppress immune responsiveness. Many of these act by interfering with cell division. Inasmuch as the response to antigen requires clonal proliferation, agents that block mitosis are effective inhibitors of the immune response. But these agents have two grave drawbacks: their immunosuppression is general, not specific, and they damage all tissues (e.g., epithelia, bone marrow) where rapid cell division is occurring. The first drawback exposes the patient to serious infections; the second leads to undesirable side effects.

### Radiation

A sufficiently large dose of radiation directed to the entire body wipes out all immune responsiveness and, if no further steps are taken, kills the animal. Many of the experiments described in this book have used mice that are lethally irradiated to destroy their own immune system and then restored with an infusion of bone marrow cells. In the early days of transplantation, high doses of radiation were tried on a few recipients. The radiation had the desired effect of totally blocking any rejection response, but the side effects were usually fatal. More recently, a modified approach called *total lymphoid irradiation* (TLI) has been used. In TLI, a series of sublethal doses of radiation is directed at the patient's lymphoid tissue (spleen, thymus, and lymph nodes in the neck, chest, and abdomen). The bone marrow and other vital organs are shielded from the radiation. TLI produces prolonged allograft survival in experimental animals and has shown promise in humans.

### Purine Analogs

Purine analogs interfere with DNA synthesis and thus are powerful antimitotic agents. In fact, their earliest clinical use was as anticancer drugs.

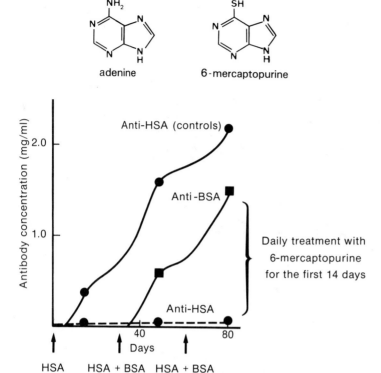

Figure 19.6 Immunosuppression by 6-mercaptopurine, an analog of adenine *(top)*. All animals were injected with horse serum albumin (HSA) on day 0. The experimental group was then given daily injections of 6-mercaptopurine for 14 days. These animals failed to respond to subsequent injections (on days 30 and 60) of HSA, although their response to BSA given at the same time was unimpaired. (The response of the controls to HSA is shown; their response to BSA was the same as that of the experimental group.) [Based on R. S. Schwartz and W. Dameshek, *Nature* 183:1682, 1959.]

But it was soon realized that their antimitotic action should make them effective immunosuppressants as well. For example, 6-mercaptopurine, an anticancer agent, also exerts a profound suppression on the immune system (Figure 19.6). Azathioprine (Imuran), another purine analog, has become one of the mainstays of all immunosuppressive regimens for transplant patients.

### Alkylating Agents

These substances introduce chemical groups into DNA and, as a result, interfere with cell proliferation. In high doses, cyclophosphamide is a powerful immunosuppressant. In small doses, however, it preferentially affects $T_s$ cells (at least in mice) and thus may actually enhance responses (see Section 15.8).

### Corticosteroids

The mode of action of corticosteroids like prednisone and prednisolone is still not understood. These substances act powerfully to suppress the inflammation that accompanies a rejection crisis. Regardless of whether they serve as anything more than antiinflammatory agents, corticoste-

514

roids are another mainstay of any regimen of immunosuppression, particularly when a rejection crisis threatens.

## Antilymphocyte Globulin (ALG)

Antilymphocyte serum (ALS) is produced by immunizing a large animal (usually a horse) with lymphocytes (human in this case). Injections of ALS into a graft recipient have a powerful suppressive effect on graft rejection. Unlike the other agents described, ALS exerts its effects more strongly on the cell-mediated branch than on the humoral branch of the immune system. The effect of ALS in the patient can be followed by monitoring the level of T cells (by SRBC rosettes, see Section 7.7) in the circulation. So long as these are kept at a low level, the chances of rejection are reduced. Unfortunately, ALS has several drawbacks; some (described in the following section) in common with all general immunosuppressants, some unique. Among the latter is the immunogenicity of the extraneous horse serum proteins in the preparation. These can elicit the production of antibodies and bring on serum sickness (see Section 18.6) and allergic responses. Purifying the gamma globulin fraction of the serum produces antilymphocyte globulin (ALG) and reduces this risk.

## Cyclosporin A

A number of antibiotics suppress cell division. Some, like actinomycin D, are too powerful to be safely used in patients. However, one fungal metabolite, called cyclosporin A, has shown great promise. It acts preferentially on T cells, probably by interfering with IL-2-driven proliferation.

## 19.7 Other Approaches to Graft Survival

Even though ALG and cyclosporin A show some selectivity in their action, all of the agents discussed above are general immunosuppressants. In suppressing the response against a set of HLA antigens, they suppress the response against all antigens. How ironic that the best tools we presently have for manipulating the immune system do not exploit the one feature so characteristic of the system: specificity. Ideally, we ought to be able to turn the specificity of the immune response back on itself and suppress only undesirable responses. In other words, we need a practical means of inducing immunological tolerance to the histocompatibility antigens on the transplant.

How might this be done? Chapters 15 and 16 examine methods for suppressing a specific immune response. Broadly speaking, these are through (1) the use of tolerogenic doses of antigen, (2) the use of antibodies directed against the antigen and (3) the formation of antibodies and/or cells directed against particular idiotypes.

Although each of these approaches has proved promising in animal models, only one has reached a point where it is of clinical value. That is to treat the potential graft recipient by giving several small blood transfusions prior to the transplant. Some transplant centers use blood from the prospective organ donor; others use pooled blood representing a broad spectrum of antigen specificities. The procedure was developed empirically; an association was noticed between prior blood transfusions and improved graft retention. But there is probably an immunological basis for the effect. In the absence of cells expressing class II antigens — and neither RBCs nor platelets do express them — the class I antigens on the transfused cells appear to give a tolerogenic rather than an immunogenic signal to the recipient's immune system. We have seen elsewhere the important role played by class II antigens in triggering both humoral (Section 12.4) and cell-mediated (Section 13.3) immune responses.

### Reducing Graft Immunogenicity

Another approach to improving the success of allografts — which has yet to move from the laboratory to the clinic — is to reduce the immunogenicity of the graft before it is implanted. If, as our earlier discussion indicates, class II-bearing cells (e.g., dendritic cells) provide a critical signal for immunity, then any method which reduces the number of these cells in the graft should reduce its potential for triggering its own rejection. Several approaches to this goal have been tried. One is to culture the tissue in vitro for a period before it is implanted. This procedure seems to reduce the number of cells expressing class II antigens in the tissue. A second method is to treat the tissue with complement and antibodies directed against its class II antigens. Both approaches have been successful with laboratory animals, especially for grafts of endocrine tissue.

Whether these results will be translated into practical gains in the clinic remains to be seen. For the present, transplant surgeons still must make do with such general immunosuppressants as azathioprine, prednisone, ALG, and cyclosporin A. By the judicious use of these materials, many people have been restored to productive lives following implantation of a new kidney or even, on a few occasions, a new heart, liver, or pancreas. But the side effects of these agents are very troublesome. Undesirable effects fall into two categories. First, the generalized immunosuppression exerted by all of these materials leaves the transplant recipient vulnerable to infection by a variety of pathogens. Bacterial infections can usually be eliminated with antibiotics, but infections by fungi and viruses are far harder to control. Many kidney recipients have succumbed to lethal infections while their new kidney continued to perform beautifully.

A more rare but equally troublesome side effect of these agents is a marked rise in the incidence of certain cancers. In a few cases, the tumor cells have been introduced as passengers in the transplant. The cure is simple: stop immunosuppression and both the transplant and the tumor are rejected. But more often the tumor is of host origin. From 5–25% of the patients who have retained a kidney transplant for longer than a year develop cancer, most often skin cancer or a lymphoma. This rate is much higher than the incidence of these cancers in the general population.

Why should this occur? There are two schools of thought. One is that immunosuppression destroys *immune surveillance.* Immune surveillance is the name given an intriguing concept first articulated by Ehrlich and later developed by Burnet, Thomas, and others. The concept postulates that one of the functions of the immune system is to patrol the body looking for the emergence of *neoplastic* (cancerous) *cells.* According to this notion, neoplastic cells arise at a relatively high frequency throughout our lives. But thanks to an efficient system of surveillance, these altered cells are almost always destroyed by the immune system before they develop into a life-threatening tumor. This theory leads to the prediction that generalized immunosuppression should allow tumor cells to escape surveillance resulting in an increased frequency of cancer.

The second school holds that the frequency of tumors in transplant recipients is the outcome of the intense immune stimulation created by the transplant, not the result of immunosuppression. In Chapter 20, we shall examine the evidence on both sides of this issue as part of our analysis of the immunobiology of tumors.

## 19.8 Bone Marrow Transplants

The transplantation of allogeneic bone marrow cells presents special immunological problems. The goal of such transplants is to colonize the recipient's bone marrow with stem cells of the donor. Currently there are two principal uses for such therapy: (1) for patients whose bone marrow fails to produce one or more types of blood cells and (2) for patients with leukemia. Examples of the first category are the severe combined immunodeficiencies (SCID — Section 18.10), where T cell function is missing, and aplastic anemia where production of red cells fails. In SCID, the immunological problem is just the reverse of the normal transplant problem. The danger is not that the patient will reject the graft but that the grafted cells will attack the patient, i.e., trigger a graft vs. host reaction (GVHR — Section 6.4). SCID patients are so susceptible to GVHR that even a transfusion of whole blood is fatal because of the immunocompetent T cells it contains.

If a SCID patient is to survive a bone marrow transplant, the donor must be carefully matched. The first successes came with the use of sibling donors who shared both HLA haplotypes with the patient. Although minor histocompatibility antigens create some GVH problems, these can usually be controlled. The donor stem cells ultimately establish residence in the recipient and provide the patient with an immune system. These patients become fully immunocompetent producing T cells (and often B cells and other blood cells as well) of the donor's genotype.

Similar successes are now being achieved using family members as donors even in the absence of a full HLA match. In these cases, life-threatening GVHR can be avoided by pretreating the donor cells to remove the T cells. Lectins and rosetting with SRBC (Section 7.7) have been used as well as complement and monoclonal antibodies directed against surface antigens of mature T cells. Some attempts have also been made to use fetal liver cells for bone marrow reconstitution. Fetal liver is the earliest source of hematopoietic stem cells but contains no T cells.

The approach taken in the case of leukemia is first to destroy the patient's leukemic cells. This is done with high doses of cytotoxic drugs and radiation—doses so high that if nothing further were done, the patient would die. Then the patient is given transplanted marrow to reconstitute his now destroyed hematopoietic system. Again, great care must be taken to avoid a lethal GVHR. An increasing number of leukemia patients have been cured by this technique. Like the former SCID patient, these people are blood cell chimeras—their blood cells have the genotype of the marrow donor.

In a substantial number of cases of SCID, the immediate problem seems to stem from an enzyme deficiency, usually a lack of adenosine deaminase (Section 18.10). The rapid progress in techniques of gene manipulation makes likely the possibility of removing marrow cells from these patients, introducing a functional adenosine deaminase gene into them, and then returning them to the patient. Such autologous bone marrow reconstitution should pose no problem of GVHR. However, some treatment of the patient with cytotoxic agents will probably be needed to make "room" in the recipient for his genetically altered stem cells.

## ADDITIONAL READING

1. Bodmer, Julia, and W. Bodmer, "Histocompatibility 1984," *Immunology Today* 5:251, 1984. Summarizes the findings presented at the 1984 workshop on the HLA system.

2. Dausset, J., "The Major Histocompatibility Complex in Man," *Science* 213:1469, 1981. The Nobel Lecture of a pioneer in the field.

3. Dixon, F. J., and D. W. Fisher, *The Biology of Immunologic Disease*, Sinauer Associates, Inc., Sunderland, MA, 1983. Includes chapters on immune suppression and enhancement (Schwartz), organ transplantation (Najarian), bone marrow transplantation (Good), and total lymphoid irradiation (Strober).

4. Faustman, D., et al., "Prevention of Allograft Rejection by Immunization with Donor Blood Depleted of Ia-Bearing Cells," *Science* 217:157, 1982.

5. Lacy, P. E., and J. M. Davie, "Transplantation of Pancreatic Islets," *Ann. Rev. Immunol.* 2:183, 1984. Includes a review of methods for reducing the immunogenicity of islet allografts.

6. Reinherz, E. L., et al., "Reconstitution after Transplantation with T-Lymphocyte-Depleted HLA Haplotype-Mismatched Bone Marrow for Severe Combined Immunodeficiency," *Proc. Natl. Acad. Sci. USA* **79:**6047, 1982.

7. Steinmetz, M., and L. Hood, "Genes of the Major Histocompatibility Complex in Mouse and Man," *Science* **222:**727, 1983.

CHAPTER **20**

# Tumor Immunology

One of the serious problems associated with organ transplantation is the elevated incidence of cancer in the recipients. The most common cancers in these patients are skin cancers and lymphomas, a cancerous proliferation of lymphoid cells. As many as 25% of those who retain a kidney transplant for longer than a year develop cancer. This incidence is some 100 times greater than in a properly matched control population.

While a lamentable situation for the transplant recipient, this finding lends support to the concept that one of the functions of the immune system is to inhibit the development of cancer. The concept is called **immune surveillance.** It dates back to Paul Ehrlich, although it was later more fully developed by Burnet and Thomas.

In its modern form, immune surveillance postulates that malignant cells appear at a relatively high frequency throughout the life of an organism. These malignant cells express new antigens which the immune system recognizes as foreign. The immune system responds to these antigens by destroying the cells expressing them. Those occasions on which a clinically observable tumor appears represent the failures of surveillance.

There is considerable indirect evidence which supports the theory of immune surveillance, and other evidence which does not. But even if surveillance does not exist, there is still a need for a better understanding of the antigenic nature of cancerous cells if current hopes of enlisting the immune system in tumor therapy are to be realized.

Later in the chapter (Sections 20.6 and 20.7) we shall examine the evidence on either side of the question of immune surveillance. We shall also examine the prospects for the specific immunotherapy of tumors (Section 20.9). But before we do, let us look at some of the properties that distinguish cancer cells from normal cells.

## 20.2   The Cancer Cell

Probably there is no cell type of the >100 that occur in humans that cannot become cancerous. As a general rule, the higher the mitotic rate of a cell type, the more likely it is to become cancerous. Thus cancers of epithelia (carcinomas) and of blood-forming cells (e.g., leukemias) are more common than cancers of such cell types as neurons and muscle cells. Despite their diversity, cancer cells share a number of properties that distinguish them from their normal counterparts.

1. **Cancer cells divide uncontrollably.** Some cancer cells divide rapidly, but this is not always the case. Whereas mitosis of normal cells is regulated by the needs of the body, the division of cancer cells is not. The mitotic rate of the normal liver is low. If a portion of the liver is surgically removed, division of the remaining cells begins at a high rate and continues until — and only until — the organ is regenerated. In some way, as

yet unknown, the organ knows when it is "full," and the mitotic rate drops to its normal low level. Cancer cells, in contrast, keep dividing in the tissue where they arise and eventually spill out beyond its boundaries. Thus cancer cells tend to invade adjacent tissues.

2. **Cancer cells thrive in a variety of microenvironments.** The process of bone marrow transplantation (described in Section 19.8) involves introducing a suspension of bone marrow cells into a vein of the recipient. These cells are carried in the blood throughout the entire body and presumably lodge in many different locations. But only those stem cells that lodge in the recipient's bone marrow will be able to establish residence and begin proliferating to form the various blood cells. No other microenvironment will do. Cancer cells, on the other hand, can grow in locations far different from the tissue in which they arose. Cancer cells shed from the primary tumor can be carried in blood and lymph to other locations where they lodge and begin to grow into secondary tumors. This is the phenomenon of **metastasis,** and it often is the cause of death in cancer patients.

3. **Cancer cells have abnormal karyotypes.** One of the first examples to be recognized was the "Philadelphia" chromosome found in the cells of one form of leukemia (chronic myelogenous leukemia). These leukemic cells have one chromosome 22 that is shorter than normal. This Philadelphia chromosome arises because a portion of chromosome 22 has been translocated to chromosome 9. As techniques of studying chromosome structure have improved, it has become apparent that many types of cancer cells have translocations or other types of chromosome abnormalities. What is remarkable about these is that these aberrations are often *recurrent;* i.e., a particular aberration is associated repeatedly with a particular kind of cancer cell. In the group of human B cell tumors known as Burkitt's lymphoma, one member of chromosome 8 is invariably translocated to one of either chromosome 14, 22, or 2 (Figure 20.1).

4. **Cancers are clones.** The presence of a unique karyotype in all the cells of a tumor but in no normal cells of the host suggests that the tumor cells arose from a single progenitor; in other words that the tumor is a clone. There are several other observations that support the notion that most tumors — no matter how massive and how widely metastasized — are clones. For example, the production of a unique immunoglobulin by all the cells of a plasmacytoma (e.g., TEPC-15, MOPC-321) indicates that these cells are the descendants of a single cell in which a unique V region had been assembled.

5. **Cancer cells grow abnormally in vitro.** The behavior of cancer cells in tissue culture is also quite different from that of normal cells. Whereas normal cells proliferate for a limited number of divisions and then die out, many cancer cells grow indefinitely. Normal cells can grow in vitro only if they can attach to the surface of the culture vessel, and when the surface fills up with an unbroken sheet of cells, proliferation ceases. Cancer cells, on the other hand, are less dependent on anchorage to a surface, and grow over each other when they become crowded.

When normal cells growing in vitro are treated with certain carcinogens, they take on the properties of cancer cells. This phenomenon is called **transformation.** Often when cells that have been transformed in vitro are introduced into an immunoincompetent host (e.g., the nude

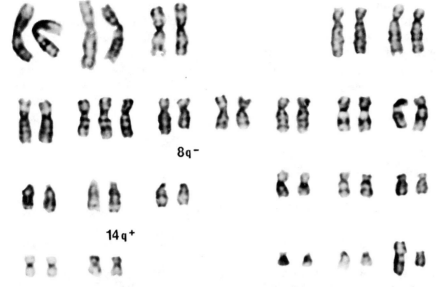

**Figure 20.1** Karyotype of a Burkitt's lymphoma cell. A reciprocal translocation has occurred between one chromosome 8 and one chromosome 14. The
long (q) arm of the resulting chromosome 8 is shorter (8q⁻) than its normal
homologue; the long arm of translocated chromosome 14 longer (14q⁺). The q
arm of chromosome 8 carries the c-*myc* gene; that of chromosome 14 carries
the genes encoding the heavy chain of antibodies. [Courtesy of Janet Finan
and C. M. Croce.]

mouse), they grow into tumors. Both radiation and chemical carcinogens
can transform mouse cells. Oncogenic retroviruses and DNA-mediated
gene transfer can transform both mouse and human cells. The ability to
transform cells in vitro provides a valuable tool for investigating the
genetic basis of carcinogenesis.

## 20.3  Causes of Cancer

Cancers are caused by radiation, certain chemicals, and some kinds of
viruses. As for radiation and chemical carcinogens, the underlying problem appears to be the generation of point mutations and/or chromosomal
aberrations. The Ames test, the most widely used test for potential chemical carcinogens, is simply a test of mutagenicity.

Several types of viruses cause cancer in animals. We shall focus our
attention on a group of retroviruses: viruses whose genetic material is
RNA. These viruses are not lytic for their host cell. Instead, once inside,
they copy their few genes (after having the cell translate their gene for
reverse transcriptase) into DNA and incorporate this DNA into the genome of their host. The process often leads to transforming the cell into a
cancer cell.

The first oncogenic retrovirus to be discovered (in 1911) was the Rous
sarcoma virus, a virus that causes cancer in chickens. A number of other

oncogenic retroviruses have been discovered since. Of particular interest to us are the simian sarcoma virus, which causes connective tissue tumors in monkeys, and the avian myelocytomatosis virus MC29 that causes a myeloid leukemia in chickens (Figure 20.2). Two retroviruses have been strongly implicated in certain rare human leukemias. These are the human T cell lymphotropic viruses types I and II (HTLV-I and HTLV-II). For obvious reasons, proof that HTLV-I and -II cause human cancer is only circumstantial.

## Viral Oncogenes (v-*onc*)

The genome of oncogenic retroviruses is quite small. The Rous sarcoma virus, for example, has only four genes. Usually only one of the genes is responsible for the cancer-causing ability of the virus. In the Rous virus, expression of a single gene, v-*src*, is all that is needed to transform the host cell. The v-*src* gene encodes a protein associated with the cell membrane of the host. While the mechanism by which expression of this protein transforms the cell is not yet understood, it is clear that the gene must be expressed continuously for the cell to remain transformed. The oncogenic potential of the simian sarcoma virus resides in an oncogene designated v-*sis;* that of avian myelocytomatosis virus in v-*myc*.

## Cellular Oncogenes (c-*onc*)

Normal cells contain within their genome genes homologous to the transforming genes of retroviruses. For example, a single-stranded cDNA copy of the v-*src* gene hybridizes with a gene in normal chicken cells. This gene is designated c-*src*. The cellular equivalents of a number of other transforming genes (e.g., c-*myc* and c-*sis*) have also been discovered. In a growing number of cases, the chromosomal location of the normal gene has been identified (Figure 20.2). Curiously, these c-*onc* genes appear to be highly conserved. Probes for cellular oncogenes can detect homologous sequences in many, often distantly related species (e.g., mouse, yeast, *Drosophila*). This suggests that these genes encode proteins with cell functions of fundamental importance.

In most cases, hybridization of v-*onc* DNA with c-*onc* DNA reveals numerous introns in the cellular version of the gene but not in the viral version. In all likelihood, viral oncogenes are "processed" versions of normal cellular genes; i.e., the DNA intermediates made by the viral reverse transcriptase occasionally include a copy of the mRNA transcript of a normal host cell c-*onc* gene. It begins to appear, then, as though the genetic potential to become cancerous is carried within the cell's own genome.

How the protein products of oncogenes produce cancer is as yet not known. Some, such as *src*, encode a kinase that phosphorylates proteins associated with the cell membrane. The product of c-*sis* seems to be one chain of platelet-derived growth factor (PDGF), a strong mitogen for

| Oncogene | Retrovirus | Chromosome location (human) | Product | Chromosome defect | Associated tumor |
|---|---|---|---|---|---|
| myc | Avian MC29 myelocytomatosis | 8 | DNA-binding protein | t: 8↔14<br>t: 8↔2<br>t: 8↔22 | Burkitt's lymphoma |
| sis | Simian sarcoma | 22 | Platelet-derived growth factor (PDGF) | t: 22↔9 | Chronic myelogenous leukemia (CML) |
| src | Rous sarcoma | 20 | Tyrosine kinase | | |
| erbB | Avian erythroblastosis | 7 | Receptor for EGF | deletion: 7 | Acute nonlymphocytic leukemia |
| abl | Abelson murine leukemia | 9 | Tyrosine kinase | t: 9↔22 | Chronic myelogenous leukemia (CML) |
| mos | Moloney murine sarcoma | 8 | Cytoplasmic protein | t: 8↔21 | Acute myelogenous leukemia |
| fes | Feline sarcoma | 15 | Tyrosine kinase | t: 15↔17 | Acute promyelocytic leukemia |

**Figure 20.2** Cellular oncogenes and the retroviruses from which their viral counterparts were first isolated. In only a few cases (e.g., c-*myc*, c-*mos*, c-*sis*) has it been demonstrated that the c-*onc* locus is involved in the chromosomal aberration (e.g., translocation) associated with a particular tumor. EGF = epidermal growth factor; *t* = translocation.

connective tissue cells. V-*erb*B, an oncogene carried by avian erythro-blastosis virus, encodes a molecule similar to part of the *receptor* on epithelial cells for epidermal growth factor (EGF). The product of c-*myc* binds to DNA in the nucleus. The level of *myc* protein in the cell becomes elevated when cells enter the cell cycle ($G_0 \rightarrow G_1$). One of the first effects seen when B or T cells are stimulated by mitogen or antigen is a rise in the concentration of the *myc* protein in the cell. The products of other cellular oncogenes appear to act later in the cell cycle.

## 20.4  The Neoplastic Event

There are two theories as to why oncogenes cause cancer.

1. A failed control mechanism causes an excessive and unregulated production of a normal cell growth stimulant. This is known as the dosage hypothesis.
2. The cancer-causing substance is a mutant version of the normal cell product and escapes the normal control mechanisms.

As it turns out, either (or both) mechanism may be at work in a particular tumor.

In some cases of tumors induced by viruses, the integration of a viral gene and its promoter into the host genome results in an overproduction of the v-*onc* product. In other cases, integration of a viral promoter alone appears to turn on excessive activity of a normal c-*onc* gene. In fact, it is possible to transform a cell by inserting into its genome one of its own normal c-*onc* genes along with a viral promoter. Here is strong evidence for the dosage hypothesis.

It is well known that radiation and chemical carcinogens induce point mutations and chromosome aberrations. And as we have seen, certain chromosome aberrations are closely associated with certain types of tumors. What makes this phenomenon particularly interesting for our story is that in an increasing number of cases, it turns out that these chromosomes, and specific sites of translocation, inversion, deletion, etc. on the chromosomes, are the sites of known cellular oncogenes.

Analysis of Burkitt's lymphomas has been particularly revealing. As we have seen, these human B cell tumors involve a recurrent pattern of reciprocal translocations. In every case, a portion of one copy of chromosome 8 has been translocated to another chromosome: most (75%) of the time to chromosome 14 (Figure 20.3), about 15% of the time to chromosome 22, the remainder (~10%) to chromosome 2. The point at which the break occurs on chromosome 8 is the location of the c-*myc* locus. The breakpoint on the second chromosome is between the V genes and the C genes of one of the immunoglobulin gene clusters: heavy chain in the case of chromosome 14, lambda light chain genes for chromosome 22, kappa light chain genes for chromosome 2. A parallel phenomenon is seen in mice. In the various mouse plasmacytomas, reciprocal translocation has occurred between chromosome 15 (where the mouse c-*myc* is located) and either chromosome 12 (heavy chain loci) or 6 (kappa chain

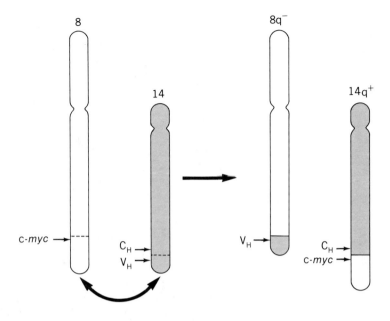

**Figure 20.3** Chromosome translocation seen in 75% of the cases of Burkitt's lymphoma. In the remainder of the cases, the portion of chromosome 8 containing the c-*myc* gene is translocated to one of the chromosomes carrying antibody light chain genes (22 for lambda, 2 for kappa). *q* refers to the long arm of the chromosome.

loci). (No mouse plasmacytomas involving the lambda genes on chromosome 16 have been identified as yet.)

There are several ways in which these reciprocal translocations might trigger an overproduction of the c-*myc* product.

1. The intron between the 3' $J_H$ gene segment and the $C_\mu$ gene contains, in addition to the switch region (Section 10.10), a region that seems to enhance — in B cells only — the rate of transcription of the rearranged antibody gene. Once the V gene segment, with its associated promoter, is joined to the $J_H$ gene segment, it comes under the influence of the enhancer (Figure 20.4). In some cases of Burkitt's lymphoma, an 8 ↔ 14 translocation brings the c-*myc* gene to a position close to the heavy chain gene enhancer (Figure 20.4). The job of a normal B cell is to transcribe and translate an assembled set of heavy chain (and light chain) gene segments. Bringing c-*myc* into this active area of the genome enhances its rate of transcription in these lymphoma cells. The c-*myc* gene on the normal chromosome 8 (chromosome 15 in mice) is unaffected.

2. In other cases of Burkitt's lymphoma, c-*myc* joins chromosome 14 within the switch region (Figure 20.4). In these cases, the enhancer is presumably translocated to chromosome 8, along with the $V_H$ gene cluster, and is unavailable to enhance the transcription of c-*myc*. In these cases, however, the first exon of c-*myc* is left behind. Perhaps this portion of c-*myc* contains a control site — analogous to the repressible operators in prokaryotes — that ordinarily keeps c-*myc* from being transcribed at inappropriate times. Removed from its control site, the translocated c-*myc* is free to be expressed constitutively. Only exons 2 and 3 are translated into the c-*myc* protein, even when c-*myc* is in its normal location, so the product of the translocated gene is normal. As before, the c-*myc* locus on the normal member of the chromosome 8 pair remains silent.

3. The translocated c-*myc* gene in some Burkitt's cells contains a number of point mutations. These occur in both exons 1 and 2. We have

**527**

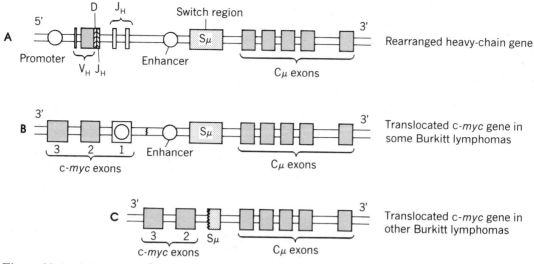

**Figure 20.4** A: Location of the transcription enhancer in a B cell synthesizing $\mu$ chains. B and C: Two types of translocation seen in Burkitt's lymphoma cells. In case **B**, the entire c-*myc* gene is translocated to a position 5′ to the enhancer. In case **C**, translocation has occurred within the switch region (S$\mu$). The translocated genes are transcribed in opposite directions. Exon 1 of c-*myc* contains promoters. The solid and hatched boxes represent exons that encode protein.

examined (in Chapter 10) the importance of somatic mutation for the generation of antibody V region diversity. The high rate of mutation of antibody V genes has suggested the operation of a hypermutation mechanism. If so, the translocation of c-*myc* into such a region of hypermutation could cause so many point mutations that (a) the first exon of the gene is no longer responsive to its normal repressor and/or (b) the translated exons produce a defective product. In these cases, then, both translocation and point mutation have teamed up to cause the neoplastic event.

Recent evidence indicates that two or more oncogenes may have to become altered before a normal cell becomes cancerous. Some oncogenic viruses do carry two oncogenes. As for radiation and chemical carcinogens, this requirement suggests that carcinogenesis is a multistep process. Laboratory, clinical, and epidemiological data support the notion that a cell must suffer two or more insults — perhaps occurring years apart — before it progresses to the stage of being a fully invasive, uncontrolled cancer cell.

## 20.5  Tumor Antigens

If the immune system is to respond to and attempt to destroy malignant cells, these cells must express tumor-specific antigens; i.e., antigens that are not found on the normal cells of the host. But how are these antigens to be demonstrated? The tumor-bearing host is soon going to die. If, as so many early workers did, we take tumor cells out of a mouse before it dies and inject them into some other outbred mouse, the tumor cells fail to grow in the new host. The failure *is* due to immune attack but the attack is directed against *normal* histocompatibility antigens (like H-2) expressed on the tumor cells. In other words, these cells behave like any other allograft. On the other hand, if we inject these cells into another mouse of the same inbred strain, the cells grow quickly and soon kill the new host.

In order to show tumor-specific antigenicity, we must find a way to immunize mice against an otherwise syngeneic tumor. In an epochal series of experiments commencing in the 1940s, Gross, Foley, Prehn, and Main, and the Kleins accomplished this goal and, in so doing, laid the foundation of tumor immunology. Let us examine Foley's work, which is depicted in Figure 20.5.

Foley worked with a chemically induced solid tumor. Methylcholan-

**Figure 20.5** Foley's demonstration of tumor-specific transplantation antigens (TSTAs). If the tumor is removed before it kills its host, the host can then be shown to be immune to a *second* injection of the same tumor cells, even though they are otherwise syngeneic to the host.

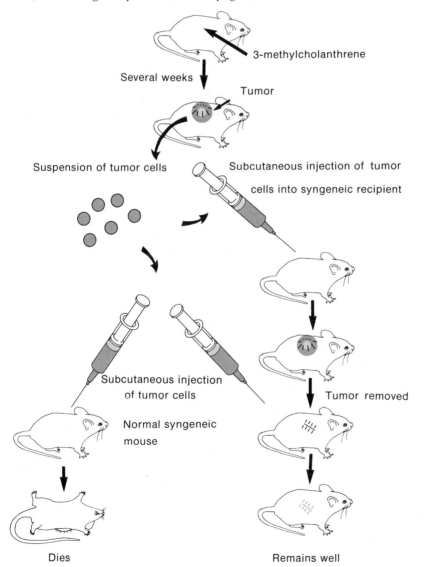

threne (MCA) is a polycyclic hydrocarbon that is highly carcinogenic in some mouse strains. Applied to the skin, it produces a high incidence of sarcoma, a solid tumor, some weeks later. The tumor can be excised and a suspension of tumor cells prepared. When these cells are injected subcutaneously into syngeneic recipients, they once again develop into localized, solid tumors. If left alone, the tumor soon kills the host. However, if the tumor is surgically removed in time, the animal recovers. The critical observation comes when this mouse is *re*injected with the tumor cells. This time, the cells fail to develop into a tumor. Prior exposure to the tumor has induced immunity. The effect is quite specific. MCA-induced tumor cells from other syngeneic donors, even from a second, independently induced tumor on the original donor, are not rejected. Evidently the primary immune response is too slow, but the secondary response is fast enough to cope with the rapidly growing tumor. Note that these tumor cells are syngeneic; they are rejected even though they share the normal histocompatibility antigens of their host. So these tumors *are* antigenic. Their antigens are called **tumor-specific transplantation antigens (TSTAs)**.

The TSTAs expressed on chemically induced tumors are extremely diverse. Every tumor produced by a single carcinogen in a single mouse strain, even in a single mouse, appears to possess unique TSTAs. Only rarely can a mouse immunized to, for example, one MCA-induced tumor go on to reject a different MCA-induced tumor. No one yet knows the molecular basis for this great diversity.

Tumors induced by oncogenic viruses also express TSTAs. However, these are not as diverse as the TSTAs of chemically induced tumors. Immunity to one tumor induced by simian virus 40 (SV40) will usually provide protection against any other SV40-induced tumor.

The molecular nature of the TSTAs in virus-induced tumors is under intense study. In the case of oncogenic DNA viruses like polyoma and SV40, the antigens expressed on the surface of the tumor cell are not components of the virion itself. Nevertheless, immunity against the virus can, in some cases, provide immunity against the tumor. For example, a mouse immunized with polyoma virus will not succumb to an injection of polyoma induced tumor cells (Figure 20.6).

Some tumors express antigens that play little or no role in rejection. These **tumor-associated antigens** are detected by the antibodies they elicit. Sometimes the antibodies appear spontaneously in the tumor-bearing host. Sometimes deliberate immunization of another animal is used to secure antisera. Two important examples of tumor-associated antigens found in humans are **alpha-fetoprotein (AFP)** and **carcinoembryonic antigen (CEA)**. Alpha-fetoprotein is associated with cancers of the liver, pancreas, testis, and occasional other organs. In the late stages of these diseases, the concentration of AFP in the patient's serum may exceed 1 mg/ml. (Elevated levels of AFP are also found in patients with nonmalignant liver disease, e.g., viral hepatitis.)

As its name suggests, alpha-fetoprotein is also present during fetal development. It is synthesized by the fetal liver and yolk sac, and it becomes a major serum protein during fetal development (probably the fetal equivalent of serum albumin) with concentrations rising to the

**Figure 20.6** Injection of an immunocompetent mouse with polyoma virus does not produce tumors, but does confer immunity against polyoma-induced syngeneic tumor cells. Presumably, the initial infection with virus led to the appearance of cells expressing polyoma-specific antigens. Although these cells failed to develop into tumors, they did immunize the host against their surface antigens.

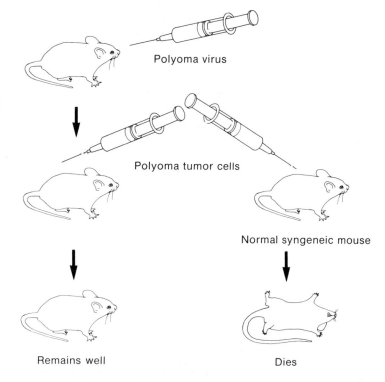

Polyoma virus

Polyoma tumor cells

Normal syngeneic mouse

Remains well

Dies

range of 1 mg/ml. The possible role of AFP in protecting the fetus from its mother's immune system is discussed in Section 16.6.

Victims of colon cancer often show high levels of carcinoembryonic antigen (CEA). The concentration of this tumor-associated antigen may rise to 1 mg/ml in the late stages of the disease. CEA is often found in patients with breast, prostate, bladder, and lung cancer as well in some nonmalignant conditions such as alcoholic cirrhosis of the liver. CEA is also found in normal fetal tissue where it is expressed by cells of endodermal origin.

Because AFP and CEA are associated both with cancer and with normal fetal development, they are often referred to as oncofetal antigens. Why should such an association exist? One popular idea is that cancer cells are dedifferentiated cells and reexpress the gene products characteristic of embryonic cells. This may well explain the reappearance of AFP. But another possibility should be considered. The cells most at risk of suffering the mysterious event that makes them cancerous are dividing cells. Dividing cells are likely to be cells that are proceeding along a pathway of differentiation from a precursor or stem cell to a fully differentiated end cell. Thus a cancerous cell may not be a *de*differentiated cell but simply an *un*differentiated cell. The presence of, for example, CEA in the fetus may simply reflect the greater proportion of dividing cells during this period of rapid growth and tissue development. If this is the case, we would expect that even adult tissues would produce some oncofetal antigens and indeed they do. Normal adults have serum concentrations of CEA (and AFP) in the range of 1–10 ng/ml.

If the second interpretation of the origin of oncofetal antigens is cor-

531

rect, it should raise a flag of warning for those who would like to exploit these antigens as targets for an attack against cancerous tissue. For if such a methodology were possible, it might well exert its cytotoxic activity not only against the cancer but against one or more kinds of normal precursor cells within the body.

In any case, little evidence now exists to offer any hope that these tumor associated antigens can be enlisted in manipulating an immune attack against cancer. Their main practical importance stems from their value in diagnosis and in monitoring the progress of cancer therapy. After surgical removal of a tumor, the serum levels of these antigens drop markedly; a subsequent rise suggests recurrence of the disease.

## 20.6   Immune Surveillance: The Evidence Against

Attractive though it may be, the concept of immune surveillance fails to explain a number of well established immune phenomena.

### Nude Mice Are No More Susceptible to Cancer Than Normal Mice

If newly arisen cancer cells are destroyed by a cell-mediated attack, then nude mice, which have few mature T cells, should be especially susceptible to cancer. But they are not. They neither suffer an unusual incidence of spontaneous tumors, nor are they more susceptible than other mice to carcinogenic chemicals and oncogenic viruses. This tends to be the case for neonatally thymectomized mice as well, although these animals sometimes show an increased susceptibility to chemical and virus-induced cancer.

On the other hand, nude mice have high levels of natural killer (NK) cells. NK cells have a well-demonstrated ability to destroy tumor cells in vitro and in vivo (see Section 14.10). If NK cells, not T cells, are the chief mediators of surveillance, then the data from nude mice are irrelevant.

### The Tumors of Immunosuppressed Patients Are Restricted to a Few Kinds

If the immune system patrols the body against all cancer cells, then immunosuppression should lead to an increase in the incidence of all kinds of cancers. But this is clearly not the case. Most of the cancers in transplant recipients (and other immunodeficient patients) are cancers of the lymphoid system (especially B cell lymphomas) and skin cancer. Cancers of the lung, breast, colon, and bladder are no more common in

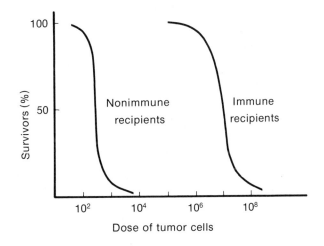

**Figure 20.7** Dose response curves for normal (nonimmune) animals and animals previously immunized against the tumor. Both groups are inoculated with graded doses of tumor cells.

immunosuppressed patients than in the general population. The high incidence of cancers of the immune system (e.g., lymphoma) in immuno-suppressed transplant recipients may not be a result of the immunosup-pression but rather of the intense antigenic stimulation provided by the allograft. Many agents that can stimulate mitotic activity in a tissue (e.g., mechanical abrasion, chemicals, hormones) have been implicated in the development of cancer in that tissue.

## "Sneaking Through"

A dose–response curve can be constructed for tumor cells just as it can for pathogens. The higher the dose of tumor cells, the more rapidly the tumor grows and the sooner the animal dies. Furthermore, in each sys-tem there is a threshold dose below which the animal is able to reject the tumor and survive (Figure 20.7). The exact value of this dose depends on such factors as the immunogenicity of the tumor and the immunocompe-tence of the recipient. Curiously, though, in some systems the dose–response curve is biphasic. That is, very *low* doses of tumor cells may also go on to kill the host. This phenomenon is called *sneaking through*. What-ever the mechanism that accounts for sneaking through (and you may be able to think of one), the phenomenon is not at all what you would expect to see if the animal is under immune surveillance. If immune surveillance works to destroy tumor cells as they arise, then you would expect it to work most effectively against small doses of tumor cells.

## Immune Stimulation

The presence of immune cells capable of destroying cancer cells can be demonstrated in the Winn assay (Figure 20.8). Graded doses of lymph-oid cells from an immunized donor are mixed with a constant number of

533

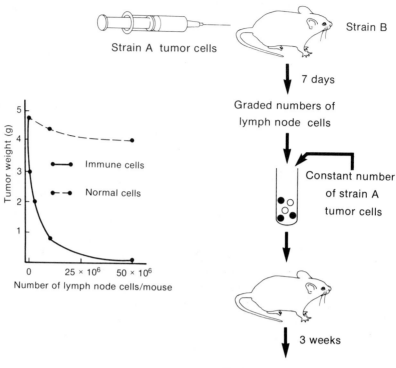

Figure 20.8   The Winn assay. In the experiments shown in the graph, graded numbers of allogeneic immune lymph node cells were mixed with 5000 strain A tumor cells and injected into strain A mice. The tumors were excised and weighed 3 weeks later. The Winn assay can also be carried out with syngeneic donor and recipient mice and allogeneic tumor cells. In this case, the dose of tumor cells must be much larger (e.g., $10^6$), the numbers of immune spleen cells somewhat smaller, and the resulting tumors are smaller. The Winn assay demonstrates the adoptive transfer of tumor immunity. [Graph from H. J. Winn, *J. Immunol.* 86:228, 1961.]

tumor cells. These mixtures are then injected into syngeneic mice (which may be normal or immunosuppressed as desired). In general, the higher the ratio of immune to tumor cells, the better the recipient is protected from tumor development. However, Prehn and his colleagues found a ratio (usually around 1:1) at which the immune spleen cells not only failed to suppress tumor growth but actually allowed more rapid tumor growth than did the normal, nonimmune spleen cells used in the control assays. While a strong immune response clearly inhibits tumor development, a weak response appears to favor it. This behavior is not what you would predict for a system of immune surveillance.

At the time Prehn's observations were made, the role of $T_S$ cells in cell-mediated responses was just beginning to be investigated. As we shall see below, $T_S$ cells can interfere with tumor-rejection responses. Possibly, the phenomenon of immune stimulation reflects the dominance of $T_S$ cells at low cell densities of immune spleen cells.

**20.7** Immune Surveillance: Supporting Evidence

**535**

*Section 20.7
Immune Surveil-
lance: Supporting
Evidence*

While Burnet's and Thomas' concept of immune surveillance may need modification, some forms of immune protection from cancer surely exist.

### The Evidence from Immunodeficiency Diseases

If the immune system protects us from cancer, then victims of inherited or acquired immunodeficiency disorders should have an increased incidence of cancer. At least this should be true for the T lymphocyte deficiencies (see Section 18.10). What is the evidence? Unfortunately it is a difficult issue to resolve because victims of such serious T cell deficiencies as *severe combined immunodeficiency* (SCID) and *DiGeorge syndrome* seldom survive long enough for cancers to appear. However, some milder forms of T cell deficiency exist, such as *Wiscott–Aldrich syndrome*, and, in adults, *ataxia telangiectasia*, in which the victims may live for a number of years. Both of these disorders are indeed characterized by a high incidence of malignancy. But like the malignancies of immunosuppressed patients, they tend to be cancers of the lymphoid system itself such as leukemias and lymphomas. A high incidence of lymphomas is also seen in patients with acquired immune deficiency syndrome (AIDS — see Section 18.10). However, these patients also develop other types of cancers such as Kaposi's sarcoma (in 30% of the cases) and skin cancers.

A clue to the role of cell-mediated immunity in cancer comes from a rare, inherited disorder known as X-linked lymphoproliferative disorder or *Duncan's syndrome.* As the first name suggests, the disease is inherited as an X-linked, recessive trait (thus it is found mostly in males) and is characterized by an excessive proliferation of lymphocytes (B lymphocytes). The disease seems to be triggered by virus infection, especially infection with Epstein–Barr virus (EBV). EBV infection in infants produces a very mild disease. In normal adolescents and young adults, the virus produces infectious mononucleosis. One of the major features of "mono" is a proliferation of B cells and enlargement of the spleen. Normally, the disease is self-limiting and the patient recovers fully. But in Duncan's syndrome, the patient seems unable to limit the proliferation of B cells. The spleen often becomes so enlarged that it bursts. In some cases, the disease progresses to a B lymphocyte lymphoma.

The picture that emerges is that a B cell lymphoma is a possible outcome of infection by EBV. In normal individuals, the patient usually recovers completely from EBV infection. In immunodeficient (and immunosuppressed) patients, the disease may progress to lymphoma. If this view is correct, then recovery from EBV infection may be an example of immune surveillance, but the surveillance is directed at virus-infected cells *before* they become transformed to malignancy. Of course, we have abundant evidence of the importance of T cells in coping with virus-infected cells (see, for example, Section 14.9). Perhaps, then, immune surveillance by T lymphocytes is incidental to their function as a mechanism for eliminating all virus-infected cells.

## Skin Cancer

Transplant recipients have an extraordinarily high incidence of skin cancer. Usually, the malignancy occurs in an area of the skin exposed to light. This suggests that the effect is the outcome of a synergism between the well-documented carcinogenic effect of ultraviolet light and the immunosuppressive therapy given the patient. Experiments with mice support this view. Mice given such T cell suppressants as antilymphocyte serum (ALS) are unusually susceptible to the induction of skin cancers by ultraviolet light. All of this strongly suggests the operation of immune surveillance.

## Natural Killer (NK) Cells

The properties of NK cells are reviewed in Section 14.10. When placed in culture, these cells are cytotoxic for tumor cells but not for the normal cells of the donor. Their activities do not show antigenic specificity in the way that $T_D$ and $T_C$ cells do. Nude mice have high levels of NK cells and this has been proposed as the reason that nude mice are no more susceptible to carcinogens than normal mice. Perhaps, then, immune surveillance does not depend upon a specific immune response by T cells so much as upon the antitumor activities of NK cells. Of course what goes on in vitro may have little relevance in vivo. However, several lines of evidence point to an important role for NK cells in the intact organism. The beige mutation in mice is associated with very low levels of NK activity. We might expect, then, that homozygous beige mice would have an elevated susceptibility to cancer, and there is considerable evidence for this. Human victims of the Chediak–Higashi syndrome also have depressed levels of NK cells and a high incidence of malignancies. But as in the other immunodeficiency disorders, the cancers generally involve cells of the lymphoid system. NK cells in mice express large amounts of an antigen called Ly-5. Cantor and his collaborators have used this feature to prepare suspensions of purified NK cells. The intravenous injection of these cells protects mice from a dose of lymphoma cells that would otherwise be uniformly fatal. Injection of NK cells has also been shown to inhibit tumor metastases in mice.

## Immune Response to Tumors

Whether or not immune surveillance occurs, the immune system can unquestionably respond to tumor antigens. Specific antitumor immunity in mice can be generated by immunization with living tumor cells (as Foley did), killed tumor cells, and even with purified preparations of TSTAs. When a tumor-bearing animal is given additional injections of the *same* tumor cells at other sites, these usually fail to develop. This phenomenon is called **concomitant immunity**. It is as if the animal has mounted an immune response to the first tumor, which is adequate to protect the animal from the development of new tumors, although inadequate to destroy the primary tumor.

Specific antitumor immunity in mice can be adoptively transferred by the intravenous injection of T cells from an immune donor. In most cases, the immune cells must be given before or simultaneously with (as in the Winn assay — Figure 20.8) the inoculum of tumor cells.

Tumor-bearing mice generate $T_C$ cells specific for their own tumor cells. Their $T_C$ cells will not lyse allogeneic tumor cells even if these carry the same TSTAs. This is because tumor-specific $T_C$ cells, like other $T_C$ cells, are restricted by the MHC. They only lyse tumor cells that express the same K and/or D antigens that were expressed on the tumor cells that induced them.

When T cells from a tumor-bearing host are cultured with antigen extracted from the tumor, they respond by proliferation and the release of lymphokines. This points to the existence of a population of $T_D$ cells sensitized to the tumor antigens. Sometimes these cells can be demonstrated in vivo as well. An intradermal injection of tumor cells or antigens extracted from these cells may elicit a DTH reaction in animals previously sensitized to the tumor. The response is most apt to occur when the recipient has been exposed to but is no longer carrying the tumor. Human leukemia patients often give a DTH reaction to an extract of their own leukemic cells but usually this occurs only during the periods when the disease is in remission. All of this suggests that $T_D$ cells are produced in response to tumor antigens but that their action may be suppressed by an actively growing tumor.

## 20.8 Why Does the System Fail?

Whether or not the immune system patrols the body on the lookout for the first appearance of a cancer cell, the system responds to the antigens on a fully developed tumor. Why, then, does the system not destroy the tumor?

### Tumor Cells May Lose Their Antigens

Chemically induced tumors, which have played such an important part in experimental tumor immunology, are strongly immunogenic. In this respect, they are quite unlike most of the tumors that arise spontaneously. Spontaneous tumors are usually only weakly immunogenic and elicit few if any signs of an immune response in the host. One possible reason for this low immunogenicity of long-established tumors is that during the development of the tumor, the immune system exerts a selective pressure for the emergence of tumor cells of reduced immunogenicity. Certain long-established tumors in mice express lower levels of class I histocompatibility antigens than recently-arisen tumors of the same type. Reduced expression of class I antigens makes the tumor cells more resistant to killing by class-I-restricted $T_C$ cells.

Leukemic cells "hide" their antigens by a mechanism known as *antigenic modulation*. Leukemic T cells in mice often express TL antigens. However, when these cells are injected into a mouse that has been immunized against the same TL antigens, the antigens are no longer seen on the cells although the cells continue to proliferate. The disappearance of TL antigens is only apparent; antibodies in the immunized mouse bind to the antigens on the cell surface and mask their presence. The binding of antibodies to tumor antigens on B cell leukemias causes the antigen–antibody complexes to be capped and engulfed by endocytosis. This is standard behavior for normal B cells exposed to antibodies directed against their surface immunoglobulins (see Section 8.7). It is uncertain whether modulation of tumor antigens is simply another example of this normal behavior or a specific mechanism for defense against detection by the immune system.

### Immunological Enhancement

With the realization that tumors can be immunogenic, it was only natural that attempts were soon made to see if experimental animals (even people) could be immunized against their own tumor. The early results were disappointing. Prior immunization, whether active or passive, not only failed to protect the host against the tumor but often caused the tumor to grow more rapidly than it would otherwise, the phenomenon of immunological enhancement. A typical protocol for demonstrating enhancement is shown in Figure 20.9. Note that there is no evidence here of the response being directed against TSTAs. Almost all tumors grow rapidly in a syngeneic host, so it is easier to demonstrate enhancement in an allogeneic situation where you would normally expect to see rejection. So what is illustrated here is simply enhancement of an allograft. Nevertheless, a few workers have been able to demonstrate enhancement directed against TSTAs.

If serum from a tumor-sensitized donor can passively transfer enhancement, could the serum of a tumor-bearing animal enhance the growth of its own tumor? Put this way, the question is difficult to test. Instead, we might ask: can the serum of a tumor-bearing animal interfere with cell mediated immune responses against that tumor? The answer is yes, sometimes.

The basic way to study this question is to choose an in vitro test of cell-mediated antitumor immunity and determine if serum from tumor-bearing animals interferes with the assay. The cell-mediated cytotoxicity (CMC) assay is one of several that can be used for this purpose. Spleen cells from tumor-sensitized animals are cultured with radiolabeled

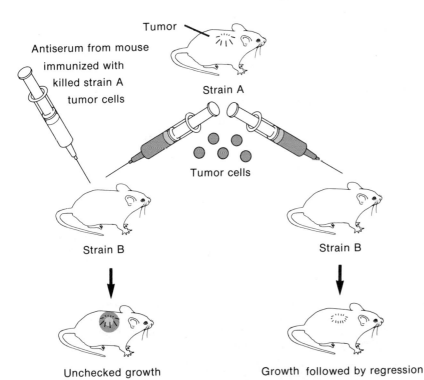

**Figure 20.9** Immunological enhancement. The presence of anti-strain A antibodies permits the tumor to grow unchecked in an allogeneic host which would otherwise reject it. Although the procedure shown here simply involves enhancement of an allograft, some workers have been able to demonstrate immunological enhancement of tumor growth with antibodies specific for tumor antigens (TSTAs).

tumor cells as their targets. The amount of cell killing is measured by the release of the isotope. The influence of serum from tumor-bearing animals can be examined by adding it to the incubation mixture. The results from many laboratories show that the serum from an animal with a rapidly growing tumor does interfere with or "block" the action of cytotoxic cells. Sometimes the effect of these "blocking factors" is specific for the particular tumor; sometimes not. Attempts to characterize the blocking factors usually reveals two or three different types of molecules at work. Some blocking factors are the size of IgG molecules; some are smaller and some are much larger. The bulk of the evidence indicates that blocking can occur through the action of (1) antibodies (of the size of IgG molecules), (2) tumor antigens (the smaller factors), and (3) complexes of tumor antigens with antibodies (the larger factors).

***Antibodies as Blocking Factors.*** One could easily picture antitumor antibodies blocking CMC in vitro by the same sort of masking mechanism that we postulated for enhancement in vivo. By binding to TSTAs on the surface of the tumor cells, they would shield the cells from attack by $T_C$ cells. Although there have been some reports of such a mechanism, uncomplexed antitumor antibodies do not usually block.

***Tumor Antigens as Blocking Factors.*** There is some evidence that tumor antigens can themselves serve as blocking factors. They might operate by filling the receptor sites on $T_C$ cells, thus preventing the cells from binding to their tumor targets.

There is considerable evidence that many growing tumors shed large quantities of tumor antigens into their surroundings. Possibly this soluble antigen could "defend" the tumor against immune attack by blocking the action of $T_C$ cells or $T_D$ cells. But the interaction of tumor antigens with circulating antitumor antibodies also gives rise to immune complexes, and these exert a different sort of blocking activity.

***Immune Complexes as Blocking Factors.*** Complexes of tumor antigen with antitumor antibodies are often present in the serum of tumor-bearing animals. These complexes have a strong blocking effect when tested in various cytotoxicity assays. For example, they interfere with the action

**Figure 20.10** A: Antibody-dependent cell-mediated cytotoxicity (ADCC) directed against tumor cells. The specificity is provided by antibodies directed against tumor antigens on the surface of the tumor cells. B: Mechanism by which complexes of soluble tumor antigen and antibody could block ADCC.

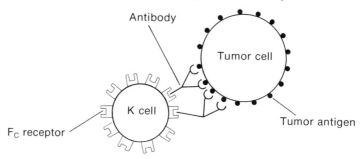

A　　　　　　　ADCC

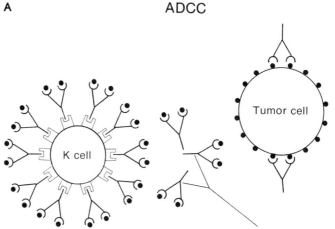

Complexes of antibody and soluble tumor antigen

B　　Blocking of ADCC by immune complexes

of $T_C$ cells. This could result from the binding of the antibody part of the complex to the target. Antigen–antibody complexes also interfere with antibody-dependent cell-mediated cytotoxicity (ADCC). Tumor cells are susceptible to ADCC; i.e., they can be destroyed by culturing them with *non*immune spleen cells and specific antitumor antibodies (Figure 20.10). Several kinds of cells can serve as the effectors of ADCC, including the K cell, which is a non-B, non-T lymphocyte (see Section 14.4). Immune complexes block ADCC by occupying the Fc receptors on K cells (Figure 20.10), and preventing the K cells from binding to antibody-coated targets and lysing them. ADCC can be demonstrated in a number of different experimental tumor systems. Whether it plays an antitumor role in the intact organism is not known.

## Tumor Cells Secrete Self-Protective Substances

Tumors may participate actively in creating favorable conditions for their own growth. They may employ specific mechanisms, like the shedding of tumor antigens, to block immune attack. They may also employ nonspecific mechanisms. A number of tumor products have been shown to have generalized immunosuppressive activity. Tumors also liberate materials that promote their own growth by inducng the blood vessels of the host to grow into them thus supplying them with their metabolic needs. A number of laboratories have reported that tumors liberate a soluble material that interferes with macrophage chemotaxis. Regressing tumors are heavily infiltrated with macrophages, suggesting that these cells play an important part in destroying tumor tissue. Thus anything that interferes with the mobilization of macrophages to the site of the tumor would be important for its survival.

## Suppressor Cells

Up to this point, you might well conclude that cell mediated immune responses work against tumors even if humoral responses are likely to be counterproductive. But this is too simplistic a view. There is a rapidly growing body of evidence that a subset of T cells — suppressor T cells — also works to enhance tumor development.

An early clue to the existence of such a mechanism is shown in Figure 20.11. Here again the tumor is a methylcholanthrene-induced sarcoma that can be transplanted indefinitely in normal syngeneic (A/J) mice. A subcutaneous injection of $10^6$ tumor cells produces a rapidly growing tumor that kills the animal in a few weeks. However, if after seven days the animal's spleen is removed, further growth of the tumor is inhibited. This suggests that the spleen contains something that enhances tumor growth. That something turns out to be a population of specific $T_S$ cells.

Tumor-specific $T_S$ cells are found in the spleen of animals with *growing* tumors. Their presence can be demonstrated by adoptive transfer. A

542

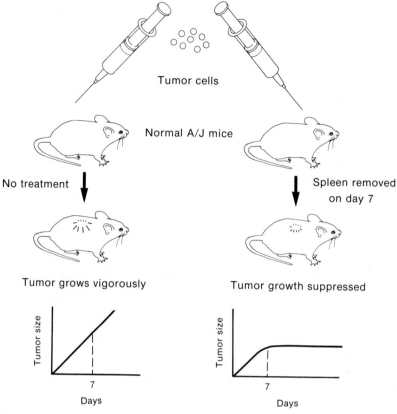

Tumor cells

Normal A/J mice

No treatment

Spleen removed
on day 7

Tumor grows vigorously

Tumor growth suppressed

**Figure 20.11** Splenectomy of the tumor-bearing host suppresses further growth of the tumor. Subsequent work (see, e.g., Figure 20.12) has shown that the spleen of a mouse harboring a growing tumor contains $T_s$ cells that suppress the animal's ability to mount an immune attack against the tumor. [Based on S. Fujimoto, M. I. Greene, and A. H. Sehon, *J. Immunol.* **116**:791, 1976.]

protocol for doing this is shown in Figure 20.12. The recipient is a mouse made immune to the tumor by injecting it with tumor cells and later surgically removing the tumor (just as Foley did — see Figure 20.5). A second injection of tumor cells starts to develop into a tumor but is then rejected. However, if *spleen* cells from a tumor-bearing mouse are mixed with *tumor* cells (a Winn-type assay), the second injection of tumor cells develops to a much greater size and is rejected more slowly. Evidently, a population of cells within the spleen has suppressed the rejection response. That these suppressor cells are T cells can be shown by treating the suspension with anti-Thy-1 serum and complement, which eliminates their influence. The suppressive effect is specific: normal spleen cells or spleen cells of animals carrying other tumors have no effect in this adoptive transfer.

The spleens of animals with *regressing* tumors contain T cells that are cytotoxic for the tumor. As we noted earlier in the chapter, these cells can adoptively transfer tumor-specific *immunity*. To be successful, the transfer must ordinarily be made before or at the time of the injection of tumor cells (as in the Winn assay — Figure 20.8). However, Berendt and

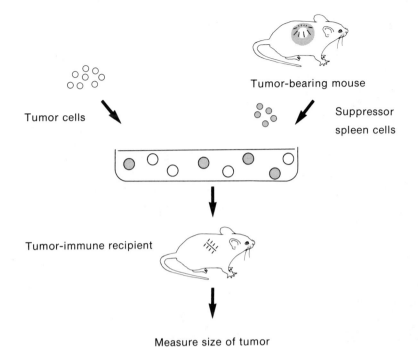

Tumor-bearing mouse

Tumor cells

Suppressor
spleen cells

Tumor-immune recipient

Measure size of tumor

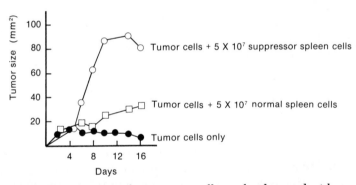

**Figure 20.12**   The presence of suppressor cells can be detected with
a Winn-type assay using an immune recipient; i.e., one that will reject
the tumor in the absence of suppressor cells. [From Linda L. Perry and
Mark I. Greene, *Fed. Proc.* **40**:39, 1981.]

North have developed a tumor system in which they are able to eliminate
*established* tumors with an injection of immune spleen cells. Their system uses an MCA-induced sarcoma propagated in "B" mice; i.e., irradiated, thymectomized mice reconstituted with bone-marrow cells. The
tumor grows unchecked in these T-deficient animals. However, an injection of *immune* spleen cells (from an animal rejecting its tumor) cures
the T-deficient recipients of their tumor (Figures 20.13 and 20.14). But
the injection of suppressor cells (from a tumor-bearing donor) along with
immune cells eliminates the rejection response. After a brief lag in
growth, the tumor begins to grow rapidly again (Figure 20.14) and goes
on to kill the host.

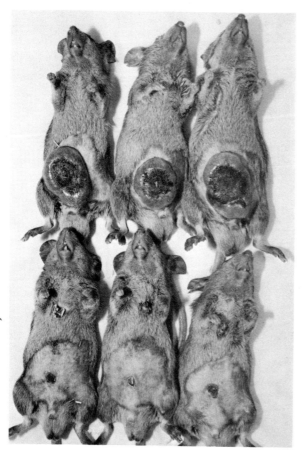

**Figure 20.13** *Top:* Tumors in otherwise normal mice 18 days after an intradermal injection of tumor cells and 12 days after receiving an injection of spleen cells from donors immunized against the tumor. The tumors have grown as rapidly as those in mice receiving nonimmune spleen cells or no spleen cells at all. *Bottom:* Regressed tumors in T-deficient mice (thymectomized, irradiated, and reconstituted with bone marrow) otherwise treated like the top group. Adoptive antitumor immunity has succeeded in this case because these T-deficient animals cannot manufacture suppressor T cells. [Courtesy of Dr. Robert J. North.]

As the details of tumor immunology are discovered, they really seem to represent no more than another example of the intricate regulatory systems that characterize all immune responses (reviewed in Chapter 15). Tumor antigens first induce a potentially protective immune response and then, as time goes on, a down regulation of that response. T-mediated suppression plays such a large part in the host's responses to a tumor because a tumor, unlike an allograft or an injection of conventional antigen, is growing continuously and releasing larger quantities of tumor antigens as it does. This massive antigenic stimulus turns on a vigorous counter response, which probably operates through the same sort of idiotype–antiidiotype network envisaged by Jerne.

## 20.9 Prospects for the Immunotherapy of Cancers

The evidence is strong that the immune system responds to a tumor growing within the organism. Concomitant immunity is one particularly forceful example. But the evidence is equally strong that—at least by the time the tumor becomes clinically evident—the immune system is

**Figure 20.14** A T-deficient mouse (irradiated, thymectomized, and reconstituted with B cells) succumbs to a syngeneic tumor unless it is given tumor-immune spleen (T) cells (see also Figure 20.13). However, the immune cells cannot save the mouse if suppressor cells are given at the same time. [From M. J. Berendt and R. J. North, *J. Exp. Med.* **151**:69, 1980.]

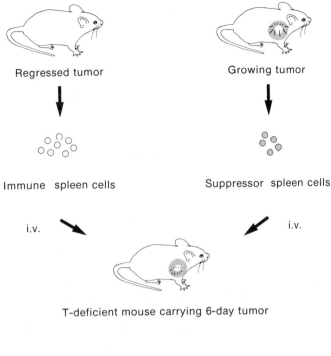

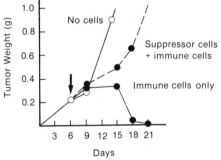

unable to protect the host. Untreated, the tumor grows until it kills the host.

We are left with the question: can we assist the immune system to tip the scales in favor of the host? Failing or beyond that, might we exploit the antigens expressed by the tumor as a means of specifically attacking the tumor through some form of pharmacological attack?

## Immunization Against Tumors

Starting with Foley's demonstration (Figure 20.5), we have seen that we can immunize an experimental animal against a particular tumor. For several reasons, this work will be difficult to apply to humans. These experiments involve syngeneic, transplantable tumors so it is known in advance which TSTAs the animal will eventually face. For many, if not most, human tumors, this is certainly not the case. Furthermore, immuni-

**545**

zation is effective only when completed prior to inoculating the animal with tumor cells. Only very rarely has it been possible to cure an already growing tumor by immunizing against it.

If human tumors express anything like the diversity of TSTAs that we find on mouse tumors, the possibility — much less the desirability — of trying to immunize humans against various types of tumors they might later develop seems unlikely. Many tumors in humans do express antigens shared by the same type of tumor in different patients. But such molecules are nonimmunogenic or weakly immunogenic at best. Furthermore, these tumor-associated molecules may occur on normal cells, like stem cells, with vital functions to perform. Immunization against antigens found on normal cells, even if it could be achieved, would be a risky undertaking.

One possibility remains: the use of vaccines to protect against tumors induced by oncogenic viruses. As we have seen, virus-induced tumors express TSTAs that occur on all tumors induced by that virus. These TSTAs are even shared by the tumors induced in different species by the same virus. In fact, an antitumor vaccine exists and is available commercially. It is used to protect chickens against Marek's disease, a lymphoma that is caused by a highly contagious herpes virus. The vaccine is prepared from attenuated virus, and the immunity it creates probably interferes with the spread of the virus within the animal. However, chicks can also be protected against Marek's disease by immunizing them with virus-transformed cells. In this case, the response is cell mediated and is directed against TSTAs on the tumor cells rather than antigens present on the virions.

One problem in applying such an approach to humans is that of identifying which, if any, human tumors are caused by viruses. Perhaps the best candidates to date are the B cell lymphomas that are so closely related to infections by the Epstein–Barr virus (EBV—see Section 20.7) and certain rare leukemias associated with HTLV-I and -II. However, the use of a future EBV or HTLV vaccine as a *tumor* preventive would seem to make sense only for persons, such as immunosuppressed transplant recipients, who are especially at risk of developing lymphoma.

Just as passive immunization is sometimes used for unprotected persons exposed to an infectious disease (see Section 2.5), so we must consider the possibility of using passive immunotherapy for those with diagnosed tumors. Unfortunately, the prospects do not seem hopeful. A little evidence suggests that the passive administration of antiserum might be helpful in leukemia and multiple myeloma. Leukemia cells seem more susceptible to damage by complement-fixing antibodies than the cells of solid tumors. Passive administration of antibodies directed against the idiotype of the immunoglobulin produced by a plasmacytoma (e.g., TEPC-15) has prolonged the survival of mice carrying the tumor.

The adoptive transfer of immune *cells* has also been effective in some experimental situations. But the possibility of applying such therapy effectively, much less safely, to humans seems remote. For example, the possibility exists that an infusion of antigen-primed T cells might greatly enhance T cell *suppression* and thus enhance rather than inhibit tumor growth.

# Immunopotentiation

Although specific immunotherapy of human malignancies remains an elusive goal, nonspecific methods have achieved some success. The introduction of BCG into such accessible tumors as melanomas and carcinomas of the skin have caused regression of the tumor in many instances. In some cases, treatment at a single site has also caused regression of distant metastases not treated directly. Other materials have had similar effects. These include preparations of killed bacteria, such as *Corynebacterium parvum* and *Bordetella pertussis*, and contact-sensitizing chemicals like oxazolone and dinitrochlorobenzene (DNCB). Oral therapy with levamisole, a drug widely used for deworming, has reportedly benefitted some cancer patients. These materials seem to share a strong stimulatory effect on all cell-mediated immune response including macrophage activity. Although these agents are nonspecific in the sense of being antigenically unrelated to the tumor, the response to their presence is probably specific. In other words, these materials have an adjuvant-like action that turns the host's specific antitumor defenses up to an effective level.

As increasing quantities of pure interferon become available, its potential as an anticancer agent will be under intense investigation. The method by which interferon exerts an antitumor effect is unknown, although its ability to enhance the in vitro activity of natural killer (NK) cells is well established.

# Immunotoxins

For the present, some mix of surgery, radiation, and chemotherapy provides the most effective method for treating cancer victims. A major problem with chemotherapy is the damage that cytotoxic drugs cause to all tissues where rapid cell division occurs. What is needed is a "magic bullet," a method of delivering a cytotoxic drug directly and specifically to tumor cells, bypassing all other types of cells. Such a magic bullet would have two parts: (1) a molecule capable of binding specifically to the desired target linked to (2) a molecule capable of killing the target. The specificity of antibodies makes them ideal candidates for the first function if they can be developed against surface antigens unique to the tumor. The cytotoxic function could be carried out by any number of agents such as chemotherapeutic drugs and toxins. All that is required is that the cytotoxic agent bind irreversibly to the antibody molecule and remain sufficiently toxic that the number of molecules delivered to each target cell will be sufficient to kill it. Several toxins are candidates for the cytotoxic function. These include diphtheria toxin and ricin (a lectin found in the castor bean). Both are proteins that are exceedingly lethal for most eukaryotic cells. Both consist of two polypeptide chains linked by disulfide bonds. One chain, the B chain, binds to the surface of cells —almost all cells—and this enables the other chain, the A chain, to

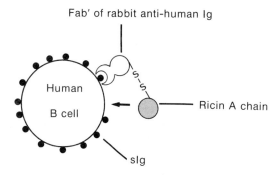

Fab' of rabbit anti-human Ig

Human

B cell

Ricin A chain

sIg

**Figure 20.15** A "magic bullet" specific for human B cells (sIg⁺). By using the Fab' fragment of the anti-Ig antibodies, a cysteine remains available for covalently linking to the ricin A chain. Once bound to the cell surface, the complex is taken into the cell by endocytosis. The ricin A chain blocks protein synthesis and kills the cell. [Based on the work of V. Raso and T. Griffin, *J. Immunol.* **125**:2610, 1980.]

enter the cytoplasm of the cell. Once inside, the A chain — even as few as one or two molecules of it — blocks the assembly of proteins on the ribosomes and eventually kills the cell.

One promising approach to a "magic bullet" is to substitute an antibody (or its Fab' fragment) for the B chain of the toxin. Without the B chain, such a complex should bind only to cells expressing the appropriate antigen. Once bound, the complex should be capped and taken into the cells by endocytosis where the A chain, if it can be released from the endosome into the cytoplasm, can do its lethal work.

Several research groups have reported success at producing in vitro cell-specific killing using this approach. For example, Raso and Griffin used a covalently linked conjugate of the ricin A chain with the Fab' fragment of rabbit antibodies directed against human IgG. Placed in cultures of various human lymphocyte cell lines, the conjugate bound only to cells expressing IgG on their surface (B cells — Figure 20.15). The binding resulted in widespread death of the cells. Human lymphocytes without sIg (e.g., T cells) neither bound the conjugate nor were harmed by it. Other laboratories have used conjugates of A chains and monoclonal antibodies directed against tumor-specific or tumor-associated antigens with which to kill — in vitro — the appropriate tumor cells without harm to other types of cells.

Many are the procedures that have worked dramatically in the laboratory only to fail in the clinic. After all, neither a tissue culture nor a mouse is a patient. But in time we should learn whether site-directed chemotherapy of tumors will become practical. Certainly one problem that remains to be solved is to use antigen–antibody systems that are truly specific for the tumor and that will not inadvertently damage small populations of vital cells. But with an increasing knowledge of tumor antigens and with the means of producing monoclonal antibodies, perhaps the dream of a magic antitumor bullet will eventually come true.

## 20.10 In Conclusion

The immunotherapy of cancer is still experimental. Whether an effective, safe, and reliable way of using the immune system to destroy tumors

548

will eventually be developed is still uncertain. I surely hope so. My hope is nourished by several considerations.

First, the need is great. The costs of malignancies to individuals and to society are huge and growing. And these costs are more than just financial, as anyone will attest who has watched a loved one battle cancer.

Second, I want to see the discipline I admire so much and that has opened so many vistas for its students once again display its power to aid humanity. Certainly the record established by immunology is already magnificent. In fact, what field of human activity can claim to have done more for humanity than immunology? Just think of its triumphs. Jenner's development of vaccination has eliminated one of humanity's greatest scourges from the earth. Immunization with diphtheria toxoid gives absolute protection from a disease that once could kill every child in a family within a fortnight. Surely many of us still remember the feelings of helplessness and panic as — in the days before Salk and Sabin — each summer brought another poliomyelitis epidemic. And no woman pregnant for the first time need fear ever having a baby that is desperately ill or even stillborn from hemolytic disease caused by Rh incompatibility. These are simply a few of the incalculable benefits that immunology has given us. There have been and will continue to be others. Let us hope that included among these new benefits will be some forms of effective tumor prevention or therapy. In fact, the successes that immunology has had against infectious disease has so increased life expectancy that age-related diseases, which include many forms of cancer, now take an ever-increasing toll.

Finally, we can hope for a successful immunotherapy of tumors for intellectual (even esthetic) reasons. The hallmark of immunity is specific adaptation. If a single theme has permeated this entire book, it has been the theme of specificity. Whether one considers the specificity of antibodies or the specificity of T cells, the ability of the immune system to discriminate between the subtlest alterations in molecular structure is dazzling. Tumor cells seem to possess identifying signals by which they could be distinguished from normal cells. How satisfying it would be to use the exquisite powers of recognition of the immune system as an adjunct to, if not a replacement for, the present nonspecific anticancer weapons of radiation and cytotoxic drugs.

## ADDITIONAL READING

1. Bishop, J. M., "Oncogenes," *Scientific American* **246**(3):80, March, 1982 (Offprint No. 1513).

2. Burnet, F. M., *Immunology, Aging, and Cancer*, W. H. Freeman and Company, San Francisco, 1976.

3. Collier, R. J., and D. A. Kaplan, "Immunotoxins," *Scientific American* **251**(1):56, July, 1984 (Offprint No. 1552).

4. Croce, C. M., and G. Klein, "Chromosome Translocations and Human Cancer," *Scientific American* **252**(3):54, March, 1985 (Offprint No. 1558).

5. Fisher, M. S., and Margaret L. Kripke, "Suppressor T Lymphocytes Control the Development of Primary Skin Cancers in Ultraviolet-Irradiated Mice," *Science* **216**:1133, 1982.

6. Foley, E. J., "Antigenic Properties of Methylcholanthrene-Induced Tumors in Mice of the Strain of Origin," *Cancer Res.* **13**:835, 1953.

7. Gross, L., "Intradermal Immunization of C3H Mice Against a Sarcoma That Originated in an Animal of the Same Line," *Cancer Res.* **3**:326, 1943.

8. Huber, S. A., and Z. J. Lucas, "Immune Response to a Mammary Adenocarcinoma. V. Sera from Tumor-Bearing Rats Contain Multiple Factors Blocking Cell-Mediated Cytotoxicity," *J. Immunol.* **121**:2485, 1978.

9. Hunter, T., "The Proteins of Oncogenes," *Scientific American* **251**(2):70, August, 1984 (Offprint No. 1553).

10. Kasai, M., et al., "Direct Evidence That NK Cells in Nonimmune Spleen Cell Populations Prevent Tumor Growth in Vivo," *J. Exp. Med.* **149**:1260, 1979.

11. Klein, G., et al., "Demonstration of Resistance Against Methylcholanthrene-Induced Sarcomas in the Primary Autochthonous Host," *Cancer Res.* **20**:1561, 1960.

12. Krolick, K. A., J. W. Uhr, S. Slavon, and Ellen S. Vitetta, "In Vivo Therapy of a Murine B Cell Tumor (BCL$_1$) Using Antibody-Ricin A Chain Immunotoxins," *J. Exp. Med.* **155**:1797, 1982.

13. Land, H. et al., "Cellular Oncogenes and Multistep Carcinogenesis," *Science* **222**:771, 1983.

14. Leder, P., et al., "Translocations Among Human Antibody Genes in Human Cancer," *Science* **222**:765, 1983.

15. Miller, R. A., et al., "Treatment of B-Cell Lymphoma with Monoclonal Anti-idiotype Antibody," *New Engl. J. Med.* **306**:517, 1982. In a human.

16. Prehn, R. T., and Joan M. Main, "Immunity to Methylcholanthrene-Induced Sarcomas" *J. Natl. Cancer Inst.* **18**:769, 1957.

17. Prehn, R. T., "The Immune Reaction as a Stimulator of Tumor Growth," *Science* **176**:170, 1972.

18. Terman, D. S., et al., "Extensive Necrosis of Spontaneous Canine Mammary Adenocarcinoma after Extracorporeal Perfusion over *Staphylococcus aureus* Cowans I. I. Description of Acute Tumoricidal Response: Morphologic, Histologic, Immunohistochemical, Immunologic, and Serologic Findings," *J. Immunol.* **124**:795, 1980.

19. Thorpe, P. E., et al., "Selective Killing of Malignant Cells in a Leukemic Rat Bone Marrow Using Antibody-Ricin Conjugate," *Nature* **297**:591, 1982.

20. Weinberg, R. A., "A Molecular Basis of Cancer," *Scientific American* **249**(5):126, November, 1983 (Offprint No. 1544).

21. Yunis, J. J. et al., "The Chromosomal Basis of Human Neoplasia," *Science* **221**:227, 1983.

# Glossary

**Adherent cell**  Cell that sticks to glass or plastic. Macrophages and dendritic cells.

**Adjuvant**  Material added to an antigen to increase its immunogenicity. Common examples are (a) alum, (b) killed *Bordetella pertussis*, (c) an oil emulsion of the antigen, either alone (Freund's incomplete adjuvant) or with killed mycobacteria (Freund's complete adjuvant).

**Adoptive transfer**  The infusion of lymphocytes, usually from an antigen-primed donor to an unprimed recipient.

**Affinity**  Strength of binding (association constant) between one site (e.g., of an antibody molecule) and a monovalent ligand.

**Allelic exclusion**  The restriction of a heterozygous B cell to the synthesis of only one of the two parental allotypes.

**Allergy**  Secondary immune response to an enviromental antigen (allergen) resulting in tissue damage. Hypersensitivity.

**Allogeneic**  Refers to genetically different members of the same species, e.g., different inbred mouse strains.

**Allograft**  Graft of tissue between genetically different members of the same species. Also called a homograft.

**Allotype**  Antigenic determinant(s) found on antibody chains of some, but not all, members of a species and which are inherited as simple Medelian traits. The Gm allotypes on human gamma chains are examples.

**Anaphylaxis**  An immediate (type I) hypersensitivity reaction following introduction of antigen into a primed individual. Mediated by reaginic antibodies, chiefly IgE.

**Anergy**  A failure to respond to antigen.

**Antigen**  Substance that (1) elicits an immune response and (2) reacts specifically with antibodies and/or T cells.

**Antiserum**  Serum containing induced antibodies.

**Autograft**  Graft of tissue from one area to another on the same individual.

**Autologous**   Derived from the same individual, e. g., the cells in the autologous mixed lymphocyte reaction (AMLR).

**Avidity**   Strength of binding between an antibody molecule (multivalent) and a multivalent antigen.

**Bence-Jones protein**   Light chains or dimers of light chains found in the serum and urine of some multiple myeloma patients.

**Capping**   Aggregation at one location on the cell surface of membrane proteins following their binding by a multivalent ligand.

**Carcinoma**   A cancer of epithelial tissue.

**Carrier**   A macromolecule (e.g., a protein like KLH) to which a hapten (e.g., DNP) can be conjugated rendering the hapten immunogenic.

**Chimera**   An animal whose body contains two (or more) genetically different cell populations.

**Class I antigen**   Histocompatibility antigen consisting of an integral membrane polypeptide associated noncovalently with $\beta_2$-microglobulin. Encoded by H-2K, -D, and -L in mice; by HLA-A, -B, and -C in humans. Found on most cells of the body.

**Class II antigen**   Histocompatibility antigen consisting of two integral membrane polypeptides encoded by loci in H-2I in mice, HLA-D in humans. Expressed on dendritic cells, B cells, and some macrophages and other cells involved in immune responses.

**Clone**   The descendants, produced asexually, of a single cell.

**Concomitant immunity**   Immunity which prevents the establishment of new tumors (or parasites) while unable to eliminate the original tumor (or parasites).

**Congenic**   Having identical genotypes except for a small segment of one chromosome pair. The inbred mouse strains B10 and B10.A are congenic; they are genetically identical except for their MHC.

**Conventional antigen**   An antigen such as DNP–KLH or SRBC as distinct from a histocompatibility antigen. Also called nominal antigen.

**Cytotoxic**   Antibodies or cells that damage target cells.

**Determinant**   A site on an antigen molecule to which an antibody (or a T-cell antigen receptor) with a complementary site binds by noncovalent interactions.

**Epitope**   Antigenic determinant.

**Exon**   Portion of a DNA molecule whose transcribed sequence is retained in mRNA.

**Flare**   A temporary reddened area of the skin because of localized vasodilation. Erythema.

**Gamma globulins**   Serum proteins that migrate least far toward the anode when serum is electrophoresed at pH 8.6. IgG antibodies are gamma globulins.

**Genome**   A complete haploid set of genes.

**Germinal center**   Region within an active follicle containing dividing B lymphocytes. Found in antigen-stimulated peripheral lymphoid tissue such as lymph nodes and spleen.

**Granulocyte**   A white blood cell (neutrophil, basophil, or eosinophil) that contains cytoplasmic granules.

**Haplotype**   The set of alleles (e.g., in the MHC) found on one chromosome.

**Hapten**   A molecule not immunogenic by itself but that, when coupled to a macromolecular carrier, can elicit antibodies directed against itself. The DNP, TNP, NP, and ABA (azobenzenearsonate) groups are commonly used haptens.

**Hemolysis**   The lysis of red blood cells.

**Heterologous**   Derived from a different source. Refers to such things as molecules (and their subunits), cells, and tissue grafts.

**Humoral**   Referring to molecules (e.g., antibodies and complement components) dissolved in such body fluids as plasma and lymph.

**Hybridoma**   Cell clone produced by fusing a lymphocyte with a tumor cell, thereby combining the function of the lymphocyte (e.g., synthesis of a monoclonal antibody of the desired specificity) with the ability of the tumor cell to grow indefinitely.

**Hypersensitivity**   Secondary immune response which causes tissue damage. May be mediated by antibodies (types I, II, and III) or cells (type IV).

**I-A**   A subregion of H-2 in mice that encodes class II antigens.

**Ia antigen**   Class II histocompatibility antigen encoded in the murine I region of the MHC (or its homologue in other species). "I-region associated" antigen.

**Idiotype**   The antigenic determinants unique to a particular $V_H$ and/or $V_L$ domain. A single idiotypic determinant is called an idiotope.

**Immunogen**   An antigen that elicits immunity.

**Immunoglobulin**   Protein with the structure of antibodies.

**Internal image**   Determinant on an antibody that resembles a determinant on an exogenous antigen and to which antibodies (or T cells) specific for that exogenous antigen can bind. The concept that internal images of antigens are expressed by the immune system prior to encounter with the antigen is central to the network theory.

**Intron**   Portion of a DNA molecule whose transcribed sequence is removed by splicing during the formation of mRNA.

**Ir gene**   Gene that controls the ability of an animal to respond to a thymus-dependent antigen. In mice, most Ir genes map to the I region of H-2.

**Isograft**   Graft between genetically identical individuals.

**Isotype**   Set of antigenic determinants found on a subset of H or L chains of all members of a species. Corresponds to the classes and subclasses of H and L chains.

**J chain**   Polypeptide covalently associated with polymeric IgM and IgA molecules.

**Karyotype**   The set of chromosomes in a cell.

**Lectin**   Glycoprotein derived from plants or animals that binds to particular sugar residues.

**Ligand**   A molecule or group that binds to another molecule or to a cell.

**Linked recognition**   The requirement that both haptenic and carrier determinants must be present on the *same* antigen molecule in order for B cells to receive help from $T_H$ cells. Also called cognate interaction.

**Lipopolysaccharide (LPS)**   Macromolecule, containing lipid and polysaccharide moieties, found in the outer membrane of gram-negative bacteria like *E. coli*. Mitogenic for murine B cells. Also called endotoxin.

**Lymphoblast** Lymphocyte in the cell cycle. Lymphoblasts are larger than resting ("small") lymphocytes.

**Lymphoid** Referring to lymphocytes or tissues, e.g., lymph nodes, in which lymphocytes are a major constituent.

**Lymphokine** Biologically active substance (e.g., IL-2) secreted by activated lymphocytes, especially T lymphocytes.

**Lymphoma** A cancer of lymphoid tissue.

**Macrophage** Phagocytic cell derived from the monocyte. Somewhat larger than and without the lobed nucleus and cytoplasmic granules of the neutrophilic phagocytes.

**Metastasis** The secondary growth of malignant cells away from the site of the primary tumor.

**Mitogen** A substance that induces cell division. Lymphocyte mitogens act polyclonally, i.e., without regard to the antigen specificity of the lymphocytes.

**Monokine** Biologically active substance secreted by monocytes and macrophages.

**Myeloma** Cancerous proliferation of a clone of plasma cells. Produces a myeloma protein. A plasmacytoma.

**Neoplastic** Cancerous.

**Oncogene** Gene that through excessive activity or a mutant product takes its cell one step of the way toward becoming cancerous. Oncogenes introduced into the cell by certain retroviruses are designated v-*onc*; their conterparts in normal cells are called proto-oncogenes or c-*onc*.

**Oncogenic** Cancer causing.

**Ontogeny** The development of an individual organism or its parts.

**Opsonin** Antibody that, after binding to the surface of a particle, enhances its phagocytosis.

**Paratope** Antigen-binding site of an antibody.

**Phagosome** Vacuole containing particulate matter engulfed by phagocytosis.

**Plasma cell** A terminally differentiated B lymphocyte chiefly occupied with antibody synthesis and secretion.

**Plasmacytoma** Cancerous proliferation of a clone of plasma cells. Causes multiple myeloma in humans.

**Primed** Previously exposed to antigen.

**Reagin** Antibody that mediates immediate hypersensitivity reactions. IgE is the major reagin in humans.

**Restriction endonuclease** Enzyme that cleaves DNA at sites defined by a particular sequence of nucleotides.

**Sarcoma** A cancer of supporting tissue such as bone or muscle.

**Serological** Pertaining to methods, tests, etc., that employ antibodies.

**Serum** Fluid left after blood has clotted. It is blood plasma minus fibrinogen and other clotting factors.

**Signal peptide** N-terminal portion ("leader") of a newly synthesized polypeptide that enables it to enter the endoplasmic reticulum after which the signal peptide is cleaved away.

**Specificity**  The ability of an antibody or lymphocyte to discriminate between two antigenic determinants.

**Stem cell**  Undifferentiated cell that divides by mitosis to produce (1) daughter cells that enter one or more differentiation pathways and (2) more stem cells.

**Syngeneic**  Having virtually the same genetic makeup, e.g., all the members (of the same sex) of one inbred mouse strain.

**Theta (θ) antigen**  Glycoprotein found on mouse T cells of all subsets. Also called Thy-1.

**Thymocyte**  Lymphocyte in the thymus.

**Titer**  Reciprocal of the highest dilution of an antiserum that gives a positive reaction in the test being used.

**Tolerogen**  Antigen that, because of its chemical nature, dose, or method of administration, elicits specific immunological tolerance.

**Toxoid**  Bacterial toxin treated (e.g., with formaldehyde) to destroy its toxicity without harming its ability to elicit protective antibodies against the undenatured toxin.

**Transformation**  (1) Conversion of a resting lymphocyte into a dividing lymphoblast following exposure to a mitogen or the antigen for which it is specific. Blast transformation. (2) The genetic modification of a cell by introducing foreign DNA into it. (3) The alteration of normal cells growing in tissue culture into cells with certain traits characteristic of cancer cells.

**Unprimed**  Having no prior exposure to the antigen. Naive. Virgin.

**Wheal**  A temporary, sharply delimited, elevated area of the surface of the skin caused by local edema (see Figure 5.17).

**Xenograft**  Graft of an organ or tissue between members of different species. Sometimes called a heterograft.

# Index

An italicized number indicates that the reference appears in a figure.

| | | | | |
|---|---|---|---|---|
| **AA** | Arachidonic acid | | **DTH** | Delayed-type hypersensitivity |
| **Ab** | Antibody | | | |
| **ABA** | Azobenzenearsonate | | **EA** | Erythrocyte-antibody |
| **ABC** | Antigen-binding cell | | **EAC** | Erythrocyte-antibody-complement |
| **A-CHO** | Group A streptococcal carbohydrate | | **EAE** | Experimental allergic encephalomyelitis |
| **AChR** | Acetylcholine receptor | | **EBV** | Epstein–Barr virus |
| **ADCC** | Antibody-dependent cell-mediated cytotoxicity | | **ELISA** | Enzyme-linked immunosorbent assay |
| **AFP** | Alpha-fetoprotein | | **EPP** | End-plate potential |

**AA** Arachidonic acid
**Ab** Antibody
**ABA** Azobenzenearsonate
**ABC** Antigen-binding cell
**A-CHO** Group A streptococcal carbohydrate
**AChR** Acetylcholine receptor
**ADCC** Antibody-dependent cell-mediated cytotoxicity
**AFP** Alpha-fetoprotein
**Ag** Antigen
**AIDS** Acquired immune deficiency syndrome
**AMLR** Autologous mixed lymphocyte reaction
**APC** Antigen-presenting cell

**BCDF** B cell differentiation factor
**BCG** Bacillus Calmette-Guérin
**BCGF** B cell growth factor
**BGG** Bovine gamma globulin
**BSA** Bovine serum albumin
**BUdR** Bromodeoxyuridine

**C** Complement
**CAD** Compound antigenic determinant
**CD** Cluster of differentiation (of human leukocyte antigens)
**cDNA** Complementary DNA
**CDR** Complementarity-determining region
**CEA** Carcinoembryonic antigen
**CFA** Complete Freund's adjuvant
**CMC** Cell-mediated cytotoxicity
**CMI** Cell-mediated immunity
**Con A** Concanavalin A
**cOVA** Chicken ovalbumin
**CRI** Cross-reacting idiotype
**CTL** Cytotoxic T lymphocyte ($T_C$)

**DNCB** Dinitrochlorobenzene
**DNP** Dinitrophenyl

**DTH** Delayed-type hypersensitivity

**EA** Erythrocyte-antibody
**EAC** Erythrocyte-antibody-complement
**EAE** Experimental allergic encephalomyelitis
**EBV** Epstein–Barr virus
**ELISA** Enzyme-linked immunosorbent assay
**EPP** End-plate potential

**FACS** Fluorescence-activated cell sorter
**FGG** Fowl gamma globulin
**FITC** Fluorescein isothiocyanate
**FR** Framework region

**GL** Poly-L-Glu-L-Lys
**GLPhe** Poly-L-Glu-L-Lys-L-Phe
**GT** Poly-L-Glu-L-Tyr
**GVHR** Graft versus host reaction

**H-2** Major histocompatibility complex of mice
**HBsAg** Hepatitis B surface antigen
**HGG** Human gamma globulin
**HLA** Major histocompatibility complex of humans
**HSA** Human serum albumin
**³H-TdR** Tritiated thymidine
**HTLV** Human T cell lymphotropic virus

**Ia** I-region associated
**IEP** Immunoelectrophoresis
**IFN** Interferon
**Ig** Immunoglobulin
**IG** Immune globulin (human)
**IL-2** Interleukin 2
**Ir** Immune response (e.g., Ir gene)